S0-BYY-946

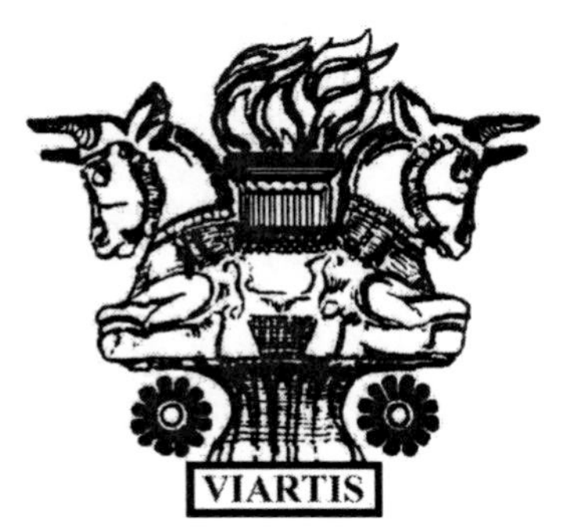
VIARTIS

THE COMPREHENSIVE GUIDE TO
PARKINSON'S DISEASE

Keith Bridgeman
Tahira Arsham

SECOND EDITION

PUBLISHING DATA

TITLE : The Comprehensive Guide to Parkinson’s Disease

AUTHORS : Keith Bridgeman, Tahira Arsham

ISBN : 978-1-906421-06-9

PUBLISHER : Viartis http://viartis.net/publishers

PUBLICATION DATE : 2017

PLACE OF PUBLICATION : London, England

LANGUAGE : English

FORMAT : Paperback

EDITION : Second

TOPICS : Parkinson's Disease, Parkinson Disease, Neurology, Medicine

LIBRARY CLASSIFICATION (Dewey decimal classification) : 616.833

SHORT DESCRIPTION : The Comprehensive Guide to Parkinson’s Disease

LONG DESCRIPTION : The Comprehensive Guide to Parkinson’s Disease, which is fully referenced, includes the history of Parkinson's Disease, famous people with Parkinson's Disease, its biochemistry, cytology and cytological effects, anatomy and anatomical effects, physiology and physiological effects, the symptoms of each system in the body (muscular, nervous, alimentary, urinary, cardiovascular, respiratory, skeletal, integumentary, sensory, endocrine, reproductive and immune), its methods of diagnosis (observational, technological and chemical), its causes (biochemical, toxic, genetic, pharmacological and medical), its treatment including its biochemical treatment, pharmacological treatments (L-dopa, dopamine agonists, MAO inhibitors, COMT inhibitors, anti-cholinergics and non-dopaminergic), surgical treatments, natural treatments, exercise methods, technological methods, and details of national and international Parkinson's Disease organisations, the most useful Parkinson's Disease web sites, and the main books concerning Parkinson's Disease nursing.

SIZE : 227 mm x 152 mm x 41mm

PAGES : 814

INTRODUCTION TO PARKINSON'S DISEASE

Parkinson's Disease is a medical disorder whose most prominent symptoms are muscular, including rigidity, tremors, and slowness of movement. Parkinson's Disease is primarily due to the insufficient formation of dopamine, which is produced in the dopaminergic neurons in the brain.

There have been descriptions and treatments of Parkinson's Disease that date back as far as 5000 BC. Descriptions continued throughout ancient times, the medieval era, and subsequent centuries. In 1690 Ferenc Pápai Páriz described all of the main symptoms of Parkinson's Disease. However, it was not until 1817 that the symptoms became well known due to James Parkinson. Later that century Parkinson's Disease was named after him. In the 1960's L-dopa became the standard treatment. It was produced as Sinemet and Madopar, which included a dopa decarboxylase inhibitor in order to maintain the levels of L-dopa. Since then, the use of L-dopa has been added to with the use of dopamine agonists, MAO inhibitors, COMT inhibitors, other formats of L-dopa, and surgical treatments including Deep Brain Stimulation.

Worldwide, there are likely to be more than ten million people with Parkinson's Disease. The prevalence differs enormously in different countries. Parkinson's Disease can occur at any age, but it is uncommon in people under the age of 30. The likelihood of somebody developing Parkinson's Disease becomes increasingly more common with age, increasing sharply at the age of 60, and peaking in those aged 85 to 90 years old. In most, but not all countries, there are more men than women with Parkinson's Disease. The incidence rate at which people with Parkinson's Disease are newly diagnosed has been declining for years.

Dopamine is produced in the dopaminergic neurons. Dopamine stimulates the dopamine receptors, which then stimulate the G proteins. Dopaminergic neurons are concentrated in dopaminergic neuronal groups in the central nervous system. Dopamine is transmitted from the dopaminergic neurons via the dopaminergic pathways to other parts of the brain where it has effect on a variety of physiological functions.

The most prominent symptoms of Parkinson's Disease are muscular, including rigidity, tremors, and bradykinesia (slowness of movement). However, Parkinson's Disease can eventually affect every system in the body. Other common symptoms can include freezing, falling, reduced arm swing, depression, apathy, fatigue, anxiety, pain, sleep disturbance, speech difficulties, reduced facial expression, constipation, swallowing difficulty, reduced handwriting size, urinary symptoms, cardiovascular symptoms, respiratory dysfunction, reduced sense of smell, and sexual dysfunction. The symptoms are different in each person, over time, and in their severity.

SPECT or PET scans, involving the scanning of the brain, are the most accurate methods of diagnosing Parkinson's Disease. However, diagnosis is usually based on physical observation and questioning of the patients. There are a number of symptom questionnaires and rating scales. The most commonly used is the Unified Parkinson Disease Rating Scale (UPDRS). There are also chemical methods for assisting with the diagnosis of Parkinson's Disease.

Parkinson's Disease is caused by the insufficient biosynthesis of dopamine. When the enzymes, substrates, coenzymes and cofactors required for dopamine biosynthesis are deficient the biosynthesis of dopamine is greatly reduced. Uncommonly, there are a variety of toxic causes, genetic causes, and certain drugs that can be a partial cause or the sole cause of Parkinson's Disease. Other medical disorders can cause symptoms, some of which coincide with those of Parkinson's Disease. Those medical disorders are usually called a Parkinsonism.

The most common basis for treating Parkinson's Disease is the use of L-dopa. L-dopa can enter the brain and then form dopamine. L-dopa is available in various formats, such as Sinemet, Madopar, Rytary and Numient. They also include a dopa decarboxylase inhibitor, which helps to maintain the levels of L-dopa. L-dopa can initially be effective, but its effects eventually wear off and lead to the disorder becoming gradually and progressively worse. Other common treatments include dopamine agonists, which mimic the action of dopamine, and MAO Inhibitors and COMT inhibitors, which help to prevent the breakdown of dopamine. Deep Brain Stimulation is the most effective surgical treatment for Parkinson's Disease. The ultimate therapy, one that was able to rid symptoms without side effects, was still to be revealed.

CONTENTS

SECTION 1 HISTORY OF PARKINSON'S DISEASE

1 1 History of Parkinson's Disease

2 25 Famous people with Parkinson's Disease

SECTION 2 PREVALENCE OF PARKINSON'S DISEASE

3 47 Prevalence of Parkinson's Disease

SECTION 3 BIOCHEMISTRY OF PARKINSON'S DISEASE

4 63 Dopamine biosynthesis

5 67 Coenzyme biosynthesis

6 71 Iron metabolism

7 83 Zinc metabolism

8 91 Manganese metabolism

9 97 Dopamine receptors

10 127 G proteins

11 156 Dopamine receptor phosphoprotein

SECTION 4 CYTOLOGY OF PARKINSON'S DISEASE

12 162 Dopaminergic neurons

13 170 Cytological effects

SECTION 5 ANATOMY OF PARKINSON'S DISEASE

14 183 Dopaminergic neuronal groups

15 188 Anatomical effects

SECTION 6 PHYSIOLOGY OF PARKINSON'S DISEASE

16 198 Dopaminergic pathways

17 206 Physiological effects

SECTION 7 SYMPTOMS OF PARKINSON'S DISEASE

18 217 Primary symptoms

19 222 Symptom progression

20 232 Muscular system

21 271 Nervous system

22 319 Alimentary system

23 329 Urinary system

24 332 Cardiovascular system

25 338 Respiratory system

26 341 Skeletal system

27 347 Integumentary system

28 352 Sensory system

29 363 Endocrine system

30 368 Reproductive system

31 373 Immune system

SECTION 8 DIAGNOSIS OF PARKINSON'S DISEASE

32 377 Observational methods

33 403 Technological methods

34 427 Chemical methods

SECTION 9 CAUSES OF PARKINSON'S DISEASE

35 433 Biochemical causes

36 440 Toxic causes

37 472 Genetic causes

38 533 Pharmacological causes

39 544 Medical causes

SECTION 10 TREATMENTS OF PARKINSON'S DISEASE

40 582 Biochemical treatment

41 592 Pharmacological : L-dopa

42 617 Pharmacological : Dopamine agonists

43 664 Pharmacological : MAO inhibitors

44 675 Pharmacological : COMT inhibitors

45 687 Pharmacological : Anti-cholinergics

46 692 Pharmacological : Non-dopaminergic

47 734 Surgical treatments

48 764 Natural treatments

49 777 Exercise methods

50 792 Technological methods

APPENDIX PARKINSON'S DISEASE RESOURCES

1 805 Parkinson's Disease organisations

2 811 Parkinson's Disease web sites

3 813 Parkinson's Disease nursing

CHAPTER 1

HISTORY OF PARKINSON'S DISEASE

Origins

Parkinson's Disease is primarily due to insufficient dopamine. There has been the potential for humans to have insufficient dopamine and to develop Parkinson's Disease since humans have existed. Consequently there have been descriptions and treatments of Parkinson's Disease since ancient times [1].

Ancient India

An ancient civilisation in India practiced their medical doctrine called Ayurveda. Ayurveda is claimed to be a divine revelation of the ancient Indian creator God Lord Brahma as he awoke to recreate the universe. They described the symptoms of Parkinson's Disease, that they called Kampavata, as far back as 5000 BC [2]. To treat Kampavata they used Atmagupta, which is a tropical legume called mucuna pruriens. The seeds of mucuna pruriens are a natural source of therapeutic quantities of L-dopa [3]. Mucuna pruriens is the oldest known method of treating the symptoms of Parkinson's Disease and is still widely used to treat Parkinson's Disease. The earliest reference to bradykinesia was in 600 BC. In 300 BC Charaka described the Parkinson's Disease symptoms tremor, rigidity, bradykinesia and gait disturbances [4].

Ancient China

The Huang di nei jing su wen, which is often known as the Su wen, is the oldest existing Chinese medical text. It was written in around 500 BC. It is composed of two texts each of 81 chapters or treatises in a question and answer format between the mythical Huang di (Yellow Emperor) and his ministers. The first text, the Suwen, which is also known as Plain Questions, covers the theoretical foundation of Chinese Medicine, diagnosis methods and treatment methods. It also describes the symptoms of Parkinson's Disease [5].

The Yellow Emperor's Internal Classic, which is considered the first Chinese medical classic, was titled with the name of the Yellow Emperor in around 425 BC to 221 BC. A 24 volume section of the Yellow Emperor's Internal Classic collected the clinical experiences of Chinese practitioners up until that period. Volume 5 on "Pulse and Essence Thesis" describes symptoms compatible with limitation of movement, postural disturbances, stiffness, and tremor as follows : A person appears with crouching of the head and with staring eyes, bending the trunk with shoulders drooped, with difficulty turning and rocking the low back, inability of the knees to flex and extend, with the back bowed, failure to stand for long periods, and tremor whilst walking [6].

The Bible

It is claimed that there are references to the symptoms of Parkinson's Disease in both the old and new testaments of the Bible. Often cited as possible references to Parkinsonism is the following depiction of old age in the Old Testament : "When the guardians of the house tremble, and the strong men are bent" (Ecclesiastes 12 : 3), and the following description in the New Testament "There was a woman who for eighteen years had been crippled by a spirit.....bent and completely incapable of standing erect" (Luke 13:11) [7].

Ancient Greece

In the Illiad, which along with the Odyssey are claimed to have been written by the Greek author Homer in the eighth century BC, the septuagenarian King Nestor describes symptoms that appear to be those of Parkinson's Disease. King Nestor remarks that, despite the fact he still partakes of the armed struggle, he can no longer compete in athletic contests : my limbs are no longer steady my friend, nor my feet, neither do my arms, as they once did, swing light from my shoulders [8, 9].

Erasistratus of Ceos (310 BC - 250 BC) was a Greek anatomist and royal physician under Seleucus I Nicator of Syria. Erasistratus of Ceos founded a school of anatomy in Alexandria with the Greek philosopher

Herophilus. Caelius Aurelianus wrote that Erasistratus of Ceos appeared to be describing the freezing that occurs in Parkinson's Disease when he termed paradoxos a type of paralysis in which a person walking along must suddenly stop and cannot go on but after a while can walk again [10].

Ancient Rome

Aulus Cornelius Celsus (c25 BC - c50 AD), although apparently not a physician himself, compiled an encyclopedia entitled De artibus (25 AD - 35 AD) that included De medicina octo libri (The Eight Books of Medicine) [11]. He advised against administering those who suffered tremor of the sinews with emetics or drugs that promoted urination, and also against baths and dry sweating. Relief from worry, rubbing of the limbs and their exercise by ball games and walking were indicated. The patient could eat whatever he wanted but sexual activity should be restricted. If he should succumb he should afterwards be rubbed in bed with olive oil by boys not men. Fine tremor was distinguished from a coarser shaking, which was independent of voluntary motion. So it resembled resting tremor. It could be alleviated by the application of heat and by bloodletting.

Pedanius Dioscorides (c40 AD - c90 AD) was an ancient Greek physician, pharmacologist and botanist from Anazarbus, Cilicia, Asia Minor, who practised in ancient Rome during the time of Nero. Dioscorides is famous for writing De Materia Medica, which is a precursor to all modern pharmacopeias, and is one of the most influential herbal books [12]. Dioscorides wrote that beaver testes, prepared with vinegar and roses was helpful not only for the "lethargicall" but was also good for tremblings and convulsions, and for all diseases of the Nerves, being either drank or anointed on, and that it had a warming faculty.

Symptoms of Parkinson's Disease were described by the ancient Greek physician Galen (129 AD - 200 AD) who worked in ancient Rome. He wrote of tremors of the hand at rest [13]. He wrote extensively on disorders of motor function including the book "On tremor, palpitation, rigor and convulsion". He distinguished between forms of shaking of the limb on the basis of origin and appearance. The aged, he noted, exhibited tremor because of a decline in their power to control the motion of their limbs. The key to overcoming tremor was to abolish the proximal cause but for the aged this was impractical. Galen related that a person suffering from "catoche" has wild, wide open eyes, that he lies rigid in bed, as if he were made of wood. He also suffers from tremor, constipation and certain psychiatric symptoms.

Medieval history

Paul of Aegina (c625-c690), the Byzantine Greek physician, wrote the medical encyclopedia "Medical Compendium in Seven Books" [14]. For many years in the Byzantine Empire this work contained the sum of all Western medical knowledge and was unrivalled in its accuracy and completeness. Paul of Aegina noted in his work "On trembling" that tremor was characteristic of alcoholism and what Mettler interpreted as "senile paralysis agitans".

An ancient Syrian medical text detailed among its prescriptions for nervous diseases a complex unguent for "pains in the excretory organs and in the joints, and in cases of gout and palsy, and for those who have the tremors, and for all the pains which take place in the nerves". It consisted of 35 components including frankincense, rosemary, several types of cypress, cardamom, peppercorns, myrrh, mandragora and frogs. The unguent was rubbed on to the paralysed or rigid limb [15].

Ibn Sina (c980-1037), the Persian polymath and foremost physician of his time, discussed the various forms of motor unrest in his chapter on nervous disorders in his book the "Canon of Medicine" [16]. Ibn Sina's description of tremor is similar to Galen's description of tremor, as it was based on previous works including that of Galen. A range of measures are proposed according to the cause of the disorder : bathing in sea-water or in mineral baths (nitrate, arsenic, asphalt, sulphur), evacuation, composite preparations including made from the excretion of the anal gland of the beaver (oleum castoreum) – a common spasmolytic – mixed with honey and cold oil to which pills formed from rue (Ruta graveolens) and scolopendrium (Scolopendrium vulgare; hart's tongue).

In Jin Dynasty China, Zhang Zihe (1151-1231), who was one of four famous medical experts during the Jin dynasty, described in "Ru Men Shi Qin" a man who had tremor in his jaw, hands and feet, inexpressive facial features, stiffness, inability to perform common motor activities, and also the loss of dexterity of finger movements. He also noted mood changes with depression. The most reasonable diagnosis was Parkinson's Disease but Zhang's medieval diagnosis was "wind shaking" [5].

Sixteenth century

The Italian artist, engineer and scientist Leonardo da Vinci (1452-1519) also studied anatomy, physiology and medicine. Leonardo da Vinci kept secret notebooks in which he wrote and sketched his ideas and observations [17]. He saw people whose symptoms coincided with the tremors seen in Parkinson's Disease. Leonardo wrote in his notebooks that "you will see.....those who.....move their trembling parts, such as their heads or hands without permission of the soul; (the) soul with all its forces cannot prevent these parts from trembling." Due to most of his notebooks being secret, his observations remained unknown for centuries. At the end of his life Leonardo was unable to paint due to the loss of control of movement in his hands. It has been suggested that, by then, Leonardo had the disorder himself.

There are examples of references to the symptoms of Parkinson's Disease in the plays of William Shakespeare (1564-1616). There is a reference to shaking palsy in the second part of Henry VI, during an exchange between Dick and Say [18]. Say explains to Dick that it is shaking palsy rather than fear that was causing his shaking. Dick asks Say : "Why dost thou quiver, man ?" Say responds : "The palsy, and not fear, provokes me."

John Gerard (1545-1611/12) was an English botanist famous for his herbal garden. He studied medicine and travelled widely as a ship's surgeon. In 1597, he published a list of plants cultivated in his garden at Holborn. It was basically a translation of a 1583 Latin herbal illustrated. In Gerard's Herball he writes of Sage that it "strengthneth the sinewes, restoreth health to those that have the palsie upon a moist cause, takes away shaking or trembling of the members". He also mentioned cabbage, pellitory and mugwort for treating trembling of the sinews [19].

Seventeenth century

Nicholas Culpeper (1616-1654) was an English botanist, herbalist, physician and astrologer. He published books, The English Physitian (1652) and Complete Herbal (1653). The Complete Herbal contains both pharmaceutical and herbal knowledge. Among recommendations in Complete Herbal, he suggests sage for "sinews, troubled with palsy and cramp". For centuries prior to this, sage had been recommended for tremor in the hands. Amongst other plant remedies Culpepper suggested for palsy and trembling were bilberries, briony (called "English mandrake"), and mistletoe. In the 1696 edition of his Pharmacopoeia Londinensis, a variety of substances were claimed to be useful in the treatment of "palsies", the "dead palsy", and "tremblings". These included "oil of winged ants" and preparations including earthworms [20].

The writer and antiquary, John Aubrey (1626-1697) wrote a biography of the philosopher Thomas Hobbes (1588-1679) titled "Life of Mr Thomas Hobbes of Malmesbury" [21]. In it, he used the term "Shaking Palsey" in his description of the progressive disability that had afflicted Thomas Hobbes. John Aubrey wrote of Thomas Hobbes that he "had the shaking Palsey in his hands.....and has grown upon him in degrees", and that ".....Mr Hobbs wase for severall yeares before he died so Paralyticall that he wase scarce able to write his name".

The Hungarian doctor Ferenc Pápai Páriz (1649-1716) described in 1690 in his medical text Pax Corporis not only individual signs of Parkinson's Disease, but all four cardinal signs : tremor, bradykinesia, rigor and postural instability [22]. This was the first time that all of the main symptoms of Parkinson's Disease had been formally described. The book was published in Hungarian, which because it is understood by so few people, had resulted in his description of Parkinson's Disease being ignored in the medical literature in favour of later descriptions of Parkinson's Disease wrongly being claimed to be the first.

EIGHTEENTH CENTURY

George Cheyne (1671-1743) was a Scottish physician, psychologist, philosopher and mathematician. It is possible to interpret a medical disorder described in chapter XII of his book The English Malady (1734) as parkinsonian [23]. The subject of his discussion is the vaguely defined "Palsy", or "Paralytick Symptoms". "Palsy" was then defined as "a disease wherein the body, or some of its members lose their motion, and sometimes their sensation of feeling. The disease is never acute, often tedious, and in old people, almost incurable; and the patient for the most part drags a miserable life.....he totters and shakes, and becomes a dismal sight; as if no longer a man, but an animal half dead".

Francois Boissier de Sauvages de la Croix (1706-1767) provided one of the clearest descriptions of a parkinsonism-like condition in 1763 [24]. He spoke of a condition that he named "sclerotyrbe festinans" in which decreased muscular flexibility led to difficulties in the initiation of walking. Both of the cases he observed were in elderly people. His observations, along with those of Jerome David Gaubius (1705-1780) and Franciscus Sylvius de la Boë (1614-1672) were subsequently cited by James Parkinson because although none of them described the whole syndrome they all described aspects of it.

John Hunter (1728-1793) was a distinguished Scottish surgeon. In his Croonian lecture in 1776, John Hunter gave a description of Lord L. that was similar to paralysis agitans. He wrote that "Lord L's hands are almost perpetually in motion, and he never feels the sensation in them of being tired. When he is asleep his hands, &c., are perfectly at rest; but when he wakes in a little time they begin to move". James Parkinson's son, John William Keys Parkinson transcribed his father's shorthand notes from John Hunter's lectures into a book, The Hunterian Reminiscences [25].

JAMES PARKINSON

James Parkinson (1755-1824) was a London physician [26]. He systematically described six individuals with symptoms of the medical disorder that eventually bore his name. He described his findings in "An Essay on the Shaking Palsy", which was published in 1817 [27]. Unusually for such a description, he did not actually examine all these patients himself but observed them on daily walks. The purpose of his essay was to document the symptoms of the disorder, which he described as "Involuntary tremulous motion, with lessened muscular power, in parts not in action and even when supported; with a propensity to bend the trunk forwards, and to pass from a walking to a running pace : the senses and intellect being uninjured." Although Parkinson's Disease was eventually named after James Parkinson, it was not until several decades after he died. So James Parkinson never knew that Parkinson's Disease was named Parkinson's Disease after him.

THE FIRST CLAIMED CURE

From 1827 to 1831, the English physician John Elliotson (1791-1868) published pamphlets concerning the disorder in the Lancet, which largely consisted of case reports, although some of those he described probably did not actually have Parkinson's Disease [28]. Amongst his preferred methods of treatment were bleeding, induction and maintenance of pus building, cauterisation, purging, low diet and mercurialisation, silver nitrate, arsenic, zinc sulphate, copper compounds, and also the administration of iron as a tonic with some porter, which is a kind of dark beer. Elliotson made the first known claimed cure. He suggested that many young patients could be cured, although unreliably, using the carbonate of iron. On another occasion, he reported that the "disease instantly and permanently gave way" when he treated with iron a patient who had proved resistant to all other forms of therapy. This was well over a century before iron was found to be essential for the formation of dopamine.

THE FIRST NAMED PATIENT

From 1828 until his death in 1835, Wilhelm von Humboldt (1767-1835), a philosopher and diplomat, described in his letters his own symptoms, which gave a more complete description of the symptoms than had James Parkinson [29]. They included resting tremor and especially problems in writing, called by him "a special clumsiness" that he attributed to a disturbance in executing rapid complex movements. In addition to lucidly describing akinesia, he was also the first to describe micrographia. He furthermore noticed his typical parkinsonian posture. There were incidental references in the following decades to what may (or may not) have been some of the symptoms of Parkinson's Disease by Toulmouche (1833), Hall (1836, 1841), Elliotson (1839), Romberg (1846) [29]. However, the syndrome still remained hardly known.

Mid nineteenth century treatments

In 1842, the first clear recommendation of a pharmacological agent following Elliotson's iron cure was that of ergot of rye (Secale cornutum). The recommendation was made by the English surgeon J.B.Thompson who saw "in the paralysis agitans or tremens in advanced life, where I have seen it of considerable benefit myself". J.B.Thompson wrote that ergot of rye conveyed "a more fixed steadiness and firmness" [30]. Over a century later ergot derived drugs began to be used as dopamine agonists in the treatment of Parkinson's Disease.

The naming of Parkinson's Disease

It was not until 1861 and 1862 that Jean-Martin Charcot (1825-1893) [31] with Alfred Vulpian (1826-1887) added more symptoms to James Parkinson's clinical description. At that time, they considered that there was nothing that could be done to halt the progression of the disease [32]. Charcot added to the list of symptoms the mask like face, various forms of contractions of the hands and feet, akathesia, and referred to rigidity. It was quite difficult to understand from his description what was meant by rigidity. It was only after Charcot gave a clinical lesson in 1868 that the difference became clear [33]. In 1876 Charcot described a patient who was suffering from "paralysis agitans" in the absence of tremor while rigidity was present. In this case there was no paralysis. So Charcot rejected the term paralysis agitans. Instead he suggested it be referred to as Parkinson's Disease after James Parkinson [34].

Early visual depictions of Parkinson's Disease

In 1880 Jean-Marie Charcot completed a full clinical description of Parkinson's Disease. The symptoms were depicted by Paul Richer in drawings and a statuette of people with Parkinson's Disease [35]. Paul Marie Louis Pierre Richer (1849-1933) was a French anatomist, physiologist, sculptor and anatomical artist. Paul Richer was an assistant to Jean-Martin Charcot at the Salpêtrière. Along with a photograph these are some of the earliest visual depictions of Parkinson's Disease.

Expanding the known symptoms

After Charcot initiated the research of incomplete forms of Parkinson's Disease, rigidity as a symptom grew in importance. Although Jean-Martin Charcot and James Parkinson pointed out that patients are moving slowly and with difficulty they did not see this as a symptom in its own right. The slowness of movement was firstly taken into account by Claveleira [36]. Jaccoud referred to this symptom in 1873 as akinesia [37]. In 1886 the neurologist and artist Sir William Richard Gowers drew an illustration as part of his documentation of Parkinson's Disease [38]. Cruchet introduced the word bradykinesia and emphasised that this symptom should be mentioned in the first place in any definition of Parkinson's Disease [39]. Jules Froment, a French neurologist from Lyon, subsequently contributed to the study of parkinsonian rigidity during the 1920s [40].

The early use of alkaloids

In 1867 Charcot had introduced treatment using an anti-cholinergic, the alkaloid drug hyoscine (or scopolamine), which is derived from the Datura plant. Emanuel Mendel abandoned the use of hyoscine in favour of duboisine, because of the lesser toxic effects and the lower dosages required, and then applied the use of duboisine in the treatment of parkinsonism in 1893, thereby greatly reducing tremor [41]. Wilhelm Heinrich Erb introduced hyoscine in to general use for Parkinson's Disease in 1898 [42] but it was not known in the English speaking world until 1906 [43]. Severe cases responded especially well to it :

tremor was markedly reduced, rigidity was reduced, sialorrhea was suspended, patients enjoyed both freer movement and increased self satisfaction. Erb also noticed there were twice as many males as females with Parkinson's Disease and that the major risk factor for Parkinson's Disease was age with the majority of cases commencing after 50 years of age.

The use of electrotherapy

In 1868, Jean-Martin Charcot wrote that the French doctor Guillame Benjamin-Amand Duchenne (1806-1875) had reported a case in which he had cured paralysis agitans by application of galvanism [34]. Duchenne had popularised the use of electrical means with his 1855 publication "On localised electrification, and on its application to pathology and therapy". The Irish physician U.S.L.Butler also claimed in 1869 that it cured a patient of paralysis agitans [44]. William Sanders had mentioned in his paper in 1865 that the application of "galvanism" was without benefit for his patient [45]. Hughlings Jackson, and William Gowers in 1893, who also tried it in paralysis agitans, were unstinting in their deprecation of the practice as "useless" [46]. Despite this, electrical stimulation in Parkinson’s disease continued to be used for decades more. In the 1924 edition of his handbook on electrotherapy, Toby Cohn commented that "remarkable results could not be expected", and that what benefits he had seen were largely psychological [47]. In his 1941 review of the "modern treatment of parkinsonism" Critchley specifically warned against electricity and other spurious claims of curing the disease [48].

Encephalitis Lethargica

In 1915 epidemics of Encephalitis Lethargica broke out around the world. It was first described in 1917 by the Austrian neurologist Constantin von Economo [49]. It started off as an influenza like fever and then developed in to symptoms such as headache, depression, delirium, confusion, motor disturbances, psychosis and stupor. Its symptoms were thought to encompass almost anything imaginable. Encephalitis Lethargica could cause death in a short period or a type of sleep that might last days, weeks or months, but could also cause insomnia. Many of those that survived developed Postencephalitic Parkinsonism [50]. Encephalitis Lethargica consequently led to a huge increase in the number of people with Parkinsonism. In the 1920's, the majority of Parkinsonian patients had Postencephalitic Parkinsonism. Encephalitis Lethargica was at its most prevalent in the early 1920's but new cases of Postencephalitic Parkinsonism were still being reported in the 1940's.

THE LATER USE OF ALKALOIDS

The first widespread use of the alkaloid atropine was in the 1920's [51, 52, 53]. Some success was reported with its use [54]. Carl Römer initiated high dosage use of atropine for post encephalitic Parkinsonism, which he first used after 1924 [55], but idiopathic Parkinson's Disease did not respond well to it. High dose atropine therapy dominated in the first half of the 1930's, achieving significant results but it was accompanied by serious side effects.

In 1926, the Bulgarian Ivan Raeff introduced in to the treatment of post encephalitic Parkinsonism what was later called the "Bulgarian treatment", which was white wine extract of the belladonna root, with a special diet and psychotherapy. Idiopathic Parkinson's Disease did not respond as well to it [56]. It was the belladonna root that was the effective part [57]. Belladonna, which is known as Deadly Nightshade, is so poisonous that just one leaf could kill an adult. The alkaloid content of the extract included varying amounts of hyoscyamine, atropine and, in lesser quantities, scopolamine and belladonnine. It was presumed that this alkaloid mixture was responsible for the relative lack of side effects in comparison to treatment with atropine alone. By the beginning of the 1940's most patients were being treated using belladonna alkaloids [58].

THE USE OF NEUROSURGERY

The first specific attempt to treat Parkinsonism surgically was reported by Leriche in 1912 via section of the posterior roots. The method relieved tremor or rigidity. Delmas-Marsalet claimed success in the treatment of rigidity with lesions of the cerebellum. Improvements in tremor were subsequently achieved by cortectomy but often at the price of other functional losses. Cordotomy was directed against unilateral tremor and rigidity and was associated with fewer side effects. Meyers reported in 1951 that sectioning of pallidofugal fibres achieved the best results for relieving tremor and rigidity but most surgeons chose to undertake a more direct attack on the pallidum with equal success and a lower fatality rate. The publication of the first stereotactic atlas of the human brain by Spiegel and Wycis in 1952 increased the popularity of stereotactic surgery. The thalamus gradually became the preferred target as the impact on tremor was greater and the operation was safer. By 1969 only 15% of patients were suitable for stereotactic operations, but up to 90% of those could expect relief from tremor and rigidity. After a sharp decline in stereotactic surgery, thalamotomy was revived in the 1970's for patients whose tremor was not helped by L-dopa. Laitinen and colleagues resumed operations on the medial pallidum in 1985 [59].

New synthetic drugs

During the 1950's, synthetic drugs became the main methods of treating Parkinson's Disease. Due to their side effects and limited efficacy the plant derived treatments were almost completely replaced by these synthetic drugs. The main type of drugs used were anti-cholinergics because of their ability to reduce muscle contraction. The most widely used of them was Benzhexol HCl, which had anti-cholinergic activity. It was marketed as Artane in the U.S.A.. It was at that time the primary choice for treating Parkinson's Disease for most medical practitioners [60]. Benztropine methane sulfonate was a potent anti-cholinergic. It was marketed in the U.S.A. as Cogentin. However, it was considered to be inferior to Benzhexol [60]. Other anti-cholinergic drugs were assessed but they were not widely used.

To a lesser extent anti- histaminergics were used for Parkinson's Disease. They lessened the effect of allergic reactions but they also reduced muscle contraction. Anti-histaminergic drugs were sold commercially, but only two of them, diphenhydramine (Benadryl) and phenindamine (Theophorin), were widely used in Parkinson's Disease [61]. Phenothiazines were sedatives that had anti-histaminergic effects.

The main phenothiazines used were diethazine HCl (Diparcol), and ethopropazine HCl (Parsidol) [62, 63]. Phenothiazines were normally used in combination with anti-cholinergics and anti-histaminergics.

Dopamine and Parkinson's Disease

During the 1950's the underlying biochemical changes in the brain were identified due largely to the work of Swedish scientist Arvid Carlsson. He demonstrated that dopamine was a neurotransmitter in the brain and not merely a precursor for noradrenaline as had been previously believed. He developed a method for measuring the amount of dopamine in brain tissues and found that dopamine levels in the basal ganglia, a brain area important for movement, were particularly high. He then showed that giving animals the drug reserpine caused a decrease in dopamine levels and a loss of movement control. These effects were similar to the symptoms of Parkinson's Disease [64]. Arvid Carlsson subsequently won the Nobel Prize in Physiology or Medicine in 2000 along with co-recipients Eric Kandel and Paul Greengard [65]. In 1960, Oleh Hornykiewicz showed that there was a lack of dopamine in Parkinson's Disease [66]. As the brain was impermeable to dopamine Hornykiewicz suggested the use of its precursor L-dopa in treating Parkinson's Disease. In 1964 it was demonstrated that L-dopa was made from L-tyrosine in the brain [67, 68].

The therapeutic use L-dopa

During the 1960's these findings led other doctors to try L-dopa with human Parkinson's patients and found it to alleviate some of the symptoms in the early stages of Parkinson's. Unlike dopamine its precursor L-Dopa could pass the blood brain barrier. The validity of the approach was shown by the transient benefit seen after injection of L-dopa. However, it was not of practical value as a treatment because of the severe toxicity associated with the injection. At this point, George C.Cotzias (1918-1977) made a critical observation that converted the transient response into a successful, large scale treatment [69, 70]. By starting with very small doses of L-Dopa, given orally every two hours under continued observation and gradually increasing the dose, he was able to stabilise patients on large enough doses to cause a dramatic remission of their symptoms. The first study reporting improvements in patients with Parkinson's Disease resulting from treatment with L-dopa was published in 1968 [71]. The result was soon confirmed by other investigators and so L-dopa became the standard treatment for Parkinsonian symptoms. L-dopa was the most effective method of relieving Parkinson's Disease symptoms there had ever been up until then but it was accompanied by widespread side effects and a long term deterioration.

Sinemet and Madopar

The dopa decarboxylase inhibitor Ro 4-4602 (benserazide) was synthesized by B. Hegedüs of Hoffmann-La Roche. Birkmayer found that Ro 4-4602 (benserazide) intensified and extended the effect of L-dopa in Parkinson's Disease by reducing its metabolism [72]. L-dopa dose could consequently be reduced by about 80%, and side effects were reduced. Hardly any Ro 4-4602 (benserazide) could pass the blood brain barrier and so it reduced the breakdown of peripheral L-dopa [73]. The combination of L-dopa with the decarboxylase inhibitor benserazide was commercially launched by Hoffmann-LaRoche in 1973 as Madopar. It was eventually also produced in a controlled release version called Madopar CR.

Cotzias tried the use of the dopa decarboxylase inhibitor MK485 (carbidopa) alongside L-dopa in his 1969 paper [74]. L-dopa combined with the decarboxylase inhibitor carbidopa was commercially launched in 1972 as Sinemet. Carbidopa made the product more effective by delaying the conversion of L-dopa into dopamine until the drug passed into the brain. The product was improved in 1991 when approval was given for Sinemet CR, which is a controlled release version of Sinemet. Marketed in both its new and older forms Sinemet became the world's leading treatment for Parkinson’s Disease [75].

MAO inhibitors

During the 1970's, MAO inhibitors were introduced in order to prolong the effect of L-dopa by delaying its breakdown. The enzyme monoamine oxidase (MAO) was first described in 1928 [76]. By inhibiting monoamine oxidase, MAO inhibitors were shown to be able to raise dopamine levels but the side effects were severe [77]. In 1968 it had been shown that there were two MAO enzymes, MAO-A and MAO-B [78]. Inhibition of MAO-B was suitable for Parkinson's Disease because its inhibition was not subject to the same risks as MAO generally. The most suitable drug for use as a MAO-B inhibitor, called at the time E-250, had already been synthesized in 1962 [79, 80]. It was eventually called deprenyl. In a clinical trial started in 1974 deprenyl was shown to be effective in Parkinson's Disease [81]. It was launched commercially in Hungary in 1977. Its use gradually spread to other countries but it was not approved in the U.S.A. until 1989. It came to be known as Selegiline. Since then, other MAO-B inhibitors such as Rasagiline have been used in Parkinson's Disease.

Dopamine agonists

Despite L-dopa initially being seen as a major breakthrough, as many as 25% of people taking L-dopa did not respond to it. Other people were being caused widespread side effects due to using it including dsykinesia. Consequently, directly stimulating the dopamine receptors using dopamine agonists appeared to some to be a better option. Apomorphine had been known since the 1950's. Schwab had used it with Parkinson's Disease in 1951 [82]. During the 1960's apomorphine was show to be similar in structure to dopamine and be capable of stimulating dopamine receptors [83, 84, 85]. Cotzias demonstrated efficacy using apomorphine in the treatment of Parkinsonism [86, 87]. When used alongside L-dopa its effects appeared to be additive. In 1974 the use of another dopamine agonist, bromocriptine, was introduced for the treatment of Parkinson's Disease with positive results [88, 89]. Other dopamine agonists were subsequently developed including cabergoline, lisuride, pergolide, pramipexole, ropinirole, and rotigotine [90]. However, all of the dopamine agonists caused side effects of their own.

From 2000 onwards

From 2000 onwards, L-dopa primarily as Sinemet and Madopar was already being widely used in the treatment of Parkinson's Disease, as were MAO-B inhibitors and dopamine agonists. Even more variants of each of them were being used, assessed or introduced. Besides these there was a proliferation of new approaches to the treatment of Parkinson's Disease that were being introduced or developed. These included Deep Brain Stimulation, COMT inhibitors, Stem cell surgery, and different formats of L-dopa.

Deep Brain Stimulation

Deep Brain Stimulation (DBS) is a surgical treatment that involves the use of electrodes that are implanted into the brain and connected to a small electrical device called a pulse generator that can be externally programmed. In 2002, The Food and Drug Administration (FDA) approved the use of Deep Brain Stimulation in Parkinson's Disease. It has normally only been approved for use in patients whose symptoms cannot be adequately controlled using drugs or whose drugs cause severe side effects [91]. Its use helped to rid or reduce symptoms but it has never rid Parkinson's Disease and has caused a variety of adverse effects [92].

COMT inhibitors

Catechol-O-methyl transferase (COMT) inhibitors had been suggested at the end of the 1960s as dopamine is metabolised not only by MAO but also by COMT, which is an enzyme [93]. During the first clinical trial in 1971 there were beneficial effects. However, its toxic effects prevented its further use [94]. Since then a number of COMT inhibitors have been developed, including the entacapone (Comtan) and tolcapone (Tasmar). Stalevo combined entacapone with L-dopa and carbidopa. It was given approval for use in 2003.

Stem cell surgery

At the beginning of the 21st century stem cell surgery was widely claimed to be capable of curing Parkinson's Disease. However, ethical objections to the method it used were delaying its use. Stem cell surgery, in which stem cells are placed inside the brain in order to replace lost cells, was claimed to be necessary for Parkinson's Disease because it was assumed that there is massive loss of the dopaminergic neurons (the cells involved in Parkinson's Disease). However, the theoretical basis of stem cell surgery in Parkinson's Disease was based on a fallacy because no studies had ever shown that there was a massive loss of the dopaminergic neurons in Parkinson's Disease. When stem cell surgery underwent formal clinical trials there was found to be little or no effect [95, 96, 97]. In a subsequent study, involving the use of bone marrow derived mesenchymal stem cells, there was also little or no effect [98].

Different forms of L-dopa

There was a proliferation of means of administering L-dopa aimed at providing advantages over the use of Sinemet and Madopar. Rytary and Numient combined the immediate release and the controlled release versions of L-dopa thereby combining the advantages of both [99]. Parcopa is an orally disintegrating tablet version of Sinemet [100]. Duodopa is Sinemet in the form of a gel. It is administered throughout the day using a portable pump directly into the small intestine through a surgically placed tube [101]. AcuForm is being added to a combination of L-dopa and carbidopa. AcuForm helps to deliver a drug like Sinemet over a longer period of time [102]. An L-dopa inhaler is also being developed. Due to problems caused by Parkinson's Disease drugs some people were even resorting back to mucuna pruriens, which is natural source of L-dopa that has been used for thousands of years [103].

Recent history

After thousands of years of describing and treating Parkinson's Disease, and despite the enormous resources used in developing new treatments, each method of treating Parkinson's Disease has been found to have serious inadequacies. They have all had either an unsound or only partially sound scientific basis. They have been aimed mostly at alleviating the symptoms in the short term rather than dealing with the cause. The treatments recently being developed for treating Parkinson's Disease have become progressively more diverse and scientifically unsound. The ultimate therapy, one that was able to rid symptoms without side effects, was still to be revealed.

[1] Beans, Roots and Leaves [2003] (Paul Bernard Foley)

[2] The four Vedas : Rik, Sama, Yajur and Atharva; Journal of the Royal Society of Medicine [1991] 84 (8) : 491-492 (M.Gourie-Devi, M.G.Ramu, B.S.Venkataram)

[3] Movement disorders [1990] 5 (91) : 47-48 (B.V.Manyam)

[4] Movement Disorders [2013] 28 (5) : 566-568 (S.Ovallath, P. Deepa)

[5] Huang Di Nei Jing Su Wen (Paul U.Unschuld)

[6] Archives of Neurology [2006] 63 : 782-784 (Z.Zhang, Z.Dong, G. C.Román)

[7] The Bible

[8] The Illiad (Homer)

[9] The Odyssey (Homer)

[10] Concerning Acute and Chronic Diseases (Caelius Aurelianus)

[11] De artibus (Aulus Cornelius Celsus)

[12] De Materia Medica (Pedanius Dioscorides)

[13] On tremor, palpitation, rigor and convulsion (Galen)

[14] Medical Compendium in Seven Books (Paul of Aegina)

[15] Syrian Anatomy, Pathology and Therapeutics or "The Book of Medicines" (E.A.W.Budge)

[16] Canon of Medicine (Ibn Sina)

[17] The notebooks of Leonardo da Vinci (Leonardo da Vinci), New England Journal of Medicine [1989] 320 (9) : 594 (D.B.Calne, A. Dubini, G.Stern)

[18] Henry VI (William Shakespeare), Movement Disorders [2005] 20 (6) : 768-769 (R.Stien)

[19] Herball, or Generall Historie of Plantes (John Gerard)

[20] Complete Herbal (Nicholas Culpeper)

[21] Life of Mr Thomas Hobbes of Malmesbury (John Aubrey)

[22] Pax Corporis (Ferenc Pápai Páriz)

[23] The English Malady (George Cheyne)

[24] Nosologia Methodica (François Boissier de Sauvages de Lacroix)

[25] The Hunterian Reminiscences (James Parkinson)

[26] James Parkinson : His life and times (A.D.Morris)

[27] An Essay on the Shaking Palsy (James Parkinson)

[28] Medico Chirurgical Transactions [1827] 13 : 232 (J.Elliotson), Lancet [1830/1831] i : 119 (J.Elliotson), Lancet [1831] i : 294, ii : 296, i : 556 (J. Elliotson)

[29] Neurology [1995] 45 (3 part 1) : 565-568 (R.Horowski, L. Horowski, S.Vogel, W.Poewe, F.W.Kielhorn)

[30] Lancet [1842] i : 616 (J.B.Thompson)

[31] Oeuvres complètes [Complete works] (by J.M.Charcot) [1885]

[32] Gazette de Hebdomadaire Medecine et Chirurgie [1861] 8 : 765, 816 (J.-M.Charcot, A.Vulpian), Gazette de Hebdomadaire Medecine et Chirurgie [1862] 9 : 54 (J.-M.Charcot, A.Vulpian)

[33] Lectures on diseases of the nervous system. Delivered at La Saltpêtrière [1877] 155 (J.-M.Charcot, translated by G.Sigerson)

[34] Lectures on diseases of the nervous system. Delivered at La Saltpêtrière [1877] 133-134, 150 (J.-M.Charcot)

[35] Lectures on the Diseases of the Nervous System, Volume 1 [1877] (J.-M.Charcot, translated by G. Sigerson)

[36] De la paralysie agitante [1872] (M.Claveleira)

[37] Traité de pathologie interne [1873] (S.Jaccoud)

[38] A Manual of Diseases of the Nervous System [1886] (William Gower)

[39] Lancet [1925] ii : 263 "The relation of paralysis agitans to the parkinsonian syndrome of epidemic encephalitis" (R.Cruchet)

[40] Movement Disorders [2007] (E.Broussolle, P.Krack, S.Thobois, J.Xie-Brustolin, P.Pollak, C.G.Goetz)

[41] Neurol.Centralbl. [1893] 12 : 89 (E.Mendel)

[42] Zeitschrift für Praktische Ärzte [1898] "Ueber Paralysis Agitans und ihre Behandlung" (Wilhelm Heinrich Erb)

[43] Paralysis agitans (Parkinson'sche Krankheit) (Wilhelm Heinrich Erb) [1906] in Die Deutsche Klinik (E.von Leyden and F.Klemperer)

[44] Practitioner [1869] 3 : 287 (U.S.L.Butler)

[45] Edinburgh Medical Journal [1865] 10 : 987 (W.R.Sanders)

[46] A manual of the diseases of the nervous system [1893] (W.R. Gowers)

[47] Leitfaden der Elektrodiagnostik und Elektrotherapie für Praktiker und Studierende [1824] (Toby Cohn)

[48] Practitioner [1941] 146 : 332 (M.Critchley)

[49] Wiener klinische Wochenschrift [1917] 30 : 581-585 (K.von Enonimo)

[50] Encephalitis Lethargica : During and After the Epidemic (Joel Vilensky)

[51] La Presse Médicale [1921] 29 : 83 (A.Radovici, J.F.Nicolesco),

[52] Schweiz Medizinische Wochenschrift [1936] 17 : 101 (M.Musella)

[53] Medizinische Klinik [1922] 18 : 41 (H.Pette)

[54] Münsch Medizinische Wochenschrift [1923] 70 : 47 (W. Szyszka)

[55] Münsch Medizinische Wochenschrift [1933] : 24 (C.Römer)

[56] Pharmaceutisch Weekblad [1937] 49 : 1456 (P.Kuiper, P.van der Vielen)

[57] QJM [1938] 7 (4) : 565-574 (N.S.Alcock, E.A.Carmichael)

[58] Psychiatrisch-neurologische Wochenschrift [1941] 43 : 465 (W.Völler)

[59] British Journal of Neurosurgery [1989] 3 : 271 (R.M.Redfern)

[60] British Medical Journal [1958] 2 : 1214 (M.Critchley)

[61] Extra Pharmacopoeia [1952] 715-730

[62] Die Geschichte der Arzneimittelforschung (B.Issekutz) [1971]

[63] Discoveries in Pharmacology [1983] 1 : 163 (P.Deniker)

[64] Nature [1957] 127 : 471 (A.Carlsson, M.Lindqvist, T.Magnusson)

[65] Nobel : A Century of Prize Winners (Michael Worek)

[66] Klinische Wochenschrift [1960] 38 : 1236 (H.Ehringer, O. Hornykiewicz)

[67] Biochemical and Biophysical Research Communications [1964] 14 : 453 (T.Nagatsu, M.Levitt, S.Udenfriend)

[68] Journal of Biological Chemistry [1964] 239 : 2910 (T.Nagatsu, M.Levitt, S.Udenfriend)

[69] Neurotoxicology [1984] 5 (1) : 5-12 "A personal and scientific biography of Dr. George C.Cotzias" (L.C.Tang)

[70] Trans Association of American Physicians [1978] 91 : 23-24 "George C.Cotzias 1918-1977" (L.Thomas)

[71] New England Journal of Medicine [1968] 278 (11) : 630 (G. Cotzias)

[72] Archiv fur Psychiatrie und Zeitschrift fur die gesamte Neurologie [1967] 210 : 29 (W.Birkmayer, M.Mentasti)

[73] Nature [1967] 215 : 852 (G.Bartholini, W.P.Burkard, A.Pletscher, H.M.Bates)

[74] New England Journal of Medicine [1969] 280 : 337 (G.C.Cotzias, P.S.Papavasilou, R.Gellene)

[75] Du Pont heritage - Sinemet (online history)

[76] Biochemical Journal [1928] 22 : 968 (M.L.C.Hare)

[77] Naunyn-Schmiedeberg's Archiv für experimentelle Pathologie und Pharmakologie [1959] 237 : 27 (G.Holzer, O.Hornykiewicz)

[78] Biochemical Pharmacology [1968] 17 : 1285 (J.P.Johnston)

[79] Magyar Tudom Akadémiai V. Tudom Osztály Közlem [1964] 15 : 231 (J.Knoll, Z.Ecseri, J.Nievel, B.Knoll)

[80] Archives Internationales de pharmacodynamie et de thérapie [1965] 155 : 154 (J.Knoll, Z.Ecseri, K.Keleman, J.Nievel, B.Knoll)

[81] Advances in Parkinsonism [1976] 381 (W.Birkmayer, P.Riederer, M.B.H.Youdim, W.Linauer)

[82] Transactions of the American Neurological Association [1951] 56 : 251-253 (R.Schwab, L.Amador, J.Lettvin)

[83] Psychopharmacologica [1965] 7 : 391 (A.M.Ernst), Experientia [1966] 22 : 837 (A.M.Ernst, P.G.Smelik)

[84] The Journal of Pharmacy and Pharmacology [1967] 19 : 627 (N.E.Andén, A.Rubenson, K.Fuxe, T.Hökfeldt)

[85] Psychopharmacologica [1967] 10 : 316 (A.M.Ernst)

[86] New England Journal of Medicine [1970] 282 : 31 (G.C.Cotzias, P.S.Papavasaliou, C.Fehling, B.Kaufman, I.Mena)

[87] New England Journal of Medicine [1970] 283 : 1289 (G.C. Cotzias, S.Duby, J.Z. Ginos, A.Steck, P.S.Papavasaliou)

[88] British Medical Journal [1974] 4 : 442 (D.B.Calne, P.F. Teychenne, L.E.Claveria, R.Eastman, J.K.Greenacre, A.Petrie)

[89] Lancet ii [1974] : 1355 (D.B.Calne, P.F.Teychenne, P.N.Leigh, A.N.Bamji, J.K. Greenacre)

[90] Journal of Neural Transmission [2007] 114 (1) : 127-134 (R. Horowski)

[91] Deep Brain Stimulation [2009] (Peter Bain, Tipu Aziz, Xuguang Liu, Dipankar Nandi)

[92] World Neurosurgery [2010] 73 (4) : 338-344 (F.Vergani, A.Landi, D.Pirillo, R.Cilia, A.Antonini, E.P.Sganzerla)

[93] Helvetica Chimica Acta [1962] 45 : 270 (A.Carlsson, M.Lindqvist, S.Filahromadko, H.Corrodi)

[94] Journal of Neurological Science [1971] 14 : 193 (A.D.Ericsson)

[95] Neurology [2000] 54 (5) : 1042-1050 (J.M.Schumacher, S.A. Ellias, E.P.Palmer, H.S.Kott, J.Dinsmore, P.K.Dempsey, A.J.Fischman, C.Thomas, R.G.Feldman, S.Kassissieh, R.Raineri, C.Manhart, et al)

[96] New England Journal of Medicine [2001] 344 (10) : 710-719 (C.R.Freed, P.E.Greene, R.E.Breeze, W.Y.Tsai, W.DuMouchel, R.Kao, S.Dillon, H.Winfield, S.Culver, J.Q.Trojanowski, D.Eidelberg, S.Fahn)

[97] Annals of Neurology [2003] 54 (3) : 403-414 (C.W.Olanow, C.G. Goetz, J.H.Kordower, A.J.Stoessl, V.Sossi, M.F.Brin, K.M.Shannon, G.M.Nauert, D.P.Perl, J.Godbold, T.B.Freeman)

[98] Translational Research [2010] 155 (2) : 62-70 (N.K. Venkataramana, S.K.Kumar, S.Balaraju, R.C.Radhakrishnan, A.Bansal, A.Dixit, D.K.Rao, M.Das, M.Jan, P.K.Gupta, S.M.Totey)

[99] Clinical Neuropharmacology [2009] 32 (4) : 189-192 (V.K. Hinson, C.G.Goetz, S.Leurgans, W.Fan, T.Nguyen, A.Hsu)

[100] Movement Disorders [2010] 25 (16) : 2724-2727 (W.G. Ondo, L.Shinawi, S. Moore)

[101] Duodopa's guide for health care givers [online]

[102] Movement Disorders [2015] 30 (9) : 1222-1228 (L.Verhagen Metman, N.Stover, C.Chen, V.E.Cowles, M.Sweeney)

[103] Panta [2010] 231 (6) : 1361-1369 (P.M.Luthra, S.Singh)

CHAPTER 2

FAMOUS PEOPLE WITH PARKINSON'S DISEASE

MUHAMMAD ALI
American boxer (1942-2016)

Muhammad Ali is a former American boxer who was three time world heavyweight champion. He became Olympic light heavyweight champion in 1960 at the Rome Olympics. In 1964 he became the youngest world heavyweight champion by beating Sonny Liston. In 1967 Muhammad Ali was stripped of his world heavyweight title for refusing to be drafted into the U.S. Army, because of his conscientious objections. He was allowed to resume boxing again in 1970. In 1974 he regained the world heavyweight title by beating George Foreman, and retained it the following year against former champion Joe Frazier. In 1978 Muhammad Ali lost the title to Leon Spinks but regained it the same year before relinquishing the title. He made a failed attempt to regain the world heavyweight title in 1980, and retired in 1981. He was diagnosed with Parkinson's Syndrome in 1984. In 1996, with Parkinsonian symptoms, he lit the flame at the Summer Olympics in Atlanta. In 1997 he set up The Muhammad Ali Parkinson Center to help people with Parkinson's Disease. In 2012, with assistance, he was a bearer of the Olympic Flag during the opening ceremonies of the London Olympics. In 2016 he was hospitalised with a respiratory condition from which he died the following day.

YASSER ARAFAT
Palestinian politician (1929-2004)

Yasser Arafat was Chairman of the Palestine Liberation Organization (PLO), President of the Palestinian National Authority (PNA), and leader and founder of the Fatah political party. He spent much of his life opposing Israel in order to try to achieve a Palestinian state. In 1994 he received the Nobel Peace Prize jointly with Yitzhak Rabin and Shimon Peres because of their peace negotiations. It was frequently speculated that Yasser Arafat had Parkinson's Disease because he exhibited the symptoms but he denied that he had it.

JIM BACKUS
American actor (1913-1989)

James Gilmore "Jim" Backus was an American actor most famous for the voice of the cartoon character Mr. Magoo. He also played James Dean's character's father in Rebel Without a Cause. Jim Backus died from complications of pneumonia, after suffering from Parkinson's Disease for many years.

ROGER BANNISTER
British athlete (1929)

Roger Bannister is a former British athlete. He is famous for breaking the world mile record by running the first sub four minute mile in 1954. Later that year he retired from athletics to become a neurologist, which included the treatment of Parkinson's Disease. He was knighted in 1975. He was diagnosed with Parkinson's Disease in 2011.

JOHN BETJEMAN
British Poet Laureate (1906-1984)

Sir John Betjeman was an English poet and writer. He wrote a lot of poetry collections as well as books on other subjects. In 1969 he received a knighthood and became Sir John Betjeman. In 1972 he was made Poet Laureate by Queen Elizabeth II. For the last decade of his life he increasingly suffered from Parkinson's Disease.

BOYI BHIMANNA
Telugu poet (1911-2005)

Boyi Bhimanna was a Telugu poet. He wrote over 70 books in total with his Gudiselu Kaalipothunnaayi (The huts are burning) being the most popular. After suffering from Parkinson's Disease for some time he died in 2005.

WHIT BISSELL
American actor (1909-1996)

Whit Bissell was an American actor, who made appearances in hundreds of films and television episodes including The Time Machine,

The Time Tunnel, The Incredible Hulk, Invasion of the Body Snatchers, The Virginian, The Caine Mutiny, and The Manchurian Candidate. He died in 1996 from the effects of Parkinson's Disease.

Margaret Bourke-White

American photographer (1904-1971)

Margaret Bourke-White was an American photographer. She was the first female to be allowed to work in combat zones during World War II. She photographed Stalin and also photographed Gandhi only hours before he was assassinated. She died from the complications of Parkinson's Disease about 18 years after she developed her first symptoms.

Antonio Cervantes

Colombian boxer (1945)

Antonio Cervantes is a former boxer from Colombia. He grew up shining shoes and selling contraband cigarettes. He became a professional boxer whilst only 18. He was world light welterweight champion from 1972 to 1976 and again from 1977 to 1980. He successfully defended his world championship title 16 times and had 21 world championship contests. He retired from boxing in 1983 having had 106 contests. He was diagnosed with Parkinson's Disease in 2011.

Owen Chamberlain

American physicist (1920-2006)

Own Chamberlain was an American physicist who is most known for his discovery, with his collaborator Emilio Segrè, of antiprotons, which are subatomic antiparticles. In 1959 they won the Nobel Prize for Physics for their discovery. Owen Chamberlain was diagnosed with Parkinson's Disease in 1985 and died from complications from Parkinson's Disease in 2006.

Prince Claus

Husband of Queen Beatrix of Netherlands (1926-2002)

Prince Claus was the prince consort of Queen Beatrix of the Netherlands. Prince Claus was born in Germany. In 1944 he was conscripted in to the German army but was captured before taking part in any military combat. In 1966 he married Princess Beatrix who subsequently became Queen of the Netherlands in 1980. Consequently, he was prince consort of the Netherlands until his death in 2002. Later in his life Prince Claus suffered from severe depression, cancer and Parkinson's Disease.

Billy Connolly

Scottish comedian and actor (1942)

Billy Connolly is a Scottish comedian, actor and musician. He is best known as a stand-up comedian and has made a lot of recordings. He was also in the films : The Last Samurai, Gulliver's Travels and The Hobbit: The Battle of the Five Armies. In 2013 it was announced that he was being treated for the initial symptoms of Parkinson's Disease.

Joe Cook

American actor (1890-1959)

Joe Cook was an American actor, comedian and entertainer most known for his work on Broadway but who also appeared in now mostly forgotten films such as Rain or Shine directed by Frank Capra. His career was prematurely ended by Parkinson's Disease in 1942.

George Coulouris

British actor (1903-1989)

George Coulouris was a British actor most famous for his role in Citizen Kane. He received an Oscar nomination for Watch on the Rhine. He also appeared in For Whom the Bell Tolls, Papillon, Joan of Arc, Mahler, and Murder on the Orient Express. He died in 1989 of heart failure following Parkinson's Disease.

Jordan Cronenweth

American cinematographer (1935-1996)

Jordan Scott Cronenweth was an American cinematographer who is probably best known for Blade Runner, for which he won major awards. He also worked on Altered States, and Peggy Sue Got Married, for which he earned an Academy Award nomination. He was misdiagnosed and treated for multiple sclerosis. However, in 1978 it was discovered that he was actually suffering from Parkinson's Disease.

SALVADOR DALÍ
Spanish artist (1904-1989)

Salvador Dalí was a Spanish surrealist artist who was famous for his eccentricity. He also wrote books and worked on films. Some of his most famous paintings are The Sacrament of the Last Supper, The Discovery of America by Christopher Columbus, Christ of Saint John of the Cross, The Persistence of Memory and Metamorphosis of Narcissus. He also created sculptures. In 1980 his hand started trembling. Consequently, in 1981 he was diagnosed with Parkinson's Disease.

BASIL D'OLIVEIRA
South African cricketer (1931-2011)

Basil D'Oliveira CBE is a former South African born cricketer. He was barred from first class cricket because he was classified as coloured under the South African apartheid regime. He emigrated to England who he represented in forty four Test matches and four One Day Internationals. The South African apartheid government refused to allow him to play for England in South Africa. In the latter part of his life he had Parkinson's Disease.

JAMES DOOHAN
Canadian actor (1920-2005)

James Doohan was a Canadian actor who is most known for his role as Scotty in the Star Trek films and television series. He also appeared in the tv series The Twilight Zone, Bewitched, Fantasy Island, The Man from U.N.C.L.E. (1964), and Bonanza. In later life he suffered from Parkinson's Disease.

ROBERT DRYDEN
American actor (1917-2003)

Robert Dryden was an American actor, who was one of radio's busiest character actors in the 1940s and 1950s, including over 200 episodes of

"CBS Radio Mystery Theater". He also appeared on television until the 1970s and in films including The Good, The Bad, and The Ugly. In 2003 he died of the complications of Parkinson's Disease.

Michael J.Fox
Canadian actor (1961)

Michael J.Fox is a Canadian born actor. He is most well known for the Back to the Future film trilogy. He acted in many other films, and also extensively on television, including the series Family Ties and Sin City. Michael J. Fox was diagnosed with Parkinson's Disease in 1991 but did not make it widely known until 1998. In 2000 He founded The Michael J.Fox Foundation for Parkinson's Research. He subsequently authored autobiographies in which he detailed his experiences with Parkinson's Disease.

Franco
Spanish dictator (1892-1975)

Francisco Franco was a Spanish dictator. He became a general in 1926 and in 1936 took part in a military coup. The coup failed and devolved into the Spanish Civil War during which Franco emerged as the leader of the Nationalists against the Popular Front government. After winning the civil war he established a right-wing authoritarian regime that lasted for the rest of his life. For a long time before he died he had Parkinson's Disease. He eventually had to give up power due to his illness.

Kirk Gibson
American baseball player (1957)

Kirk Gibson is a retired American baseball player. He played Major League baseball for Detroit Tigers, Los Angeles Dodgers, Kansas City Royals, Pittsburgh Pirates, and then again for Detroit Tigers. He won the Baseball World Series twice, with the Detroit Tigers in 1984, and the Los Angeles Dodgers in 1988. In the 1988 World Series, despite being injured, he hit a game winning home run. After being a baseball coach and manager he retired from baseball in 2014. He was diagnosed with Parkinson's Disease in 2015.

Carlos Antonio Gomes

Portuguese footballer (1932-2005)

Carlos António do Carmo Costa Gomes was a Portuguese goalkeeper. He won the Portuguese championship with Sporting Lisbon in 1952, 1953, 1954 and 1958, and the Portuguese Cup in 1958. He played for Portugal 18 times, from 1953 to 1958. He went in to exile because of his opposition to the dictatorial regime in Portugal. He returned to Portugal in 2005 suffering from Parkinson's Disease and died soon after.

Reverend Billy Graham

American evangelist (1918)

William Franklin "Billy" Graham is an American evangelical Christian evangelist. He rose to celebrity status as his sermons were broadcast on radio and television. It is claimed that Graham has preached the Gospel in person to more people than any other person in history. He has suffered from Parkinson's Disease since his late seventies.

Brian Grant

American basketball player (1972)

Brian Grant is a retired American basketball player. He began his career in the NBA in 1994 with the Sacramento Kings. He went on to play with Portland Trail Blazers, Miami Heat, Los Angeles Lakers, Phoenix Suns, and Boston Celtics. He retired from basketball in 2006. He was diagnosed with Parkinson's Disease soon after retiring in 2008. He set up The Brian Grant Foundation to help Parkinson's Disease.

Forrest Gregg

American football player (1933)

Forrest Gregg is a former American football player and coach. He played for the Green Bay Packers and the Dallas Cowboys. He was part of the Green Bay Packers team that won the first two Super Bowls, and won the 1972 Super Bowl with the Dallas Cowboys. He was a coach from 1972 until 1995 taking the Cincinnati Bengals to the Super Bowl in 1982. He was entered in to the Pro Football hall of fame in 1977. In 2011 Forrest Gregg was diagnosed with Parkinson's Disease.

NATHAN HEARD
American novelist (1937-2004)

Nathan Heard, sometimes known as Nathan C.Heard, was an American author. He wrote his most famous book, Howard Street, while serving time in the Trenton State Penitentiary for armed robbery. His other books include A Cold Fire Burning, House of Slammers, To Reach a Dream and When Shadows Fall. He died in 2004 of complications from Parkinson's Disease.

GEORGE ROY HILL
American film director (1921-2002)

George Roy Hill was an American film director. He directed films including The Sting (for which he won an Oscar), Butch Cassidy and the Sundance Kid (for which he was nominated for an Oscar). Both starred the acting duo Paul Newman and Robert Redford. He also directed Slaughterhouse-Five, The Great Waldo Pepper, The World According to Garp, and Thoroughly Modern Millie. He died in 2002 of complications of Parkinson's Disease.

PHIL HILL
American motor racing driver (1927-2008)

Philip Toll Hill was an American motor racing driver. In 1961 he won the Formula One World Drivers' Championship. He also won the Le Mans 24 hour race three times, in 1958, 1961, 1962. He died in 2008 after a short illness from the complications of Parkinson's Disease.

ADOLF HITLER
German dictator (1889-1945)

The Nazi leader, Adolf Hitler, was known to have Parkinson's Disease from 1933 until his suicide in 1945. At the end of the Second World War he was largely confined to his bunker in Berlin. In his final days in the bunker he shuffled around his room mumbling to himself, repeating the same phrases, sometimes pointing to his hand and saying repeatedly "Look it is getting better. It's not trembling so much, and I can keep it still". He had trembling hands and stooped shoulders. He also had tremor in his left leg. The right arm trembled more than the left. With his hand extended and fingers spread he did not tremor. His shaking was related to emotional upsets. When the military situation became far worse his left hand tremor was stronger. At the end of his life he had a stooped back, could barely walk, had a shuffling gait, his right leg was dragging, and he had head shaking. His left hand violently trembled on a limply dangling arm. He had developed the appearance of an old man. The Nazi hierarchy had tried to conceal his Parkinson's Disease. There are two films of Adolf Hitler's last public appearance, one that was shown in which he displayed no symptoms of Parkinson's Disease, and another that was not shown in which he had the symptoms of Parkinson's Disease. Hitler was treated by his personal physician Dr Theo Morrell, who was well known for his unconventional, holistic and alternative treatments. Dr Morell kept detailed diaries of his treatment of Hitler's Parkinson's Disease. Hitler was being given 28 different pills a day along with numerous injections every few hours. Dr Morell saw Hitler every day, sometimes 2 or 3 times daily. Dr Morell made an attempt at temporarily influencing Hitler's Parkinson's Disease by subcutaneous injections of Harmin (a MAO inhibitor). On April 22nd, 1945 Hitler dismissed Morell from his Berlin bunker saying that he didn't need any more medical help. Dr Morell's methods still continued after he went because he left behind a lot of pre-prepared medicines including those for Parkinson's Disease. However, just a week later Hitler committed suicide.

Bob Hoskins
British actor (1942-2014)

Bob Hoskins was an English film and television actor. He appeared in films such as The Long Good Friday (1980), The Cotton Club (1984), Mona Lisa (1986), Who Framed Roger Rabbit (1988), Mermaids (1990), Hook (1991), and Neverland (2011). He retired from acting when he was diagnosed with Parkinson's Disease in 2012. In 2014 he died of pneumonia.

Alexander Issigonis
British car designer (1906-1988)

Alexander Issigonis was a British car designer who was born in a Greek community in the Ottoman Empire. He is most famous for his creation of the Mini. He designed other cars including the Morris Minor and the Austin Maxi. He was knighted by Queen Elizabeth II for his work. He died in 1998 due to the complications of Parkinson's Disease.

Mary Jackson

American actress (1910-2005)

Mary Jackson was an American actress who is best known for her role in The Waltons. She also had roles in the tv series Route 66, The Fugitive, Barnaby Jones, Columbo, Hart to Hart, Quincy, Hill Street Blues, and Magnum P.I.. She died at the age of 95 because of Parkinson's Disease.

Ba Jin

Chinese writer (1904-2005)

Ba Jin, was the pen name of the Chinese writer Li Yaotang. He wrote collections of short stories, novels, novellas, and a lot of non-fiction. The work he is best known for is The Family, The Love Trilogy Fog, Rain, Lightning, and the novellas Autumn in Spring and A Dream of the Sea. During the Cultural Revolution he was heavily persecuted as a counter revolutionary. He suffered from Parkinson's Disease from 1983. It eventually confined him to a hospital and left him unable to speak and walk. He died of cancer when he was 100.

Pope John Paul II

Polish Pope (1920-2005)

Pope John Paul II was Pope of the Catholic Church and Sovereign of The Holy See from 1978 until his death in 2005. He was born in Poland and was originally called Karol Józef Wojtyla. He became a priest in 1946, a bishop in 1958, the Archbishop of Krakow in 1964, and a cardinal in 1967. He was elected Pope in 1978. Whilst Pope he travelled to 129 countries and was involved in numerous social, political and religious issues. Although he was suspected of having Parkinson's Disease it was not disclosed until 2001. It was not confirmed by the Vatican until 2003, 12 years after he developed it. He was beatified in 2011.

RAY KENNEDY
British footballer (1951)

Ray Kennedy is an English former football player. With Arsenal and Liverpool he won every domestic trophy, and six European trophies. He also played for England. He was forced to retire when he was 32, due to the early symptoms of Parkinson's Disease. Parkinson's Disease was confirmed when he was 35. He has spent the majority of his life since retirement and diagnosis working towards publicising and raising funds for the research and treatment of Parkinson's Disease.

DEBORAH KERR
British actress (1921-2007)

Deborah Kerr was a British actress known for her films The King and I, An Affair to Remember, From Here to Eternity, Quo Vadis, The Innocents, Black Narcissus, Heaven Knows, Mr. Allison, The Life and Death of Colonel Blimp, and Separate Tables. She was nominated six times for the Academy Award for best actress. She died from the effects of Parkinson's Disease in 2007.

JANSHER KHAN
Pakistani squash player (1969)

Jansher Khan is widely considered to be one of the greatest squash players of all time. During his career he won the World Open a record eight times, and the British Open six times. Jansher Khan officially announced his retirement from squash in 2001. He had won 99 professional squash titles and was ranked the World No.1 squash player for over six years. He came out of retirement in 2007. In 2011, after developing sudden shaking of hands and a loss of mental stability, he was diagnosed with Parkinson's Disease.

GUY KIBBEE
American actor (1882-1956)

Guy Kibbee was an American stage and film actor. After beginning his career on Mississippi riverboats he became a successful Broadway actor. He subsequently appeared on television and in films including 42nd Street, Captain Blood, Our Town and Mr. Smith Goes to

Washington. He died from complications arising from Parkinson's Disease in 1956.

Jimmy Knepper

American jazz trombonist (1927-2003)

Jimmy Knepper was an American jazz trombonist. He worked extensively with bassist and composer Charlie Mingus, until Charlie Mingus ended their working relationship by assaulting him. Jimmy Knepper also recorded with Kenny Burrell, Gil Evans, George Adams, Thad Jones, and Mel Lewis. Jimmy Knepper died in 2003 after a long battle with Parkinson's Disease.

Ted Kroll

American golfer (1919–2002)

Ted Kroll was an American golfer. In 1949 he began a 34 year career on the PGA Tour career in which he won eight tournaments. He topped the earnings list in 1956 by winning three tournaments, and finishing second in the PGA Championship, which is one of the major golf tournaments. He also played three times in the Ryder Cup, in 1953, 1955 and 1957. In his later years he suffered from Parkinson's Disease.

Udo Lattek

German football coach (1935-2015)

After Udo Lattek's career as a player ended he became the assistant coach of the German national team that played in the 1966 World Cup final. He went on to manage football clubs including Bayern Munich, Borussia Mönchengladbach, Borussia Dortmund and Barcelona. He won the European Champions Cup, European Cup Winners Cup, UEFA Cup, German championships and cups, and Spanish cups before retiring in 2000. In 2013 he was diagnosed with Parkinson's Disease.

Walter Lord

American author (1917–2002)

Walter Lord was an American author. He was best known for A Night to Remember, which is about the sinking of the Titanic. He also wrote best selling books on subjects such as Pearl Harbor (Day of Infamy), the Battle of Midway (Incredible Victory), the Battle of the Alamo (A Time to Stand), and Arctic exploration (Peary to the Pole). He died in 2002 after a long struggle with Parkinson's Disease.

Ferdy Mayne
German actor (1916-1998)

Ferdy Mayne was a German actor. Because his family was Jewish he was sent to Britain in 1932 to protect him from the Nazis. He made over 200 films and television programmes. Those films he appeared in included Barry Lyndon, Conan the Destroyer, Where Eagles Dare, and Dance of the Vampires. During the 1990s he suffered from Parkinson's Disease from which he died in 1998.

Eugene McCarthy
American politician (1916–2005)

Eugene McCarthy served in the U.S. House of Representatives from 1949 to 1959 and the U.S. Senate from 1959 to 1971. He unsuccessfully ran for the U.S. Presidency five times. In the 1968 election his success caused the then President Lyndon B.Johnson to withdraw from the Democratic nomination for the Presidency. He died of complications from Parkinson's Disease at the age of 89.

Ralph McQuarrie
American film artist (1929-2012)

Ralph McQuarrie designed the original Star Wars trilogy (Star Wars, The Empire Strikes Back, Return of the Jedi), the original Battlestar Galactica TV series, E.T. the Extra-Terrestrial, and also Cocoon, for which he won the 1985 Academy Award for Visual Effects. He also worked on Close Encounters of the Third Kind, Raiders of the Lost Ark, and Star Trek IV. Ralph McQuarrie died aged 82 from the complications of Parkinson's Disease.

Alois Mock
Austrian politician (1934)

Alois Mock was a politician of the Austrian People's Party. He was the Vice Chancellor of Austria from 1987 to 1989, and the Austrian foreign minister from 1987 to 1995. As Austrian foreign minister he helped take Austria into the European Union. In 1989 he opened the fortified border with Hungary, enabling East Germans to emigrate to Austria and West Germany, thereby facilitating the fall of Communism. In 1999 he retired from the Austrian parliament because of Parkinson's Disease.

Eugenio Monti

Italian bobsledder (1928-2003)

Eugenio Monti is one of the most successful bobsledders in the history of the sport. He competed in the two man and four man bobsleigh events. He won nine World Championships. He also won six Olympic medals, at the 1956, 1964 and 1968 Olympics, of which two were gold. Whilst suffering from Parkinson's Disease he committed suicide by a self inflicted gunshot to the head in 2003.

Kenneth More

British actor (1914-1982)

Kenneth More was an English film, television and theatre actor. He made films including Reach for the Sky, A Night to Remember, The Admirable Crichton, Genevieve, Sink the Bismarck!, The Longest Day, The Thirty-Nine steps, Battle of Britain, North West Frontier and Oh! What a Lovely War. His most well known television roles were in The Forsyte Saga, and Father Brown. He died in 1982 from Parkinson's Disease at the age of 67.

Giulio Natta

Italian chemist (1903-1979)

Giulio Natta was an Italian chemist. His work led to the development of the Ziegler-Natta catalyst. He won the Nobel Prize for Chemistry in 1963 with Karl Ziegler for their work on high polymers. He was diagnosed with Parkinson's Disease in 1956. In 1963, due to the deterioration in his symptoms, he required the assistance of his son and his four colleagues to present his speech when he received the Nobel Prize in Stockholm. He died when he was 76 after having had Parkinson's Disease for 23 years.

ANNA NEAGLE
British actress (1904-1986)

Anna Neagle was an English film actress and singer. She was renowned for her portrayals of real-life heroines, including Nell Gwynn, Queen Victoria (in Victoria the Great, and Sixty glorious years) and Edith Cavell. She made her last film appearance in 1957. She suffered from Parkinson's Disease in her later years.

NORMAN PANAMA
American writer, producer and director (1914-2003)

Norman Panama was an American screenwriter and film director. He collaborated with Melvin Frank in a writing partnership that lasted for three decades. He wrote films including White Christmas, The Court Jester, and Not with My Wife You Don't!. He also wrote gags for comedians such as Bob Hope and Groucho Marx. He received three Oscar nominations. He died in 2003 from complications due to Parkinson's Disease.

DAVE PARKER
American baseball player (1951)

Dave Parker is a retired American baseball player. He began his career in the Major League in 1973 with the Pittsburgh Pirates, where he spent ten years. He went on to play with Cincinnati Reds, Oakland Athletics, Milwaukee Brewers, California Angels, and Toronto Blue Jays. He won the World Series twice, in 1979 and 1989, and played in the All Star game seven times. He retired from baseball in 1991. He was diagnosed with Parkinson's Disease in 2013.

JOE PASTERNAK
American film producer (1901–1991)

Joseph Pasternak was a Hungarian born American film producer. After a successful career in Germany he moved to the U.S.A.. There he produced films such as Anchors Aweigh, The Great Caruso, and Destry Rides Again. He received two Oscar nominations. He died from complications arising from Parkinson's Disease only a few days before his 90th birthday.

Mervyn Peake
British author (1911-1968)

Mervyn Peake was an English author and artist. He was born in China a few months before the revolution. He is best known for a series of novels usually referred to as the Gormenghast series : Titus Groan (1946), Gormenghast (1950), and Titus Alone (1959). He eventually developed the early symptoms of Parkinson's Disease for which he was given electroconvulsive therapy without gaining any beneficial effect from it.

Enoch Powell
British politician (1912-1998)

John Enoch Powell was a British politician, who served as a Conservative Party MP from 1950 until 1974, as Minister of Health from 1960 to 1963, and as the Shadow Defence Secretary from 1965 to 1968. He was most famous for his anti-immigration "Rivers of Blood" speech made in 1968. In 1974 he suddenly left the Conservative Party. From 1974 until 1987 he was an Ulster Unionist Party MP. At the age of 80, he was diagnosed with Parkinson's Disease.

Vincent Price
American actor (1911-1993)

Vincent Price was an American actor. He made his film debut in 1938. He is most well known for his films such as The Fall of the House of Usher, House on Haunted Hill, The Last Man on Earth, Edward Scissorhands, as well as television series, and his voice on the pop video Thriller. He is mainly associated with horror films. He had Parkinson's Disease for a long time. He was a life long smoker and died of lung cancer.

Michael Redgrave
British actor (1908-1985)

Sir Michael Redgrave was an English actor most known for films such as The Lady Vanishes, The Dam Busters, The Importance of Being Earnest, The Loneliness of the Long Distance Runner, 1984, The Hill, Battle of Britain, and Oh! What a Lovely War. He also had children and grandchildren who were famous actors. He was knighted in 1959. His career came to an end in 1975 after developing Parkinson's Disease, which contributed to his death.

JANET RENO
American politician (1938-2016)

Janet Reno was the U.S. Attorney General from 1993 until 2001. She was the first Attorney General to be a woman. She was nominated to be Attorney General by President Bill Clinton. In 1995, while serving as Attorney General, she announced that she had Parkinson's Disease. In 2002 she failed to become the Governor of Florida and retired from public office. She died from the complications of Parkinson's Disease.

FREDERICK ROACH
American boxing trainer (1960)

"Freddie" Roach is an American boxing trainer and a former boxer. Freddie Roach suffers from Parkinson's Disease. He has trained more than twenty world champions including Oscar De La Hoya, Virgil Hill, Mike Tyson, Wladimir Klitschko, Michael Moorer, Amir Khan, Bernard Hopkins, Marlon Starling, and Manny Pacquiao. He has also trained mixed martial arts fighters.

LINDA RONSTADT
American singer (1946)

Linda Ronstadt is a former American singer. She won 11 Grammy Awards and has gold, platinum and multi-platinum albums. She has recorded with artists including Frank Zappa, Rosemary Clooney, The Chieftains, Emmylou Harris, Dolly Parton, Aaron Neville, Neil Young, and Johnny Cash. She could no longer sing after being diagnosed with Parkinson's Disease when she was 66. She began to show symptoms eight years earlier.

SONIA RYKIEL
French fashion designer (1930-2016)

Sonia Rykiel was a French fashion designer. In 1968 she founded the Sonia Rykiel label. Her knitwear designs and new fashion techniques led her to be dubbed the "Queen of Knitwear". She also wrote several novels. In 2012, she revealed she had been diagnosed with Parkinson's Disease 15 years earlier. She eventually died from the complications of Parkinson's Disease.

Frank Sherwood Rowland

American chemist (1927-2012)

Frank Sherwood Rowland was a Nobel Prize winning chemist. His research was on atmospheric chemistry and chemical kinetics. His best known work was the discovery, in 1974, that chlorofluorocarbons contribute to the depletion of the ozone layer. In 1995 he won the Nobel Prize for Chemistry along with Mario Molina and Paul Crutzen for their contribution towards various fields. He died of complications from Parkinson's Disease.

Leonid Shamkovich

Russian chess grandmaster (1923-2005)

Leonid Aleksandrovich Shamkovich was a chess Grandmaster. He was the five times champion of the Soviet Union. He left the Soviet Union in 1975, moving first to Israel, then Canada, and finally the U.S.A., where he lived for the rest of his life. After his emigration he became the U.S. champion. He died of complications from Parkinson's Disease and cancer in 2005.

Walter Sisulu

South African politician (1912-2003)

Walter Sisulu was a South African anti-apartheid activist and member of the African National Congress (ANC). He was Secretary General of the ANC from 1949 until 1954. He was repeatedly jailed for his activism until 1964 when he received a life sentence. He remained in prison, mostly on Robben Island, at the same time as Nelson Mandela until 1989 when he was released from prison. In 1991 he became the ANC deputy president. He remained as ANC deputy president until after South Africa's first democratic election in 1994, when ill health forced him to retire from active politics. In later life he had Parkinson's Disease.

TERRY THOMAS
British actor (1911-1990)

Terry Thomas was an English actor most known for films such as It's a Mad, Mad, Mad, Mad World, Those Magnificent Men in Their Flying Machines, Monte Carlo or Bust, I'm all right Jack, and Jules Verne's Rocket to the Moon. He was diagnosed with Parkinson's Disease in 1971, which eventually brought his career to an end. His last film role was in 1980. At the time of his death he was very ill with Parkinson's Disease and living in virtual poverty.

JEREMY THORPE
British politician (1921-2014)

Jeremy Thorpe is a former British politician. He was a Member of Parliament from 1959 to 1979, and leader of the Liberal Party from 1967 to 1976. He was accused of having a homosexual relationship when homosexuality was still illegal, and of conspiring to murder the accuser. Although he was acquitted the trial ended his political career. Soon after his acquittal Jeremy Thorpe was found to have Parkinson's Disease and retired from public life.

PIERRE TRUDEAU
Canadian politician (1919-2000)

Pierre Trudeau was the Canadian Prime Minister from 1968 to 1979, and then again from 1980 to 1984. He was a member of the Canadian Parliament from 1965 until 1984 and leader of the Liberal Party of Canada from 1968 to 1984. During this period his personality dominated the political scene to an extent never seen before in Canada. In the last years of his life he was afflicted with Parkinson's Disease and prostate cancer. Yet he continued to work at his law practice up until his death.

JOHN WALKER
New Zealand athlete (1952)

John Walker is a former middle distance runner. He broke the world record for the mile in 1975. In 1976, he became Olympic 1500 metre champion at the Munich Olympics. The same year he broke the 2000 metre world record. In 1979 he broke the 1500 metre indoor world record. In 1985 he became the first man in history to run 100 sub 4 minute miles and eventually ran 135 sub 4 minute miles. In 1996, he announced that he had Parkinson's Disease.

Tim Wall
Australian cricketer (1904-1981)

Thomas Wall, who was known as Tim Wall, was an Australian cricketer. He played eighteen Test matches for Australia between 1929 and 1934. He was primarily a bowler. His 10 wickets for 36 runs was the best first-class figures recorded in Australia. He died in 1981 after a long battle with Parkinson's Disease.

George Wallace
American politician (1919-1998)

George Wallace was the Governor of Alabama, serving four terms : 1963-1967, 1971-1975, 1975-1979 and 1983-1987. He was known for being in favour of racial segregation, which he eventually renounced. As a Democrat he unsuccessfully ran for the U.S. Presidency four times. An assassination attempt in 1972 left him paralysed requiring him to use a wheelchair. At the end of his life he had Parkinson's Disease.

Ed Weinberger
American furniture designer (1942)

Ed Weinberger is an American furniture designer. He began designing furniture in 1988. Some of his unique furniture designs include a Cubist-Constructivist set of drawers and a mysterious tension-rod credenza. He developed Parkinson's Disease when he was 40 years old. Sometimes, having Parkinson's Disease would cause him to collapse and lay frozen.

Maurice White
American singer and songwriter (1941-2016)

Maurice White was an American singer and songwriter. He was best known for the music he produced with Earth, Wind & Fire. Their songs included September, Fantasy, Shining Star, and Boogie Wonderland. He also worked with singers including Barbra Streisand and Neil Diamond. He largely stopped touring with Earth, Wind & Fire in the early 1990s for health reasons that included Parkinson's Disease, that he had until his death in 2016.

Albert Whitlock

American matte artist (1915-1999)

Albert Whitlock was an American matte artist who was responsible for the visual effects in over 500 films. He worked on films such as The 39 steps, The Sting, Dune, The Birds, and Greystoke : The Legend of Tarzan. He won Academy awards for Earthquake and The Hindenburg. His work was cut short when he developed Parkinson's Disease.

Edward Winter

American actor (1937-2001)

Edward Winter was an American actor best known for his role in M*A*S*H. He also appeared in Cabaret, Murder She Wrote, Cagney & Lacey, Dallas, Falcon Crest, and Soap. He died from the complications of Parkinson's Disease.

Deng Xiaoping

Chinese politician (1904-1997)

Deng Xiaoping was a Chinese politician. As leader of the Communist Party of China Deng Xiaoping was a reformer who led China towards a market economy. He was a major supporter of Mao Zedong in the early 1950s. He was a member of the People's National Congress from 1959 to 1964 and again from 1978 to 1997. He was Paramount leader of the People's Republic of China from 1978 to 1992. He helped to develop China into one of the fastest-growing economies in the world. He died in 1997 at the age of 92 from a lung infection and Parkinson's Disease.

Lee Kuan Yew

Singapore politician (1923-2015)

Lee Kuan Yew was the first Prime Minister of Singapore. He was Prime Minister from 1959 to 1980. He was a member of Parliament for

60 years from 1955 until his death in 2015. He had Parkinson's Disease for the last few years of his life. Parkinson's Disease severely limited his mobility but he refused to use a wheelchair or a walking stick. He instead walked aided by his security officers.

MAO ZEDONG
Chinese politician (1893-1976)

Chairman Mao Zedong was the leader of the Chinese revolution. He led the Communist Party to victory against Kuomintang in the Chinese Civil War and was a founder of the People's Republic of China in 1949. In 1966 he introduced the Cultural revolution, which aimed to advance socialism, but declared it at an end in 1969. He retained political control of China until his death in 1976. His theoretical contributions are collectively known as Maoism. In the last years of his life Chairman Mao was faced with declining health, which included Parkinson's Disease. However, in China his Parkinson's Disease is rarely mentioned.

CHAPTER 3

PREVALENCE OF PARKINSON'S DISEASE

History of prevalence

As life expectancies have improved, the number and proportion of people with Parkinson's Disease has probably been increasing for centuries. However, in recent decades, the rate at which people with Parkinson's Disease have been newly diagnosed has been declining. The annual rate of decline is somewhere between 1% and 6%. A rate of decline of 1% was obtained when symptoms and Parkinson's Disease drugs were included. A decline of 6% was obtained when only Parkinson's Disease diagnosis was considered [1]. An assessment of the incidence rates between 1990 and 2010 found a reduction in 2000 down to 55% of what the incidence rate was in 1990. The incidence of Parkinson's Disease in 2010 was found to be only 39% of what it was in 1990. Therefore, the incidence of Parkinsonism in general, and Parkinson's Disease in particular, decreased substantially between 1990 and 2011, and is continuously declining [2]. However, in another study, there was found to be a very gradual increase in the incidence of Parkinson's Disease between 1976 and 2005 but only in men [3].

World prevalence

There are up to 10 million or more people in the world who have Parkinson's Disease. There may be many more than this due to the incompleteness and inconsistencies of prevalence studies, no precise definition of Parkinson's Disease, and so many people with Parkinson's Disease not being diagnosed. The actual number of people in the world with Parkinson's Disease is not known.

World's highest prevalence

China is the country with the world's greatest number of people with Parkinson's Disease. In China there are probably more than 1.7 million people who have Parkinson's Disease [4].

The world's highest prevalence of Parkinson's Disease is along the River Nile in Egypt, south of Cairo, amongst illiterate Egyptians in rural areas. They have a prevalence rate of 1,103 per 100,000. The high prevalence of Parkinson's Disease is probably related to poverty rather than illiteracy [5].

The world's second highest prevalence of Parkinson's Disease has been found among the Amish religious community [6]. The Amish are primarily in the North East of the U.S.A.. They are a devoutly religious community who believe in the literal interpretation of the Bible. They usually segregate themselves from other communities, wear traditional clothes, and live a traditional lifestyle that does not permit the use of electricity, television, radio, or telephones. For transport they use horses and carriages instead of cars, which they are not allowed to use. The prevalence of Parkinson's Disease among the Amish aged 60 or older has been found to be 5,703 per 100,000. According to U.N. Data, 17% of the U.S. population is aged 60 or older. So the prevalence of Parkinson's Disease in the Amish community as a whole is around 970 per 100,000. The Amish refuse to take out health insurance. They are also afflicted by genetic disorders. However, the more closely related the Amish were the less likely they were to be affected by Parkinson's Disease, suggesting that genetics is not the cause. The Amish are primarily involved in agriculture, and most of them use pesticides, but the effect of pesticides on the Amish has not been assessed.

Albania is the country with the world's highest prevalence of Parkinson's Disease by far. The prevalence figures for Parkinsonism were found to be 800 per 100,000. Parkinsonism includes some other medical disorders. So the Albanian figure for only Parkinson's Disease would be lower but still far higher than any other country. The prevalence of neurological disorders in Albania was found to be high generally [7].

The world's highest prevalence of Parkinson's Disease of any specific area is in the vicinities of ferromanganese plants near Brescia in Italy, where 407 people per 100,000 population have Parkinson's Disease [8]. Manganese concentrations in settled dust were found to be significantly higher in the surroundings and downwind from the ferromanganese plants. In high concentrations, manganese is a known cause of Parkinson's Disease.

Native Americans, including American Indian and Alaska Native peoples have a prevalence rate of 355 per 100,000, which is well beyond that of the general population [9]. Amongst the Navajo Indians it is 261-336 per 100,000 and the incidence is 35.9 per 100,000 [10, 11]. The highest prevalence rate of any region of North America is Nebraska, in the U.S.A. with 329 people per 100,000 population having Parkinson's Disease. It is possible that the prevalence of Parkinson's Disease in Nebraska is due to the heavy use of insecticides in what is largely a farming area [12].

The Parsi community of Bombay, India have a prevalence of Parkinson's Disease of 328 per 100,000 population [13]. This is despite India as a whole having a low prevalence of Parkinson's Disease. The Parsi practice Zoroastrianism, a religion based on the teachings of Zoroaster. As part of their religion, the Parsis in Mumbai burn Aspand seeds on charcoal to rid their children of the Evil Eye, which is the name for a sickness transmitted, usually without intention, by someone who is envious, jealous, or covetous. The fumes are often inhaled. Aspand seed is the richest natural source of two alkaloids, harmine and harmaline [14]. They are MAO Inhibitors, which are a type of drug used in Parkinson's Disease. Long term use of drugs such as MAO inhibitors eventually has the opposite effect and so may cause the high prevalence of Parkinson's Disease amongst the Parsi.

World's lowest prevalence

Ethiopia has the world's lowest recorded prevalence of Parkinson's Disease. At a rate of only 7 per 100,000 it is far below the world's highest prevalence rate of 1,103 per 100,000 that exists just south of Cairo [15]. As Parkinson's Disease tends to be more common in older people the very low prevalence in Ethiopia may result from the very low life expectancy in Ethiopia. For most African countries the prevalence rates are not known. If they were, other countries in the same region as Ethiopia or even in other parts of Africa may produce even lower prevalence figures than those of Ethiopia.

Prevalence by country

The prevalence for each country per 100,000 of population, in those countries in which it is known, from highest to lowest is : Albania 800 [7], China 797-16 [16-19], Egypt 557-213 [5, 20], France 410-308 [21], U.S.A. 329-107 [12, 22], Canada 317-125 [23, 24], Italy 294-104 [25-29], Iran 285 [30], Navajo Indians 261 [11], Israel 256 [31], Faeroe Islands 206-183 [32, 33], Turkey 202 [34], Japan 192-76 [35-40], San Marino 185 [41], Germany 183 [42], Finland 166-120 [43, 44], Bulgaria 164-137 [45, 46], Estonia 152 [47], Taiwan 147 [48], Australia 146-104 [49, 50], England 142-121 [51, 52, 53], Wales 142 [54], Portugal 180-135 [55, 125], Cuba 135 [56], Scotland 129-103 [57, 58], Spain 122 [59], Norway 102 [60], Thailand 95 [61], Sweden 76 [62], New Zealand 76 [57], Nigeria 67 [63], Poland 66 [64], Jordan 59 [65], India 52 [66], Bolivia 50 [67], Israel (muslims) 43 [68], Libya 31 [69], Colombia 31 [70], Sub Saharan Africa 20-7 [71], Korea 19 [72], Ethiopia 7 [15].

The prevalence of Parkinson's Disease can even differ a lot within the same country among different peoples. The prevalence amongst Bulgarian Gypsies is only one tenth of that found amongst other Bulgarians [46]. The prevalence in the U.S.A. tends to differ according to race, with Hispanics, then Whites, then Asians, then Blacks being more prone in one study [73], and Whites then Blacks then Asians in another [74]. Other studies in the U.S.A. gave different results [75, 76].

Incidence by country

The rate at which people with Parkinson's Disease are newly diagnosed differs greatly according to the country. The incidence for each country, in which it is known, per 100,000 of population per year, from highest to lowest is : France 49-36 [21], Navajo Indians 35.9 [11], Argentina 31.2 [77], Taiwan 28 [48], Italy 23-10 [29, 78], Sweden 22.5-7.9 [62, 79], Faeroe Islands 21.1 [31], U.S.A. 20.5-13.0 [73, 75, 80], Japan 16.9 - 10.2 [35, 37, 39, 81], Estonia 16.8 [82], Finland 16.6-14.9 [43, 44], Scotland 16.0-14.6 [83, 84], Norway 12.6 [85], England 12 [53, 86], Bulgaria 11.6 [87], Netherlands 11.5 [88], Russia 9.0 [89], China 8.7-1.5 [18, 19], India 5.7 [66], Libya 4.5 [69] .

Age distribution

In 1875, Henri Huchard (1844-1911) detailed the first case of Juvenile Parkinson's Disease. He described a 3 year old child who had all the clinical features of Parkinson's Disease. The youngest reported case of Parkinson's Disease is that of a 10 year old girl from Oklahoma, who showed her first symptoms of Parkinson's Disease at only 2 years old. However, although there are teenagers and people in their twenties with Parkinson's Disease it is very uncommon for people under the age of 30 to develop Parkinson's Disease. The likelihood of somebody developing Parkinson's Disease becomes increasingly more common with age [90-96]. The average age at which symptoms usually begin differs from country to country, with the latest average onset being in Sweden 65.6 [62], and Estonia 66.9 [47]. The likelihood of Parkinson's Disease increases sharply at the age of 60 and peaks in those aged 85 to 90 years old [83, 97, 98]. The likelihood of developing Parkinson's Disease then starts to decline at 90 years of age [97], and reduces even further after that. Consequently, Parkinson's Disease is rare amongst the very oldest people - those people that are over 100 years old [99], and is even rare in those people who are 110 to 119 years old [100].

Gender differences

There are more men than women with Parkinson's Disease. However, the ratio of males to females who have Parkinson's Disease differs a lot according to the country. In Nigeria there are far more men than women who have Parkinson's Disease. In Japan more women than men have Parkinson's Disease. The ratio of males to females, in those countries in which it is known, from highest to lowest is : Nigeria 3.3 [101], Spain 2.55-2.06 [90, 102], Taiwan 2.4 [103], U.S.A. 1.91-1.0 [73, 76, 104], Scotland 1.9 [83], Finland 1.7 [43], Egypt 1.7 [5], Iran 1.62 [30], Norway 1.58-1.35 [60, 85], Canada 1.56-1.16 [23, 58], Netherlands 1.54 [105], France 1.48-1.4 [106, 107], China (Uygurs) 1.31 [108], Argentina 1.31-1.0 [77, 109], China 1.29 [18], Israel (muslims) 1.17 [68], Portugal 1.08 [55], Italy 1.06-0.98 [28, 91], San Marino 1.02 [41], Sweden >1.0 [62], Netherlands 1.00-0.92 [110, 88], Estonia <1.0 [82], Finland <1.0 [44], Russia 0.87 [78], Japan 0.71-0.67 [81].

Occupational differences

Parkinson's Disease was found to be far more common amongst welders [111, 112]. Prevalence was also significantly higher amongst physicians, dentists, teachers, lawyers, scientists, and religion-related jobs [113]. Computer programmers had a younger age at diagnosis, and risk of diagnosis [113]. Clerical occupations were also positively associated with Parkinson's Disease [114]. Agricultural workers were more prone to Parkinson's Disease [88, 113] than people who were involved in hunting and forestry [72, 115]. Parkinson's Disease tends to be more common in rural areas but it differs according to the country. The ratio of rural to urban cases in those countries in which it is known, from highest to lowest is : Italy 2.03-1.14 [91, 88], Sweden 1.3 [76], Estonia 1.14 [47], Taiwan 0.5 [116]. Another study found that the risk of developing Parkinson's Disease was not significantly affected by farming work, by metal work, or by exposure to pesticides, metals, or solvents [117]. A previous history of evening work increased the risk of Parkinson's Disease [118].

People involved in manufacturing and transportation were less likely to develop Parkinson's Disease [114]. Outdoor work also reduced the risk of Parkinson's Disease [119]. The lowest risk of Parkinson's Disease, which is only 14% of normal, is in men with an artistic occupation late in life. Being an artist as a first occupation made the likelihood of developing Parkinson's Disease 72% less likely than normal [120]. Although artistic occupations later in life are associated with a greatly reduced risk of developing Parkinson's Disease it is probable that because higher dopamine levels are required for visual creativity that people whose dopamine levels are low, as they are in Parkinson's Disease, would be less inclined to be artistic visually.

Birth

No significant relationship with Parkinson's Disease was observed for : birth weight, paternal age, pre-term birth, multiple birth, and having been breastfed. Older maternal age at birth increased the risk of developing Parkinson's Disease by 75% among those with mothers aged 30 years and older versus those with mothers younger than 20 years old. Left handed women are 62% more likely to develop Parkinson's Disease than right handed women. Men are not affected according to whether they are right or left handed [121]. People born during winter and spring have a higher capacity to produce dopamine compared to people born during the summer and autumn [122]. A modest association was suggested for season of birth as there was a 30% higher risk of developing Parkinson's Disease in those born in Spring rather than Winter [121]. However, in another study Parkinson's Disease was not associated with the season of birth [123].

Hair colour

The risk of developing Parkinson's Disease increases according to hair colour [124]. People with black hair are least prone to developing Parkinson's Disease. People with brown hair are 40% more likely than them to develop Parkinson's Disease. People with blonde hair are around 60% more likely to develop Parkinson's Disease. Worst at risk are people with red hair for whom the risk of Parkinson's Disease is nearly double those with black hair [124, 126]. Hair colour and Parkinson's Disease have a similar biochemistry. The dopamine needed to relieve Parkinson's Disease is initially made from L-tyrosine turning in to L-dopa. Melanin, the pigment that colours hair and skin, is also initially made by turning L-tyrosine in to L-dopa. However, in skin cells, L-dopa then turns in to melanin instead of dopamine in order to darken the hair and the skin.

[1] Journal of Neurology [2012] 260 (5) : 1351-1357 (L.Horsfall, I.Petersen, K.Walters, A.Schrag)

[2] American Journal of Epidemiology [2016] 183 (11) : 1018-1026 (S.K.Darweesh, P.J.Koudstaal, B.H.Stricker, A.Hofman, M.A.Ikram)

[3] JAMA Neurology [2016] Jun 20 [Epub ahead of print] (R.Savica, B.R.Grossardt, J.H.Bower, J.E.Ahlskog, W.A.Rocca)

[4] Lancet [2005] 365 (9459) : 595-597 (Z.X.Zhang, G.C.Roman, Z. Hong, C.B.Wu, Q.M.Qu, J.B.Huang, B.Zhou, Z.P.Geng, J.X.Wu, H.B. Wen, H.Zhao)

[5] Neuroepidemiology [2012] 38 (3) : 154-163 (E.M.Khedr, G.S.Al Attar, M.R.Kandil, N.F.Kamel, N.Abo Elfetoh, M.A.Ahmed)

[6] Neuroepidemiology [2009] 33 (3) : 225-230 (B.A.Racette, L.M. Good, A.M.Kissel, S.R.Criswell, J.S.Perlmutter)

[7] Neuroepidemiology [2012] 38 (3) : 138-147 (J.Kruja, E.Beghi, D. Zerbi, D.Dobi, A.Kuqo, I.Zekja, S.Mijo, M.Kapisyzi, P.Messina)

[8] American Journal of Industrial Medicine [2007] 50 (11) : 788-800 (R.G.Lucchini, E.Albini, L.Benedetti, S.Borghesi, R.Coccaglio, E.C. Malara, G.Parrinello, S.Garattini, S.Resola, L.Alessio)

[9] Movement Disorders [2012] 27 (11) : 1456-1459 (P.H.Gordon, J.M. Mehal, R.C.Holman, A.S.Rowland, J.E.Cheek)

[10] Journal of Parkinsons Disease [2013] 3 (2) : 193-198 (P.H. Gordon, H.Zhao, D.Bartley, L.J.Sims, M.G.Begay, S.Pirio Richardson, J.Lewis, A.S.Rowland)

[11] Movement Disorders [2015] 30 (5) : 714-720 (P.H.Gordon, J.M. Mehal, R.C.Holman, M.L.Bartholomew, J.E.Cheek, A.S. Rowland)

[12] Movement Disorders [2004] 19 (3) : 318-323 (D.Strickland, J.M. Bertoni)

[13] Archives of Neurology [1988] 45 (12) : 1321-1323 (N.E. Bharucha, E.P.Bharucha, A.E.Bharucha, A.V.Bhise, B.S.Schoenberg)

[14] http://www.luckymojo.com/aspand.html [2007]

[15] Neuroepidemiology [1990] 9 (5) : 263-277 (R.Tekle-Haimanot, M. Abebe, A.Gebre-Mariam, L.Forsgren, J.Heijbel, G.Holmgren, J. Ekstedt)

[16] Archives of Neurology [1996] 53 (1) : 66-71 (S.J.Wang, J.L.Fuh, E.L.Teng, C.Y.Liu, K.P.Lin, H.M.Chen, C.H.Lin, P.N.Wang, Y.C. Ting, H.C.Wang, K.N.Lin, P.Chou, E.B.Larson, H.C.Liu)

[17] Archives of Neurology [1985] 42 (7) : 655-657 (S.C.Li, B.S. Schoenberg, C.C.Wang, X.M.Cheng, D.Y.Rui, C.L.Bolis, D.G. Schoenberg)

[18] Journal of Neural Transmission [2014] 43 (31) : 12037-12043 (C. L.Ma, L.Su, J.J.Xie, J.X.Long, P.Wu, L.Gu)

[19] Neuropsychiatric Disease and Treatment [2015] 11 : 1467-1472 (Y.M.Zou, J.Liu, Z.Y.Tian, D.Lu, Y.Y.Zhou)

[20] Neuropsychiatric Disease and Treatment [2013] 9 : 1821-1826 (H. N.El-Tallawy, W.M.Farghaly, G.A.Shehata, T.A.Rageh, N.M.Hakeem, M.A.Hamed, R.Badry)

[21] European Journal of Neurology [2015] 22 (3) : 464-471 (P.Blin, C.Dureau-Pournin, A.Foubert-Samier, A.Grolleau, E. Corbillon, J.Jové, R.Lassalle, P.Robinson, N.Poutignat, C.Droz- Perroteau, N.Moore)

[22] American Journal of Epidemiology [1995] 142 (8) : 820-827 (R. Mayeux, K.Marder, L.J.Cote, J.Denaro, N.Hemenegildo, H.Mejida, M. X.Tang, R.Lantigua, D.Wilder, B.Gurland, et al)

[23] Parkinsonism & Related Disorders [2012] 18 (4) : 327-331 (C. Allyson Jones, W.R.Martin, M.Wieler, P.King-Jesso, D.C.Voaklander)

[24] Parkinsonism & Related Disorders [2003] 9 (4) : 233-238 (B.C. Lai, M.Schulzer, S.Marion, K. Teschke, J.K.Tsui)

[25] Movement Disorders [1998] 13 (3) : 400-405 (A.Chio, C.Magnani, D.Schiffer)

[26] Parkinsonism & Related Disorders [2008] 14 (7) : 572-575 (L. Morgante, A.Nicoletti, A.Epifanio, D.Contrafatto, R.Savica, S. Lanzafame, R.Musolino, P.La Spina, U.Bonuccelli, R.Marconi, et al)

[27] Parkinsonism & Related Disorders [2008] 14 (7) : 572-575 (L. Morgante, A.Nicoletti, A.Epifanio, D.Contrafatto, R.Savica, S. Lanzafame, R.Musolino, P.La Spina, U.Bonuccelli, R.Marconi, et al)

[28] Journal of Neural Transmission [2015] 123 (4) : 415-420 (A.Di Napoli, S.Scalmana, F.Franco, D.Di Lallo, E.Lacorte, N.Vanacore)

[29] Neuroepidemiology [2016] 47 (1) : 38-45 (E.Pupillo, C.Cricelli, F.Mazzoleni, I.Cricelli, A.Pasqua, S.Pecchioli, F.Lapi, E.Beghi)

[30] Neuropsychiatric Disease and Treatment [2015] 11 : 321-332 (S. M.Fereshtehnejad, M.Shafieesabet, A.Rahmani, A.Delbari, J.Lökk)

[31] Journal of Parkinson's Disease [2011] 1 (1) 35-47 (O.Chillag-Talmor, N.Giladi, S.Linn, T.Gurevich, B.El-Ad, B.Silverman, N. Friedman, C.Peretz)

[32] Acta Neurologica Scandinavica [2008] 118 (2) : 126-131 (L. Wermuth, S.Bech, M.Skaalum Petersen, P.Joensen, P.Weihe, P. Grandjean)

[33] Neurology [1997] 49 (2) : 426-432 (L.Wermuth, P.Joensen, N. Bunger, B.Jeune)

[34] Neurological Science [2015] 36 (3) : 411-413 (H.Durmus, M.A. Gokalp, H.A.Hanagasi)

[35] Neuroepidemiology [1996] 15 (4) : 201-207 (M.Kusumi, K. Nakashima, H.Harada, H.Nakayama, K.Takahashi)

[36] Gerontology [1990] 36 (5-6) : 340-344 (K.Okada, S.Kobayashi, T. Tsunematsu)

[37] Archives of Neurology [1983] 40 (3) : 151-154 (H.Harada, S. Nishikawa, K.Takahashi)

[38] Neuroepidemiology [2003] 22 (5) : 313 (H.Kimura, M.Kurimura, M.Wada, T.Kawanami, K.Kurita, Y.Suzuki, T.Katagiri, M.Daimon, T. Kayama, T.Kato)

[39] Neuroepidemiology [2009] 32 (4) : 263-269 (M.Yamawaki, M. Kusumi, H.Kowa, K.Nakashima)

[40] Acta Neurologica Scandinavica [2011] 124 (3) : 182-187 (Y. Osaki, Y.Morita, T.Kuwahara, I.Miyano, Y.Doi)

[41] Neurology [1987] 37 (10) 1679-1682 (R.D'Alessandro, G. Gamberini, E.Granieri, G.Benassi, S.Naccarato, D.Manzanoli)

[42] Das Offentliche Gesundheitswesen [1990] 52 (4) : 181-190 (J. Kleinhenz, P.Vieregge, H.Fassl, J.Jorg)

[43] Neurology [1999] 52 (2) : 302-308 (A.M.Kuopio, R.J.Marttila, H. Helenius, U.K.Rinne

[44] Acta Neurologica Scandinavica [1976] 53 (2) : 81-102 (R.J. Marttila, U.K.Rinne)

[45] Neuroepidemiology [2001] 20 (3) : 212-214 (I.Milanov, K. Kmetska, B.Karakolev, E.Nedialkov)

[46] Neuoepidemiology [2000] 19 (4) 206-209 (I.Milanov, T.S. Kmetski, K.E.Lyons, W.C.Koller)

[47] Acta Neurologica Scandinavica [2002] 106 (5) 276-281 (P.Taba, T.Asser)

[48] Journal of the Formosan Medical Association [2016] 115 (7) : 531-538 (W.M.Liu, R.M.Wu, J.W.Lin, Y.C.Liu, C.H.Chang, C.H.Lin)

[49] Journal of Clinical Neuroscience [2006] 13 (3) : 343-348 (C.M. Peters, C.E.Gartner, P.A.Silburn, G.D.Mellick)

[50] Internal Medicine Journal [2007] 37 (12) : 812-814 (P.Mehta, A. Kifley, J.J.Wang, E.Rochtchina, P.Mitchell, C.M.Sue)

[51] Neuroepidemiology [2006] 26 (3) : 156-161 (B.Porter, R. Macfarlane, N.Unwin, R.Walker)

[52] Acta Neurologica Scandinavica [1995] 92 (6) : 443-450 (R.L. Sutcliffe, J.R.Meara)

[53] Parkinsonism & Related Disorders [2010] 16 (9) : 572-575 (R.W. Walker, A.Hand, C.Jones, B.H.Wood, W.K.Gray)

[54] Journal of Neurology, Neurosurgery, and Psychiatry [2009] 80 (7) : 805-807 (M.M.Wickremaratchi, D.Perera, C.O'Loghlen, D.Sastry, E. Morgan, A.Jones, P.Edwards, N.P.Robertson, C.Butler, et al)

[55] European Journal of Epidemiology [1994] 10 (6) : 763-767 (J.A. Dias, M.M.Felgueiras, J.P.Sanchez, J.M.Goncalves, J.M.Falcao, Z.P. Pimenta)

[56] Neurologia [2000] 15 (7) : 269-273 (J.L.Giroud Benitez, F. Collado- Mesa, E.M.Esteban)

[57] Movement Disorders [2009] 24 (3) : 401-406 (E.J.Newman, K.A. Grosset, D.G.Grosset)

[58] Acta Neurologica Scandinavica [1992] 86 (1) : 40-44 (T.H. Caradoc-Davies, M.Weatherall, G.S.Dixon, G.Caradoc-Davies, P. Hantz)

[59] Movement Disorders [1999] 14 (4) : 596-604 (J.M.Errea, J.R.Ara, C.Aibar, J.de Pedro-Cuesta)

[60] Movement Disorders [1995] 10 (5) : 541-549 (E.Landberg, J.P. Larsen, E.G.Nessler, T.Riise, J.A.Aarli)

[61] Neuroepidemiology [2011] 37 (3-4) : 222-230 (R.Bhidayasiri, N. Wannachai, S.Limpabandhu, S.Choeytim, Y.Suchonwanich, S. Tananyakul, C.Tharathep, P.Panjapiyakul, R.Srismith, et al)

[62] Journal of Clinical Epidemioogy [1996] 49 (6) : 637-641 (P.A.Fall, O.Axelson, M.Fredriksson, G.Hansson, J.E.Olsson, A.K. Granerus)

[63] Neurology [1988] 38 (4) : 645-646 (B.S.Schoenberg, A.O.Adeuja, B.O.Osuntokun, O.Bademosi, V.Nottidge, D.W.Anderson, A.F.Haerer)

[64] Przeglad Epidemiologiczny [1989] 43 (2) : 150-155 (M.Wender, D.Pruchnik, P.Kowal, J.Florczak, M.Zalejski)

[65] Clinical Neurology and Neurosurgery [2009] 111 (10) : 812-815 (A.Alrefai, M.Habahbih, M.Alkhawajah, M.Darwish, W.Batayha, Y. Khader, K.El-Salem)

[66] Neurology [2010] 75 (15) : 1362-1369 (S.K.Das, A.K.Misra, B.K. Ray, A.Hazra, M.K.Ghosal, A.Chaudhuri, T.Roy, T.K.Banerjee, D.K. Raut)

[67] Parkinsonism & Related Disorders [2003] 10 (1) : 19-21 (P. Nicoletti, V.Sofia, A.Bartoloni, F.Bartalesi, H.Gamboa Barahon, S. Giuffrida, A. Reggio)

[68] The Israel Medical Association Journal [2010] 12 (1) : 32-35 (R. Masalha, E.Kordysh, G.Alpert, M.Hallak, M.Morad, M.Mahajnah, P. Farkas, Y.Herishanu)

[69] Clinical Neurology and Neurosurgery [1986] 88 (2) : 109-113 (P.P. Ashok, K.Radhakrishnan, R. Sridharan, M.E.Mousa)

[70] International Journal of Neuroscience [2004] 114 (2) : 175-182 (J. L.Sanchez, O.Buritica, D.Pineda, C.S.Uribe, L.G.Palacio)

[71] Journal of Neurological Science [2013] 335 (1-2) : 22-25 (J. Blanckenberg, S.Bardien, B.Glanzmann, N.U.Okubadejo, J.A.Carr)

[72] Parkinsonism & Related Disorders [2003] (Supplement 2) : S99-S104 (J.S.Kim, Y.H.Sohn)

[73] American Journal of Epidemiology [2003] 157 (11) : 1015-1022 (S.K.Van Den Eeden, C.M.Tanner, A.L.Bernstein, R.D.Fross, A. Leimpeter, D.A.Bloch, L.M.Nelson)

[74] Neuroepidemiology [2010] 34 (3) : 143-151 (W.A.Wright, B.A. Evanoff, M.Lian, S.R.Criswell, B.A.Racette)

[75] American Journal of Epidemiology [1995] 142 (8) : 820-827 (R. Mayeux, K.Marder, L.J.Cote, J.Denaro, N.Hemenegildo, H.Mejida, M. X.Tang, R.Lantigua, D.Wilder, B.Gurland, et al)

[76] Neurology [1985] 35 (6) : 841-845 (R.S.Schoenberg, D.W. Anderson, A.F.Haerer)

[77] European Journal of Neurology [2012] 19 (8) : 1108-1113 (D.J. Bauso, J.P.Tartari, C.V.Stefani, J.I.Rojas, D.H.Giunta, E.Cristiano)

[78] Movement Disorders [2010] 25 (3) : 349-356 (Y.Winter, Y. Bezdolnyy, E.Katunina, G.Avakjan, J.P.Reese, J.Klotsche, W.H.Oertel, R.Dodel, E.Gusev)

[79] Movement Disorders [2010] 25 (3) : 341-348 (J.Linder, H. Stenlund, L.Forsgren)

[80] The Canadian Journal of Neurological Sciences [1984] 11 (1 Supplement) : 156-159 (A.H.Rajput)

[81] Journal of Epidemiology [2002] 12 (6) : 403-407 (S.Morioka, K. Sakata, S.Yoshida, E.Nakai, M.Shiba, N.Yoshimura, T.Hashimoto)

[82] Neuroepidemiology [2003] 22 (1) : 41-45 (P.Taba, T.Asser)

[83] Journal of Neurology, Neurosurgery, and Psychiatry [2010] 81 (11) : e21 (C.Counsell, J.Gordon, W.Primrose, C.Harris, R.Caslake)

[84] Parkinsonism & Related Disorders [2013] 19 (5) : 515-521 (R. Caslake, K.Taylor, N.Scott, J.Gordon, C.Harris, K.Wilde, A.Murray, C.Counsell)

[85] Journal of Neurology, Neurosurgery, and Psychiatry [2009] 80 (8) : 851-857 (G.Alves, B.Müller, K.Herlofson, I.Hogenesch, W.Telstad, D.Aarsland, O.B.Tysnes, J.P.Larsen)

[86] Age and Ageing [2014] 43 (2) : 257-263 (G.W.Duncan, T.K. Khoo, S.Y.Coleman, C.Brayne, A.J.Yarnall, J.T.O'Brien, R.A.Barker, D.J.Burn)

[87] Neuroepidemiology [2009] 34 (2) : 76-82 (D.Hristova, Z. Zachariev, N.Mateva, I.Grozdev)

[88] Neuroepidemiology [1989] 8 (6) : 296-299 (A.Hofman, H.J. Collette, A.L.Bartelds)

[89] Archives of Neurology [1991] 48 (8) : 854-857 (E.Granieri, M. Carreras, I.Casetta, V.Govoni, M.R.Tola, E.Paolino, V.C.Monetti, P.De Bastiani)

[90] Movement Disorders [2002] 17 (2) 242-249 (L.E.Claveria, J. Duarte, M.D.Sevillano, A.Perez-Sempere, C.Cabezas, F.Rodriguez, J. de Pedro-Cuesta)

[91] Acta Neurologica Scandinavica [2005] 112 (1) : 24-28 (R. Totaro, C.Marini, F.Pistoia, S.Sacco, T.Russo, A.Carolei)

[92] Acta Neurologica Scandinavica [2005] 112 (1) : 29-35 (L.Zhang, Z.Y.Nie, Y.Liu, W.Chen, S.M.Xin, X.D.Sun, J.H.Fan, Y.H.Liu, X.H. Gao, L.Q.Lu, P.Como, M.P.McDermott, Y.L.Qiao, K. Kieburtz)

[93] Neuroepidemiology [2003] 22 (1) : 41-45 (P.Taba, T.Asser)

[94] Pharmacoepidemiology and drug safety [2001] 10 (6) : 549-554 (D.A.Van de Vijver, R.A.Roos, P.A.Jansen, A.J.Porsius, A.de Boer)

[95] Neurology [1999] 52 (6) : 1214-1220 (J.H.Bower, D.M. Maraganore, S.K.McDonell, W.A.Rocca)

[96] Movement Disorders [2014] 29 (13) : 1583-1590 (T.Pringsheim, N.Jette, A.Frolkis, T.D.Steeves)

[97] Neurology [2009] 72 (5) : 432-438 (J.A.Driver, G.Logroscino, J. M.Gaziano, T.Kurth)

[98] European Review for Medical Pharmacological Sciences [2014] 18 (24) : 3908-3915 (Y.M.Zou, J.P.Tan, N.Li, J.S.Yang, B.C.Yu, J.M.Yu, W.Du, W.J.Zhang, L.Q.Cui, Q.S.Wang, X.N.Xia, J.J.Li, et al)

[99] The Journal of Rural Health [2009] 25 (3) : 320-325 (J.Kaye, Y. Michael, J.Calvert, M.Leahy, D.Crawford, P.Kramer)

[100] Journal of American Geriatric Society [2006] 54 (8] : 1237-1240 (E.A.Schoenhofen, D.F.Wyszynski, S.Andersen, J.Pennington, R. Young, D.F.Terry, T.T.Perls)

[101] BMC Neurology [2010] 10 (1) : 1 (N.U.Okubadejo, O.O.Ojo, O.O.Oshinaike)

[102] Neurology [2004] 62 (5) : 734-741 (J.Benito-Leon, F.Bermejo-Pareja, J.M.Morales-Gonzalez, J.Porta-Etessam, R.Trincado, S.Vega, E. D.Louis)

[103] Neuroepidemiology [1992] 11 (3) : 113-120 (L.G.Chia, L.H.Liu)

[104] Journal of Neurology, Neurosurgery and Psychiatry [2004] 75 (4) : 637-639 (G.F.Wooten, L.J.Currie, V.E.Bovbjerg, J.K.Lee, J.Patrie)

[105] Neurology [2004] 63 (7) : 1240-1244 (L.M.de Lau, P.C. Giesbergen, M.C.de Rijk, A.Hofman, P.J.Koudstaal, M.M.Breteler)

[106] Acta Neurologica Scandinavica [1994] 90 (2) : 111-115 (F. Tison, J.F.Dartigues, L.Dubes, M.Zuber, A.Alperovitch, P.Henry)

[107] Journal of Neurology, Neurosurgery and Psychiatry [2015] Dec 23 [Epub ahead of print] (F.Moisan, S.Kab, F.Mohamed, M.Canonico, M.LeGuern, C.Quintin, L.Carcaillon, J.Nicolau, N.Duport, et al)

[108] Genetics and Molecular Research [2015] 14 (3) : 8539-8546 (X.L.Yang, Q.Luo, H.X.Song, Y.L.Wang, Y.N.Yao, H.Xia)

[109] Movement disorders [1997] 12 (2) : 197-205 (M.O.Melcom, D.W.Anderson, R.H.Vergara, W.A.Rocca)

[110] Neurology [2000] 54 (11 Supplement 5) : S21-S23 (M.C.de Rijk, L.J.Launer, K.Berger, M.M.Breteler, J.F.Dartigues, M.Baldereshi, L. Fratiglioni, A.Lobo, J.Martinez-Lage, C.Trenkwalder)

[111] Neurology [2005] 64 (2) : 230-235 (B.A.Racette, S.D.Tabbal, D. Jennings, L.Good, J.S.Perlmutter, B.Evanoff)

[112] Neurotoxicology [2012] 33 (5) : 1356-1361 (B.A.Racette, S.R. Criswell, J.I.Lundin, A.Hobson, N.Seixas, P.T.Kotzbauer, B.A.Evanoff, J.S.Perlmutter, J.Zhang, L.Sheppard, H.Checkoway)

[113] Neurology [2005] 65 (9) : 1430-1435 (S.M.Goldman, C.M. Tanner, C.W.Olanow, R.L.Watts, R.D.Field, J.W.Langston)

[114] Industrial Health [2004] 42 (3) : 352-358 (J.Park, C.I.Yoo, C.S. Sim, J.W.Kim, Y.Li, K.Y.Jung, S.E.Chung, Y.Kim)

[115] Neurotoxicology [2005] 26 (1) : 99-105 (J.Park, C.I.Yoo, C.S. Sim, H.K.Kim, J.W.Kim, B.S.Jeon, K.R.Kim, O.Y.Bang, W.Y.Lee, Y.Yi, K.Y.JUng, S.E.Chung, Y.Kim)

[116] Neuroepidemiology [2009] 33 (4) : 350-357 (C.C.Chen, T.F. Chen, Y.C.Hwang, Y.R.Wen, Y.H.Chiu, C.Y.Wu, R.C.Chen, J.J.Tai, T. H.Chen, H.H.Liou)

[117] American Journal of Industrial Medicine [2010] 53 (3) : 217-223 (J.A.Firestone, J.I.Lundin, K.M.Powers, T.Smith-Weller G.M.Franklin, P.D.Swanson, W.T.Longstreth Jr, H.Checkoway)

[118] Journal of Neurology [2012] 259 (11) : 2447-2451 (M.Wolz, C. Schleiffer, L.Klingelhöfer, C.Schneider, F.Proft, U.Schwanebeck, H. Reichmann, P.Riederer, A.Storch)

[119] Occupational and Environmental Medicine [2011] 68 (4) : 273-278 (L.Kenborg, C.F.Lassen, B.Ritz, E.S.Schernhammer, J. Hansen, N.M. Gatto, J.H.Olsen)

[120] Journal of Neurology [2015] 262 (9) : 2171-2176 (C.A.Haaxma, G.F.Borm, D.van der Linden, A.C.Kappelle, B.R.Bloem)

[121] Movement Disorders [2010] 25 (11) : 1560-1567 (H.Gardener, X. Gao, H.Chen, M.A.Schwarzschild, D.Spiegelman, A.Ascherio)

[122] Neuroscience Letters [2102] 530 (1) : 80-84 (V.Kaasinen, P. Jokinen, J.Joutsa, O.Eskola, J.O.Rinne)

[123] Movement Disorders [2007] 22 (8) : 1097-1101 (R.B.Postuma, C. Wolfson, A.Rajput, A.J.Stoessl, W.R.Martin, O.Suchowersky, S. Chouinard, M.Panisset, M.S.Jog, D.A.Grimes, C.Marras, A.E.Lang)

[124] Annals of Neurology [2009] 65 (1) : 76-82 (X.Gao, K.C.Simon, J. Han, M.A.Schwarzschild, A.Ascherio)

[125] European Journal of Neurology [2017] Mar 2 [Epub ahead of print] (J.J.Ferreira, N.Gonçalves, A.Valadas, C.Januário, M.R.Silva, L.Nogueira, J.L.Vieira, A.B.Lima)

[126] Annals of Clinical and Translational Neurology [2017] 4 (3) : 212-216 (X.Chen, D.Feng, M.A.Schwarzschild, X.Gao)

CHAPTER 4

BIOCHEMISTRY OF PARKINSON'S DISEASE

DOPAMINE BIOSYNTHESIS

DOPAMINE BIOSYNTHESIS

Parkinson's Disease is primarily due to the insufficient formation of dopamine. Therefore, in order to treat Parkinson's Disease effectively it is essential to increase the biosynthesis of dopamine. Dopamine is biosynthesized in the dopaminergic neurons, in the brain, from L-tyrosine via L-dopa : L-tyrosine > L-dopa > dopamine.

FIRST STEP

The first step in the biosynthesis of dopamine requires L-tyrosine, ferrous iron as a cofactor, and the coenzyme tetrahydrofolic acid, for the enzyme tyrosine 3-monoxygenase, which catalyzes the formation of L-dopa [1-4]. In studies on the enzyme tyrosine 3-monoxygenase the biosynthesis of L-dopa rose or fell according to the concentrations of L-tyrosine, ferrous iron and tetrahydrofolic acid [1-4].

enzyme name : tyrosine 3-monooxygenase
enzyme classification : EC 1.14.16.2
cofactor : ferrous iron (Fe^{2+})
substrate : L-tyrosine + tetrahydrofolic acid + O_2
product : L-dopa + dihydrofolic acid + H_20

SECOND STEP

The second step in the biosynthesis of dopamine requires pyridoxal phosphate as a coenzyme for the enzyme aromatic L-amino acid decarboxylase (dopa decarboxylase) which catalyzes the formation of dopamine from L-dopa [5-9]. In studies on the enzyme L-amino acid decarboxylase the biosynthesis of dopamine rose or fell according to the concentrations of pyridoxal phosphate [5-9].

enzyme name : L-aromatic amino acid decarboxylase
enzyme classification : EC 4.1.1.28
coenzyme : pyridoxal phosphate
substrate : L-dopa
product : dopamine + CO_2

DOPAMINE METABOLISM

Dopamine is metabolised and inactivated by two means, via the enzyme monoamine oxidase (MAO) [10-17], and via the enzyme catechol-O-methyl transferase (COMT) [18, 19, 20]. These enzymes are not necessary for treating Parkinson's Disease because they are not responsible for increasing dopamine biosynthesis. Dopamine is metabolised via two routes (1) via monoamine oxidase (MAO) and then catechol-O-methyl transferase (COMT), and (2) via catechol-O-methyl transferase (COMT) and then monoamine oxidase (MAO).

VIA MAO THEN COMT

The enzyme monoamine oxidase (MAO) metabolises dopamine to 3,4-dihydroxyphenylacetic acid, which is then metabolised to homovanillic acid by the enzyme catechol-O-methyl transferase (COMT).

MONOAMINE OXIDASE

enzyme name : monoamine oxidase (MAO-A and MAO-B)
enzyme number : EC 1.4.3.4
substrate : dopamine + H_2O + O_2
product : 3,4-dihydroxyphenylacetic acid + H_2O_2

CATECHOL-O-METHYL TRANSFERASE

enzyme name : catechol-O-methyl transferase (COMT)
enzyme number : EC 2.1.1.6
substrate : dihydroxyphenylacetic acid + S-adenosyl-L-homocysteine
product : homovanillic acid + S-adenosyl-L-homocysteine

VIA COMT THEN MAO

The enzyme catechol-O-methyl transferase (COMT) metabolises dopamine to 3-methoxytyramine, which is then metabolised to homovanillic acid by the enzyme monoamine oxidase (MAO).

CATECHOL-O-METHYL TRANSFERASE

enzyme name : catechol-O-methyl transferase (COMT)
enzyme number : EC 2.1.1.6
substrate : dopamine + S-adenosyl-L-methionine
product : 3-methoxytyramine + S-adenosyl-L-homocysteine

MONOAMINE OXIDASE

enzyme name : monoamine oxidase (MAO-A and MAO-B)
enzyme number : EC 1.4.3.4
substrate : 3-methoxytyramine + H_2O + O_2
product : homovanillic acid + H_2O_2

Homovanillic acid is the primary, but not the only, breakdown product of dopamine. From the bloodstream, it is excreted in the urine [21].

[1] Nature [1983] 302 : 830-832 (S.El Mestikawy, J.Glowinski, M. Hamon)

[2] Archives of Biochemistry and Biophysics [1967] 120 : 420-427 (M.Ikeda, M.Levitt, S.Udenfriend)

[3] Journal of Biological Chemistry [1964] 239 : 2910-2917 (T. Nagatsu, M.Levitt, S.Udenfriend)

[4] Comptes Rendue des Academie Sciences Series 3 [1986] 302 : 435-438 (D. Pigeon, R.Drissi-Daoudi, F.Gros, J.Thibault)

[5] Proceedings of the National Academy of Sciences, USA [1972] 69 : 343-347 (J.G.Christenson, W.Dairman, S.Udenfriend)

[6] Journal of Biological Chemistry [1962] 237 : 89-93 (W.Lovenberg, H.Weissbach, S.Udenfriend)

[7] Journal of Biological Chemistry [1957] 227 : 617-624 (H. Weissbach, D.F.Bogdanski, B.G.Redfield, S.Udenfriend)

[8] Journal of Biological Chemistry [1948] 174 : 813-816 (R.W. McGilvery, P.P.Cohen)

[9] Hoppe-Seyler's Zeitschrift fur Physiologie Chemie [1963] 332 : 70-78 (C.E.Sekeris)

[10] The Enzymes, Volume 8 [1963] : 337-351 (H.Blaschko)

[11] Medical Care Research and Review [1989] 9 : 45-89 (P.L.Dostert, M.Strolin Benedetti, K.F.Tipton)

[12] Current Medicinal Chemistry [2004] 11 : 1983-1993 (D.E. Edmondson, A.Mattevi, C.Binda, M.Li, F.Hubálek)

[13] Current Medicinal Chemistry [2004] 11 : 1995-2005 (J.C.Shih, K. Chen)

[14] Current Medicinal Chemistry [2004] 11 : 1965-1982 (K.F.Tipton, S.Boyce, J.O'Sullivan, G.P.Davey, J.Healy)

[15] Proceedings of the National Academy of Sciences, USA [2005] 102 : 12684-12689 (L.De Colibus, M.Li, C.Binda, A.Lustig, D.E. Edmondson, A.Mattevi)

[16] Nature Reviews Neuroscience [2006] 7 : 295-309 (M.B.Youdim, D.E.Edmondson, K.F.Tipton)

[17] British Journal of Pharmacology [2006] 147 (Supplement 1) : S287-S296 (M.B.Youdim, Y.S.Bakhle)

[18] Journal of Biological Chemistry [1958] 233 : 702-705 (J.Axelrod, R.Tomchick)

[19] Journal of Neurochemistry [1979] 32 : 1525-1529 (P.A.Gulliver, K.F.Tipton)

[20] Journal of Biological Chemistry [1979] 254 : 299-308 (M.M.Huh, A.J.Friedhoff)

[21] British Journal of Pharmacology [1996] 117 (6) : 1193-1198 P.Soares-da-Silva, M.A.Vieira-Coelho, M.Pestana)

CHAPTER 5

BIOCHEMISTRY OF PARKINSON'S DISEASE

COENZYME BIOSYNTHESIS

COENZYME BIOSYNTHESIS

Coenzymes are essential for the biosynthesis of dopamine. The coenzymes that are necessary for dopamine biosynthesis are : tetrahydrofolic acid, pyridoxal phosphate and the nicotinamide coenzymes NADP and NADPH. The vitamins folic acid, pyridoxine and nicotinamide are essential for their formation.

TETRAHYDROFOLIC ACID

The first step in the biosynthesis of dopamine requires tetrahydrofolic acid in order to turn L-tyrosine into L-dopa. Tetrahydrofolic acid cannot be administered in order to facilitate dopamine biosynthesis as it is not easily absorbed intact. Folic acid can be administered instead of tetrahydrofolic acid as it readily forms tetrahydrofolic acid [1-4] : folic acid > dihydrofolic acid > tetrahydrofolic acid

FIRST STEP

enzyme name : dihydrofolate reductase
enzyme classification : EC 1.5.1.3
substrate : folic acid + NADPH + H^+
product : dihydrofolic acid + $NADP^+$

SECOND STEP

enzyme name : dihydrofolate reductase
enzyme classification : EC 1.5.1.3
substrate : dihydrofolic acid + NADPH + H^+
product : tetrahydrofolic acid + $NADP^+$

Pyridoxal phosphate

The second step in the biosynthesis of dopamine requires pyridoxal phosphate in order to turn L-dopa in to dopamine. However, pyridoxal phosphate is not absorbed intact. Pyridoxine can be administered instead as it readily forms pyridoxal phosphate [5, 6, 7]. This requires zinc [6, 7] : pyridoxine > pyridoxal > pyridoxal phosphate

First step

enzyme name : pyridoxine 4-dehydrogenase
enzyme classification : EC 1.1.1.65
substrate : pyridoxine + $NADP^+$
product : pyridoxal + NADPH + H^+

Second step

enzyme name : pyridoxal kinase
enzyme classification : EC 2.7.1.35
cofactor : zinc (Zn^{2+})
substrate : pyridoxal + ATP
product : pyridoxal 5'-phosphate + ADP

Nicotinamide coenzymes

Dopamine biosynthesis requires tetrahydrofolic acid, which requires NADPH, and pyridoxal phosphate, which requires NADP. However, NADP and NADPH are not absorbed intact. Nicotinamide can be administered instead as it readily forms the nicotinamide coenzymes [8-18]. This requires manganese [19-20] : nicotinamide > NMN > NAD > NADP > NADPH

First step

enzyme name : nicotinamide phosphoribosyltransferase
enzyme classification : EC 2.4.2.12
substrate : nicotinamide + 5-phospho-a-D-ribose 1-diphosphate
product : nicotinamide ribonucleotide + diphosphate

SECOND STEP

enzyme name : nicotinamide-nucleotide adenylyltransferase
enzyme classification : EC 2.7.7.1
substrate : nicotinamide ribonucleotide + ATP
product : NAD^+ + diphosphate

THIRD STEP

enzyme name : NAD^+ kinase
enzyme classification : EC 2.7.1.23
cofactor : manganese (Mn^{2+})
substrate : NAD^+ + ATP
product : $NADP^+$ + ADP

FOURTH STEP

enzyme name : NAD^+ kinase
enzyme classification : EC 2.7.1.23
cofactor : manganese (Mn^{2+})
substrate : $NADP^+$ + ATP
product : $NADPH^+$ + ADP

[1] Journal of Biological Chemistry [1961] 1163 (R.L.Blakley, B.M. MacDougall)

[2] Journal of Biological Chemistry [1982] 257 : 13650-13662 (J.T. Bolin, D.J.Filman, D.A.Matthews, J.Kraut)

[3] Journal of Biological Chemistry [1966] 241 : 1319-1328 (B.T. Kaufman, R.C.Gardiner)

[4] Biochimica et Biophysica Acta [1969] 177 : 401-411 (I.G.Young, F.Gibson)

[5] Biochimica et Biophysica Acta [1961] 48 : 71-76 (H.Holzer, S. Schneider)

[6] Journal of Biological Chemistry [1961] 236 : 2076-2084 D.B. McCormick, M.E.Gregory, E.E.Snell)

[7] Biulleten Eksperimental noi Biologii i Meditsiny [1946] 22 (6) 40-43 (A.F.Trufanov, J.A.Krisanova)

[8] Journal of Biological Chemistry [1957] 225 : 759-770 (J.Preiss, P.Handler)

[9] Biochemical Journal [1961] 80 : 318-323 (M.R.Atkinson, J.F. Jackson, R.K.Morton)

[10] Archives of Biochemistry and Biophysics [1967] 120 : 440-450 (W.Dahmen, B.Webb, J.Preiss)

[11] Journal of Biological Chemistry [1951] 191 : 535-541 (A. Kornberg, W.E.Pricer)

[12] Biochemistry [1990] 29 (10) : 2501 (S.Ruggieri, L.Gregori, P. Natalini, A.Vita, M.Emanuelli, N.Raffaelli, G.Magni)

[13] International Journal of Biochemistry [1982] 14 : 839-844 (J.R. Butler, E.T.McGuinness)

[14] Journal of Biological Chemistry [1967] 242 : 1182-1186 (A.E. Chung)

[15] Journal of Biological Chemistry [1950] 182 : 805-813 (A. Kornberg)

[16] Journal of Biological Chemistry [1954] 206 : 311-325 (T.P.Wang, N.O.Kaplan)

[17] The Pyridine Nucleotide Coenzymes (J.Everse, B.M.Anderson, K.You) [1982] : 279 (R.R. Fisher, S.R.Earle)

[18] CRC Critical Reviews in Biochemistry [1985] 17 : 313 (K.S.You)

[19] Analytical Biochemistry [1986] 154 (1) : 64 (S.J.Berger, N.A. Berger)

[20] Enzyme and Microbial Technology [1994] 16 (3) : 236 (L.M. Simon, M.Kotorman, B.Szajani)

CHAPTER 6

BIOCHEMISTRY OF PARKINSON'S DISEASE

IRON METABOLISM

FERROUS IRON COFACTOR

The first step in the biosynthesis of dopamine requires ferrous iron as a cofactor. The activity of the enzyme increases or decreases according to the concentration of ferrous iron [1-4].

enzyme name : tyrosine 3-monooxygenase
enzyme classification : EC 1.14.16.2
cofactor : ferrous iron (Fe^{2+})
substrate : L-tyrosine + tetrahydrofolic acid + O_2
product : L-dopa + dihydrofolic acid + H_20

TRANSFERRIN BIOSYNTHESIS

The transport of iron requires the secretion of transferrin from the hepatocytes of the liver. Transferrin is biosynthesized from amino acids, which via translation first form a single chain polypeptide in the ribosomes. With the addition of two molecules of water, leader peptidase removes the signal peptide to produce transferrin in the endoplasmic reticulum. Serotransferrin glycan is added to transferrin in the golgi complex. Iron is attached to the transferrin in the plasma [5-13].

TRANSFERRIN STRUCTURE

Transferrin is a protein consisting of a chain of 679 amino acids [5]. There are two known variants of transferrin. One has isoleucine replaced by asparagine at position 378 or 381 [14]. The other has glycine replaced by arginine at position 394 [15].

NH$_2$ – Val – Pro – Asp – Lys – Thr – Val – Arg – Trp – Cys

1 |

Cys – Lys – Thr – Ala – Glu – His – Glu – Ser – Val – Ala

| 10

Gln – Ser – Phe – Arg – Asp – His – Met – Lys – Ser – Val

20 |

Cys – Ala – Val – Ser – Pro – Gly – Asp – Ser – Pro – Ile

| 30

Val – Lys – Lys – Ala – Ser – Tyr – Leu – Asp – Cys – Ile

40 |

Ala – Asp – Ala – Glu – Asn – Ala – Ala – Ile – Ala – Arg

| 50

Val – Thr – Leu – Asp – Ala – Gly – Leu – Val – Tyr – Asp

60 |

Pro – Lys – Leu – Asn – Asn – Pro – Ala – Leu – Tyr – Ala

| 70

Val – Val – Ala – Glu – Phe – Tyr – Gly – Ser – Lys – Glu

80 |

Ala – Val – Ala – Tyr – Tyr – Phe – Thr – Gln – Pro – Asp

| 90

Val – Val – Lys – Lys – Asp – Ser – Gly – Phe – Gln – Met

100 |

His – Cys – Ser – Lys – Lys – Gly – Arg – Leu – Gln – Asn

| 110

Thr – Gly – Leu – Gly – Arg – Ser – Ala – Gly – Trp – Asn

120 |

Leu – Asp – Cys – Tyr – Leu – Leu – Gly – Ile – Pro – Ile

| 130

Pro – Glu – Pro – Arg – Lys – Pro – Leu – Glu – Lys – Ala

140 |

Ala – Cys – Ser – Gly – Ser – Phe – Phe – Asn – Ala – Val

| 150

Pro – Cys – Ala – Asp – Gly – Thr – Asp – Phe – Pro – Gln

160 |

```
Cys – Gly – Cys – Gly – Pro – Cys – Leu – Gln – Cys – Leu
|                                                   170
Ser – Thr – Leu – Asn – Gln – Tyr – Phe – Gly – Tyr – Ser
180                                                   |
Ala – Gly – Asp – Lys – Leu – Cys – Lys – Phe – Ala – Gly
|                                                   190
Gly – Asp – Val – Ala – Phe – Val – Lys – His – Ser – Thr
200                                                   |
Asp – Ala – Lys – Asn – Ala – Leu – Asn – Glu – Phe – Ile
|                                                   210
Arg – Asp – Gln – Tyr – Glu – Leu – Leu – Cys – Leu – Asp
220                                                   |
Lys – Tyr – Glu – Asp – Val – Pro – Lys – Arg – Thr – Asn
|                                                   230
Asp – Cys – His – Leu – Ala – Glu – Val – Pro – Ser – His
240                                                   |
Lys – Gly – Gly – Met – Ser – Arg – Ala – Val – Val – Thr
|                                                   250
Glu – Asp – Leu – Ile – Trp – Glu – Leu – Leu – Asn – Gln
260                                                   |
Ser – Lys – Asp – Lys – Gly – Phe – His – Glu – Gln – Ala
|                                                   270
Lys – Glu – Phe – Gln – Leu – Phe – Ser – Ser – Pro – His
280                                                   |
Ala – Ser – Asp – Lys – Phe – Leu – Leu – Asp – Lys – Gly
|                                                   290
His – Gly – Phe – Leu – Lys – Val – Pro – Pro – Arg – Met
300                                                   |
Tyr – Glu – Tyr – Gly – Leu – Tyr – Met – Lys – Ala – Asn
|                                                   310
Val – Thr – Ala – Ile – Arg – Asn – Leu – Arg – Glu – Gly
320                                                   |
Cys – Glu – Asp – Thr – Pro – Ala – Glu – Pro – Cys – Thr
|                                                   330
```

Lys – Pro – Val – Lys – Trp – Cys – Ala – Leu – Ser – His
340

Ser – Trp – Glu – Asp – Cys – Lys – Leu – Arg – Glu – His
350

Val – Ser – Asp – Val – Gly – Lys – Ile – Glu – Cys – Val
360

Ala – Ile – Cys – Asp – Glu – Thr – Thr – Glu – Ala – Ser
370

Lys – Ile – Met – Asn – Gly – Glu – Ala – Asp – Ala – Met
380

Ala – Ile – Tyr – Val – Phe – Gly – Gly – Asp – Leu – Ser
390

Gly – Lys – Cys – Gly – Leu – Val – Pro – Val – Leu – Ala
400

Glu – Cys – Asp – Asp – Ser – Lys – Asn – Tyr – Asn – Glu
410

Asp – Thr – Pro – Glu – Ala – Gly – Tyr – Phe – Ala – Val
420

Leu – Asp – Ser – Ala – Ser – Lys – Lys – Val – Val – Ala
430

Thr – Trp – Asp – Asn – Leu – Lys – Gly – Lys – Lys – Ser
440

Gly – Ala – Thr – Arg – Gly – Val – Ala – Thr – His – Cys
450

Trp – Asn – Ile – Pro – Met – Gly – Leu – Leu – Tyr – Asn
460

Phe – Glu – Asp – Phe – Arg – Cys – His – Asn – Ile – Lys
470

Phe – Ser – Glu – Gly – Cys – Ala – Pro – Gly – Ser – Lys
480

Met – Cys – Leu – Lys – Cys – Leu – Ser – Ser – Asp – Lys
490

Gly – Ser – Gly – Leu – Asn – Leu – Cys – Glu – Pro – Asn
500

Gly – Thr – Tyr – Gly – Tyr – Tyr – Gly – Glu – Lys – Asn
510

Ala – Phe – Arg – Cys – Leu – Val – Glu – Lys – Gly – Asp
520

Thr – Val – Thr – Gln – His – Lys – Val – Phe – Ala – Val
530

Gln – Asn – Pro – Gly – Gly – Lys – Asn – Pro – Asp – Pro
540

Tyr – Asp – Lys – Glu – Asn – Leu – Asn – Lys – Ala – Trp
550

Glu – Leu – Leu – Cys – Leu – Asp – Gly – Thr – Arg – Lys
560

Leu – His – Cys – Asn – Ala – Tyr – Glu – Gln – Val – Pro
570

Ala – Arg – Ala – Pro – Asn – His – Ala – Val – Val – Thr
580

Lys – His – Val – Cys – Ala – Glu – Lys – Asp – Lys – Arg
590

Ile – Leu – Arg – Gln – Gln – Gln – His – Leu – Phe – Gly
600

Phe – Asn – Gly – Ser – Cys – Asp – Thr – Val – Asn – Ser
610

Cys – Leu – Phe – Arg – Ser – Glu – Thr – Lys – Asp – Leu
620

Ala – Leu – Cys – Val – Thr – Asp – Asp – Arg – Phe – Leu
630

Lys – Leu – His – Asp – Arg – Asn – Thr – Tyr – Glu – Lys
640

Val – Ala – Lys – Val – Tyr – Glu – Gln – Gly – Leu – Tyr
650

Gly – Asn – Leu – Arg – Lys – Cys – Ser – Thr – Ser – Ser
660

Pro – Arg – Arg – Phe – Thr – Cys – Ala – Glu – Leu – Leu
COOH 670

SEROTRANSFERRIN GLYCAN

This is the structure of serotransferrin glycan [16]. It is attached to serotransferrin via asparagine residues [16]. It is not needed for the delivery of iron [17].

NeuAc (alpha2-6) - Gal (beta1-4) - GlcNAc (beta1-2) - Man (alpha1-3)
|
Asn - (beta1) GlcNAc - (beta1-4) GlcNAc - (beta1-4) Man
|
NeuAc (alpha2-6) - Gal (beta1-4) - GlcNAc (beta1-2) - Man (alpha1-3)

TRANSFERRIN RECEPTORS

Whilst attached to transferrin in the plasma, iron is delivered to the target cells [18]. Transferrin receptor protein is needed to transfer iron into the cell. It does this primarily via transferrin receptor 1. It is biosynthesized by similar means to transferrin except for the addition of serotransferrin glycan [5-13].

TRANSFERRIN RECEPTOR PROTEIN 1 STRUCTURE

Transferrin receptor protein 1 is a protein consisting of a chain of 760 amino acids [19, 20]. Transferrin receptor protein 2 is a lesser receptor protein that is not essential for the transfer of iron in to the cells [21].

NH_2 – Met – Met – Asp – Gln – Ala – Arg – Ser – Ala – Phe
1 |
Ser – Leu – Phe – Glu – Gly – Gly – Phe – Leu – Asn – Ser
| 10
Tyr – Thr – Arg – Phe – Ser – Leu – Ala – Arg – Gln – Val
20 |
Lys – Met – Glu – Val – His – Ser – Asn – Asp – Gly – Asp
| 30

Leu – Ala – Val – Asp – Glu – Glu – Glu – Asn – Ala – Asp

40 |

Phe – Lys – Thr – Val – Asn – Ala – Lys – Thr – Asn – Asn

| 50

Lys – Arg – Cys – Ser – Gly – Ser – Ile – Cys – Tyr – Gly

60 |

Ile – Leu – Phe – Phe – Val – Ile – Val – Ala – Ile – Thr

| 70

Gly – Phe – Met – Ile – Gly – Tyr – Leu – Gly – Tyr – Cys

80 |

Glu – Cys – Glu – Thr – Lys – Phe – Glu – Val – Gly – Lys

| 90

Arg – Leu – Ala – Gly – Thr – Glu – Ser – Phe – Val – Arg

100 |

Ala – Ala – Phe – Phe – Asp – Glu – Gly – Phe – Glu – Glu

| 110

Arg – Arg – Leu – Tyr – Trp – Asp – Asp – Leu – Lys – Arg

120 |

Asp – Thr – Ser – Asp – Leu – Lys – Glu – Ser – Leu – Lys

| 130

Phe – Thr – Gly – Thr – Ile – Lys – Leu – Leu – Asn – Glu

140 |

Ser – Gly – Ala – Glu – Arg – Phe – Val – Tyr – Ser – Asn

| 150

Gln – Lys – Asp – Glu – Asn – Leu – Ala – Leu – Tyr – Val

160 |

Ser – Leu – Lys – Phe – Glu – Arg – Phe – Gln – Asn – Glu

| 170

Lys – Val – W – Arg – Asp – Gln – His – Phe – Phe – Lys

180 |

Ser – Asn – Gln – Ala – Ser – Asp – Lys – Val – Gln – Ile

| 190

Val – Ile – Ile – Val – Asp – Lys – Asn – Gly – Arg – Leu

200 |

Tyr – Gly – Gly – Phe – Asn – Glu – Val – Leu – Tyr – Val
210

Val – Ala – Tyr – Ser – Lys – Ala – Ala – Thr – Val – Thr
220

Thr – Gly – Phe – Asn – Ala – His – Val – Leu – Lys – Gly
230

Lys – Lys – Asp – Phe – Glu – Asp – Leu – Tyr – Thr – Pro
240

Ala – Arg – Val – Ile – Val – Ile – Ser – Gly – Asn – Val
250

Gly – Lys – Ile – Thr – Phe – Ala – Glu – Lys – Val – Ala
260

Val – Gly – Ile – Ala – Asn – Leu – Ser – Glu – Ala – Asn
270

Leu – Ile – Tyr – Met – Asp – Gly – Thr – Lys – Phe – Pro
280

Gly – Phe – Phe – Ser – Leu – Glu – Ala – Asn – Val – Ile
290

H – Ala – His – Leu – Gly – Thr – Gly – Asp – Phe – Tyr
300

Thr – His – Asn – Phe – Ser – Phe – Phe – Gly – Phe – Thr
310

Gln – Phe – Phe – Phe – Ser – Arg – Ser – Ser – Gly – Leu
320

Arg – Ser – Ile – Thr – Gln – Val – Phe – Ile – Asn – Pro
330

Ala – Ala – Ala – Glu – Lys – Leu – Phe – Gly – Asn – M
340

Thr – Lys – Trp – Asp – Ser – Phe – Cys – Asp – Gly – Glu
350

Asp – Ser – Thr – Cys – Arg – Met – Val – Thr – Ser – Glu
360

Asn – Ser – Val – Thr – Leu – Lys – Val – Asn – Lys – Ser
370

Val – Leu – Lys – Glu – Ile – Lys – Ile – Leu – Asn – Ile

380 |

Pro – Glu – Val – Phe – Gly – Lys – Ile – Val – Gly – Phe

| 390

Asp – His – Tyr – Val – Val – Val – Gly – Ala – Gln – Arg

400 |

Ser – Lys – Ala – Ala – Gly – Phe – Gly – Trp – Ala – Asp

| 410

Gly – Val – Gly – Thr – Ala – Leu – Leu – Leu – Lys – Leu

420 |

Lys – Leu – Val – Met – Asp – Ser – Phe – Met – Gln – Ala

| 430

Asp – Gly – Val – Gln – Phe – Ser – Arg – Ser – Ile – Ile

440 |

Gly – Phe – Asp – Gly – Ala – Ser – Trp – Ser – Ala – Phe

| 450

Ser – Val – Gly – Ala – Thr – Glu – Trp – Leu – Glu – Gly

460 |

Phe – Ala – Lys – Leu – His – Leu – Ser – Ser – Leu – Tyr

| 470

Thr – Tyr – Ile – Asn – Leu – Asp – Lys – Ala – Val – Leu

480 |

Ser – Ala – Ser – Val – Lys – Phe – Asn – Ser – Thr – Gly

| 490

Pro – Leu – Leu – Tyr – Thr – Leu – Ile – Glu – Lys – Thr

500 |

Gly – Thr – Val – Phe – His – Lys – Val – Asn – Gln – Met

| 510

Gln – Phe – Leu – Tyr – Gln – Asp – Ser – Asn – Trp – Ala

520 |

Asn – Asp – Leu – Thr – Leu – Lys – Glu – Val – Lys – Ser

| 530

Ala – Ala – Phe – Phe – Phe – Leu – Ala – Tyr – Ser – Gly

540 |

Glu – Cys – Phe – Cys – Phe – Ser – Val – Ala – Phe – Ile 550
|
560 Asp – Thr – Asp – Tyr – Phe – Tyr – Leu – Gly – Thr – Thr
|
Arg – Glu – Ile – Leu – Glu – Lys – Tyr – Thr – Asp – Met 570
|
580 Ile – Phe – Glu – Leu – Asn – Lys – Val – Ala – Arg – Ala
|
Ile – Val – Phe – Gln – Gly – Ala – Val – Glu – Ala – Ala 590
|
600 Lys – Leu – Thr – His – Asp – Val – Glu – Leu – Asn – Leu
|
Leu – Leu – Gln – Ser – Asn – Tyr – Arg – Glu – Tyr – Asp 610
|
620 Ser – Phe – Val – Arg – Asp – Leu – Asn – Gln – Tyr – Arg
|
Leu – Ser – Leu – Gly – Met – Glu – Lys – Ile – Asp – Ala 630
|
640 Gln – W – Leu – Tyr – Ser – Ala – Arg – Gly – Asp – Phe
|
Asp – Thr – Thr – Leu – Arg – Ser – Thr – Ala – Arg – Phe 650
|
660 Phe – Gly – Asn – Ala – Glu – Lys – Thr – Asp – Arg – Phe
|
Met – Val – Arg – Asp – Asn – Leu – Lys – Lys – Met – Val 670
|
680 Arg – Val – Glu – Tyr – His – Phe – Leu – Ser – Phe – Tyr
|
His – Arg – Phe – Phe – Ser – Glu – Lys – Phe – Ser – Val 690
|
700 Val – Phe – Trp – Gly – Ser – Gly – Ser – His – Thr – Leu
|
Arg – Leu – Lys – Leu – Asn – Glu – Leu – Leu – Ala – Pro 710
|

Lys – Gln – Asn – Asn – Gly – Ala – Phe – Asn – Glu – Thr
720
|
Thr – Ala – Leu – Ala – Leu – Gln – Asn – Arg – Phe – Leu
|
730

Trp – Thr – Ile – Gln – Gly – Ala – Ala – Asn – Ala – Leu
740
|
Glu – Asn – Asp – Ile – Asp – Trp – Val – Asp – Gly – Ser
|
750

Phe – COOH
760

[1] Nature [1983] 302 : 830-832 (S.El Mestikawy, J.Glowinski, M. Hamon)

[2] Archives of Biochemistry and Biophysics [1967] 120 : 420-427 (M.Ikeda, M.Levitt, S.Udenfriend)

[3] Journal of Biological Chemistry [1964] 239 : 2910-2917 (T. Nagatsu, M.Levitt, S.Udenfriend)

[4] Comptes Rendue des Academie Sciences Series 3 [1986] 302 : 435-438 (D.Pigeon, R.Drissi-Daoudi, F.Gros, J.Thibault)

[5] Journal of Biological Chemistry [1983] 258 : 3543 (R.T.A. MacGillivray, E.Mendez, J.G.Schewale, S.K.Sinha, J.Lineback-Zins, K. Brew)

[6] Journal of Biological Chemistry [1983] 258 : 12073 (P.B.Wolfe, W.Wickner, J.M.Goodman)

[7] Journal of Biological Chemistry [1981] 256 : 3593 (C.Zwizinski, T. Date, W.Wickner)

[8] Nucleic Acids Research [1986] 14 : 4683 (G.von Heijne)

[9] Journal of Bioenergetics and Biomembranes [1990] 22 : 271 (I.K. Dev, P.H.Ray)

[10] Journal of Biological Chemistry [1989] 264 : 15813 (M.P. Caulfield, L.T.Duong, R.K.Baker, M.Rosenblatt, M.O.Lively)

[11] EMBO Journal [1986] 5 : 427 (R.Dierstein, W.Wickner)

[12] Journal of Biological Chemistry [1989] 264 : 15762 (G.Greenburg, G.S.Shelness, G.Blobel)

[13] Protein Biosynthesis [1992] (H.R.V.Arnstein, R.A.Cox)

[14] International Journal of Biochemistry [1990] 22 (3) : 275 (S. Welch, L.Langmead)

[15] Biochemistry [1994] 33 (41) : 12512 (R.W.Evans, J.B.Crawley, R.C.Garratt, J.G.Grossmann, M.Neu, A.Aitken, K.J.Patel, A.Meilak, C.Wong, J.Singh, A.Bomford, S. Hasnain)

[16] FEBS Letters [1975] 50 : 296 (G.Spik, G.Strecker, B.Fournet, S.Bouquelet, J. Montreuil)

[17] Comparative Biochemistry [1983] 74B : 603 (A.Stratil, P. Bobak, M.Valenta, V.Tomasek)

[18] Cell [2004] 116 : 565-576 (Y,Cheng, O.Zak, P.Aisen, S.C. Harrison, T.Walz)

[19] Cell [1984] 39 (2 Part 1) : 267-274 (A.McClelland, L.C.Kühn, F.H.Ruddle)

[20] EMBO Journal [1986] 5 (7) : 1543-1550 (M.Zerial, P.Melancon, C.Schneider, H.Garoff)

[21] Journal of Biological Chemistry [1999] 274 (30) : 20826-20832 (H.Kawabata, R.Yang, T.Hirama, P.T.Vuong, S.Kawano, A.F. Gombart, H.P.Koeffler)

CHAPTER 7

BIOCHEMISTRY OF PARKINSON'S DISEASE

ZINC METABOLISM

Zinc cofactor

The second step in the biosynthesis of dopamine requires pyridoxal phosphate. The biosynthesis of pyridoxal phosphate requires zinc as a cofactor. The activity of the enzyme increases or decreases according to the concentration of zinc [1, 2].

enzyme name : pyridoxal kinase
enzyme classification : EC 2.7.1.35
cofactor : zinc (Zn^{2+})
substrate : pyridoxal + ATP
product : pyridoxal 5'-phosphate + ADP

Metallothionein biosynthesis

The transport of zinc requires the secretion of metallothionein. Metallothionein is biosynthesized from amino acids, which via translation first form a single chain polypeptide in the ribosomes. With the addition of two molecules of water, leader peptidase removes the signal peptide to produce metallothionein in the endoplasmic reticulum [3-11]. In the golgi complex zinc is added to metallothionein to form zinc-thionein in the plasma. Zinc is then detached from apothionein in the plasma making it available to the target cells [12, 13].

Metallothionein structure

There are eleven forms of Metallothionein : Metallothionein MT-2, MT-3, MT-1a, MT-1b, MT-1e, MT-1f, MT-1g, MT-1h, MT-1j, MT-1k, and MT-1l.

METALLOTHIONEIN MT-2 [14]

NH_2 – Met – Asp – Pro – Asn – Cys – Ser – Cys – Ala – Ala

1 |

Cys – Ser – Gly – Ala – Cys – Thr – Cys – Ser – Asp – Gly

| 10

Lys – Cys – Lys – Glu – Cys – Lys – Cys – Thr – Ser – Cys

20 |

Val – Pro – Cys – Cys – Ser – Cys – Cys – Ser – Lys – Lys

| 30

Gly – Cys – Ala – Lys – Cys – Ala – Gln – Gly – Cys – Ile

40 |

Cys – Ser – Cys – Lys – Asp – Ser – Ala – Gly – Lys – Cys

| 50

Cys – Ala – COOH

60 61

METALLOTHIONEIN MT-3 [15]

NH_2 – Met – Asp – Pro – Glu – Thr – Cys – Pro – Cys – Pro

1 |

Ser – Asp – Ala – Cys – Thr – Cys – Ser – Gly – Gly – Ser

| 10

Cys – Lys – Cys – Glu – Gly – Cys – Lys – Cys – Thr – Ser

20 |

Pro – Cys – Cys – Ser – Cys – Cys – Ser – Lys – Lys – Cys

| 30

Ala – Glu – Cys – Glu – Lys – Cys – Ala – Lys – Asp – Cys

40 |

Ala – Glu – Ala – Ala – Glu – Gly – Gly – Lys – Cys – Val

| 50

Glu – Ala – Glu – Lys – Cys – Ser – Cys – Cys – Gln 68

60 |

COOH

Metallothionein MT-1a [16]

NH_2 – Met – Asp – Pro – Asn – Cys – Ser – Cys – Ala – Thr
1
|
Cys – Ser – Gly – Ala – Cys – Thr – Cys – Ser – Gly – Gly
| 10
Lys – Cys – Lys – Glu – Cys – Lys – Cys – Asn – Ser – Cys
20 |
Met – Pro – Cys – Cys – Ser – Cys – Cys – Ser – Lys – Lys
| 30
Ser – Cys – Ala – Lys – Cys – Ala – Gln – Gly – Cys – Ile
40 |
Cys – Ser – Cys – Lys – Glu – Ser – Ala – Gly – Lys – Cys
| 50
Cys – Ala – COOH
60 61

Metallothionein MT-1b [17]

NH_2 – Met – Asp – Pro – Asn – Cys – Ser – Cys – Thr – Thr
1
|
Cys – Ser – Gly – Ala – Cys – Ala – Cys – Ser – Gly – Gly
| 10
Lys – Cys – Lys – Glu – Cys – Lys – Cys – Thr – Ser – Cys
20 |
Val – Pro – Cys – Cys – Ser – Cys – Cys – Cys – Lys – Lys
| 30
Gly – Cys – Ala – Lys – Cys – Ala – Gln – Gly – Cys – Val
40 |
Cys – Arg – Cys – Lys – Glu – Ser – Ser – Gly – Lys – Cys
| 50
Cys – Ala – COOH
60 61

METALLOTHIONEIN MT-1e [18]

NH_2 – Met – Asp – Pro – Asn – Cys – Ser – Cys – Ala – Thr

1

Cys – Ser – Gly – Ala – Cys – Thr – Cys – Ser – Gly – Gly

10

Lys – Cys – Lys – Glu – Cys – Lys – Cys – Thr – Ser – Cys

20

Val – Pro – Cys – Cys – Ser – Cys – Cys – Ser – Lys – Lys

30

Gly – Cys – Ala – Lys – Cys – Ala – Gln – Gly – Cys – Val

40

Cys – Ser – Cys – Lys – Glu – Ser – Ala – Gly – Lys – Cys

50

Cys – Ala – COOH

60 61

METALLOTHIONEIN MT-1f [18]

NH_2 – Met – Asp – Pro – Asn – Cys – Ser – Cys – Ala – Ala

1

Cys – Ser – Gly – Ala – Cys – Thr – Cys – Ser – Val – Gly

10

Lys – Cys – Lys – Glu – Cys – Lys – Cys – Thr – Ser – Cys

20

Val – Pro – Cys – Cys – Ser – Cys – Cys – Ser – Lys – Lys

30

Gly – Cys – Ser – Lys – Cys – Ala – Gln – Gly – Cys – Val

40

Cys – Ser – Cys – Lys – Glu – Ser – Ala – Gly – Lys – Cys

50

Cys – Asp – COOH

60 61

METALLOTHIONEIN MT-1g [19]

NH_2 – Met – Asp – Pro – Asn – Cys – Ser – Cys – Ala – Ala
1
|
Cys – Ser – Ser – Ala – Cys – Thr – Cys – Ser – Val – Gly
10
|
Lys – Cys – Lys – Glu – Cys – Lys – Cys – Thr – Ser – Cys
20
|
Val – Pro – Cys – Cys – Ser – Cys – Cys – Ser – Lys – Lys
30
|
Gly – Cys – Ala – Lys – Cys – Ala – Gln – Gly – Cys – Ile
40
|
Cys – Ser – Cys – Lys – Glu – Ser – Ala – Gly – Lys – Cys
50
|
Cys – Ala – COOH
60 61

METALLOTHIONEIN MT-1h [13]

NH_2 – Met – Asp – Pro – Asn – Cys – Ser – Cys – Ala – Ala
1
|
Cys – Ser – Gly – Ala – Cys – Thr – Cys – Ser – Asp – Gly
10
|
Lys – Cys – Lys – Glu – Cys – Lys – Cys – Thr – Ser – Cys
20
|
Leu – Pro – Cys – Cys – Ser – Cys – Cys – Ser – Lys – Lys
30
|
Gly – Cys – Ala – Ser – Lys – Cys – Ala – Gln – Gly – Cys
40
|
Ser – Cys – Lys – Glu – Ser – Ala – Gly – Lys – Cys – Ile
50
|
Cys – Cys – Ala – COOH
60 62

METALLOTHIONEIN MT-1j [13]

NH_2 – Met – Asp – Pro – Asn – Cys – Ser – Cys – Ala – Ala
1 |
Cys – Ser – Gly – Ala – Cys – Thr – Cys – Ser – Val – Gly
| 10
Lys – Cys – Lys – Glu – Cys – Lys – Cys – Thr – Ser – Cys
20 |
Val – Pro – Cys – Cys – Ser – Cys – Cys – Ser – Lys – Lys
| 30
Gly – Cys – Ala – Lys – Cys – Ala – Gln – Gly – Cys – Ile
40 |
Cys – Ser – Cys – Lys – Glu – Ser – Ala – Gly – Lys – Cys
| 50
Cys – Ala – COOH
60 61

METALLOTHIONEIN MT-1k [13]

NH_2 – Met – Asp – Pro – Asn – Cys – Ser – Cys – Ala – Ala
1 |
Ser – Ser – Ala – Cys – Thr – Cys – Ser – Val – Gly – Ala
| 10
Cys – Lys – Cys – Lys – Glu – Cys – Lys – Cys – Thr – Ser
20 |
Pro – Cys – Cys – Ser – Cys – Cys – Ser – Lys – Lys – Cys
| 30
Val – Gly – Cys – Ala – Lys – Cys – Ala – Gln – Gly – Cys
40 |
Ser – Cys – Lys – Glu – Ser – Ala – Gly – Lys – Cys – Ile
| 50
Cys – Cys – Ala – COOH
60 62

METALLOTHIONEIN MT-1l [13]

NH_2 – Met – Asp – Pro – Asn – Cys – Ser – Cys – Ser – Pro
(Met = 1)

Cys – Ser – Gly – Ala – Cys – Ala – Cys – Ser – Gly – Val
(Val = 10)

Lys – Cys – Lys – Glu – Cys – Lys – Cys – Thr – Ser – Cys
(Lys = 20)

Val – Pro – Cys – Cys – Ser – Cys – Cys – Ser – Lys – Lys
(Lys = 30)

Gly – Cys – Ala – Lys – Cys – Ala – Gln – Gly – Cys – Ile
(Gly = 40)

Cys – Ser – Cys – Lys – Asp – Ser – Thr – Gly – Lys – Cys
(Cys = 50)

Cys – Ala – COOH
(Cys = 60, Ala = 61)

[1] Journal of Biological Chemistry [1961] 236 : 2076-2084 (D.B. McCormick, M.E.Gregory, E.E.Snell)

[2] Biulleten Eksperimental noi Biologii i Meditsiny [1946] 22 (6) : 40-43 (A.F.Trufanov, J.A.Krisanova)

[3] Journal of Biological Chemistry [1981] 256 : 3593 (C.Zwizinski, T.Date, W.Wickner)

[4] Journal of Biological Chemistry [1989] 264 : 15813 (M.P.Caulfield, L.T.Duong, R.K.Baker, M.Rosenblatt, M.O.Lively)

[5] Journal of Bioenergetics and Biomembranes [1990] 22 : 271 (I.K. Dev, P.H.Ray)

[6] EMBO Journal [1986] 5 : 427 (R.Dierstein, W.Wickner)

[7] Journal of Biological Chemistry [1989] 264 : 15762 (G.Greenburg, G.S.Shelness, G.Blobel)

[8] Nucleic Acids Research [1986] 14 : 4683 (G.von Heijne)

[9] Journal of Biological Chemistry [1983] 258 : 12073 (P.B.Wolfe, W.Wickner, J.M.Goodman)

[10] Protein Biosynthesis [1992] (H.R.V.Arnstein, R.A.Cox)

[11] Biochemical Journal [1975] 149 : 733 (I.Bremner, N.T.Davies)

[12] Biochemical Pharmacology [1979] 28 : 2852 (K.T.Suzuki, M. Yamamura)

[13] Experientia [1987] (supplement 52) : 25 (J.H.R.Kägi, Y.Kojima)

[14] Nature [1982] 299 : 797 (M.Karin, R.I.Richards)

[15] Proceedings, National Academy of Science USA [1992] 89 (14) : 6333 (R.D.Palmiter, S.D. Findley, T.E.Whitmore, D.M.Durnam)

[16] Cell [1984] 37 : 263 (R.I.Richards, A.Heguy, M.Karin)

[17] Molecular and Cellular Biology [1986] 6 : 2149 (A.Heguy, A. West, R.I.Richards, M.Karin)

[18] Journal of Biological Chemistry [1985] 260 : 7731 (C.J.Schmidt, M.F.Jubier, D.H.Hamer)

[19] Experienta Supplementum [1987] 52 : 361 (L.Gedamu, U. Varshney, N.Jahroudi, R.Foster, N.W.Shworak)

CHAPTER 8

BIOCHEMISTRY OF PARKINSON'S DISEASE

MANGANESE METABOLISM

MANGANESE COFACTOR

Dopamine biosynthesis requires tetrahydrofolic acid, which requires NADPH, and also pyridoxal phosphate, which requires NADP. NADP and NADPH are biosynthesized from nicotinamide. Their biosynthesis requires manganese as a cofactor. The activity of the enzymes increases or decreases according to the concentration of manganese [1-8].

enzyme name : NAD^+ kinase
enzyme classification : EC 2.7.1.23
cofactor : manganese (Mn^{2+})
substrate : NAD^+ (or $NADP^+$) + ATP
product : $NADP^+$ (or $NADPH^+$) + ADP

DMT1 BIOSYNTHESIS

The transport of manganese requires the secretion of DMT1 (divalent metal transporter 1) [9]. DMT1 is biosynthesized from amino acids, which, via translation form a single chain polypeptide in the ribosomes. With the addition of two molecules of water, leader peptidase removes the signal peptide to produce DMT1 in the endoplasmic reticulum. Glycosylation takes place in the Golgi Complex [10-17]. Manganese is added in the plasma. Manganese is then detached from DMT1 in the plasma making it available to the target cells [9].

DMT1 STRUCTURE

DMT1 (divalent metal transporter 1) is a protein consisting of a chain of 568 amino acids [9]. Its known variants are inactive.

NH_2 – Met – Val – Leu – Gly – Pro – Glu – Gln – Lys – Met
1
Gly – His – Asp – Gly – Ser – Val – Ser – Asp – Asp – Ser
10
Glu – Ser – Ala – Ser – Leu – Gly – Asn – Ile – Asn – Pro
20
Ser – Gln – Ser – Leu – Ser – Pro – Asn – Ser – Tyr – Ala
30
Pro – Gly – Asp – Ser – Glu – Glu – Tyr – Phe – Ala – Thr
40
Glu – Pro – Ile – Ser – Ile – Lys – Glu – Asn – Phe – Tyr
50
Glu – Glu – Tyr – Ser – Cys – Phe – Ser – Phe – Arg – Lys
60
Leu – Phe – Gly – Pro – Gly – Thr – Phe – Ala – Trp – Leu
70
Met – Ser – Ile – Ala – Tyr – Leu – Asp – Pro – Gly – Asn
80
Val – Ala – Gly – Ser – Gln – Leu – Asp – Ser – Glu – Ile
90
Ala – Gly – Phe – Lys – Leu – Leu – Trp – Ile – Leu – Leu
100
Gln – Leu – Leu – Leu – Gly – Val – Leu – Thr – Ala – Leu
110
Arg – Leu – Ala – Ala – Arg – Leu – Gly – Val – Val – Thr
120
Arg – His – Cys – Val – Glu – Ala – Leu – His – Leu – Gly
130
Gln – Tyr – Pro – Lys – Val – Pro – Arg – Val – Ile – Leu
140
Gly – Ile – Ile – Ala – Leu – Glu – Val – Met – Leu – Trp
150
Ser – Asp – Met – Gln – Glu – Val – Ile – Gly – Ser – Ala
160

Arg – Gly – Val – Ser – Leu – Leu – Asn – Ile – Ala – Ile
| 170

Ile – Pro – Leu – Trp – Gly – Gly – Val – Leu – Ile – Thr
180 |

Leu – Phe – Leu – Phe – Val – Phe – Thr – Asp – Ala – Ile
| 190

Asp – Lys – Tyr – Gly – Leu – Arg – Lys – Leu – Glu – Ala
200 |

Ala – Met – Ile – Thr – Ile – Leu – Phe – Gly – Phe – Phe
| 210

Leu – Thr – Phe – Gly – Tyr – Glu – Tyr – Val – Thr – Val
220 |

Gly – Lys – Leu – Val – Gln – Ser – Gln – Ser – Pro – Lys
| 230

Met – Phe – Val – Pro – Ser – Cys – Ser – Gly – Cys – Arg
240 |

Ile – Gly – Val – Ala – Gln – Glu – Ile – Gln – Pro – Thr
| 250

Val – Gly – Ala – Val – Ile – Met – Pro – His – Asn – Met
260 |

Arg – Ser – Lys – Val – Leu – Ala – Ser – His – Leu – Tyr
| 270

Gln – Val – Asn – Arg – Asn – Asn – Lys – Gln – Glu – Val
280 |

Glu – Ile – Phe – Phe – Tyr – Lys – Asn – Ala – Glu – Arg
| 290

Ser – Cys – Ile – Ala – Leu – Phe – Val – Ser – Phe – Ile
300 |

Ala – Phe – Val – Ser – Val – Val – Phe – Val – Asn – Ile
| 310

Glu – Ala – Phe – Phe – Gly – Lys – Thr – Asn – Glu – Gln
320 |

Ser – Ser – Thr – Asn – Thr – Cys – Val – Glu – Val – Val
| 330

Pro – His – Ala – Gly – Leu – Phe – Pro – Lys – Asp – Asn
340 |

Gly – Lys – Tyr – Ile – Asp – Val – Ala – Leu – Thr – Ser
| 350

Gly – Val – Val – Leu – Gly – Cys – Tyr – Phe – Gly – Pro
360 |

Ile – Gly – Val – Ala – Trp – Ile – Tyr – Leu – Ala – Ala
| 370

Leu – Ala – Ala – Gly – Gln – Ser – Ser – Thr – Met – Thr
380 |

Glu – Met – Val – Phe – Gln – Gly – Ser – Tyr – Thr – Gly
| 390

Gly – Phe – Leu – Asn – Leu – Lys – Trp – Ser – Arg – Phe
400 |

Ala – Ile – Ser – Arg – Thr – Leu – Val – Val – Arg – Ala
| 410

Ile – Ile – Pro – Thr – Leu – Leu – Val – Ala – Val – Phe
420 |

Asn – Met – Gly – Thr – Leu – His – Glu – Val – Asp – Gln
| 430

Asp – Phe – Leu – Asn – Val – Leu – Gln – Ser – Leu – Gln
440 |

Thr – Leu – Ile – Pro – Ile – Leu – Ala – Phe – Pro – Leu
| 450

Phe – Thr – Ser – Leu – Arg – Pro – Val – Met – Ser – Asp
460 |

Ala – Ile – Arg – Trp – Gly – Leu – Gly – Asn – Ala – Phe
| 470

Gly – Gly – Ile – Leu – Val – Leu – Ile – Ile – Cys – Ser
480 |

Val – Tyr – Val – Val – Val – Phe – Tyr – Met – Asn – Ile
| 490

Arg – Asp – Leu – Gly – His – Val – Ala – Leu – Tyr – Val
500 |

```
Leu – Tyr – Ala – Val – Ser – Val – Val – Ala – Ala – Val
 |                                                   510
Gly – Phe – Val – Phe – Tyr – Leu – Gly – Trp – Gln – Cys
520                                                   |
Asp – Leu – Phe – Ser – Met – Gly – Leu – Ala – Ile – Leu
 |                                                   530
Cys – Gly – His – Thr – Cys – His – Leu – Gly – Leu – Thr
540                                                   |
Thr – Asn – Leu – Leu – Tyr – Leu – Glu – Pro – Gln – Ala
 |                                                   550
Met – Asp – Ala – Asp – Ser – Leu – Val – Ser – Arg  568
560                                              |
                                                COOH
```


[1] International Journal of Biochemistry [1982] 14 : 839-844 (J.R. Butler, E.T.McGuinness)

[2] Journal of Biological Chemistry [1967] 242 : 1182-1186 (A.E. Chung)

[3] Journal of Biological Chemistry [1950] 182 : 805-813 (A.Kornberg)

[4] Journal of Biological Chemistry [1954] 206 : 311-325 (T.P.Wang, N.O.Kaplan)

[5] The Pyridine Nucleotide Coenzymes (J.Everse, B.M.Anderson, K.You) [1982] : 279 (R.R.Fisher, S.R.Earle)

[6] CRC Critical Reviews in Biochemistry [1985] 17 : 313 (K.S.You)

[7] Analytical Biochemistry [1986] 154 (1) : 64 (S.J.Berger, N.A. Berger)

[8] Enzyme and Microbial Technology [1994] 16 (3) : 236 (L.M. Simon, M.Kotorman, B.Szajani)

[9] Poultry Science [2008] 87 (4) : 768-776 (S.P.Bai, L.Lu, X.G.Luo, B.Liu)

[10] Journal of Biological Chemistry [1981] 256 : 3593 (C.Zwizinski, T.Date, W.Wickner)

[11] Journal of Biological Chemistry [1989] 264 : 15813 (M.P. Caulfield, L.T.Duong, R.K.Baker, M.Rosenblatt, M.O.Lively)

[12] Journal of Bioenergetics and Biomembranes [1990] 22 : 271 (I.K. Dev, P.H.Ray)

[13] EMBO Journal [1986] 5 : 427 (R.Dierstein, W. Wickner)

[14] Journal of Biological Chemistry [1989] 264 : 15762 (G. Greenburg, G.S.Shelness, G.Blobel)

[15] Nucleic Acids Research [1986] 14 : 4683 (G.von Heijne)

[16] Journal of Biological Chemistry [1983] 258 : 12073 (P.B.Wolfe, W.Wickner, J.M.Goodman),

[17] Protein Biosynthesis [1992] (H.R.V.Arnstein, R.A.Cox)

CHAPTER 9

BIOCHEMISTRY OF PARKINSON'S DISEASE

DOPAMINE RECEPTORS

Dopamine secretion

When dopamine has been biosynthesized it is secreted from the dopaminergic neurons, and then stored in synaptic vesicles before being released to the synaptic cleft. The synaptic cleft is the gap between the dopaminergic neuron and the receptive cell whose dopamine receptors it stimulates.

Dopamine receptor biosynthesis

Dopamine, via translation, stimulates the biosynthesis in the receptive cells of the dopamine receptors [1-8]. Dopamine causes amino acids to form Pre Dopamine Receptor Protein in the ribosomes. In the endoplasmic reticulum, the addition of two molecules of H_20 enables leader peptidase to remove the signal peptide of Pre Dopamine Receptor Protein. Sugars are then added in the golgi complex. Glycosylation has little effect on the activity of this type of receptor [9]. Secretory vesicles then transport the dopamine receptors to the plasma membrane [1-8].

Types of dopamine receptor

There are five types of dopamine receptor : D1, D2, D3, D4, D5. Dopamine receptors D1, D5 are stimulatory. Dopamine receptors D2, D3, D4 are inhibitory. The overall effect of the dopamine receptors is inhibitory because the combined effect of the inhibitory dopamine receptors (D2, D3, D4) is far more powerful than the combined effect of the stimulatory dopamine receptors (D1, D5) [10-15].

Dopamine receptor D1

Dopamine receptor D1 is a protein consisting of a chain of 446 amino acids [16-18].

N_2 – Met – Arg – Thr – Leu – Asn – Thr – Ser – Ala – Met

1 CHO

Asp – Arg – Glu – Val – Val – Leu – Gly – Thr – Gly – Asp

10

Phe – Ser – Val – Arg – Ile – Leu – Thr – Ala – Cys – Phe

20

Leu – Leu – Thr – Ser – Leu – Ile – Leu – Leu – Ser – Leu

30

Gly – Asn – Thr – Leu – Val – Cys – Ala – Ala – Val – Ile

40

Thr – Val – Lys – Ser – Arg – Leu – His – Arg – Phe – Arg

50

Asn – Phe – Phe – Val – Ile – Ser – Leu – Ala – Val – Ser

60

Pro – Met – Val – Leu – Val – Ala – Val – Leu – Leu – Asp

70

Trp – Lys – Ala – Val – Ala – Glu – Ile – Ala – Gly – Phe

80

Trp – Ile – Asn – Cys – Phe – Ser – Gly – Phe – Pro – Trp

90

Val – Ala – Phe – Asp – Ile – Met – Cys – Ser – Thr – Ala

100

Val – Ser – Ile – Val – Cys – Leu – Asn – Leu – Ile – Ser

110

Asp – Arg – Tyr – Trp – Ala – Ile – Ser – Ser – Pro – Phe

120

Ala – Lys – Pro – Thr – Met – Lys – Arg – Glu – Tyr – Arg

130

Ala – Phe – Ile – Leu – Ile – Ser – Val – Ala – Trp – Thr

140

Val – Pro – Ile – Phe – Ser – Ile – Leu – Val – Ser – Leu

150

Gln – Leu – Ser – Trp – His – Lys – Ala – Lys – Pro – Thr

160

Leu – Ser – Thr – Ala – Asn – Gly – Asp – Ser – Pro – Ser

CHO 170

Ala – Glu – Thr – Ile – Asp – Asn – Cys – Asp – Ser – Ser

180

Ser – Ser – Ser – Ile – Ala – Tyr – Thr – Arg – Ser – Leu

190

Val – Ile – Ser – Phe – Tyr – Ile – Pro – Val – Ala – Ile

200

Arg – Tyr – Ile – Arg – Thr – Tyr – Thr – Val – Ile – Met

210

Ile – Ala – Gln – Lys – Gln – Ile – Arg – Arg – Ile – Ala

220

Lys – Ala – His – Val – Ala – Ala – Arg – Glu – Leu – Ala

230

Asn – Cys – Gln – Thr – Thr – Thr – Gly – Asn – Gly – Lys

240

Ser – Ser – Glu – Pro – Gln – Ser – Cys – Glu – Val – Pro

250

Phe – Lys – Met – Ser – Phe – Lys – Arg – Glu – Thr – Lys

260

Gly – Met – Ile – Val – Ser – Leu – Thr – Lys – Leu – Val

270

Val – Phe – Val – Cys – Cys – Trp – Leu – Pro – Phe – Phe

280

Gly – Cys – Phe – Pro – Leu – Ile – Cys – Asn – Leu – Ile

290

Ser – Gly – Glu – Thr – Gln – Pro – Phe – Cys – Ile – Asp

300

Phe – Trp – Val – Phe – Val – Asp – Phe – Thr – Asn – Ser

| 310

Gly – Trp – Ala – Asn – Ser – Ser – Leu – Asn – Pro – Ile

320 |

Lys – Arg – Phe – Asp – Ala – Asn – Phe – Ala – Tyr – Ile

| 330

Ala – Phe – Ser – Thr – Leu – Leu – Gly – Cys – Tyr – Arg

340 |

Glu – Ile – Ala – Asn – Asn – Thr – Ala – Pro – Cys – Leu

| 350

Thr – Val – Ser – Ile – Asn – Asn – Asn – Gly – Ala – Ala

360 |

Gly – Arg – Pro – Glu – His – His – Ser – Ser – Phe – Met

| 370

Ser – Ile – Ser – Lys – Glu – Cys – Asn – Leu – Val – Tyr

380 |

Glu – Ser – Ser – Gly – Val – Ala – His – Pro – Ile – Leu

| 390

Asp – Leu – Lys – Lys – Glu – Glu – Ala – Ala – Gly – Ile

400 |

Ala – Pro – Ser – Leu – Lys – Glu – Leu – Pro – Arg – Ala

| 410

Leu – Ser – Val – Ile – Leu – Asp – Tyr – Asp – Thr – Asp

420 |

Thr – Ile – Pro – Gln – Ile – Lys – Glu – Leu – Ser – Val

| 430

Gln – Asn – Gly – Gln – His – Pro – Thr – COOH

440 446

There are carbohydrate links at amino acids 5 and 175 [16-18].

Putative location of transmembrane helical segments : 29-49, 60-78, 82-102, 139-159, 194-214, 277-297, 313-333 [16-18]

Intracellular segments : 50-59, 103-138, 215-276, 333-446 [16-18]

Dopamine receptor D2

Dopamine receptor D2 is a protein that has two forms - a short version (D2Sh) consisting of a chain of 414 amino acids [19], and a long version (D2Lh) consisting of a chain of 443 amino acids [20].

Dopamine receptor D2Sh

Dopamine receptor D2Sh is the short version of Dopamine receptor D2. It consists of a chain of 414 amino acids [19].

N_2 – Met – Asp – Pro – Leu – Asn – Leu – Ser – Trp – Tyr
1 |

Ser – Trp – Asn – Gln – Arg – Glu – Leu – Asp – Asp – Asp
| 10

Arg – Pro – Phe – Asn – Gly – Ser – Asp – Gly – Lys – Ala
20 |

Thr – Ala – Tyr – Tyr – Asn – Tyr – His – Pro – Arg – Asp
| 30

Leu – Leu – Thr – Leu – Leu – Ile – Ala – Val – Ile – Val
40 |

Val – Ala – Met – Cys – Val – Leu – Val – Asn – Gly – Phe
| 50

Ser – Arg – Glu – Lys – Ala – Leu – Gln – Thr – Thr – Thr
60 |

Ala – Val – Ala – Leu – Ser – Val – Ile – Leu – Tyr – Asn
| 70

Asp – Leu – Leu – Val – Ala – Thr – Leu – Val – Met – Pro
80 |

Glu – Gly – Val – Val – Glu – Leu – Tyr – Val – Val – Trp
| 90

Trp – Lys – Phe – Ser – Arg – Ile – His – Cys – Asp – Ile
100 |

Thr – Cys – Met – Met – Val – Asp – Leu – Thr – Val – Phe
| 110
Ala – Ser – Ile – Leu – Asn – Leu – Cys – Ala – Ile – Ser
120 |
Pro – Met – Ala – Val – Ala – Thr – Tyr – Arg – Asp – Ile
| 130
Met – Leu – Tyr – Asn – Thr – Arg – Tyr – Ser – Ser – Lys
140 |
Val – Ile – Ser – Ile – Met – Val – Thr – Val – Arg – Arg
| 150
Trp – Val – Leu – Ser – Phe – Thr – Ile – Ser – Cys – Pro
160 |
Gln – Asp – Ala – Asn – Asn – Leu – Gly – Phe – Leu – Leu
| 170
Asn – Glu – Cys – Ile – Ile – Ala – Asn – Pro – Ala – Phe
180 |
Tyr – Phe – Ser – Val – Ile – Ser – Ser – Tyr – Val – Val
| 190
Val – Pro – Phe – Ile – Val – Thr – Leu – Leu – Val – Tyr
200 |
Arg – Arg – Arg – Leu – Val – Ile – Tyr – Ile – Lys – Ile
| 210
Arg – Lys – Arg – Val – Asn – Thr – Lys – Arg – Ser – Ser
220 |
Pro – Ala – Arg – Leu – His – Ala – Arg – Phe – Ala – Arg
| 230
Leu – Lys – Gly – Asn – Cys – Thr – His – Pro – Glu – Asp
240 |
Ser – Lys – Met – Ile – Val – Thr – Cys – Leu – Lys – Met
| 250
Asn – Gly – Ser – Phe – Pro – Val – Asn – Arg – Arg – Arg
260 |
Leu – Glu – Gln – Ala – Arg – Arg – Ala – Ala – Glu – Val
| 270

Glu – Met – Glu – Met – Leu – Ser – Ser – Thr – Ser – Pro
280

Pro – Ile – Pro – Ser – Tyr – Arg – Thr – Arg – Glu – Pro
290

Pro – Ser – His – His – Gln – Leu – Thr – Leu – Pro – Asp
300

Pro – Thr – Ser – His – Leu – Gly – His – His – Ser – Pro
310

Asp – Ser – Pro – Ala – Lys – Pro – Glu – Lys – Asn – Gly
320

Lys – Ala – Ile – Lys – Pro – His – Asp – Lys – Ala – His
330

Ile – Phe – Glu – Ile – Gln – Thr – Met – Pro – Asn – Gly
340

Ser – Met – Thr – Lys – Leu – Ser – Thr – Arg – Thr – Lys
350

Arg – Arg – Lys – Leu – Ser – Gln – Gln – Lys – Glu – Lys
360

Leu – Val – Ile – Ala – Leu – Met – Gln – Thr – Ala – Lys
370

Gly – Val – Phe – Ile – Ile – Cys – Trp – Leu – Pro – Phe
380

Cys – His – Ile – Asn – Leu – Ile – His – Thr – Ile – Phe
390

Asp – Cys – Asn – Ile – Pro – Pro – Val – Leu – Tyr – Ser
400

COOH – Leu – Trp – Thr – Phe – Ala
414 410

Putative location of transmembrane helical segments : 39-59, 72-92, 109-129, 154-174, 195-215, 375-395, 406-426 [15]

DOPAMINE RECEPTOR D2LH

Dopamine receptor D2Lh is the long version of Dopamine receptor D2. It consists of a chain of 443 amino acids [20]. It has the same structure as Dopamine receptor D2Sh apart from an additional 29 amino acids on the end of the protein [20].

N_2 – Met – Asp – Pro – Leu – Asn – Leu – Ser – Trp – Tyr
1 |
Ser – Trp – Asn – Gln – Arg – Glu – Leu – Asp – Asp – Asp
| 10
Arg – Pro – Phe – Asn – Gly – Ser – Asp – Gly – Lys – Ala
20 |
Thr – Ala – Tyr – Tyr – Asn – Tyr – His – Pro – Arg – Asp
| 30
Leu – Leu – Thr – Leu – Leu – Ile – Ala – Val – Ile – Val
40 |
Val – Ala – Met – Cys – Val – Leu – Val – Asn – Gly – Phe
| 50
Ser – Arg – Glu – Lys – Ala – Leu – Gln – Thr – Thr – Thr
60 |
Ala – Val – Ala – Leu – Ser – Val – Ile – Leu – Tyr – Asn
| 70
Asp – Leu – Leu – Val – Ala – Thr – Leu – Val – Met – Pro
80 |
Glu – Gly – Val – Val – Glu – Leu – Tyr – Val – Val – Trp
| 90
Trp – Lys – Phe – Ser – Arg – Ile – His – Cys – Asp – Ile
100 |
Thr – Cys – Met – Met – Val – Asp – Leu – Thr – Val – Phe
| 110
Ala – Ser – Ile – Leu – Asn – Leu – Cys – Ala – Ile – Ser
120 |
Pro – Met – Ala – Val – Ala – Thr – Tyr – Arg – Asp – Ile
| 130

Met – Leu – Tyr – Asn – Thr – Arg – Tyr – Ser – Ser – Lys
140 |

Val – Ile – Ser – Ile – Met – Val – Thr – Val – Arg – Arg
| 150

Trp – Val – Leu – Ser – Phe – Thr – Ile – Ser – Cys – Pro
160 |

Gln – Asp – Ala – Asn – Asn – Leu – Gly – Phe – Leu – Leu
| 170

Asn – Glu – Cys – Ile – Ile – Ala – Asn – Pro – Ala – Phe
180 |

Tyr – Phe – Ser – Val – Ile – Ser – Ser – Tyr – Val – Val
| 190

Val – Pro – Phe – Ile – Val – Thr – Leu – Leu – Val – Tyr
200 |

Arg – Arg – Arg – Leu – Val – Ile – Tyr – Ile – Lys – Ile
| 210

Arg – Lys – Arg – Val – Asn – Thr – Lys – Arg – Ser – Ser
220 |

Pro – Ala – Arg – Leu – His – Ala – Arg – Phe – Ala – Arg
| 230

Leu – Lys – Gly – Asn – Cys – Thr – His – Pro – Glu – Asp
240 |

Ser – Lys – Met – Ile – Val – Thr – Cys – Leu – Lys – Met
| 250

Asn – Gly – Ser – Phe – Pro – Val – Asn – Arg – Arg – Arg
260 |

Leu – Glu – Gln – Ala – Arg – Arg – Ala – Ala – Glu – Val
| 270

Glu – Met – Glu – Met – Leu – Ser – Ser – Thr – Ser – Pro
280 |

Pro – Ile – Pro – Ser – Tyr – Arg – Thr – Arg – Glu – Pro
| 290

Pro – Ser – His – His – Gln – Leu – Thr – Leu – Pro – Asp
300 |

Pro – Thr – Ser – His – Leu – Gly – His – His – Ser – Pro
| 310
Asp – Ser – Pro – Ala – Lys – Pro – Glu – Lys – Asn – Gly
320 |
Lys – Ala – Ile – Lys – Pro – His – Asp – Lys – Ala – His
| 330
Ile – Phe – Glu – Ile – Gln – Thr – Met – Pro – Asn – Gly
340 |
Ser – Met – Thr – Lys – Leu – Ser – Thr – Arg – Thr – Lys
| 350
Arg – Arg – Lys – Leu – Ser – Gln – Gln – Lys – Glu – Lys
360 |
Leu – Val – Ile – Ala – Leu – Met – Gln – Thr – Ala – Lys
| 370
Gly – Val – Phe – Ile – Ile – Cys – Trp – Leu – Pro – Phe
380 |
Cys – His – Ile – Asn – Leu – Ile – His – Thr – Ile – Phe
| 390
Asp – Cys – Asn – Ile – Pro – Pro – Val – Leu – Tyr – Ser
400 |
Ser – Asn – Val – Tyr – Gly – Leu – Trp – Thr – Phe – Ala
| 410
Ala – Val – Asn – Pro – Ile – Ile – Tyr – Thr – Thr – Phe
420 |
Lys – Leu – Phe – Ala – Lys – Arg – Phe – Glu – Ile – Asn
| 430
Ile – Leu – His – Cys – COOH
440 443

Putative location of transmembrane helical segments : 39-59, 72-92, 109-129, 154-174, 195-215, 375-395, 406-426 [20]

Dopamine receptor D3

Dopamine receptor D3 is a protein consisting of a chain of 400 amino acids [21].

N_2 – Met – Ala – Ser – Leu – Ser – Gln – Leu – Ser – Ser
1
|
Asn – Glu – Ala – Gly – Cys – Thr – Tyr – Asn – Leu – His
CHO CHO 10
|
Ser – Thr – Gly – Ala – Ser – Gln – Ala – Arg – Pro – His
20
|
Leu – Ala – Cys – Tyr – Ser – Leu – Ala – Tyr – Tyr – Ala
| 30
Ile – Leu – Ala – Ile – Val – Phe – Gly – Asn – Gly – Leu
40
|
Ala – Arg – Glu – Lys – Leu – Val – Ala – Met – Cys – Val
| 50
Leu – Gln – Thr – Thr – Thr – Asn – Tyr – Leu – Val – Val
60
|
Ala – Val – Leu – Leu – Asp – Ala – Val – Ala – Leu – Ser
| 70
Thr – Leu – Val – Met – Pro – Trp – Val – Val – Tyr – Leu
80
|
Ser – Phe – Asn – Trp – Val – Gly – Gly – Thr – Val – Glu
| CHO 90
Arg – Ile – Cys – Cys – Asp – Val – Phe – Val – Thr – Leu
100
|
Leu – Ile – Ser – Ala – Thr – Cys – Met – Met – Val – Asp
| 110
Asn – Leu – Cys – Ala – Ile – Ser – Ile – Asp – Arg – Tyr
120
|
Gln – Tyr – His – Val – Pro – Met – Val – Val – Ala – Thr
| 130

His – Gly – Thr – Gly – Gln – Ser – Ser – Cys – Arg – Arg
140
|
Val – Trp – Val – Ala – Thr – Ile – Met – Leu – Ala – Val
| 150
Leu – Ala – Phe – Ala – Val – Ser – Cys – Pro – Leu – Leu
160
|
Thr – Pro – Asp – Gly – Thr – Thr – Asn – Phe – Gly – Phe
| CHO 170
Val – Cys – Ser – Ile – Ser – Asn – Pro – Asp – Phe – Val
180
|
Leu – Tyr – Phe – Ser – Val – Val – Ser – Ser – Tyr – Ile
| 190
Pro – Phe – Gly – Val – Thr – Val – Leu – Val – Tyr – Ala
200
|
Arg – Arg – Gln – Lys – Leu – Val – Val – Tyr – Ile – Arg
| 210
Arg – Lys – Arg – Ile – Leu – Thr – Arg – Gln – Asn – Ser
220
|
Pro – Phe – Gly – Pro – Arg – Val – Ser – Asn – Cys – Gln
| 230
Gln – Gln – Thr – Leu – Ser – Pro – Asp – Pro – Ala – His
240
|
Cys – Ile – Ser – Tyr – Tyr – Arg – Lys – Leu – Glu – Leu
| 250
Gln – Asp – Thr – Ala – Leu – Gly – Gly – Pro – Gly – Phe
260
|
Glu – Arg – Lys – Leu – Glu – Gly – Gly – Arg – Glu – Gln
| 270
Glu – Lys – Thr – Arg – Asn – Ser – Leu – Ser – Pro – Thr
280
|
Arg – Val – Glu – Leu – Ser – Leu – Lys – Pro – Ala – Ile
| 290
Lys – Leu – Ser – Asn – Gly – Arg – Leu – Ser – Thr – Ser
300
|

Gly – Arg – Pro – Gln – Leu – Pro – Gly – Leu – Lys – Leu
| 310
Val – Pro – Leu – Arg – Glu – Lys – Lys – Ala – Thr – Gln
320 |
Ile – Phe – Ala – Gly – Leu – Val – Ile – Ala – Val – Met
| 330
Val – Cys – Trp – Leu – Pro – Phe – Phe – Leu – Thr – His
340 |
His – Cys – Thr – Gln – Cys – His – Thr – Asn – Leu – Val
| 350
Val – Ser – Pro – Glu – Leu – Tyr – Ser – Ala – Thr – Thr
360 |
Asn – Leu – Ala – Ser – Asn – Val – Tyr – Gly – Leu – Arg
| 370
Pro – Val – Ile – Tyr – Thr – Thr – Phe – Asn – Ile – Glu
380 |
Ser – Leu – Ile – Lys – Leu – Phe – Ala – Lys – Arg – Phe
| 390
Cys – COOH
400

Putative location of transmembrane helical segments : 33-55, 67-91, 105-126, 150-172, 186-209, 330-354, 367-388 [21]. There are carbohydrate links at amino acids 12, 19, 97 and 173 [21].

Dopamine receptor D4

Dopamine receptor D4 is a protein that has a common form that is referred to as Dopamine receptor D4, and also Dopamine receptor D4.2 [14].

Dopamine receptor D4 also has a number of less common variants : D4.3a, D4.3b, D4.4a, D4.4b, D4.4c, D4.4d, D4.4e, D4.5a, D4.5b, D4.6a, D4.6b, D4.7a, D4.7b, D4.7c, D.4.7d, D4.8, D4.10 [22].

DOPAMINE RECEPTOR D4.2

Dopamine receptor D4, which is also referred to as Dopamine receptor D4.2, is a protein consisting of a chain of 387 amino acids. It has two similar 16 amino acid sequences between amino acids 248 and 281.

N_2 – Met – Gly – Asn – Arg – Ser – Thr – Ala – Asp – Ala
1 CHO
|
Ala – Pro – Gly – Arg – Gly – Ala – Leu – Leu – Gly – Asp
| 10
Ala – Gly – Ala – Ser – Ala – Gly – Ala – Ser – Ala – Gly
20 |
Val – Leu – Ala – Ala – Ala – Gly – Gln – Gly – Ala – Leu
| 30
Gly – Gly – Val – Leu – Leu – Ile – Gly – Ala – Val – Leu
40 |
Val – Ser – Val – Cys – Val – Leu – Ser – Asn – Gly – Ala
| 50
Ala – Thr – Glu – Arg – Ala – Leu – Gln – Thr – Pro – Thr
60 |
Ala – Ala – Ala – Leu – Ser – Val – Ile – Phe – Ser – Asn
| 70
Asp – Leu – Leu – Leu – Ala – Leu – Leu – Val – Leu – Pro
80 |
Gly – Gly – Gln – Val – Glu – Ser – Tyr – Val – Phe – Leu
| 90
Ala – Trp – Leu – Leu – Ser – Pro – Arg – Leu – Cys – Asp
100 |
Cys – Leu – Met – Val – Asp – Met – Ala – Met – Leu – Ala
| 110
Thr – Ala – Ser – Ile – Phe – Asn – Leu – Cys – Ala – Ile
120 |
Val – Ala – Val – Ala – Val – Phe – Arg – Asp – Val – Ser
| 130

Pro – Leu – Arg – Tyr – Asn – Arg – Gln – Gly – Gly – Ser
140

Thr – Ala – Gly – Ile – Leu – Leu – Leu – Gln – Arg – Arg
150

Trp – Leu – Leu – Ser – Ala – Ala – Val – Ala – Ala – Pro
160

Gly – Arg – Val – Asp – Asn – Leu – Gly – Cys – Leu – Val
170

Arg – Asp – Pro – Ala – Val – Cys – Arg – Leu – Glu – Asp
180

Cys – Val – Ser – Ser – Tyr – Val – Val – Tyr – Asp – Arg
190

Ser – Phe – Phe – Leu – Pro – Cys – Pro – Leu – Met – Leu
200

Leu – Gly – Arg – Phe – Thr – Ala – Trp – Tyr – Leu – Leu
210

Gln – Arg – Trp – Glu – Val – Ala – Arg – Arg – Ala – Lys
220

Ser – Pro – Arg – Arg – Pro – Ala – Arg – Gly – His – Leu
230

Gly – Pro – Gly – Pro – Pro – Ser – Pro – Thr – Pro – Pro
240

Gly – Cys – Pro – Asp – Gln – Pro – Leu – Arg – Pro – Ala
250

Pro – Asp – Cys – Ala – Pro – Pro – Ala – Pro – Gly – Leu
260

Ala – Cys – Asn – Ser – Gly – Cys – Pro – Asp – Pro – Pro
270

Pro – Pro – Asp – Ala – Val – Arg – Ala – Ala – Ala – Leu
280

Arg – Arg – Thr – Gln – Pro – Pro – Thr – Gln – Pro – Pro
290

Arg – Arg – Arg – Ala – Lys – Ile – Thr – Gly – Arg – Glu
300

Val – Val – Pro – Leu – Val – Arg – Met – Ala – Lys – Arg
| 310
Val – Gly – Ala – Phe – Leu – Leu – Cys – Trp – Thr – Pro
320 |
Leu – Ala – Gln – Thr – Ile – His – Val – Val – Phe – Phe
| 330
Cys – Pro – Ala – Cys – Ser – Val – Pro – Pro – Arg – Leu
340 |
Val – Tyr – Gly – Leu – Trp – Thr – Val – Ala – Ser – Val
| 350
Asn – Ser – Ala – Leu – Asn – Pro – Val – Ile – Tyr – Thr
360 |
Phe – Val – Asn – Arg – Phe – Glu – Ala – Asn – Phe – Val
| 370
Arg – Lys – Ala – Leu – Arg – Ala – Cys – Cys – COOH
380 387

Putative location of transmembrane helical segments : 30-50, 72-92, 111-131, 154-174, 193-212, 315-335, 351-371 [14]

There is a carbohydrate link at amino acid 3 [14].

Dopamine receptor D4.3a

Dopamine receptor D4.3a has the following 16 amino acid sequence inserted after amino acid 264, thereby making Dopamine receptor D4.3a a chain of 403 amino acids [22] :

Pro – Ala – Pro – Gly – Leu – Pro – Gln – Asp – Pro – Cys
265 270 |
– Pro – Ala – Cys – Asp – Pro – Gly
280

Dopamine receptor D4.3b

Dopamine receptor D4.3b has the following 16 amino acid sequence inserted after amino acid 264, thereby making Dopamine receptor D4.3b a chain of 403 amino acids [22] :

Pro – Ala – Pro – Gly – Leu – Pro – Arg – Gly – Pro – Cys
265 270

– Pro – Ala – Cys – Asp – Pro – Gly
280

Dopamine receptor D4.4a

Dopamine receptor D4.4a has the following 32 amino acid sequence inserted after amino acid 264, thereby making Dopamine receptor D4.4a a chain of 419 amino acids [22] :

Pro – Ala – Pro – Gly – Leu – Pro – Arg – Gly – Pro – Cys
265 270

Ser – Pro – Ala – Ala – Pro – Ala – Cys – Asp – Pro – Gly
280

Leu – Pro – Gln – Asp – Pro – Cys – Gly – Pro – Asp – Cys
290

– Pro – Ala
296

Dopamine receptor D4.4b

Dopamine receptor D4.4b has the following 32 amino acid sequence inserted after amino acid 264, thereby making Dopamine receptor D4.4b a chain of 419 amino acids [22] :

Pro – Ala – Pro – Gly – Leu – Pro – Arg – Gly – Pro – Cys
265 270

Gly – Pro – Ala – Ala – Pro – Ala – Cys – Asp – Pro – Gly

```
|                    280
Leu – Pro – Gln – Asp – Pro – Cys – Gly – Pro – Asp – Cys
                              290                      |
                                               – Pro – Ala
                                                 296
```

DOPAMINE RECEPTOR D4.4C

Dopamine receptor D4.4c has the following 32 amino acid sequence inserted after amino acid 264, thereby making Dopamine receptor D4.4c a chain of 419 amino acids [22] :

```
Pro – Ala – Pro – Gly – Leu – Pro – Pro – Asp – Pro – Cys
265                           270                      |
Ser – Pro – Ala – Ala – Pro – Ala – Cys – Asn – Ser – Gly
|                       280
Leu – Pro – Gln – Asp – Pro – Cys – Gly – Pro – Asp – Cys
                              290                      |
                                               – Pro – Ala
                                                 296
```

DOPAMINE RECEPTOR D4.4D

Dopamine receptor D4.4d has the following 32 amino acid sequence inserted after amino acid 264, thereby making Dopamine receptor D4.4d a chain of 419 amino acids [22] :

```
Pro – Ala – Pro – Cys – Leu – Pro – Arg – Gly – Pro – Cys
265                           270                      |
Ser – Pro – Ala – Ala – Pro – Ala – Cys – Asn – Pro – Gly
|                       280
Leu – Pro – Gln – Asp – Pro – Cys – Gly – Pro – Asp – Cys
                              290                      |
                                               – Pro – Ala
                                                 296
```

Dopamine receptor D4.4e

Dopamine receptor D4.4e has the following 32 amino acid sequence inserted after amino acid 264, thereby making Dopamine receptor D4.4e a chain of 419 amino acids [22] :

Pro – Ala – Pro – Gly – Leu – Pro – Gln – Gly – Pro – Cys
265 270
|
Ser – Pro – Ala – Ala – Pro – Ala – Cys – Asp – Pro – Gly
| 280
Leu – Pro – Gln – Asp – Pro – Cys – Gly – Pro – Asp – Cys
290
|
– Pro – Ala
296

Dopamine receptor D4.5a

Dopamine receptor D4.5a has the following 48 amino acid sequence inserted after amino acid 264, thereby making Dopamine receptor D4.5a a chain of 435 amino acids [22] :

Pro – Ala – Pro – Gly – Leu – Pro – Arg – Gly – Pro – Cys
265 270
|
Gly – Pro – Ala – Ala – Pro – Ala – Cys – Asp – Pro – Gly
| 280
Leu – Pro – Pro – Asp – Pro – Cys – Gly – Pro – Asp – Cys
290
|
Asp – Gln – Pro – Leu – Gly – Pro – Ala – Pro – Pro – Ala
| 300
Pro – Cys – Gly – Pro – Asp – Cys – Ala – Pro –
310 312

Dopamine receptor D4.5b

Dopamine receptor D4.5b, which is 435 amino acids, has the following 48 amino acids inserted after amino acid 264 [22] :

Pro – Ala – Pro – Ser – Leu – Pro – Gln – Asp – Pro – Cys
265 (Pro), 270 (Pro)
|
Gly – Pro – Ala – Pro – Pro – Ala – Cys – Asp – Pro – Gly
280 (Pro)
|
Leu – Pro – Arg – Gly – Pro – Cys – Gly – Pro – Asp – Cys
290 (Cys)
|
Asp – Gln – Pro – Leu – Ser – Pro – Ala – Ala – Pro – Ala
300 (Ser)
|
Pro – Cys – Gly – Pro – Asp – Cys – Ala – Pro –
310 (Cys), 312 (Pro)

Dopamine receptor D4.6a

Dopamine receptor D4.6a, which is 451 amino acids, has the following 64 amino acids inserted after amino acid 264 [22] :

Pro – Ala – Pro – Gly – Leu – Pro – Arg – Gly – Pro – Cys
265 (Pro), 270 (Pro)
|
Gly – Pro – Ala – Ala – Pro – Ala – Cys – Asp – Pro – Gly
280 (Pro)
|
Leu – Pro – Pro – Asp – Pro – Cys – Gly – Pro – Asp – Cys
290 (Cys)
|
Asp – Gln – Pro – Leu – Gly – Pro – Ala – Pro – Pro – Ala
300 (Gly)
|
Pro – Cys – Gly – Pro – Asp – Cys – Ala – Pro – Pro – Ala
310 (Cys)
|
Pro – Gly – Cys – Pro – Gly – Arg – Pro – Leu – Gly – Pro
320 (Gly)
|
Asp – Cys – Ala – Pro –
328 (Pro)

Dopamine receptor D4.6b

Dopamine receptor D4.6b, which is 451 amino acids, has the following 64 amino acids inserted after amino acid 264 [22] :

```
Pro – Ala – Pro – Gly – Leu – Pro – Arg – Gly – Pro – Cys
265                         270                          |
Ser – Pro – Ala – Ala – Pro – Ala – Cys – Asp – Pro – Gly
 |                      280
Leu – Pro – Gln – Asp – Pro – Cys – Gly – Pro – Asp – Cys
                              290                        |
Gly – Arg – Pro – Leu – Gly – Pro – Ala – Pro – Pro – Ala
 |                      300
Pro – Cys – Gly – Pro – Asp – Cys – Ala – Pro – Ala – Ala
                              310                        |
Pro – Gly – Cys – Pro – Asp – Gln – Pro – Leu – Ser – Pro
 |                      320
Asp – Cys – Ala – Pro –
                  328
```

Dopamine receptor D4.7a

Dopamine receptor D4.7a, which is 467 amino acids, has the following 80 amino acids inserted after amino acid 264 [22] :

```
Pro – Ala – Pro – Gly – Leu – Pro – Arg – Gly – Pro – Cys
265                         270                          |
Gly – Pro – Ala – Ala – Pro – Ala – Cys – Asp – Pro – Gly
 |                      280
Leu – Pro – Pro – Asp – Pro – Cys – Gly – Pro – Asp – Cys
                              290                        |
Asp – Gln – Pro – Leu – Gly – Pro – Ala – Pro – Pro – Ala
 |                      300
Pro – Cys – Gly – Pro – Asp – Cys – Ala – Pro – Pro – Ala
```

310 |

Pro – Gly – Cys – Pro – Gly – Arg – Pro – Leu – Gly – Pro

| 320

Asp – Cys – Ala – Pro – Pro – Ala – Pro – Gly – Leu – Pro

330 |

Pro – Ala – Cys – Asp – Pro – Gly – Cys – Pro – Asp – Gln

344 340

Dopamine receptor D4.7b

Dopamine receptor D4.7b, which is 467 amino acids, has the following 80 amino acids inserted after amino acid 264 [22] :

Pro – Ala – Pro – Gly – Leu – Pro – Arg – Gly – Pro – Cys

265 270 |

Gly – Pro – Ala – Ala – Pro – Ala – Cys – Asp – Pro – Gly

| 280

Leu – Pro – Pro – Asp – Pro – Cys – Gly – Pro – Asp – Cys

290 |

Asp – Gln – Pro – Leu – Gly – Pro – Ala – Pro – Pro – Ala

| 300

Pro – Cys – Gly – Pro – Asp – Cys – Ala – Pro – Pro – Ala

310 |

Pro – Gly – Cys – Pro – Gly – Arg – Pro – Leu – Gly – Pro

| 320

Asp – Cys – Ala – Pro – Ala – Ala – Pro – Ser – Leu – Pro

330 |

Pro – Ala – Cys – Asp – Pro – Gly – Cys – Pro – Asp – Gln

344 340

Dopamine receptor D4.7c

Dopamine receptor D4.7c, which is 467 amino acids, has the following 80 amino acids inserted after amino acid 264 [22] :

Pro – Ala – Pro – Gly – Leu – Pro – Arg – Gly – Pro – Cys
265 270 |
Ser – Pro – Ala – Ala – Pro – Ala – Cys – Asp – Pro – Gly
| 280
Leu – Pro – Gln – Asp – Pro – Cys – Gly – Pro – Asp – Cys
290 |
Asp – Gln – Pro – Leu – Gly – Pro – Ala – Pro – Pro – Ala
| 300
Pro – Cys – Gly – Pro – Asp – Cys – Ala – Pro – Pro – Ala
310 |
Pro – Gly – Cys – Pro – Gly – Arg – Pro – Leu – Gly – Pro
| 320
Asp – Cys – Ala – Pro – Pro – Ala – Pro – Gly – Leu – Pro
330 |
Pro – Ala – Cys – Asp – Pro – Gly – Cys – Pro – Asp – Gln
344 340

Dopamine receptor D4.7d

Dopamine receptor D4.7d, which is 467 amino acids, has the following 80 amino acids inserted after amino acid 264 [22] :

Pro – Ala – Pro – Gly – Leu – Pro – Arg – Gly – Pro – Cys
265 270 |
Ser – Pro – Ala – Ala – Pro – Ala – Cys – Asp – Pro – Gly
| 280
Leu – Pro – Gln – Asp – Pro – Cys – Gly – Pro – Asp – Cys
290 |
Asp – Pro – Pro – Leu – Gly – Pro – Ala – Pro – Pro – Ala

| 300

Pro – Cys – Gly – Ser – Asn – Cys – Ala – Pro – Pro – Ala

310 |

Pro – Gly – Cys – Pro – Gly – Arg – Pro – Leu – Gly – Pro

| 320

Asp – Cys – Ala – Pro – Pro – Ala – Pro – Gly – Leu – Pro

330 |

Pro – Ala – Cys – Asp – Pro – Gly – Cys – Pro – Asp – Gln

344 340

Dopamine receptor D4.8

Dopamine receptor D4.8, which is 483 amino acids, has the following 96 amino acids inserted after amino acid 264 [22] :

Pro – Ala – Pro – Gly – Leu – Pro – Arg – Gly – Pro – Cys

265 270 |

Gly – Pro – Ala – Ala – Pro – Ala – Cys – Asp – Pro – Gly

| 280

Leu – Pro – Pro – Asp – Pro – Cys – Gly – Pro – Asp – Cys

290 |

Asp – Gln – Pro – Leu – Gly – Pro – Ala – Pro – Pro – Ala

| 300

Pro – Cys – Gly – Pro – Asp – Cys – Ala – Pro – Pro – Ala

310 |

Pro – Gly – Cys – Pro – Asp – Gln – Pro – Leu – Gly – Pro

| 320

Asp – Cys – Ala – Pro – Pro – Ala – Pro – Gly – Leu – Pro

330 |

Pro – Ala – Cys – Asp – Pro – Gly – Cys – Pro – Asp – Gln

| 340

Ala – Ala – Pro – Ser – Leu – Pro – Gln – Asp – Pro – Cys

350 |

– Pro – Ala – Cys – Asp – Pro – Gly

Dopamine receptor D4.10

Dopamine receptor D4.10, which is 511 amino acids, has the following 128 amino acids inserted after amino acid 264 [22] :

Pro – Ala – Pro – Gly – Leu – Pro – Arg – Gly – Pro – Cys
265 270

Gly – Pro – Ala – Ala – Pro – Ala – Cys – Asp – Pro – Gly
280

Leu – Pro – Arg – Asp – Pro – Cys – Gly – Pro – Asp – Cys
290

Asp – Pro – Pro – Leu – Gly – Pro – Ala – Ala – Pro – Ala
300

Pro – Cys – Gly – Pro – Asp – Cys – Ala – Pro – Pro – Ala
310

Pro – Gly – Cys – Pro – Gly – Arg – Pro – Leu – Gly – Pro
320

Asp – Cys – Ala – Pro – Ala – Ala – Pro – Gly – Leu – Pro
330

Pro – Ala – Cys – Asp – Pro – Gly – Cys – Pro – Asp – Pro
340

Pro – Ala – Pro – Gly – Leu – Pro – Gln – Asp – Pro – Cys
350

Gly – Pro – Ala – Pro – Pro – Ala – Cys – Asp – Pro – Gly
360

Leu – Pro – Arg – Gly – Pro – Cys – Gly – Pro – Asp – Cys
370

Asp – Gln – Pro – Leu – Gly – Pro – Ala – Pro – Pro – Ala
380

Pro – Cys – Gly – Pro – Asp – Cys – Ala – Pro –
390 392

Dopamine receptor D5

Dopamine receptor D5 is a protein consisting of a chain of 477 amino acids [15].

N_2 – Met – Leu – Pro – Pro – Gly – Ser – Asn – Gly – Thr
1 (Met); CHO (Asn)
|
Gln – Tyr – Leu – Ala – Phe – Gln – Gly – Pro – Tyr – Ala
| 10
Gln – Leu – Ala – Gln – Gly – Asn – Ala – Val – Gly – Gly
20 |
Ser – Pro – Gly – Leu – Pro – Pro – Ala – Gly – Ala – Ser
| 30
Gln – Val – Val – Thr – Ala – Cys – Leu – Leu – Thr – Leu
40 |
Val – Asn – Gly – Leu – Leu – Thr – Trp – Ile – Ile – Leu
| 50
Leu – Val – Cys – Ala – Ala – Ile – Val – Arg – Ser – Arg
60 |
Phe – Val – Asn – Thr – Met – Asn – Ala – Arg – Leu – His
| 70
Ile – Val – Ser – Leu – Ala – Val – Ser – Asp – Leu – Phe
80 |
Ala – Lys – Trp – Pro – Met – Val – Leu – Leu – Ala – Val
| 90
Val – Ala – Glu – Val – Ala – Gly – Tyr – Trp – Pro – Phe
100 |
Phe – Ala – Val – Trp – Val – Asp – Cys – Phe – Ala – Gly
| 110
Asp – Ile – Met – Cys – Ser – Thr – Ala – Ser – Ile – Leu
120 |
Tyr – Arg – Asp – Val – Ser – Ile – Val – Cys – Leu – Asn
| 130
Trp – Ala – Ile – Ser – Arg – Pro – Phe – Arg – Tyr – Lys

140

Val – Leu – Ala – Met – Arg – Gln – Thr – Met – Lys – Arg

150

Met – Val – Gly – Leu – Ala – Trp – Thr – Leu – Ser – Ile

160

Asn – Leu – Gln – Val – Pro – Ile – Phe – Ser – Ile – Leu

170

Trp – His – Arg – Asp – Gln – Ala – Ala – Ser – Trp – Gly

180

Asn – Ala – Leu – Asn – Asn – Pro – Leu – Asp – Leu – Gly

190

Trp – Thr – Pro – Trp – Glu – Glu – Asp – Phe – Trp – Glu

200

Ser – Asp – Cys – Asn – Glu – Ala – Phe – Val – Asp – Pro

210

Ser – Leu – Asn – Arg – Thr – Tyr – Ala – Ile – Ser – Ser

220 CHO

Ala – Val – Pro – Ile – Tyr – Phe – Ser – Ile – Leu – Ser

230

Ile – Met – Ile – Val – Thr – Tyr – Thr – Arg – Ile – Tyr

240

Ile – Arg – Arg – Ile – Gln – Val – Gln – Ala – Ile – Arg

250

Ser – Ser – Leu – Glu – Arg – Ala – Ala – Glu – His – Ala

260

Ala – Cys – Ala – Ala – Ser – Ser – Arg – Cys – Ser – Gln

270

Pro – Asp – Thr – Ser – Leu – Arg – Ala – Ser – Ile – Lys

280

Ser – Leu – Thr – Lys – Leu – Val – Lys – Thr – Glu – Lys

290

Val – Ile – Met – Gly – Val – Phe – Val – Cys – Cys – Trp

300

Val – Met – Cys – Asn – Leu – Ile – Phe – Phe – Pro – Leu

310

Pro – Phe – Cys – Ser – Gly – His – Pro – Glu – Gly – Pro

320

Thr – Glu – Ser – Val – Cys – Pro – Phe – Gly – Ala – Pro

330

Thr – Phe – Asp – Val – Phe – Val – Trp – Phe – Gly – Trp

340

Tyr – Ile – Val – Pro – Asn – Leu – Ser – Ser – Asn – Ala

350

Ala – Phe – Asn – Ala – Asp – Phe – Gln – Lys – Val – Phe

360

Cys – Phe – His – Ser – Lys – Gly – Leu – Leu – Gln – Ala

370

Ser – Arg – Thr – Pro – Val – Glu – Thr – Val – Asn – Ile

380

Asp – Gln – Asn – tyr – Ser – Ile – Leu – Glu – Asn – Ser

390

Ile – Val – Phe – His – Lys – Glu – Ile – Ala – Ala – Ala

400

Thr – Val – Ala – Asn – Pro – Met – Met – His – Ile – Tyr

410

Pro – Gly – Asn – Arg – Glu – Val – Asp – Asn – Asp – Glu

420

Gln – Phe – Met – Arg – Asp – Phe – Pro – Gly – Glu – Glu

430

Ile – Tyr – Gln – Thr – Ser – Pro – Asp – Gly – Asp – Pro

440

Cys – Asp – Leu – Glu – Trp – Val – Ser – Glu – Ala – Val

450

Glu – Gly – Glu – Ile – Ser – Leu – Asp – Lys – Ile – Thr

460

COOH – His – Phe – Gly – Asn – Pro – Thr – Phe – Pro

477 470

There are carbohydrate links at amino acids 7 and 222 [15].

Putative location of transmembrane helical segments : 45-66, 77-97, 99-119, 156-176, 225-245, 301-321, 341-361 [15]

[1] Journal of Biological chemistry [1989] 264 : 15813 (M.P. Caulfield, L.T.Duong, R.K.Baker, M.Rosenblatt, M.O.Lively)

[2] Journal of Bioenergetics and Biomembranes [1990] 22 : 271 (I.K.Dev, P.H.Ray)

[3] EMBO Journal [1986] 5 : 427 (R.Dierstein, W.Wickner)

[4] Journal of Biological Chemistry[1989] 264 : 15762 (G.Greenburg, G.S.Shelness, G.Blobel)

[5] Nucleic Acids Research [1986] 14 : 4683 (G.von Heijne)

[6] Journal of Biological Chemistry [1983] 258 : 12073 (P.B.Wolfe, W. Wickner, J.M.Goodman)

[7] Journal of Biological Chemistry [1981] 256 : 3593 (C.Zwizinski, T.Date, W.Wickner)

[8] Protein Biosynthesis [1992] (H.R.V.Arnstein, R.A.Cox)

[9] Annual Review of Neuroscience [1989] 12 : 67 (B.Phe.O'Dowd, R.J. Lefkowitz, M.G.Caron)

[10] Nature [1990] 347 : 80 (R.K.Sunahara, H.Niznik, D.M. Weiner, Stormann, M.R.Brann, J.L.Kennedy, J.E.Gelernter, P. Rozmahel, Y.Yang, Y.Israel, P.Seeman, B.F.O'Dowd)

[11] Nature [1988] 336 : 783 (J.R.Bunzow, H.M.Van Tol, D.K. Grandy, P.Albert, J.Salon, M.Chrisre, C.A.Machida, K.A.Neve, O. Civelli)

[12] Nature [1990] 347 : 146 (P.Sokoloff, B.Giros, M.-P.Martres, M.L.Bouthenet, J.-C. Schwartz)

[13] Arnzeimittel Forschung [1992] 42 : 224 (P.Sokoloff, B.Giros, M.-P.Martres, M.Andrieux, A.Besancon, C.Alon, M.L.Bouthenet, E.Souil, J.-C. Schwartz)

[14] Nature [1991] 350 : 610 (H.M.Van Tol, J.R.Bunzow, H.-G. Guan, R.K.Sunahara, P. Seeman, H.Niznik, O.Civelli)

[15] Nature [1991] 350 : 614 (R.K.Sunahara, H.-C.Guan, B.F. O'Dowd, P.Seeman, L.G. Laurier, S.R.George, J.Torchia, H.M.Van Tol, H.Niznik)

[16] Nature [1990] 347 : 72 (A.Dearry, J.A.Gingrich, P. Falardeau, R.T.Fremeau Jnr, M.D.Bates, M.G.Caron)

[17] Nature [1990] 347 : 76 (Q-Y.Zhou, D.K.Grandy, L.Thambi, J.A.Kushner, H.H.M.Van Tol, R.Cone, D.Pribnon, J.Salon, J.R.Bunzon, O. Civelli)

[18] Nature [1990] 347 : 80 (R.K.Sunahara, H.M.Niznik, D.M. Weiner, T.M. Stormann, M.R.Brann, J.L.Kennedy, J.E.Gelernter, R.Rozmahel, Y.Yang, Y.Israel, P.Seeman, B.F.O'Dowd)

[19] Molecular Pharmacology [1990] 37 : 1 (T.M.Stormann, D.C. Gdula, D.M.Weiner, M.R.Brann)

[20] Nucleic Acids Research [1990] 18 : 1299 (N.K.Robakis, M. Mohamadi, D.Y.Fu, K.Sambamurti, L.M.Refolo)

[21] Comptes Rendue Academie des Sciences [1990] 311 : 501 (B.Giros, M.P.Martres, P.Sokoloff, J.C.Schwartz)

[22] Human Molecular Genetics [1993] 2 (6) : 769 (J.B.Lichter, C.L.Barr, J.L.Kennedy, H.H.M.Van Tol, K.K.Kidd, K.J.Livak)

CHAPTER 10

BIOCHEMISTRY OF PARKINSON'S DISEASE

G PROTEINS

G PROTEIN STIMULATION

The dopamine receptors D1, D2, D3, D4 and D5, affect the G proteins [1, 2]. There are three types of G protein : Gs, Go and Gi. Dopamine receptors D1 and D5 stimulate the activity of the G protein Gs [3]. D1 and D5 stimulate the activity of the G protein Go [4]. D2, D3 and D4 stimulate the activity of the G protein Gi [5].

TYPES OF G PROTEIN SUBUNITS

There are three subunits in G proteins : alpha, beta and gamma. The alpha subunits of the G proteins are : Gs 1 alpha, Gi 1 alpha, Gi 2 alpha, Gi 3 alpha, Go alpha. The beta subunits of the G proteins are : beta one, beta two, beta four. The gamma subunits of the G proteins are : gamma 2, gamma 3, gamma 4, gamma 5, gamma 7, gamma 10, and gamma 11.

G PROTEIN BIOSYNTHESIS

The G proteins are formed from a combination of the three types of subunit (alpha, beta and gamma) [6]. Dopamine receptors stimulate the formation of the pro alpha, pro beta and pro gamma subunits in the ribosomes. With the addition of $2H_20$, leader peptidase removes the signal peptide of each of the subunits to form the alpha, beta and gamma subunits in the endoplasmic reticulum [6]. The alpha subunits in the biosynthesis of the Gs, Go and Gi proteins then undergo palmitoylation by adding palmitic acid in the endoplasmic reticulum [7]. The alpha subunits of the Go [8] and Gi [9] proteins undergo myristoylation by adding myristic acid in the endoplasmic reticulum.

The gamma subunits of the G proteins are isoprenylated [10, 11]. They also undergo carboxymethylation and COOH terminal processing [12]. The gamma unit combines with the beta unit in the endoplasmic reticulum to form a beta gamma complex [6]. An alpha subunit is added to the beta gamma complex in the Golgi complex to form the G protein, which then attaches to the membrane [6].

G PROTEIN ACTIVATION

Via nucleoside diphosphate kinase [13-18], dopamine receptors cause the separation of the beta and gamma regulatory subunits of the G proteins, from the alpha regulatory subunits of the G proteins, whilst maintaining the connection between the beta and gamma regulatory subunits [19, 20]. Manganese is required for the optimal functioning of this action [21].

enzyme name : nucleoside diphosphate kinase
enzyme classification : EC 2.7.4.6
cofactor : manganese (Mn^{2+})
substrate : G protein (alpha-beta-gamma) + GTP + ADP
product : G protein (alpha and beta-gamma) + GDP + ADP + PPi

G PROTEIN STRUCTURES

STRUCTURE OF ALPHA SUBUNITS

Gs 1 ALPHA

Gs 1 alpha is a protein consisting of a chain of 394 amino acids [22]. PA is palmitic acid [23].

```
                        (PA)
N2 – Met – Gly – Cys – Leu – Gly – Asn – Ser – Lys – Thr
      1                                                |
Asp – Arg – Glu – Val – Val – Leu – Gly – Thr – Gly – Asp
```

| 10
Phe – Ser – Val – Arg – Ile – Leu – Thr – Ala – Cys – Phe
20 |
Leu – Leu – Thr – Ser – Leu – Ile – Leu – Leu – Ser – Leu
| 30
Gly – Asn – Thr – Leu – Val – Cys – Ala – Ala – Val – Ile
40 |
Thr – Val – Lys – Ser – Arg – Leu – His – Arg – Phe – Arg
| 50
Asn – Phe – Phe – Val – Ile – Ser – Leu – Ala – Val – Ser
60 |
Pro – Met – Val – Leu – Val – Ala – Val – Leu – Leu – Asp
| 70
Trp – Lys – Ala – Val – Ala – Glu – Ile – Ala – Gly – Phe
80 |
Trp – Ile – Asn – Cys – Phe – Ser – Gly – Phe – Pro – Trp
| 90
Val – Ala – Phe – Asp – Ile – Met – Cys – Ser – Thr – Ala
100 |
Val – Ser – Ile – Val – Cys – Leu – Asn – Leu – Ile – Ser
| 110
Asp – Arg – Tyr – Trp – Ala – Ile – Ser – Ser – Pro – Phe
120 |
Ala – Lys – Pro – Thr – Met – Lys – Arg – Glu – Tyr – Arg
| 130
Ala – Phe – Ile – Leu – Ile – Ser – Val – Ala – Trp – Thr
140 |
Val – Pro – Ile – Phe – Ser – Ile – Leu – Val – Ser – Leu
| 150
Gln – Leu – Ser – Trp – His – Lys – Ala – Lys – Pro – Thr
160 |
Leu – Ser – Thr – Ala – Asn – Gly – Asp – Ser – Pro – Ser
| 170
Ala – Glu – Thr – Ile – Asp – Asn – Cys – Asp – Ser – Ser

180

Ser – Ser – Ser – Ile – Ala – Tyr – Thr – Arg – Ser – Leu

190

Val – Ile – Ser – Phe – Tyr – Ile – Pro – Val – Ala – Ile

200

Arg – Tyr – Ile – Arg – Thr – Tyr – Thr – Val – Ile – Met

210

Ile – Ala – Gln – Lys – Gln – Ile – Arg – Arg – Ile – Ala

220

Lys – Ala – His – Val – Ala – Ala – Arg – Glu – Leu – Ala

230

Asn – Cys – Gln – Thr – Thr – Thr – Gly – Asn – Gly – Lys

240

Ser – Ser – Glu – Pro – Gln – Ser – Cys – Glu – Val – Pro

250

Phe – Lys – Met – Ser – Phe – Lys – Arg – Glu – Thr – Lys

260

Gly – Met – Ile – Val – Ser – Leu – Thr – Lys – Leu – Val

270

Val – Phe – Val – Cys – Cys – Trp – Leu – Pro – Phe – Phe

280

Gly – Cys – Phe – Pro – Leu – Ile – Cys – Asn – Leu – Ile

290

Ser – Gly – Glu – Thr – Gln – Pro – Phe – Cys – Ile – Asp

300

Phe – Trp – Val – Phe – Val – Asp – Phe – Thr – Asn – Ser

310

Gly – Trp – Ala – Asn – Ser – Ser – Leu – Asn – Pro – Ile

320

Lys – Arg – Phe – Asp – Ala – Asn – Phe – Ala – Tyr – Ile

330

Ala – Phe – Ser – Thr – Leu – Leu – Gly – Cys – Tyr – Arg

340

Glu – Ile – Ala – Asn – Asn – Thr – Ala – Pro – Cys – Leu

| 350

Thr – Val – Ser – Ile – Asn – Asn – Asn – Gly – Ala – Ala

360 |

Gly – Arg – Pro – Glu – His – His – Ser – Ser – Phe – Met

| 370

Ser – Ile – Ser – Lys – Glu – Cys – Asn – Leu – Val – Tyr

380 |

COOH – Ala – His – Pro – Ile – Leu

394 390

Gi 1 ALPHA

Gi 1 alpha is a protein consisting of a chain of 354 amino acids [23]. PA is palmitic acid. MA is myristic acid [23].

(MA) (PA)

N_2 – Met – Gly – Cys – Thr – Leu – Ser – Ala – Glu – Asp

1 |

Ile – Met – Lys – Ser – Arg – Glu – Val – Ala – Ala – Lys

| 10

Asp – Arg – Asn – Leu – Arg – Glu – Asp – Gly – Glu – Lys

20 |

Leu – Leu – Leu – Leu – Lys – Val – Glu – Arg – Ala – Ala

| 30

Gly – Ala – Gly – Glu – Ser – Gly – Lys – Ser – Thr – Ile

40 |

Ala – Glu – His – Ile – Ile – Lys – Met – Gln – Lys – Val

| 50

Gly – Tyr – Ser – Glu – Glu – Glu – Cys – Lys – Gln – Tyr

60 |

Gln – Ile – Thr – Asn – Ser – Tyr – Val – Val – Ala – Lys

| 70

Ser – Ile – Ile – Ala – Ile – Ile – Arg – Ala – Met – Gly

80 |

Ala – Ser – Asp – Gly – Phe – Asp – Ile – Lys – Leu – Arg

| 90

Arg – Ala – Asp – Asp – Ala – Arg – Gln – Leu – Phe – Val

100 |

Met – Phe – Gly – Glu – Glu – Ala – Ala – Gly – Ala – Leu

| 110

Thr – Ala – Glu – Leu – Ala – Gly – Val – Ile – Lys – Arg

120 |

Cys – Ala – Gln – Val – Gly – Ser – Asp – Lys – Trp – Leu

| 130

Phe – Asn – Arg – Ser – Arg – Glu – Tyr – Gln – Leu – Asn

140 |

Leu – Asp – Asn – Leu – Tyr – Tyr – Ala – Ala – Ser – Asp

| 150

Asp – Arg – Ile – Ala – Gln – Pro – Asn – Tyr – Ile – Pro

160 |

Val – Arg – Thr – Arg – Leu – Val – Asp – Gln – Gln – Thr

| 170

Lys – Thr – Thr – Gly – Ile – Val – Glu – Thr – His – Phe

180 |

Phe – Met – Lys – Phe – His – Leu – Asp – Lys – Phe – Thr

| 190

Asp – Val – Gly – Gly – Gln – Arg – Ser – Glu – Arg – Lys

200 |

Thr – Val – Gly – Glu – Phe – Cys – His – Ile – Trp – Lys

| 210

Ala – Ile – Ile – Phe – Cys – Val – Ala – Leu – Ser – Asp

220 |

Glu – Glu – Asp – Glu – Ala – Leu – Val – Leu – Asp – Tyr

| 230

Met – Asn – Arg – Met – His – Glu – Ser – Met – Lys – Leu

240 |

Phe – Trp – Lys – Asn – Asn – Cys – Ile – Ser – Asp – Phe

| 250

Thr – Asp – Thr – Ser – Ile – Ile – Leu – Phe – Leu – Asn

260 |

Lys – Ile – Lys – Glu – Glu – Phe – Leu – Asp – Lys – Lys

| 270

Lys – Ser – Pro – Leu – Thr – Ile – Cys – Thr – Pro – Glu

280 |

Ala – Glu – Glu – Tyr – Thr – Asn – Ser – Gly – Ala – Tyr

| 290

Ala – Ala – Tyr – Ile – Gln – Cys – Gln – Phe – Glu – Asp

300 |

Ile – Glu – Lys – Thr – Asp – Lys – Arg – Lys – Asn – Leu

| 310

Tyr – Thr – His – Phe – Thr – Cys – Ala – Thr – Asp – Thr

320 |

Val – Ala – Asp – Phe – Val – Phe – Gln – Val – Asn – Lys

| 330

Thr – Asp – Val – Ile – Ile – Lys – Asn – Asn – Leu – Lys

340 |

COOH – Phe – Leu – Gly – Cys – Asp

354 350

Gi 2 ALPHA

Gi 2 alpha is a protein consisting of a chain of 355 amino acids [23]. PA is palmitic acid. MA is myristic acid [23].

(MA) (PA)

N_2 – Met – Gly – Cys – Thr – Val – Ser – Ala – Glu – Asp

1 |

Ile – Met – Lys – Ser – Arg – Glu – Ala – Ala – Ala – Lys

| 10

Asp – Lys – Asn – Leu – Arg – Glu – Asp – Gly – Glu – Lys

20 |

Leu – Leu – Leu – Leu – Lys – Val – Glu – Arg – Ala – Ala

| 30

Gly – Ala – Gly – Glu – Ser – Gly – Lys – Ser – Thr – Ile

40

Asp – Glu – His – Ile – Ile – Lys – Met – Gln – Lys – Val

50

Gly – Tyr – Ser – Glu – Glu – Glu – Cys – Arg – Gln – Tyr

60

Gln – Ile – Thr – Asn – Ser – Tyr – Val – Val – Ala – Arg

70

Ser – Ile – Met – Ala – Ile – Val – Lys – Ala – Met – Gly

80

Ser – Pro – Asp – Ala – Phe – Asp – Ile – Gln – Leu – Asn

90

Arg – Ala – Asp – Asp – Ala – Arg – Gln – Leu – Phe – Ala

100

Val – Gly – Gln – Glu – Glu – Ala – Thr – Cys – Ser – Leu

110

Leu – Pro – Asp – Asp – Leu – Ser – Gly – Val – Ile – Arg

120

Ala – Gln – Val – Gly – His – Asp – Ala – Trp – Leu – Arg

130

Cys – Phe – Gly – Arg – Ser – Arg – Glu – Tyr – Gln – Leu

140

Asp – Asn – Leu – Tyr – Tyr – Ala – Ala – Ser – Asp – Asn

150

Leu – Glu – Arg – Ile – Ala – Gln – Ser – Asp – Tyr – Ile

160

Arg – Thr – Arg – Leu – Val – Asp – Gln – Gln – Thr – Pro

170

Val – Lys – Thr – Thr – Gly – Ile – Val – Glu – Thr – His

180

Met – Lys – Phe – His – Leu – Asp – Lys – Phe – Thr – Phe

190

Phe – Asp – Val – Gly – Gly – Gln – Arg – Ser – Glu – Arg

200

Val – Gly – Glu – Phe – Cys – His – Ile – Trp – Lys – Lys

```
                                                              210
 |
Thr – Ala – Ile – Ile – Phe – Cys – Val – Ala – Leu – Ser
220                                                     |
Glu – Asp – Glu – Ala – Leu – Val – Leu – Asp – Tyr – Ala
 |                                                      230
Glu – Met – Asn – Arg – Met – His – Glu – Ser – Met – Lys
240                                                     |
Trp – Lys – Asn – Asn – Cys – Ile – Ser – Asp – Phe – Leu
 |                                                      250
Phe – Thr – Asp – Thr – Ser – Ile – Ile – Leu – Phe – Leu
260                                                     |
Ile – Lys – Glu – Glu – Phe – Leu – Asp – Lys – Lys – Asn
 |                                                      270
Thr – His – Ser – Pro – Leu – Thr – Ile – Cys – Phe – Pro
280                                                     |
Glu – Asp – Tyr – Lys – Asn – Ala – Gly – Tyr – Tyr – Glu
 |                                                      290
Ala – Ala – Ser – Tyr – Ile – Gln – Ser – Lys – Phe – Glu
300                                                     |
Glu – Lys – Thr – Asp – Lys – Arg – Lys – Asn – Leu – Asp
 |                                                      310
Ile – Tyr – Thr – His – Phe – Thr – Cys – Ala – Thr – Asp
320                                                     |
Ala – Aap – Phe – Val – Phe – Gln – Val – Asn – Lys – Thr
 |                                                      330
Val – Thr – Asp – Val – Ile – Ile – Lys – Asn – Asn – Leu
340                                                     |
              COOH – Phe – Leu – Gly – Cys – Asp – Lys
                     355                              350
```

Gi 3 ALPHA

Gi 3 alpha is a protein consisting of a chain of 354 amino acids [23]. PA is palmitic acid. MA is myristic acid [23].

(MA) (PA)

N_2 – Met – Gly – Cys – Thr – Leu – Ser – Ala – Glu – Asp
1
|
Ile – Met – Lys – Ser – Arg – Glu – Val – Ala – Ala – Lys
| 10
Asp – Arg – Asn – Leu – Arg – Glu – Asp – Gly – Glu – Lys
20 |
Leu – Leu – Leu – Leu – Lys – Val – Glu – Lys – Ala – Ala
| 30
Gly – Ala – Gly – Glu – Ser – Gly – Lys – Ser – Thr – Ile
40 |
Asp – Glu – His – Ile – Ile – Lys – Met – Gln – Lys – Val
| 50
Gly – Tyr – Ser – Glu – Asp – Glu – Cys – Lys – Gln – Tyr
60 |
Gln – Ile – Thr – Asn – Ser – Tyr – Val – Val – Val – Lys
| 70
Ser – Ile – Ile – Ala – Ile – Ile – Arg – Ala – Met – Gly
80 |
Ala – Ala – Glu – Gly – Phe – Asp – Ile – Lys – Leu – Arg
| 90
Arg – Ala – Asp – Asp – Ala – Arg – Gln – Leu – Phe – Val
100 |
Met – Val – Gly – Glu – Glu – Ala – Ser – Gly – Ala – Leu
| 110
Thr – Pro – Glu – Leu – Ala – Gly – Val – Ile – Lys – Arg
120 |
Cys – Ala – Gln – Val – Gly – Gly – Asp – Arg – Trp – Leu
| 130
Phe – Ser – Arg – Ser – Arg – Glu – Tyr – Gln – Leu – Asn
140 |
Leu – Asp – Asn – Leu – Tyr – Tyr – Ser – Ala – Ser – Asp
| 150
Asp – Arg – Ile – Ser – Gln – Ser – Asn – Tyr – Ile – Pro

160

Val – Arg – Thr – Arg – Leu – Val – Asp – Gln – Gln – Thr

170

Lys – Thr – Thr – Gly – Ile – Val – Glu – Thr – His – Phe

180

Phe – Met – Lys – Phe – Tyr – Leu – Asp – Lys – Phe – Thr

190

Asp – Val – Gly – Gly – Gln – Arg – Ser – Glu – Arg – Lys

200

Thr – Val – Gly – Glu – Phe – Cys – His – Ile – Trp – Lys

210

Ala – Ile – Ile – Phe – Cys – Val – Ala – Leu – Ser – Asp

220

Glu – Glu – Asp – Glu – Ala – Leu – Val – Leu – Asp – Tyr

230

Met – Asn – Arg – Met – His – Glu – Ser – Met – Lys – Leu

240

Phe – Trp – Lys – Asn – Asn – Cys – Ile – Ser – Asp – Phe

250

Thr – Glu – Thr – Ser – Ile – Ile – Leu – Phe – Leu – Asn

260

Lys – Ile – Lys – Glu – Glu – Phe – Leu – Asp – Lys – Lys

270

Arg – Ser – Pro – Leu – Thr – Ile – Cys – Tyr – Pro – Glu

280

Ala – Glu – Glu – Tyr – Thr – Asn – Ser – Gly – Thr – Tyr

290

Ala – Ala – Try – Ile – Gln – Cys – Gln – Phe – Glu – Asp

300

Ile – Glu – Lys – Thr – Asp – Lys – Arg – Arg – Asn – Leu

310

Tyr – Thr – His – Phe – Thr – Cys – Ala – Thr – Asp – Thr

320

Thr – Ala – Asp – Phe – Val – Phe – Gln – Val – Asn – Lys

```
|                                                        330
Thr – Asp – Val – Ile – Ile – Lys – Asn – Asn – Leu – Lys
340                                                      |
                         COOH – Tyr – Leu – Gly – Cys – Glu
                                354                     350
```

GO ALPHA

Go alpha is a protein consisting of a chain of 354 amino acids [24]. PA is palmitic acid. MA is myristic acid [24].

```
              (MA)  (PA)
N2  – Met – Gly – Cys – Thr – Leu – Ser – Ala – Glu – Glu
       1                                              |
Ile – Ala – Lys – Gly – Arg – Glu – Leu – Ala – Ala – Arg
|                                                     10
Glu – Lys – Asn – Leu – Lys – Glu – Asp – Gly – Ile – Ser
20                                                    |
Leu – Leu – Leu – Leu – Lys – Val – Asp – Lys – Ala – Ala
|                                                     30
Gly – Ala – Gly – Glu – Ser – Gly – Lys – Ser – Thr – Ile
40                                                    |
Asp – Glu – His – Ile – Ile – Lys – Met – Gln – Lys – Val
|                                                     50
Gly – Phe – Ser – Gly – Glu – Asp – Val – Lys – Gln – Tyr
60                                                    |
Gln – Ile – Thr – Asn – Ser – Tyr – Val – Val – Pro – Lys
|                                                     70
Ser – Leu – Ala – Ala – Ile – Val – Arg – Ala – Met – Asp
80                                                    |
Glu – Lys – Asp – Gly – Tyr – Glu – Ile – Gly – Leu – Thr
|                                                     90
Arg – Lys – Ala – Asp – Ala – Lys – Met – Val – Cys – Asp
100                                                   |
Pro – Glu – Thr – Asp – Glu – Met – Arg – Ser – Val – Val
```

| 110

Phe – Ser – Ala – Glu – Leu – Leu – Ser – Ala – Met – Met

120 |

Glu – Gln – Ile – Gly – Ser – Asp – Gly – Trp – Leu – Arg

| 130

Cys – Phe – Asn – Arg – Ser – Arg – Glu – Tyr – Gln – Leu

140 |

Ser – Asp – Leu – Tyr – Tyr – Lys – Ala – Ser – Asp – Asn

| 150

Leu – Asp – Arg – Ile – Gly – Ala – Ala – Asp – Tyr – Gln

160 |

Arg – Thr – Arg – Leu – Ile – Asp – Gln – Gln – Leu – Pro

| 170

Val – Lys – Thr – Thr – Gly – Ile – Val – Glu – Thr – His

180 |

Leu – Arg – Phe – His – Leu – Asn – Lys – Phe – Thr – Phe

| 190

Phe – Asp – Val – Gly – Gly – Gln – Arg – Ser – Glu – Arg

200 |

Val – Glu – Glu – Phe – Cys – His – Ile – Trp – Lys – Lys

| 210

Thr – Ala – Ile – Ile – Phe – Cys – Val – Ala – Leu – Ser

220 |

Glu – Asp – Glu – His – Leu – Val – Gln – Asp – Tyr – Gly

| 230

Thr – Thr – Asn – Arg – Met – His – Glu – Ser – Leu – Met

240 |

Phe – Lys – Asn – Asn – Cys – Ile – Ser – Asp – Phe – Leu

| 250

Phe – Ile – Asp – Thr – Ser – Ile – Ile – Leu – Phe – Leu

260 |

Ile – Lys – Glu – Gly – Phe – Leu – Asp – Lys – Lys – Asn

| 270

Lys – Lys – Ser – Pro – Leu – Thr – Ile – Cys – Phe – Pro

280

Asp – Glu – Tyr – Thr – Asn – Pro – Gly – Thr – Tyr – Glu

290

Ala – Ala – Ala – Tyr – Ile – Gln – Ala – Gln – Phe – Glu

300

Ile – Glu – Lys – Asn – Pro – Ser – Arg – Asn – Lys – Ser

310

Tyr – Cys – His – Met – Thr – Cys – Ala – Thr – Asp – Thr

320

Val – Ala – Asp – Phe – Val – Val – Gln – Ile – Asn – Asn

330

Thr – Asp – Ile – Ile – Ile – Ala – Asn – Asn – Leu – Arg

340

COOH – Thr – Leu – Gly – Cys – Gly

354 350

STRUCTURE OF BETA SUBUNITS

BETA ONE

Beta one is a protein consisting of a chain of 340 amino acids [25].

N_2 – Met – Ser – Glu – Leu – Asp – Gln – Leu – Arg – Gln

1

Arg – Ile – Gln – Asn – Lys – Leu – Gln – Glu – Ala – Glu

10

Asp – Ala – Arg – Lys – Ala – Cys – Ala – Asp – Ala – Thr

20

Pro – Asp – Ile – Asn – Asn – Thr – Ile – Gln – Ser – Leu

30

Val – Gly – Arg – Ile – Gln – Met – Arg – Thr – Arg – Arg

40

Tyr – Ile – Lys – Ala – Leu – His – Gly – Arg – Leu – Thr

| 50

Ala – Met – His – Trp – Gly – Thr – Asp – Ser – Arg – Leu

60 |

Leu – Lys – Gly – Asp – Gln – Ser – Ala – Ser – Val – Leu

| 70

Ile – Ile – Trp – Asp – Ser – Tyr – Thr – Thr – Asn – Lys

80 |

Trp – Ser – Ser – Arg – Leu – Pro – Ile – Ala – His – Val

| 90

Val – Met – Thr – Cys – Ala – Tyr – Ala – Pro – Ser – Gly

100 |

Asn – Asp – Leu – Gly – Gly – Cys – Ala – Val – Tyr – Asn

| 110

Ile – Cys – Ser – Ile – Tyr – Asn – Leu – Lys – Thr – Arg

120 |

Leu – Glu – Arg – Ser – Val – Arg – Val – Asn – Gly – Glu

| 130

Ala – Gly – His – Thr – Gly – Tyr – Leu – Ser – Cys – Cys

140 |

Thr – Val – Ile – Gln – Asn – Asp – Asp – Leu – Phe – Arg

| 150

Ser – Ser – Gly – Asp – Thr – Thr – Cys – Ala – Leu – Trp

160 |

Thr – Thr – Thr – Gln – Gln – Gly – Thr – Glu – Ile – Asp

| 170

Phe – Thr – Gly – His – Thr – Gly – Asp – Val – Met – Ser

180 |

Phe – Leu – Arg – Thr – Asp – Pro – Ala – Leu – Ser – Leu

| 190

Val – Ser – Gly – Ala – Cys – Asp – Ala – Ser – Ala – Lys

200 |

Arg – Cys – Met – Gly – Glu – Arg – Val – Asp – Trp – Leu

| 210

Gln – Thr – Phe – Thr – Gly – His – Glu – Ser – Asp – Ile

220 |

Asn – Gly – Asn – Pro – Phe – Phe – Cys – Ile – Ala – Asn

| 230

Ala – Phe – Ala – Thr – Gly – Ser – Asp – Asp – Ala – Thr

240 |

Gln – Asp – Ala – Arg – Leu – Asp – Phe – Leu – Arg – Cys

| 250

Glu – Leu – Met – Thr – Tyr – Ser – His – Asp – Asn – Ile

260 |

Ser – Phe – Ser – Val – Ser – Thr – Ile – Gly – Cys – Ile

| 270

Lys – Ser – Gly – Arg – Leu – Leu – Leu – Ala – Gly – Tyr

280 |

Ala – Asp – Trp – Val – Asn – Cys – Asn – Phe – Asp – Asp

| 290

Leu – Lys – Ala – Asp – Arg – Ala – Gly – Val – Leu – Ala

300 |

Gly – Leu – Cys – Ser – Val – Arg – Asn – Asp – His – Gly

| 310

Val – Thr – Asp – Asp – Gly – Met – Ala – Val – Ala – Thr

320 |

Trp – Ile – Lys – Leu – Phe – Ser – Asp – Trp – Ser – Gly

| 330

Asn – COOH

340

Beta two

Beta two is a protein consisting of a chain of 340 amino acids [26].

N_2 – Met – Ser – Glu – Leu – Glu – Gln – Leu – Arg – Gln

1 |

Arg – Ile – Gln – Asn – Arg – Leu – Gln – Glu – Ala – Glu

| 10

Asp – Ala – Arg – Lys – Ala – Cys – Gly – Asp – Ser – Thr

20 |

Pro – Asp – Leu – Gly – Ala – Thr – Ile – Gln – Thr – Leu

| 30

Val – Gly – Arg – Ile – Gln – Met – Arg – Thr – Arg – Arg

40 |

Tyr – Ile – Lys – Ala – Leu – His – Gly – Arg – Leu – Thr

| 50

Ala – Met – His – Trp – Gly – Thr – Asp – Ser – Arg – Leu

60 |

Leu – Lys – Gly – Asp – Gln – Ser – Ala – Ser – Val – Leu

| 70

Ile – Ile – Trp – Asp – Ser – Tyr – Thr – Thr – Asn – Lys

80 |

Trp – Ser – Ser – Arg – Leu – Pro – Ile – Ala – His – Val

| 90

Val – Met – Thr – Cys – Ala – Tyr – Ala – Pro – Ser – Gly

100 |

Asn – Asp – Leu – Gly – Gly – Cys – Ala – Val – Phe – Asn

| 110

Ile – Cys – Ser – Ile – Tyr – Ser – Leu – Lys – Thr – Arg

120 |

Leu – Glu – Arg – Ser – Val – Arg – Val – Asn – Gly – Glu

| 130

Pro – Gly – His – Thr – Gly – Tyr – Leu – Ser – Cys – Cys

140 |

Thr – Ile – Ile – Gln – Asn – Asp – Asp – Leu – Phe – Arg

| 150

Ser – Ser – Gly – Asp – Thr – Thr – Cys – Ala – Leu – Trp

160 |

Gla – Val – Thr – Gln – Gln – Gly – Thr – Glu – Ile – Asp

| 170

Phe – Ala – Gly – His – Ser – Gly – Asp – Val – Met – Ser

180

Phe – Thr – Arg – Gly – Asp – Pro – Ala – Leu – Ser – Leu

190

Val – Ser – Gly – Ala – Cys – Asp – Ala – Ser – Ile – Lys

200

Arg – Cys – Met – Ser – Asp – Arg – Val – Asp – Trp – Leu

210

Gln – Thr – Phe – Ile – Gly – His – Glu – Ser – Asp – Ile

220

Tyr – Gly – Asn – Pro – Phe – Phe – Ala – Val – Ala – Asn

230

Ala – Phe – Thr – Thr – Gly – Ser – Asp – Asp – Ala – Thr

240

Gln – Asp – Ala – Arg – Leu – Asp – Phe – Leu – Arg – Cys

250

Glu – Leu – Leu – Met – Tyr – Ser – His – Asp – Asn – Ile

260

Ser – Phe – Ala – Val – Ser – Thr – Ile – Gly – Cys – Ile

270

Lys – Ser – Gly – Arg – Leu – Leu – Leu – Ala – Gly – Tyr

280

Ala – Asp – Trp – Ile – Asn – Cys – Asn – Phe – Asp – Asp

290

Met – Lys – Gly – Asp – Arg – Ala – Gly – Val – Leu – Ala

300

Gly – Leu – Cys – Ser – Val – Arg – Asn – Asp – His – Gly

310

Val – Thr – Asp – Asp – Gly – Met – Ala – Val – Ala – Thr

320

Trp – Ile – Lys – Leu – Phe – Ser – Asp – Trp – Ser – Gly

330

Asn – COOH

340

Page 145

Beta four

Beta four is a protein consisting of a chain of 340 amino acids [27].

N_2 – Met – Ser – Glu – Leu – Glu – Gln – Leu – Arg – Gln
1

Gln – Ile – Gln – Asn – Arg – Leu – Gln – Glu – Ala – Glu
10

Asp – Ala – Arg – Lys – Ala – Cys – Asn – Asp – Ala – Thr
20

Ser – Asp – Met – Asn – Ser – Thr – Ile – Gln – Val – Leu
30

Val – Gly – Arg – Ile – Gln – Met – Arg – Thr – Arg – Arg
40

Tyr – Ile – Lys – Ala – Leu – His – Gly – Arg – Leu – Thr
50

Ala – Met – His – Trp – Gly – Tyr – Asp – Ser – Arg – Leu
60

Leu – Lys – Gly – Asp – Gln – Ser – Ala – Ser – Val – Leu
70

Ile – Ile – Trp – Asp – Ser – Tyr – Thr – Thr – Asn – Lys
80

Trp – Ser – Ser – Arg – Leu – Pro – Ile – Ala – His – Met
90

Val – Met – Thr – Cys – Ala – Tyr – Ala – Pro – Ser – Gly
100

Asn – Asp – Leu – Gly – Gly – Cys – Ala – Val – Tyr – Asn
110

Ile – Cys – Ser – Ile – Tyr – Asn – Leu – Lys – Thr – Arg
120

Leu – Glu – Arg – Ser – Val – Arg – Val – Asp – Gly – Glu
130

Ala – Gly – His – Thr – Gly – Tyr – Leu – Ser – Cys – Cys

140

Thr – Ile – Ile – Gln – Gly – Asp – Asp – Leu – Phe – Arg
150

Ser – Ser – Gly – Asp – Thr – Thr – Cys – Ala – Leu – Trp
160

Thr – Thr – Thr – Gln – Gln – Gly – Thr – Glu – Ile – Asp
170

Phe – Thr – Gly – His – Ser – Gly – Asp – Val – Met – Ser
180

Phe – Thr – Lys – Leu – Asp – Pro – Ser – Leu – Ser – Leu
190

Val – Ser – Gly – Ala – Cys – Asp – Ala – Ser – Ser – Lys
200

Arg – Cys – Met – Gly – Asp – Arg – Ile – Asp – Trp – Leu
210

Gln – Ser – Phe – Thr – Gly – His – Ile – Ser – Asp – Ile
220

Tyr – Gly – Ser – Pro – Phe – Phe – Ser – Val – Ala – Asn
230

Ala – Phe – Ala – Thr – Gly – Ser – Asp – Asp – Ala – Thr
240

Gln – Asp – Ala – Arg – Leu – Asp – Phe – Leu – Arg – Cys
250

Glu – Leu – Leu – Leu – Tyr – Ser – His – Asp – Asn – Ile
260

Ser – Phe – Ala – Val – Ser – Thr – Ile – Gly – Cys – Ile
270

Lys – Ser – Gly – Arg – Leu – Leu – Leu – Ala – Gly – Tyr
280

Ala – Asp – Trp – Val – Ser – Cys – Asn – Phe – Asp – Asp
290

Leu – Lys – Gly – Gly – Arg – Ser – Gly – Val – Leu – Ala
300

Gly – Leu – Cys – Ser – Val – Arg – Asn – Asp – His – Gly

| 310

Val – Thr – Asp – Asp – Gly – Met – Ala – Val – Ala – Thr

320 |

Trp – Ile – Arg – Leu – Phe – Ser – Asp – Trp – Ser – Gly

| 330

Asn – COOH

340

Structure of gamma subunits

Gamma 2

Gamma 2 is a protein consisting of a chain of 71 amino acids [28]. GG is all-trans geranyl geranyl cysteine methyl ester [29].

N_2 – Met – Ala – Ser – Asn – Asn – Thr – Ala – Set – Ile

1 |

Leu – Gln – Glu – Val – Leu – Lys – Arg – Ala – Gln – Ala

| 10

Lys – Met – Glu – Ala – Asn – Ile – Asp – Arg – Ile – Lys

20 |

Ala – Met – Leu – Asp – Ala – Ala – Ala – Lys – Ser – Val

| 30

Tyr – Cys – Glu – Ala – His – Ala – Lys – Glu – Asp – Pro

40 |

Asn – Glu – Ser – Ala – Pro – Val – Pro – Thr – Leu – Leu

| 50

Pro – Phe – Arg – Glu – Lys – Lys – Phe – Phe – Cys – Ala

60 GG |

COOH – Leu – Ile

71 70

Gamma 3

Gamma 3 is a protein consisting of a chain of 75 amino acids [30]. GG is all-trans geranyl geranyl cysteine methyl ester [29].

N_2 – Met – Lys – Gly – Glu – Thr – Pro – Val – Asn – Ser

1 |

Met – Lys – Arg – Ala – Gln – Gly – Ile – Ser – Met – Thr

| 10

Val – Glu – Gln – Leu – Lys – Ile – Glu – Ala – Ser – Leu

20 |

Ala – Ala – Ala – Lys – Ser – Val – Lys – Ile – Arg – Cys

| 30

Asp – Leu – Met – Thr – Tyr – Cys – Asp – Ala – His – Ala

40 |

Pro – Val – Pro – Thr – Ile – Leu – Pro – Asp – Glu – Cys

| 50

Thr – Ser – Glu – Asn – Pro – Phe – Arg – Glu – Lys – Lys

60 |

COOH – Leu – Leu – Ala – Cys – Phe – Phe

75 GG 70

Gamma 4

Gamma 4 is a protein consisting of a chain of 75 amino acids [31]. GG is all-trans geranyl geranyl cysteine methyl ester [29].

N_2 – Met – Lys – Glu – Gly – Met – Ser – Asn – Asn – Ser

1 |

Ala – Lys – Arg – Ala – Gln – Ser – Ile – Ser – Thr – Thr

| 10

Val – Glu – Gln – Leu – Lys – Met – Glu – Ala – Cys – Met

20 |

Ala – Ala – Ala – Gln – Ser – Val – Lys – Val – Arg – Asp

| 30

Asp – Leu – Leu – Ala – Tyr – Cys – Glu – Ala – His – Val
40
|
Pro – Val – Pro – Ile – Ile – Leu – Pro – Asp – Glu – Arg
|
50
Ala – Ser – Glu – Asn – Pro – Phe – Arg – Glu – Lys – Lys
60
|
COOH – Leu – Ile – Thr – Cys – Phe – Phe
75 GG 70

Gamma 5

Gamma 5 is a protein consisting of a chain of 68 amino acids [32]. GG is all-trans geranyl geranyl cysteine methyl ester [29].

N_2 – Met – Ser – Gly – Ser – Ser – Ser – Val – Ala – Ala
1
|
Leu – Arg – Leu – Gln – Gln – Val – Val – Lys – Lys – Met
|
10
Glu – Ala – Gly – Leu – Asn – Arg – Val – Lys – Val – Ser
20
|
Cys – Phe – Gln – Lys – Leu – Asp – Ala – Ala – Ala – Gln
|
30
Leu – Gln – Asn – Ala – Gln – His – Asp – Pro – Leu – Leu
40
|
Phe – Pro – Asn – Thr – Ser – Ser – Ser – Val – Gly – Thr
|
50
Arg – Pro – Gln – Lys – Val – Cys – Ser – Phe – Leu 68
60 GG
|
COOH

Gamma 7

Gamma 7 is a protein consisting of a chain of 68 amino acids [33]. GG is all-trans geranyl geranyl cysteine methyl ester [29].

```
N2  – Met – Ser – Ala – Thr – Asn – Asn – Ile – Ala – Gln
       1                                                 |
Ile – Arg – Leu – Gln – Glu – Val – Leu – Lys – Arg – Ala
 |                                                     10
Glu – Ala – Gly – Ile – Glu – Arg – Ile – Lys – Val – Ser
20                                                       |
Cys – Tyr – Ser – Met – Leu – Glu – Ser – Ser – Ala – Lys
 |                                                     30
Glu – Gln – His – Ala – Arg – Asn – Asp – Pro – Leu – Leu
40                                                       |
Phe – Pro – Asn – Glu – Ser – Ala – Pro – Val – Gly – Val
 |                                                     50
Lys – Asp – Lys – Lys – Pro – Cys – Ile – Ile – Leu 68
60                            GG                 |
                                                COOH
```

GAMMA 10

Gamma 10 is a protein consisting of a chain of 68 amino acids [31]. GG is all-trans geranyl geranyl cysteine methyl ester [29].

```
N2  – Met – Ser – Ser – Gly – Ala – Ser – Ala – Ser – Ala
       1                                                 |
Leu – Lys – Leu – Gln – Glu – Val – Leu – Arg – Gln – Leu
 |                                                     10
Glu – Ala – Gly – Val – Glu – Arg – Ile – Lys – Val – Ser
20                                                       |
Cys – Tyr – Gln – Gln – Leu – Glu – Ala – Ala – Ala – Gln
 |                                                     30
Met – Gln – Asn – Ala – Cys – Lys – Asp – Ala – Leu – Leu
40                                                       |
Phe – Pro – Asn – Ser – Gly – Ala – Pro – Val – Gly – Val
 |                                                     50
```

Arg – Glu – Pro – Arg – Ser – Cys – Ala – Leu – Leu 68
60 GG | COOH

GAMMA 11

Gamma 11 is a protein consisting of a chain of 73 amino acids [31]. GG is all-trans geranyl geranyl cysteine methyl ester [29].

N_2 – Met – Pro – Ala – Leu – His – Ile – Glu – Asp – Leu
1 |
Val – Glu – Met – Lys – Leu – Lys – Glu – Lys – Glu – Pro
| 10
Glu – Gln – Leu – Arg – Lys – Glu – Val – Lys – Leu – Gln
20 |
Glu – Glu – Ser – Cys – Lys – Ser – Val – Gln – Gln – Arg
| 30
Ile – Lys – Asn – Tyr – Ile – Glu – Glu – Arg – Ser – Gly
40 |
Glu – Pro – Ile – Gly – Lys – Val – Leu – Pro – Asp – Glu
| 50
Asp – Lys – Asn – Pro – Phe – Lys – Glu – Lys – Gly – Ser
60 |
COOH – Ser – Ile – Val – Cys
73 GG

G PROTEIN ACTION

GS PROTEIN

The action of the G protein Gs alpha is to stimulate adenylate cyclase in the cholinergic neurons [34]. This requires manganese [35].

enzyme name : adenylate cyclase

enzyme classification : EC 4.6.1.1
cofactor : manganese (Mn $^{2+}$)
substrate : ATP
product : 3',5'-cyclic AMP + diphosphate

Gi protein

The action of the G protein Gs alpha is to inhibit adenylate cyclase in the cholinergic neurons [36]. This requires manganese [35].

enzyme name : adenylate cyclase
enzyme classification : EC 4.6.1.1
cofactor : manganese (Mn $^{2+}$)
substrate : ATP
product : 3',5'-cyclic AMP + diphosphate

Go protein

The action of the G protein Gs alpha is to inhibit Ca^{2+} channels in the cholinergic neurons [37, 38]. This requires calcium [39, 40, 41].

enzyme name : Ca^{2+} - transporting ATPase
enzyme classification : EC 3.6.3.8
cofactor : calcium (Ca $^{2+}$)
substrate : ATP + H_20 + Ca^{2+} (outside)
product : ADP + phosphate + Ca^{2+} (inside)

[1] American Journal of Physiology [1987] C411 : 139 (R.B.Innis, Aghajanian)

[2] Brain Research [1990] 533 : 263 (P.Bickford-Wimer, M.Kim, C.Boyajian, F.M.F.Cooper, R.Freedman)

[3] Science [1971] 174 : 1346 (J.W.Kebabian, P.Greengard)

[4] Molecular Pharmacology [1985] 28 : 138 (P.Onali, M.C.Olianas, G.L.Gessa)

[5] Proceedings National Academy of Science USA [1992] 89 : 12093 (A.I.Cohen et al)

[6] Nature [1991] 252 : 802 (M.I.Simon, M.P.Strathmann, N.Gautam)

[7] Proceedings National Academy of Science USA [1993] 90 : 3675 (M.E.Linder, P.Middleton, J.R.Hepler)

[8] Biochemical and Biophysical Research Communications [1987] 146 : 1234 (A.M.Schultz, S.-C.Tsai, H-F Kung, et al)

[9] Proceedings National Academy of Science USA [1990] 87 : 568 (T.L.Z.Jones, W.F. Simonds, J.Merendino, et al)

[10] Proceedings National Academy of Science USA [1990] 87 : 5873 (S.M. Mumby, P.J.Casey, A.G.Gilman, et al)

[11] Biochemistry [1995] 34 (4) : 1344 (K. Yokoyama, P.McGeady, M.H.Gelb)

[12] Journal of Biological Chemistry [1990] 265 : 15572 (P.S. Backlund, W.F.Simonds, A.M.Spiegel)

[13] Journal of Biological Chemistry [1954] 210 : 657 (P.Berg, W.K.Joklik)

[14] Biochimica et Biophysica Acta [1956] 21 : 86 (D.M.Gibson, P.Ayengar, D.R.Sanadi)

[15] Biochemical Journal [1959] 72 : 716 (R.J.A.Kirkland, J.F.Turner)

[16] Biochimica et Biophysica Acta [1953] 12 : 172 (H.A.Krebs, R. Hems)

[17] Journal of Biological Chemistry [1966] 241 : 4917 (H.Nakamura, Y.Sugino)

[18] Journal of Biological Chemistry [1964] 239 : 301 (R.L.Ratliff, R.H.Weaver, H.A.Lardy, S.A.Kuby)

[19] Science [1988] 241 : 800 (A. Levitzki)

[20] Nature [1990] 348 : 125 (H.R.Bourne, D.A.Sanders, F. McCormick)

[21] Biochemical and Biophysical Research Communications [1985] 128 (3): 1440 (V.Manne, H.F.Kung)

[22] Proceedings National Academy of Science USA [1988] 85 : 2081 (T.Kozasa, H.Itoh, T.Tsukamoto, Y.Kaziro)

[23] Journal of Biological Chemistry [1988] 263 : 6656 (H.Itoh, R.Toyama, T . Kozasa, T.Tsukamoto, M . Matsuoka, Y.Kaziro)

[24] Biochemical and Biophysical Research Communications [1988] 150 : 811 (S.Lavu, J.Clark, R.Swarup, K.Matsushima, K.Paturu, J.Moss, H.-F.Kung)

[25] Proceedings National Academy of Science USA [1986] 83 : 2162 (H.K.Fong, J.B.Hurley, R.S.Hopkins, et al)

[26] Proceedings National Academy of Science USA [1987] 84 : 6122 (B.Gao, A.G.Gilman, J.D.Robishaw)

[27] Biochemical and Biophysical Research Communications [1992] 183 : 350 (E.Von Weizsãcker, M.P.Strathmann, M.I.Simon)

[28] Journal of Biological Chemistry [1989] 264 : 15758 (J.D. Robishaw, V.K.Kalman, C.R. Moomaw, et al)

[29] Proceedings National Academy of Science USA [1990] 87 : 5865 (H.K.Yamane, C.C.Farnsworth, H.Y.Xie, et al)

[30] Proceedings National Academy of Science USA [1990] 87 : 7973 (N.Gautam, J.Northup, H.Tamir, et al)

[31] Journal of Biological Chemistry [1995] 270 (37) : 21765 (K.Ray, C.Kunsch, L.M.Bonner, J.D.Robishaw)

[32] Molecular and Cellular Biology [1992] 12 : 1585 (K.J.Fisher, N.N.Aronson)

[33] Journal of Biological Chemistry [1992] 267 : 24023 (J.J.Cali, E.A.Balcueva, I.Rybalkin, et al)

[34] Cell [1992] 68 (5) : 911 (C.H. Berlot, H.R.Bourne)

[35] Journal of Biological Chemistry [1969] 244 : 6363 (J.G.Hardman, E.W.Sutherland)

[36] Science [1993] 261 : 218 (R.I.Taussig, J.A.Niguez-Lluhi, A.G. Gilman)

[37] Journal of Biological Chemistry [1990] 265 : 8243 (M.E.Linder, D.A.Ewald, R.J.Miller, A.G.Gilman)

[38] Proceedings National Academy of Science USA [1988] 85 (10) : 3633 (D.A.Ewald, P.C.Sternweis, R.J.Miller)

[39] Journal of Biological Chemistry [1981] 256 : 3263 (P.Caroni, E. Carafoli)

[40] Biochimica et Biophysica Acta [1978] 515 : 23 (W.Hasselbach)

[41] Journal of Biological Chemistry [1970] 245 : 4508 (D.H. MacLennan)

CHAPTER 11

BIOCHEMISTRY OF PARKINSON'S DISEASE

DOPAMINE RECEPTOR PHOSPHOPROTEIN

Biosynthesis of DARPP-32

G proteins increase the levels of 3',5'-Cyclic AMP [1, 2] and also Calcium [3, 4]. 3',5'-Cyclic AMP and Calcium both, by different means, stimulate the biosynthesis of Dopamine Receptor Phosphoprotein (DARPP-32).

CYCLIC AMP STIMULATED BIOSYNTHESIS

Dopamine Receptor Phosphoprotein (DARPP-32) is biosynthesized from amino acids. The amino acids, via translation first form Pre-DARPP-32 in the ribosomes. Pre-DARPP-32 is a single chain polypeptide. With the addition of two molecules of water, leader peptidase removes the signal peptide of Pre-DARPP-32 to produce unphosphorylated DARPP-32 in the endoplasmic reticulum. In the golgi complex, with the addition of ATP and the formation of ADP, 3',5'-Cyclic AMP stimulates protein kinase [5]. Protein kinase stimulates the formation of DARPP-32 in the cytosol [6].

CALCIUM STIMULATED BIOSYNTHESIS

Dopamine Receptor Phosphoprotein (DARPP-32) is biosynthesized from amino acids. The amino acids, via translation first form Pre-DARPP-32 in the ribosomes. Pre-DARPP-32 is a single chain polypeptide. With the addition of two molecules of water, leader peptidase removes the signal peptide of Pre-DARPP-32 to produce unphosphorylated DARPP-32 in the endoplasmic reticulum. In the golgi complex, with the addition of ATP and the formation of ADP, Calcium stimulates Calcium/Calmodulin dependent protein kinase [7]. Calcium/Calmodulin dependent protein kinase stimulates the formation of DARPP-32 in the cytosol [6].

DARPP-32 STRUCTURE

Dopamine receptor phosphoprotein (DARPP-32) is a protein consisting of a chain of 202 amino acids [8]. This is the bovine structure of dopamine receptor phosphoprotein (DARPP-32) because the human structure of Darpp-32 is not completely known.

```
N2  – Met – Asp – Pro – Lys – Asp – Arg – Lys – Lys – Ile
       1                                               |
Gln – Ser – Pro – Pro – Ala – Pro – Val – Ser – Phe – Gln
 |                                                     10
Leu – Asp – Pro – Arg – Gln – Val – Glu – Met – Ile – Arg
20                                                     |
Phe – Leu – Met – Ala – Pro – Thr – Pro – Arg – Arg – Arg
 |                                                     30
Arg – Leu – Ser – Glu – His – Ser – Ser – Pro – Glu – Glu
40                                                     |
Gly – Ser – Ala – Arg – Gln – His – Pro – Ser – Ala – Glu
 |                                                     50
Glu – Gly – His – His – Leu – Lys – Ser – Lys – Arg – Ser
60                                                     |
Leu – Ser – Pro – Pro – Thr – Tyr – Ala – Cys – Pro – Asn
 |                                                     70
Lys – Ala – Val – Gln – Arg – Ile – Ala – Glu – Ser – His
80                                                     |
Asn – Glu – Gly – Leu – Asn – Ser – Ile – Ser – Gln – Leu
 |                                                     90
Gln – Ala – Ser – Glu – Glu – Glu – Asp – Glu – Leu – Gly
100                                                    |
Glu – Arg – Pro – Tyr – Gly – Leu – Glu – Arg – Leu – Glu
 |                                                     110
Glu – Glu – Glu – Glu – Glu – Glu – Glu – Glu – Asp – Glu
120                                                    |
Val – Glu – Ala – Gln – Ser – Asp – Glu – Glu – Glu – Glu
```

```
|                                                                 130
Leu – Lys – Gly – Ser – Arg – Gly – Ser – Ala – Gly – Gln
140                                                                  |
Gly – Glu – Leu – Gly – Gln – Gly – Tyr – Thr – Thr – Lys
|                                                                 150
Pro – Trp – Glu – Arg – Pro – Pro – Pro – Leu – Asp – Gly
160                                                                  |
Gln – Asp – Glu – Ser – Ser – Gly – Asp – Arg – Gln – Pro
|                                                                 170
Val – Glu – Asp – Pro – Ala – Leu – Asn – Glu – Pro – Gly
180                                                                  |
Glu – Pro – His – Ala – Pro – Arg – Gln – Pro – Glu – Glu
|                                                                 190
Pro – Gly – Thr – COOH
200         202
```

PROTEIN PHOSPHORYLATION

DARPP-32 increases the phosphorylation of proteins by means of three different enzymes : protein phosphatase 1, protein kinase, and calcium / calmodulin dependent protein kinase. These three enzymes affect the phosphorylation of proteins by three different means.

PROTEIN PHOSPHATASE 1

DARPP-32 inhibits the enzyme protein phosphatase 1 [9]. Protein phosphatase 1 stimulates the desphosphorylation of proteins [10-13]. So the inhibition of protein phosphatase 1 by DARPP-32 increases the phosphorylation of proteins.

enzyme name : protein phosphatase 1
enzyme classification : EC 3.1.3.16
substrate : phosphoprotein + H_20
product : protein + Pi

PROTEIN KINASE

Protein kinase is stimulated by 3',5'-Cyclic AMP and so also has a direct effect on the phosphorylation of proteins [14-22].

enzyme name : protein kinase
enzyme classification : EC 2.7.11.1
substrate : protein + ATP
product : phosphoprotein + ADP

CALCIUM/CALMODULIN DEPENDENT PROTEIN KINASE

Ca2+/calmodulin-dependent protein kinase is stimulated by calcium and so also has a direct effect on the phosphorylation of proteins [23-26].

enzyme name : Ca2+/calmodulin-dependent protein kinase
enzyme classification : EC 2.7.11.17
cofactor : calcium (Ca^{2+})
substrate : protein + ATP
product : phosphoprotein + ADP

[1] Cell [1992] 68 (5) : 911 (C.H. Berlot, H.R.Bourne)

[2] Science [1993] 261 : 218 (R.I.Taussig, J.A.Niguez-Lluhi, A.G. Gilman)

[3] Journal of Biological Chemistry [1990] 265 : 8243 (M.E.Linder, D.A.Ewald, R.J.Miller, A.G.Gilman)

[4] Proceedings National Academy of Science, USA [1988] 85 (10) : 3633 (D.A.Ewald, P.C.Sternweis, R.J.Miller)

[5] Reviews in Biochemical Toxicology [1985] 54 : 931 (A.C.Nairn, H.C.Hemmings, P. Greengard)

[6] Nature [1983] 301 : 69 (S.I.Walaas, D.W.Aswad, P.Greengard)

[7] Annual Review of Biochemistry [1985] 54 : 931 (A.C.Nairn, H.C. Hemmings, P.Greengard)

[8] Journal of Biological Chemistry [1986] 261 : 1890 (K.R.Williams, H.C.Hemmings, W.H. Konigsberg, P. Greengard)

[9] Nature [1984] 310 : 503 (H.C.Hemmings, P.Greengard, H.Y. L. Tung, P.Cohen)

[10] Journal of Bacteriology [1985] 163 : 1203 (J.Deutscher, U. Kessler, W.Hengstenberg)

[11] European Journal of Biochemistry [1983] 132 : 255 (T.S. Ingebritsen, P.Cohen)

[12] Biochemical Journal [1959] 71 : 537 (T.A. Sundarajan, P.S.Sarma)

[13] European Journal of Biochemistry [1984] 145 : 65 (N.K.Tonks, P.Cohen)

[14] Biochimica et Biophysica Acta [1973] 315 : 347 (B.Baggio, V. Moret)

[15] Journal of Biological Chemistry [1985] 260 : 7094 (J.L.Benovic, L.J.Pike, R.A.Cerione, C.Staniszewski, T.Yoshimasha, J. Codina, M.G. Caron, R.J. Lefkowitz)

[16] FEBS Letters [1981] 124 : 145 (R.W.Brownsey, G.J.Belsham, R.M.Denton)

[17] Biochimica et Biophysica Acta [1975] 377 : 271 (M.V.Nesterova, L.P.Sashchenko, V.Y.Vasiliev, E.S.Severin)

[18] Journal of Biological Chemistry [1960] 235 : 1043 (M. Rabinowitz, F.Lipmann)

[19] FEBS Letters [1981] 124 : 140 (S. Ramakrishna, N.B.Benjamin)

[20] Biochimica et Biophysica Acta [1969] 191 : 272 (K.K.Schlender, S.H.Wei, C.Villar-Palasi)

[21] Journal of Biological Chemistry [1968] 243 : 3763 (D.A.Walsh, J.P.Perkins, E.G. Krebs)

[22] Biochimica et Biophysica Acta [1973] 315 : 333 (K.Yoshikawa, K.Adachi)

[23] Biochemistry [1985] 24 : 5320-5327 (H.Schulman, J.Kuret, A.B. Jefferson, P.S.Nose, K.H.Spitzer)

[24] Journal of Biological Chemistry [1998] 273 : 31880-31889 (K.A. Anderson, R.L.Means, Q.H.Huang, B.E.Kemp, E.G.Goldstein, M.A. Selbert, A.M.Edelman, R.T.Fremeau, A.R.Means)

[25] Journal of Biological Chemistry [1998] 273 : 21473-21481 (M. Matsushita, A.C.Nairn)

[26] Journal of Biological Chemistry [1989] 264 : 5866-5875 (C.A. Ohmstede, K.F.Jensen, N.E.Sahyoun)

CHAPTER 12

CYTOLOGY OF PARKINSON'S DISEASE

DOPAMINERGIC NEURONS

STRUCTURE

The dopaminergic neurons are cells that occur in a variety of sizes and shapes [1]. Dopaminergic neurons have dendrites, which are branched projections that act to propagate electrical stimulation. Electrical stimulation is transmitted on to dendrites via synapses, which are located on the dendrites [2]. The dopaminergic neurons also have axons, which are slender projections from the neurons. They are more consistent in shape and greater in length than dendrites.

BIOSYNTHESIS

The dopaminergic neurons, unlike most cells, do not reproduce by undergoing mitosis (cell division) in adults [3, 4]. So the number of dopaminergic neurons tends to decline with age. Although it is often claimed that there is a massive loss of dopaminergic neurons in Parkinson's Disease no research has ever shown this. The study from which these claims originate assessed the enzyme levels in the dopaminergic neurons not the number of the dopaminergic neurons. Enzyme levels determine cell activity not cell loss [5].

FUNCTION

The unique function of the dopaminergic neurons is the biosynthesis and secretion of dopamine [6]. The functions of the dopaminergic neurons are otherwise similar to those of other neurons. In dopaminergic neurons, axons and dendrites are both sites of dopamine release [6]. Insufficient biosynthesis and secretion of dopamine is the primary cause of Parkinson's Disease. In Parkinson's Disease the activity of the enzymes involved in dopamine biosynthesis, not the number of dopaminergic neurons, is greatly reduced [7, 8].

Cytological features

Cytological features of the dopaminergic neurons are the : cytoplasm, cytosol, nucleus, nucleoli, mitochondrion, smooth endoplasmic reticulum, rough endoplasmic reticulum, ribosomes, Nissl substance, the golgi complex, lysosomes, lipofuscin, endosomes, centrosomes, neurofilaments, cytoskeleton, microtubules, vesicles, and cell membrane.

Cytoplasm

The cytoplasm is the content of the fluid-filled space inside cells, which is a jelly-like substance. It is within the cytoplasm that most cellular activities occur, including many metabolic pathways. The concentrated inner area is called the endoplasm and the outer layer is called the cell cortex or the ectoplasm.

Cytosol

The cytosol is the liquid found inside cells that constitutes most of the intracellular fluid. Water forms the large majority of the cytosol. The cytosol is within the cell membrane and is part of the cytoplasm. Many of the metabolic pathways occur in the cytosol, including the biosynthesis of dopamine [9, 10].

Nucleus

The nucleus is a membrane enclosed organelle that contains most of the genetic material of the cells, including chromosomes composed of DNA. The nucleus maintains the integrity of these genes and controls the activities of the cell by regulating gene expression. Nucleolar damage can occur in Parkinson's Disease [11].

Nucleolus

The nucleolus is the largest structure within the nucleus. It is the site of rRNA transcription and processing, and of ribosome biosynthesis and assembly. Cells require large numbers of ribosomes to meet their needs for protein biosynthesis. Altered nucleolar function and morphology, including decreased nucleolar volume, have been observed in people with Parkinson's Disease [12].

Mitochondria

The mitochondria is the major energy-producing organelle. It releases energy in the form of ATP. ATP is produced by the mitochondria in the terminal respiratory chain cycle. Their dysfunction can lead to a decline in energy production, and the generation of reactive oxygen species [13, 14]. There are a large number of mitochondrion in the cells.

Smooth endoplasmic reticulum

The smooth endoplasmic reticulum has functions in several metabolic processes, including the biosynthesis of lipids and phospholipids, the metabolism of carbohydrates, and the attachment of receptors on cell membrane proteins. The L-dopa biosynthesizing enzyme, tyrosine 3-monooxygenase is localised to microtubules and smooth endoplasmic reticulum that approach the postsynaptic membrane [15].

Rough endoplasmic reticulum

The endoplasmic reticulum forms an interconnected network of flattened, membrane enclosed tube-like structures known as cisternae. The outer (cytosolic) face of the rough endoplasmic reticulum has ribosomes attached to it that are the sites of protein biosynthesis. Much of the cytoplasm of the dopaminergic neurons is densely filled with free ribosomes associated with large, well organised complexes of rough endoplasmic reticulum [16].

Ribosomes

Ribosomes are where translation (protein biosynthesis) occurs in the cells. Ribosomes link amino acids together in the order specified by messenger RNA (mRNA). In the dopaminergic neurons much of the cytoplasm is densely filled with free ribosomes associated with large complexes of rough endoplasmic reticulum [16].

Nissl substance

Nissl substance is a granular body found in dopaminergic neurons. These granules are of rough endoplasmic reticulum and free ribosomes, and are the site of protein biosynthesis. Dopaminergic neurons can be distinguished from non-dopaminergic neurons by their cytological features, and particularly by the pattern of Nissl substance [16].

Golgi complex

The Golgi complex (Golgi apparatus) packages proteins into membrane bound vesicles. The Golgi complex is of particular importance in processing proteins for secretion, containing glycosylation enzymes that attach various sugars to proteins as the proteins move through the Golgi complex [17].

Lysosomes

Lysosomes are membrane-bound cell organelle of very varying sizes. They are spherical vesicles containing hydrolytic enzymes capable of breaking down virtually all kinds of biomolecules, including proteins, nucleic acids, carbohydrates, lipids, and cellular debris. Consequently, lysosomes act as a waste disposal system by digesting unwanted materials in the cytoplasm [18, 19].

Lipofuscin

Lipofuscin are finely granular yellow-brown pigment granules that consist of lipid containing residues of lysosomal digestion. Consequently, lipofuscin accumulation is implicated in cellular degeneration. Lipofuscin granular aggregations are observed in Parkinson's Disease [20].

Endosomes

Endosomes are vesicles that traffic membrane and intra and extra cellular contents for recycling or degradation by lysosomes. Endosomes are membrane-bound compartments inside the cells.

Molecules internalised from the plasma membrane can follow this pathway all the way to lysosomes for degradation or they can be recycled back to the plasma membrane. Endosomes were mostly found in somatodendritic regions of dopaminergic neurons. Endosomes containing recycling markers are primarily found in axons [21].

Centrosomes

Centrosomes are an associated pair of cylindrical shaped protein structures (centrioles) that organize microtubules and aid in forming the mitotic spindle during cell division. Aggregation of proteins in the centrosome is associated with the pathophysiology of Parkinson's Disease. However, the relevance of the centrosome is not known [22].

Neurofilaments

Neurofilaments are the filaments found in neurons. They are a major component of the neuronal cytoskeleton. They are believed to function primarily to provide structural support for the axon and to regulate axon diameter. Neurofilaments are composed of polypeptide chains or subunits. The filamentous component of Lewy Bodies in Parkinson's Disease contains biochemically altered neurofilaments [23].

Cytoskeleton

The cytoskeleton is a complex network of interlinking neurofilaments and tubules that extend throughout the cytoplasm from the nucleus to the plasma membrane. The cytoskeleton helps cells maintain their shape and internal organisation, and provides mechanical support enabling cells to carry out essential functions. Cytoskeleton impairment can occur in Parkinson's Disease [24].

Microtubules

The microtubule system is important for many aspects of neuronal function including motility, differentiation, and cargo trafficking. Microtubules are very important in a number of cellular processes. They are involved in maintaining the structure of the cell and, together with microfilaments and intermediate filaments, form the cytoskeleton. Alteration of microtubules is an early event in Parkinson's Disease [25].

Vesicles

Vesicles are small structures within the cell consisting of fluid enclosed by a lipid bilayer. Vesicles can form naturally during the processes of secretion (exocytosis), uptake (phagocytosis and endocytosis), and during the transport of materials within the cytoplasm. Dopamine is stored in intracellular vesicles awaiting release [26].

Cell membrane

The cell membrane is the part of the cell that separates the cells from the outside environment. It protects the cell and regulates what enters and leaves the cell. It consists of the phospholipid bilayer with embedded proteins. Dopamine is transported across the cell membrane after being stored in vescicles [27].

[1] Neuroscience [1983] 8 (4) : 743-765 (V.B.Domesick, L.Stinus, P.A. Paskevich)

[2] Acta Neurobiologiae Experimentalis [2008] 68 (2) : 264-288 (M. Urbanska, M.Blazejczyk, J.Jaworski)

[3] Development [2008] 135 (20) : 3401-3413 (N.Russek-Blum, A. Gutnick, H.Nabel-Rosen, J.Blechman, N.Staudt, R.I.Dorsky, C.Houart, G.Levkowitz)

[4] Annual, New York Academy of Sciences [2003] 991 : 36-47 (H.H. Simon, L.Bhatt, D.Gherbassi, P.Sgadó, L.Alberí)

[5] Neuropathology [1999] 19 (1) : 10-13 (T.Fukuda, J.Takahashi, J. Tanaka)

[6] Journal of Neuroscience [2007] 27 (8) : 1892-1901 (L.J.Gentet, S.R.Williams)

[7] Klinische Wochenschrift [1960] 38 : 1236-1239 (H.Ehringer, O. Hornykiewicz)

[8] Journal of Neural Transmission (Supplement) [1978] (14) : 121-131 (P.Riederer, W.D.Rausch, W.Birkmayer, K.Jellinger, D. Seemann)

[9] Synapse [2007] 61 (9) : 715-723 (L.J.Wallace)

[10] Cell Communication and Signalling [2013] 11 (1) : 34 (J.Meiser, D.Weindl, K.Hiller)

[11] Journal of Neuroscience [2011] 31 (2) : 453-460 (C.Rieker, D. Engblom, G.Kreiner, A.Domanskyi, A.Schober, S.Stotz, M.Neumann, X.Yuan, I.Grummt, G.Schütz, R.Parlato)

[12] Neuroscience Letters [2013] 546 : 26-30 (M.Healy-Stoffel, S.O. Ahmad, J.A.Stanford, B.Levant)

[13] Progress in Neurobiology [2013] 106-107 : 17-32 (S.R. Subramaniam, M.F.Chesselet)

[14] Cold Spring Harbor Perspectives in Medicine [2012] 2 (2) : a009332 (C.Perier, M.Vila)

[15] Brain Research [1979] 170 (1) : 71-83 (T.Hattori, P.L.McGeer, E.G.McGeer)

[16] Neuroscience [1983] 8 (4) : 743-765 (V.B.Domesick, L.Stinus, P.A.Paskevich)

[17] ACS Chemical Neuroscience [2010] 1 (3) : 194-203 (A.Carmona, G.Devès, S.Roudeau, P.Cloetens, S.Bohic, R.Ortega)

[18] Ageing Research Reviews [2016] Mar 3 [Epub ahead of print] (M.Bourdenx, B.Dehay)

[19] Journal of Neuroscience [2010] 30 (37) : 12535-12544 (B. Dehay, J.Bové, N.Rodríguez-Muela, C.Perier, A.Recasens, P.Boya, M.Vila)

[20] Journal of Neural Transmission [2011] 118 (3) : 361-369 (Z.Lv, H.Jiang, H.Xu, N.Song, J.Xie)

[21] Molecular and Cellular Neurosciences [2011] 46 (1) : 148-158 (A. Rao, D.Simmons, A.Sorkin)

[22] Neurotoxicity Research [2008] 14 (4) : 295-305 (F.J.Diaz-Corrales, M.Asanuma, I.Miyazaki, K.Miyoshi, N.Hattori, N.Ogawa)

[23] Journal of Neuropathology and Experimental Neurology [1995] 54 (3) : 311-319 (T.J.Montine, D.B.Farris, D.G.Graham)

[24] Proteomics [2014] 14 (6) : 784-794 (V.Licker, N.Turck, E. Kövari, K.Burkhardt, M.Côte, M.Surini-Demiri, J.A.Lobrinus, J.C. Sanchez, P.R.Burkhard)

[25] Scientific Reports [2013] 3 : 1837 (D.Cartelli, F.Casagrande, C.L. Busceti, D.Bucci, G.Molinaro, A.Traficante, D.Passarella, E. Giavini, G.Pezzoli, G.Battaglia, G.Cappelletti)

[26] Current Neurology and Neuroscience Reports [2013] 13 (7) : 362 (S.P.Alter, G.M.Lenzi, A.I.Bernstein, G.W.Miller)

[27] Frontiers in Bioscience [2012] 17 : 2740-2767 (D.B.Pereira, D. Sulzer)

CHAPTER 13

CYTOLOGY OF PARKINSON'S DISEASE

CYTOLOGICAL EFFECTS

CYTOLOGICAL EFFECTS

When L-dopa or dopamine is not biosynthesized properly in the dopaminergic neurons, as occurs in Parkinson's Disease, certain cytological effects can occur. This can result in the formation of Superoxide anion [PAGE 170], Neuromelanin formation [PAGE 172], Iron accumulation [PAGE 175], the accumulation of Alpha-synuclein [PAGE 176], and the formation of Lewy bodies [PAGE 179].

SUPEROXIDE ANION

The first step in the formation of dopamine is the biosynthesis of L-dopa from L-tyrosine [1-4]. In Parkinson's Disease, largely due to inadequate cofactors, L-tyrosine and molecular oxygen do not completely form L-dopa. Consequently, the toxic partial reduction product of oxygen, the superoxide anion can be formed instead. Superoxide (O_2^-) is formed by the oxidation of ferrous ions (Fe^{2+}) by dioxygen (O_2) [5].

enzyme name : tyrosine 3-monooxygenase
enzyme classification : EC 1.14.16.2
cofactor : ferrous iron (Fe^{2+})
substrate : L-tyrosine + O_2 + Fe^{2+}
product : L-tyrosine + O_2^- + Fe^{3+}

Superoxide is the origin of most reactive oxygen species. It undergoes a chain reaction in cells playing a central role in the reactive oxygen species system. Increased oxidative stress on an organism causes damage to cells [6]. The Superoxide anion is a major inducer of neurodegenerative damage in Parkinson's Disease. There is a high oxidative status in the brains of people with Parkinson's Disease [7]. There are various pathways via which superoxide anion can manifest toxic effects.

In order to nullify its harmful effects, Superoxide is broken down to hydrogen peroxide (H_2O_2) by the enzyme Superoxide Dismutase [8, 9, 10], and is then rendered harmless by the enzyme Catalase [11-15].

enzyme name : superoxide dismutase
enzyme classification : EC 1.15.1.1
substrate : $2O_2^- + H^+$
product : $O_2 + H_2O_2$

enzyme name : catalase
enzyme classification : EC 1.11.1.6
substrate : 2 H_2O_2
product : $O_2 + H_2O$

[1] Journal of Biological Chemistry [1964] 239 : 2910 (T.Nagatsu, M. Levitt, S.Udenfriend)

[2] Archives of Biochemistry and Biophysics [1967] 120 : 420 (M. Ikeda, M.Levitt, S.Udenfriend)

[3] Nature [1983] 302 : 830 (S.El Mestikawy, J.Glowinski, M.Hamon)

[4] Comptes Rendus Academie des Sciences [1986] 302 : 435 (D. Pigeon, R.Drissi-Daoudi, F.Gros, J.Thibault)

[5] Proceedings of the Royal Society [1934] A147 : 332 (F.Haber, J.Weiss)

[6] Journal of Clinical Biochemistry and Nutrition [2015] 56 (1) : 1-7 (H.P.Indo, H.C.Yen, I.Nakanishi, K.Matsumoto, M.Tamura, Y.Nagano, H.Matsui, O.Gusev, R.Cornette, T.Okuda, Y.Minamiyama, et al)

[7] ACS Chemical Neuroscience [2013] 4 (11) : 1439-1445 (Z.Zhelev, R.Bakalova, I.Aoki, D.Lazarova, T.Saga)

[8] Journal of Biological Chemistry [1971] 246 : 2875-2880 (B.B. Keele, J.M.McCord, I.Fridovich)

[9] Biochimica Biophysica Acta [1972] 268 : 305-312 (Y.Sawada, T.Ohyama, I.Yamazaki)

[10] Journal of Biological Chemistry [1972] 247 : 4782-4786 (P.G. Vance, B.B.Keele, K.V.Rajagopalan)

[11] Biochemical Journal [1948] 43 : 193-202 (D.Herbert, J.Pinsent)

[12] Biochemical Journal [1948] 43 : 203-205 (D.Herbert, J.Pinsent)

[13] Proceedings of the Royal Society of London, Series B - Biological Science [1936] 119 : 141-159 (D.Keilin, E.F.Hartree)

[14] Journal of Biological Chemistry [1983] 258 : 6015-6019 (Y.Kono, I.Fridovich)

[15] The Enzymes [1963] 8 : 147-225 (P.Nicholls, G.R.Schonbaum)

Neuromelanin

When L-Dopa is unable to form dopamine it may instead lead to the formation and accumulation of neuromelanin, which is similar to the pigment melanin found in skin. It can do this via the enzyme peroxidase [1, 2] instead of the enzyme tyrosinase, which is usually responsible for melanin production, because tyrosinase does not occur in the dopaminergic neurons [3].

Pigmentation of the dopaminergic neurons in the substantia nigra pars compacta, which is the area of the brain most affected by Parkinson's Disease, is due to the presence of neuromelanin [4]. Neuromelanin stores iron ions as oxyhydroxide iron clusters. The iron levels are lower in Parkinson's Disease [5].

Neuromelanin is not present at birth. Initiation of pigmentation usually begins at around three years of age. There is usually a period of increasing pigment granule number and increasing pigment granule colouration until around the age of twenty. In middle and later life the colour of the pigment granules continues to darken but the darker colour is not associated with a substantial growth in pigment volume [4]. The low levels of L-dopa in Parkinson's Disease can instead cause a depletion of neuromelanin, which is typically indicated by a relative lack of brown colour in the dopaminergic neurons [6].

FIRST STEP

enzyme name : tyrosine 3-monooxygenase
enzyme classification : EC 1.14.16.2
cofactor : ferrous iron (Fe^{2+})
substrate : L-tyrosine + tetrahydrofolic acid + O_2
product : L-dopa + dihydrofolic acid + H_20

SECOND STEP

enzyme name : peroxidase
enzyme classification : EC 1.11.1.7
substrate : L-dopa + H_2O_2
product : dopaquinone + 2 H_20

THIRD STEP

enzyme name : non enzymatic
enzyme classification : non enzymatic
substrate : dopaquinone
product : leucodopachrome

FOURTH STEP

enzyme name : peroxidase
enzyme classification : EC 1.11.1.7
substrate : leucodopachrome + H_2O_2
product : dopachrome + 2 H_20

FIFTH STEP

enzyme name : non enzymatic
enzyme classification : non enzymatic
substrate : dopachrome
product : 5,6-dihydroxyindole + CO_2

SIXTH STEP

enzyme name : peroxidase
enzyme classification : EC 1.11.1.7
substrate : 5,6-dihydroxyindole + H_2O_2
product : indole 5,6-quinone + 2 H_20

SEVENTH STEP

enzyme name : non enzymatic
enzyme classification : non enzymatic
substrate : 2 indole 5,6-quinone + 2 CO_2
product : melanochrome + 2 O_2

EIGHTH STEP

enzyme name : non enzymatic
enzyme classification : non enzymatic
substrate : melanochrome
product : neuromelanin

[1] Physiological Chemistry and Physics Medical NMR [1997] 29 (1) : 15-22 (M.R.Okun)

[2] Advances in Experimental Medicine and Biology [2003] 527 : 723-730 (G.Allegri, S.Vogliardi, A.Bertazzo, C.V.Costa, R.Seraglia, P. Traldi)

[3] Neuroscience Letters [1998] 253 (3) : 198-200 (K.Ikemoto, I. Nagatsu, S.Ito, R.A.King, A.Nishimura, T.Nagatsu)

[4] Journal of Neural Transmission [2006] 113 (6) : 721-728 (G.M. Halliday, H.Fedorow, C.H.Rickert, M.Gerlach, P.Riederer, K.L. Double)

[5] Journal of Neural Transmission [2006] 113 (6) : 769-774 (M. Fasano, B.Bergamasco, L.Lopiano)

[6] Neurochemistry International [2003] 42 (7) : 603-606 (M.Fasano, S.Giraudo, S.Coha, B.Bergamasco, L.Lopiano)

Iron accumulation

Iron is essential for the formation of L-dopa. So the deficiency of iron can cause insufficient L-dopa. Insufficient formation of L-dopa is the primary biochemical fault in Parkinson's Disease.

enzyme name : tyrosine 3-monooxygenase
enzyme classification : EC 1.14.16.2
cofactor : ferrous iron (Fe^{2+})
substrate : L-tyrosine + tetrahydrofolic acid + O_2
product : L-dopa + dihydrofolic acid + H_20

In Parkinson's Disease there is a tendency for increased levels of iron in the substantia nigra, which is the main area of the brain involved in Parkinson's Disease [1-10]. The increased iron levels were related to the severity of Parkinson's Disease but not the duration or age of onset [8]. However, the Substantia nigra pars compacta, which is the area of the brain most affected by Parkinson’s Disease, is only affected in this respect in early Parkinson’s Disease. Some other areas of the brain are only affected in advanced stages of Parkinson’s Disease [9].

Iron accumulation at its worst occurs in Hereditary Hemochromatosis. If iron accumulation caused Parkinson's Disease everybody with Hereditary Hemochromatosis would have Parkinson's Disease but hardly any of them do [11]. When ferrous iron was administered to people with Parkinson's Disease there was a considerable improvement, not a considerable decline, in their Parkinson's Disease symptoms [12]. Also, instead of causing Parkinson's Disease, a higher intake of iron is associated with a reduced risk of Parkinson's Disease [13].

Iron is essential for the formation of dopamine. It is a common compensatory mechanism in biochemistry for a cofactor such as ferrous iron to accumulate when the substance it facilitates the formation of is deficient. That is why instead of iron accumulation causing Parkinson's Disease, Parkinson's Disease can cause an accumulation of iron.

[1] Archives of Neurology [2009] 66 (3) 371-374 (S.Brar, D. Henderson, J.Schenck, E.A.Zimmerman)

[2] Neurobiology of Disease [2008] 32 (2) : 183-195 (S.L.Rhodes, B. Ritz)

[3] Brain [1999] 122 (4) : 667-673 (P.D.Griffiths, B.R.Dobson, G.R. Jones, D.T.Clarke)

[4] Lancet [1987] 2 : 1219-1220 (D.T.Dexter, F.R.Wells, F.Agid, Y. Agid, A.J.Lees, P.Jenner)

[5] Journal of Neural Transmission [1988] 74 : 199-205 (E.Sofic, P. Riederer, H.Heinsen, H.Beckmann, G.P.Reynolds, G.Hebenstreit, M. B.Youdim)

[6] Journal of Neurochemistry [1989] 52 : 515-520 (P.Riederer, E. Sofic, W.D.Rausch, B.Schmidt, G.P.Reynolds, K.Jellinger, M.B. Youdim)

[7] Dementia [1993] 4 : 61-65 (P.D.Griffiths, A.R.Crossman)

[8] Brain Research [2010] 1330 : 124-130 (J.Zhang, Y.Zhang, J.Wang, P.Cai, C.Luo, Z.Qian, Y.Dai, H.Feng)

[9] NMR in Biomedicine [2016] Feb 8 [Epub ahead of print] (X.Guan, M.Xuan, Q.Gu, P.Huang, C.Liu, N.Wang, X.Xu, W.Luo, M.Zhang)

[10] Brain Research [2016] Jun 29 [Epub ahead of print] (J.Jiao, H.Guo, Y.He, J.Wang, J.Yuan, W.Hu)

[11] Journal of Neurology, Neurosurgery and Psychiatry [2004] 75 (4) : 631-633 (D.J.Costello, S.L.Walsh, H.J.Harrington, C.H.Walsh)

[12] Annals of Clinical and Laboratory Science [1987] 17 (1) : 32-35 (J.G.Birkmayer, W.Birkmayer)

[13] Journal of Neurological Science [2011] 306 (1-2) : 98-102 (Y. Miyake, K.Tanaka, W.Fukushima, S.Sasaki, C.Kiyohara, Y.Tsuboi, T. Yamada, T.Oeda, T.Miki, N.Kawamura, N.Sakae, et al)

Alpha-Synuclein

Alpha-synuclein is encoded by the PARK 1 (SNCA) gene. Alpha-synuclein is the best known form of the synuclein proteins, which include alpha-synuclein, beta-synuclein and gamma-synuclein [1]. Alpha-synuclein is a protein that is 140 amino acids in length. Alpha-synuclein is an intrinsically disordered protein as it lacks a fixed three-dimensional structure [2].

NH_2 – Met – Asp – Val – Phe – Met – Lys – Gly – Leu – Ser
1 |

Ala – Ala – Ala – Val – Val – Gly – Glu – Lys – Ala – Lys
| 10

Glu – Lys – Thr – Lys – Gln – Gly – Val – Ala – Glu – Ala
20 |

Tyr – Leu – Val – Gly – Glu – Lys – Thr – Lys – Gly – Ala
| 30

Val – Gly – Ser – Lys – Thr – Lys – Glu – Gly – Val – Val
40 |

Thr – Lys – Glu – Ala – Val – Thr – Ala – Val – Gly – His
| 50

Lys – Glu – Gln – Val – Thr – Asn – Val – Gly – Gly – Ala
60 |

Gln – Ala – Val – Ala – Thr – Val – Gly – Thr – Val – Val
| 70

Lys – Thr – Val – Glu – Gly – Ala – Gly – Ser – Ile – Ala
80 |

Gln – Asp – Lys – Lys – Val – Phe – Gly – Thr – Ala – Ala
| 90

Leu – Gly – Lys – Asn – Glu – Glu – Gly – Ala – Pro – Gln
100 |

Asp – Val – Pro – Met – Asp – Glu – Leu – Ile – Gly – Glu
| 110

Pro – Asp – Asn – Glu – Ala – Tyr – Glu – Met – Pro – Ser
120 |

Glu – Pro – Glu – Tyr – Asp – Gln – Tyr – Gly – Glu – Glu
| 130

Ala – COOH
140

Alpha-synuclein can accumulate under certain conditions. Medical disorders in which there is an abnormal accumulation of alpha-synuclein are called alpha-synucleinopathies. There are three main alpha-synucleinopathies : Parkinson's Disease, dementia with Lewy bodies, and multiple system atrophy. There are other medical disorders in which alpha-synucleinopathies can occur such as Alzheimer's Disease and neuroaxonal dystrophies. Small amounts of alpha-synuclein can also occur in individuals who do not have neurological disorders. Therefore, an accumulation of alpha-synuclein does not indicate that somebody has Parkinson's Disease [3, 4].

Iron accumulation can occur as a result of Parkinson's Disease when L-dopa is formed insufficiently. Alpha-synuclein aggregation is often accompanied by abnormal accumulation of iron [5], which also increases the aggregation of alpha-synuclein [6, 7]. Alpha-synuclein expression is regulated by iron mainly at the translational level [8].

The superoxide anion can also be produced as a result of Parkinson's Disease when L-dopa is formed insufficiently. Superoxide is broken down to hydrogen peroxide (H_2O_2) by the enzyme Superoxide Dismutase. Hydrogen peroxide (H_2O_2) plays a dominant role in the aggregation of alpha-synuclein [9].

So it is Parkinson's Disease, due to insufficient formation of L-dopa, that causes the aggregation of alpha-synuclein. Alpha-synuclein inhibits tyrosine 3-monooxygenase [10, 11, 12], which is the enzyme needed to form dopamine, which is essential for the relief of Parkinson's Disease. So when alpha-synuclein is inadvertently produced, it can worsen Parkinson's Disease symptoms even further by reducing dopamine biosynthesis.

[1] Neuropsychopharmacolica Hungarica [2014] 16 (2) : 77-84 (I. Miklya, N.Pencz, F.Hafenscher, P.Göltl)

[2] Open Journal of Biophysics [2013] 3 (1A) : 28323 A.Gonzalez-Horta, B.Gonzalez Hernandez, A.Chavez-Montes)

[3] Parkinsonism and Related Disorders [2014] 20 (Supplement 1) : S62-S67 (H.McCann, C.H.Stevens, H.Cartwright, G.M.Halliday)

[4] Alzheimers Research and Therapy [2014] 6 (5) : 73 (W.S.Kim, K.Kågedal, G.M.Halliday)

[5] Sheng Li Ke Xue Jin Zhan [2015] 46 (3) : 180-184 (J.Wang, N. Song, H.M.Xu, H.Jiang, J.X.Xie)

[6] Journal of Biological Chemistry [2002] 277 (18) : 16116-16123 (N.Golts, H.Snyder, M.Frasier, C.Theisler, P.Choi, B.Wolozin)

[7] International Journal of Biochemistry and Cell Biology [2013] 45 (6) : 1019-1030 (Q.He, N.Song, F.Jia, H.Xu, X.Yu, J.Xie, H.Jiang)

[8] Neuroreport [2012] 23 (9) : 576-580 (F.Febbraro, M.Giorgi, S. Caldarola, F.Loreni, M.Romero-Ramos)

[9] Free Radical Biology and Medicine [2002] 32 (6) : 544-550 (K.S. Kim, S.Y.Choi, H.Y.Kwon, M.H.Won, T.C.Kang, J.H.Kang)

[10] Neuroscience Bulletin [2007] 23 (1) : 53-57 (N.Gao, Y.H.Li, X.Li, S.Yu, G.L.Fu, B.Chen)

[11] Journal of Neurochemistry [2004] 89 (6) : 1318-1324 (R.G.Perez, T.G.Hastings)

[12] Journal of Neuroscience [2002] 22 (8) : 3090-3099 (R.G.Perez, J.C.Waymire, E.Lin, J.J.Liu, F.Guo, M.J.Zigmond)

LEWY BODIES

Lewy bodies can occur in Parkinson's Disease [1]. At the time of death around 85% of people with Parkinson's Disease have Lewy bodies [2]. However, whilst having Parkinson's Disease a lot of people with Parkinson's Disease do not have Lewy bodies [2]. Lewy bodies can also occur in other medical disorders including : multiple system atrophy [1], Lewy body disease [1], Parkinson's Disease dementia [2], progressive supranuclear palsy [3], and in old people who do not have any of these medical disorders [4, 5]. Therefore, Lewy bodies do not indicate that somebody has Parkinson's Disease.

Lewy bodies are characterised by abnormal intraneuronal deposits (Lewy bodies) and intraneuritic deposits (Lewy neurites) of fibrillary aggregates and Lewy grains [6]. Aggregated alpha-synuclein is the major component of Lewy bodies, Lewy neurites and Lewy grains and the primary cause of Lewy body formation [6-9].

The deposits of alpha-synuclein in Lewy bodies colocalize with ubiquitin, which is the second major component of Lewy bodies. Ubiquitin is central to proteosome mediated protein degeneration [9]. Besides alpha-synuclein and ubiquitin, more than 70 other molecules have been found in Lewy bodies [10]. Lewy body alpha-synuclein develops an altered three dimensional structure. There is a direct intermolecular interaction between ubiquitin and the N-terminus of alpha-synuclein in Lewy bodies, which undergoes ubiquitination [11]. In order to eliminate the effects of alpha-synuclein, alpha-synuclein is broken down by ubiquitination by a series of three biochemical reactions, via the enzymes E1 ubiquitin-activating enzyme [12-15], E2 ubiquitin-conjugating enzyme [16-20], and RING-type E3 ubiquitin transferase [21-25].

FIRST STEP

enzyme name : E1 ubiquitin-activating enzyme
enzyme classification : EC 6.2.1.45
substrate : ubiquitin + E1 - L-cysteine + ATP
product : S-ubiquitinyl-E1-L-cysteine + AMP + PPi

SECOND STEP

enzyme name : E2 ubiquitin-conjugating enzyme
enzyme classification : EC 2.3.2.23
substrate : S-ubiquitinyl-E1-L-cysteine + E2-L-cysteine
product : S-ubiquitinyl-E2-L-cysteine + E1-L-cysteine

THIRD STEP

enzyme name : RING-type E3 ubiquitin transferase
enzyme classification : EC 2.3.2.27
substrate : S-ubiquitinyl-E2-L-cysteine + alpha-synuclein-L-lysine
product : N6-ubiquitinyl-[alpha-synuclein]-L-lysine + E2-L-cysteine

Page 181

[1] Journal of Neuropathology and Experimental Neurology [2015] 74 (12) : 1158-1169 (D.R.Jones, M.Delenclos, A.T.Baine, M.DeTure, M.E.Murray, D.W.Dickson, P.J.McLean)

[2] JAMA Neurology [2013] 70 (11) : 1396-1402 (R.Savica, B.R. Grossardt, J.H.Bower, B.F.Boeve, J.E.Ahlskog, W.A.Rocca)

[3] Journal of Neuropathology and Experimental Neurology [2006] 65 (4) : 387-395 (H.Uchikado, A.DelleDonne, Z.Ahmed, D.W.Dickson)

[4] Annals Neurology [2012] 71 (2) : 258-266 (A.S.Buchman, J.M. Shulman, S.Nag, S.E.Leurgans, S.E.Arnold, M.C.Morris, J.A. Schneider, D.A.Bennett)

[5] Neurobiology of Aging [2011] 32 (5) : 857-863 (R.Frigerio, H. Fujishiro, T.B.Ahn, K.A.Josephs, D.M.Maraganore, A.DelleDonne, J.E.Parisi, K.J.Klos, B.F.Boeve, D.W.Dickson, J.E.Ahlskog)

[6] Neuropathology and Applied Neurobiology [2016] 42 (1) : 77-94 (A.Bellucci, N.B.Mercuri, A.Venneri, G.Faustini, F.Longhena, M. Pizzi, C.Missale, P.Spano)

[7] Protein Journal [2015] 34 (4) : 291-303 (M.Khalife, D.Morshedi, F.Aliakbari, A.Tayaranian Marvian, H.Mohammad Beigi, S.Azimzadeh Jamalkandi, F.Pan-Montojo)

[8] Journal of Neural Transmission [2014] 121 (2) : 171-181 (R.A. Armstrong, P.T.Kotzbauer, J.S.Perlmutter, M.C.Campbell, K.M.Hurth, R.E.Schmidt, N.J.Cairns)

[9] Neurotoxicity Research [2011] 19 (4) : 592-602 (R.E.Musgrove, A.E.King, T.C.Dickson)

[10] Neuropathology [2007] 27 (5) : 494-506 (K.Wakabayashi, K. Tanji, F.Mori, H.Takahashi)

[11] Acta Neuropatholigica [2001] 102 (4) : 329-334 (N.Sharma, P.J. McLean, H.Kawamata, M.C.Irizarry, B.T.Hyman)

[12] Journal of Biological Chemistry [1982] 257 : 2543-2548 (A.L. Haas, J.V.Warms, A.Hershko, L.A.Rose)

[13] Journal of Biological Chemistry [2007] 282 : 37454-37460 (J.T. Huzil, R.Pannu, C.Ptak, G. Garen, M.J. Ellison)

[14] Molecular Biology Reports [2010] 37 : 1413- 1419 (M.Zheng, J.Liu, Z.Yang, X.Gu, F.Li, T.Lou, C.Ji, Y.Mao)

[15] Molecular Biotechnology [2012] 51 : 254-261 (A.F.Carvalho, M.P.Pinto, C.P.Grou, R.Vitorino, P.Domingues, F.Yamao, C.Sa-Miranda, J.E.Azevedo)

[16] FASEB Journal [2010] 24 : 981-993 (S.J.Van Wijk, H.T.Timmers)

[17] Journal of Biological Chemistry [2010] 285 : 8595-8604 (Y.David, T. Ziv, A.Admon, A.Navon)

[18] PLoS One 7 [2012] e40786 (E.Papaleo, N.Casiraghi, A.Arrigoni, M.Vanoni, P.Coccetti, L.De Gioia)

[19] Biochemical Journal [2012] 445 : 167-174 (B.W.Cook, G.S.Shaw)

[20] Acta Crystallographica (Section F) [2013] 69 : 153-157 (D.F.Li, L.Feng, Y. J.Hou, W.Liu)

[21] FEBS Letters [2008)] 582 : 4143-4146 (F.Eisele, D.H.Wolf)

[22] Journal of Cell Science [2012] 125 : 531-537 (M.B.Metzger, V.A. Hristova, A.M.Weissman)

[23] Nature [2012] 489 : 115-120 (A.Plechanovova, E.G.Jaffray, M.H. Tatham, J.H.Naismith, R.T.Hay)

[24] Molecular Cell [2012] 47 : 933-942 (J.N.Pruneda, P.J.Littlefield, S.E.Soss, K.A.Nordquist, W.J.Chazin, P.S.Brzovic, R.E.Klevit)

[25] Biochimica et Biophysica Acta [2014] 1843 : 47-60 (M.B. Metzger, J.N.Pruneda, R.E.Klevit, A.M.Weissman)

CHAPTER 14

ANATOMY OF PARKINSON'S DISEASE

DOPAMINERGIC NEURONAL GROUPS

DOPAMINERGIC NEURONAL GROUPS

The term dopaminergic neuronal groups refers to collections of neurons in the central nervous system that have been found to contain dopamine. Ten dopaminergic neuronal groups have been recognised. They are classified as groups A8 to A17. The cell aggregations (A8, A9 and A10) are in the mesenchephalon [1]. The cell aggregations (A11, A12, A13 and A14) are in the diencephalon [2, 3]. A single group of dopaminergic neurons (A15) has been found in the hypothalamus [4, 5]. A single group of dopaminergic neurons (A16) has been found in the olfactory bulb [6]. A single group of dopaminergic neurons (A17) has been found in the retina [7].

MESENCEPHALON

The mesencephalon (the midbrain) comprises the tectum (corpora quadrigemina), the tegmentum, the cerebral aqueduct (ventricular mesocoelia), the cerebral peduncles, and several nuclei and fasciculi. It is near the centre of the brain, below the cerebral cortex and above the hindbrain. Prominent cell groups of the mesencephalon include the motor nuclei of the trochlear and oculomotor nerves, the red nucleus, and the substantia nigra. Three dopaminergic cell aggregations (A8, A9 and A10) are in the mesenchephalon. They are the main dopaminergic neuronal groups [1].

GROUP A8

Group A8, which is part of the mesencephalic reticular formation, is located in the retrorubral field [1]. It is also known as the substantia nigra pars lateralis [8].

GROUP A9

Group A9, which is part of the mesencephalic reticular formation, is located in the substantia nigra [1]. Group A9 constitutes the whole of the substantia nigra pars compacta [9].

GROUP A10

Group A10 is part of the mesencephalic reticular formation. Group 10 is located in the ventral tegmental area [1], the nucleus paranigralis, the interfascicular nucleus, and the central linear nucleus [10, 11].

DIENCEPHALON

Five dopaminergic cell aggregations (A11, A12, A13, A14 and A15) are in the diencephalon. Groups A11, 13 and 14 are considered together since their axons are relatively short and remain within the confines of the diencephalon. The diencephalon is part of the prosencephalon (forebrain), which develops from the foremost primary cerebral vesicle. The prosencephalon differentiates into a caudal diencephalon and rostral telencephalon. The cerebral hemispheres develop from the sides of the telencephalon, each containing a lateral ventricle. The diencephalon consists of structures that are lateral to the third ventricle, and include the thalamus, the hypothalamus, the epithalamus and the subthalamus.

GROUP A11

Group A11, which is part of the diencephalic reticular formation [2], is in the periventricular grey matter of the caudal thalamus [12] and the posterior hypothalamic area [13].

GROUP A12

Group A12, which is part of the diencephalic reticular formation [2], includes the tuberoinfundibular (arcuate) nucleus [14] and the dorsal arcuate region, which are in the hypothalamus [15].

GROUP A13

Group A13, which is part of the diencephalic reticular formation [3], is a small group of dopaminergic neurons that is located in the zona incerta, which is in the subthalamus [16].

GROUP A14

Group A14, which is part of the diencephalic reticular formation [2], is a group of neurons located in the periventricular nucleus of the hypothalamus [17].

GROUP A15

Group A15, is a single group of neurons in the hypothalamus. It is located in ventral and dorsal components of the preoptic periventricular nucleus and adjacent parts of the anterior hypothalamic region [4, 5].

OLFACTORY BULB

A single group of dopaminergic neurons (A16) has been found in the olfactory bulb, which is located in the forebrain. The olfactory bulb receives neural input about odours detected by cells in the nasal cavity. The axons of olfactory receptor cells extend directly into the olfactory bulb where the information concerning odours is processed.

GROUP A16

Dopaminergic neurons (A16) have been found in the olfactory bulb. The majority of the dopaminergic neurons are distributed in the glomerular layer of the olfactory bulb [6].

RETINA

A single group of dopaminergic neurons (A17) has been found in the retina [7]. The retina is the innermost of the three coats of the eye, surrounding the vitreous body and continuous posteriorly with the optic nerve. The retina is composed of light-sensitive neurons arranged in three layers. The first layer is made up of rods and cones. The other two layers transmit impulses from the rods and cones to the optic nerve. The rods are sensitive in dim light. The cones are sensitive in bright light and are responsible for colour vision. In the middle of the retina is the fovea centralis, which is the centre of the eye's sharpest vision and the location of most colour perception.

GROUP A17

Dopaminergic neurons (A17) are also found outside the brain, in the retina. The majority of the dopaminergic neurons in the retina are distributed in the proximal inner nuclear layer and the upper part of inner plexiform layer of the retina. They are characterised with the appearance of amacrine cells [7].

[1] Brain Structure and Function [2012] 217 (2) : 591-612 (Y.Fu, Y.Yuan, G.Halliday, Z.Rusznák, C.Watson, G.Paxinos)

[2] Brain Behavior and Evolution [2004] 64 (1) : 42-60 (P.R. Manger, K.Fuxe, S.H.Ridgway, J.M.Siegel)

[3] Journal of Neuroscience [1994] 14 (8) : 4903-4914 (D.Lorang, S.G.Amara, R.B.Simerly)

[4] Acta Physiologica Scandinavica Supplement [1977] 452 : 31-34 (A.Ljungdahl, T.Hökfelt, N.Halasz, O.Johansson, M.Goldstein)

[5] Histology and Histopathology [1998] 13 (4) : 1163-1177 (Y.Tillet, K.Kitahama)

[6] Brain Research [1999] 842 (2) : 491-495 (T.Hida, Y.Hasegawa, R.Arai)

[7] Brain Research [2000] 885 (1) : 122-127 (L.W.Chen, L.C.Wei, H.L. Liu, L.Duan, G.Ju, Y.S.Chan)

[8] Neuroreport [1994] 5 (4) : 429-432 (J.L.Venero, K.D.Beck, F. Hefti)

[9] Journal of Chemical Neuroanatomy [2016] Feb 6 [Epub ahead of print] (Y.Fu, G.Paxinos, C.Watson, G.M.Halliday)

[10] Brain Research [1998] 780 (1) : 148-152 (L.W.Chen, Z.L.Guan, Y.Q.Ding)

[11] Neuroscience [1996] 75 (2) : 523-533 (C.L.Liang, C.M.Sinton, D.C.German)

[12] Brain Research [1999] 842 (2) : 491-495 (T.Hida, Y.Hasegawa, R.Arai)

[13] Brain Research Bulletin [1993] 30 (5-6) : 551-559 (C.Yokoyama, H.Okamura, Y.Ibata)

[14] Journal of Chemical Neuroanatomy [1998] 16 (1) : 43-55 (K. Kitahama, K.Ikemoto, A.Jouvet, I.Nagatsu, N.Sakamoto, J.Pearson)

[15] Endocrinology [1992] 131 (1) : 509-517 (S.G.Kohama, F.Freesh, C.L.Bethea)

[16] Cell Reports [2015] 13 (5) : 1003-1015 (A.D.Bolton, Y.Murata, R.Kirchner, S.Y.Kim, A.Young, T.Dang, Y.Yanagawa, M.Constantine-Paton)

[17] Brain Research - Developmental Brain Research [2001] 126 (1) : 21-30 (G.P.Demyanenko, Y.Shibata, P.F.Maness)

CHAPTER 15

ANATOMY OF PARKINSON'S DISEASE

ANATOMICAL EFFECTS

Anatomical effects

Most of the anatomical effects in Parkinson's Disease originate from the insufficient formation of dopamine. When there is insufficient dopamine, there is often an effect on each of the anatomical structures that dopamine normally stimulates via the various dopaminergic pathways.

Nervous system

The dopaminergic neurons are one of only four cell types that can not reproduce in adults. However, when compared to people of a similar age, there is hardly any difference in the number of dopaminergic neurons in people with Parkinson's Disease [1]. There is also no difference in the volume of the relevant part of the brain either [1]. The volume of the part of the brain in which dopaminergic neurons are common does not decline as Parkinson's Disease gets worse as it would if there was a loss of these cells. People with Parkinson's Disease do not differ in this way from those people who do not have Parkinson's Disease [2].

Although it is often claimed that there is a massive loss of the dopaminergic neurons in Parkinson's Disease, no studies have ever shown this to be true. Studies making such claims have measured the enzyme activity of the dopaminergic neurons instead of the loss of the dopaminergic neurons [3]. Enzyme activity determines the activity of the cells not the number of cells. Research has always shown that there is a major reduction in cell activity in people with Parkinson's Disease rather than an actual major loss of the cells involved in Parkinson's Disease.

[1] Movement Disorders [2005] 20 (2) : 164-171 (K.M.Pedersen, L. Marner, H.Pakkenberg, B.Pakkenberg)

[2] JAMA Neurology [2013] 70 (2) : 241-247 (D.A.Ziegler, J.S. Wonderlick, P.Ashourian, L.A.Hansen, J.C.Young, A.J. Murphy, C.K. Koppuzha, J.H.Growdon, S.Corkin)

[3] Brain [2013] 136 (Part 8) : 2419-2431 (J.H.Kordower, C.W. Olanow, H.B.Dodiya, Y.Chu, T.G.Beach, C.H.Adler, G.M.Halliday, R. T.Bartus)

Muscular system

Muscle changes that occur during in Parkinson's Disease can occur as a consequence of the modified pattern of motor unit activation and rigidity, which are characteristic of Parkinson's Disease.

In people with Parkinson's Disease there is a tendency towards hypertrophy of type I muscle fibers and, in some instances, the atrophy of type II muscle fibers. Muscle modifications can be evaluated by measuring muscle fiber conduction velocity (CV) and median frequency (MDF). The main difference observed in people with Parkinson's Disease is the rate of conduction velocity (CV) and median frequency (MDF) during muscle contraction. People with Parkinson's Disease sustained a smaller fatigue related decrease in both parameters. The conduction velocity (CV) is directly related to the type I fiber diameter [1].

[1] Electroencephalography and Clinical Neurophysiology [1996] 101 (3) : 211-218 (B.Rossi, G.Siciliano, M.C.Carboncini, M.L.Manca, R. Massetani, P.Viacava, A.Muratorio)

Alimentary system

Pharyngeal sensation normally triggers the swallowing reflex. Pharyngeal sensory nerves are directly affected by pathologic processes in Parkinson's Disease. These abnormalities may decrease pharyngeal sensation, thereby impairing swallowing and airway protective reflexes and contributing to dysphagia and aspiration [1]. Gastrointestinal motility, which is the function of gastrointestinal smooth muscle, is controlled by both the intrinsic and extrinsic nerves of the gastrointestinal tract. Parkinson's Disease causes enteric nerve dysfunction, which at its worst can cause functional obstruction of the gastrointestinal tract [2].

[1] Journal of Neuropathology and Experimental Neurology [2013] 72 (7) : 614-623 (L.Mu, S.Sobotka, J.Chen, H.Su, I.Sanders, T.Nyirenda, C.H.Adler, H.A.Shill, J.N.Caviness, J.E.Samanta, L.I.Sue, T.G.Beach)

[2] American Journal of the Medical Sciences [1991] 301 (3) : 201-214 (S.Chokhavatia, S.Anuras)

Urinary system

Bladder capacity is reduced in both men and women with Parkinson's Disease in comparison with similar people without neurological disease [1, 2] in about half of people with Parkinson's Disease [3]. Bladder capacity was most noticeably decreased in the progressive cases of Parkinson's Disease [2].

The bladder is a muscular organ. Consequently the bladder could be reduced in its capacity because of the excessive muscular contraction that occurs in Parkinson's Disease. Consistent with this, bladder capacity increases in response to dopaminergic treatment [4].

[1] Age and Ageing [1995] 24 (6) : 499-504 (R.Gray, G.Stern, J. Malone-Lee)

[2] Hinyokika Kiyo [1993] 39 (6) : 523-528 (A.Wakatsuki, M. Tsujihata, O.Miyake, H.Ito, H.Itatani, F.Udaka)

[3] Japanese Journal of Psychiatry and Neurology [1992] 46 (1) : 181-186 (T.Hattori, K.Yasuda, K.Kita, K.Hirayama)

[4] Neurourology and Urodynamics [2004] 23 (7) : 689-696 (K.Winge, L.M.Werdelin, K.K.Nielsen, H.Stimpel)

Cardiovascular system

There is a cardiovascular dysfunction, which occurs solely in people with Parkinson's Disease, that the researchers describe as "Parkinsonian Heart". Parkinsonian Heart is characterised by a severe loss of the physiological noradrenergic innervation and a slight impairment of central autonomic control of the heart. Both of these prevent the heart's proper functioning [1]. The capillaries of people with Parkinson's Disease are less in number, shorter in length, and larger in diameter [2].

[1] Current Medicinal Chemistry [2007] 14 (23) : 2421-2428 (F. Fornai, R.Ruffoli, P.Soldani, S.Ruggieri, A.Paparelli)

[2] Brain Pathology [2013] 23 (2) : 154-164 (J.Guan, D.Pavlovic, N. Dalkie, H.J.Waldvogel, S.J.O'Carroll, C.R.Green, L.F.Nicholson)

Respiratory system

Over 25% of people with Parkinson's Disease have reduced total lung capacity down to less than 85% of normal. The majority of people with Parkinson's Disease had upper airway obstruction. Bradykinesia was higher in people with upper airway obstruction [1].

[1] Journal of Neurological Science [1996] 138 (1-2) : 114-119 (M.Sabaté, I.González, F.Ruperez, M.Rodríguez)

Skeletal system

In about a third of people with Parkinson's Disease there is a curvature and rotation of the spine. The deviation of the spine can be ten degrees or more [1]. It is seven times more likely in women than it is in men [2]. The excessive muscle contraction that occurs in Parkinson's Disease can cause the upper body to bend towards one side rather than the other [2]. Around 28% of people with Parkinson's Disease had cervical positive sagittal malalignment (CPSM), which was more common in males and in more severe Parkinson's Disease [3].

[1] Journal of Neurology, Neurosurgery and Psychiatry [2013] 84 (12) : 1400-1403 (K.M.Doherty, I.Davagnanam, S.Molloy, L.Silveira-Moriyama, A.J.Lees)

[2] Journal of Clinical Neurology [2009] 5 (2) : 91-94 (J.S.Baik, J.Y. Kim, J.H.Park, S.W.Han, J.H.Park, M.S.Lee)

[3] Journal of Neurosurgery - Spine [2016] 24 (4) : 527-534 (B.J.Moon, J.S.Smith, C.P.Ames, C.I.Shaffrey, V.Lafage, F.Schwab, M. Matsumoto, J.S.Baik, Y.Ha)

Integumentary system

In people with Parkinson's Disease the skin is more prone to being wrinkled when assessed using skin response tests. This is not solely due to Parkinson's Disease more commonly occurring when people are older. It is primarily due to autonomic dysfunction, which can even occur in early Parkinson's Disease [1].

[1] Biomedicine and Pharmacotherapy [2001] 55 (8) : 475-478 (R. Djaldetti, E.Melamed, N.Gadoth)

Reproductive system

Although the volume of the prostate gland is greater in men with Parkinson's Disease when compared to men of a similar age who do not have Parkinson's Disease, there is no significant difference in volume [1]. Both unilateral and bilateral oophorectomy (removal of the ovaries) performed prior to menopause increases the risk of developing Parkinson's Disease. The risk increased with younger age at the time of the oophrectomy [2].

[1] Prostate International [2015] 3 (2) : 62-64 (Y.S.Shin, H.Choi, M.W.Cheon, S.C.Park, J.K.Park, H.J.Kim, Y.B.Jeong)

[2] Neurology [2008] 70 (3) : 200-209 (W.A.Rocca, J.H.Bower, D.M. Maraganore, J.E.Ahlskog, B.R.Grossardt, M.de Andrade, L.J.Melton)

ENDOCRINE SYSTEM

Dopamine regulates the secretion of melatonin from the pineal gland [1]. Melatonin regulates the circadian rhythms, which are alterations of functions of the endocrine system [2]. The neural structures controlling pineal function are especially the suprachiasmatic nuclei of the anterior hypothalamus. In Parkinson's Disease there is a significant reduction in the volume of the hypothalamus. Melatonin levels were significantly associated with hypothalamic grey matter volume [3].

[1] PLoS Biology [2012] 10 (6) : e1001347 (S.González, D.Moreno-Delgado, E.Moreno, K.Pérez-Capote, R.Franco, J.Mallol, A.Cortés, V. Casadó, C.Lluís, J.Ortiz, S.Ferré, E.Canela, P.J.McCormick)

[2] JAMA Neurology [2014] 71 (4) : 463-469 (A.Videnovic, C.Noble, K.J.Reid, J.Peng, F.W.Turek, A.Marconi, A.W. Rademaker, T.Simuni, C.Zadikoff, P.C.Zee)

[3] Movement Disorders [2016] Mar 12 [Epub ahead of print] (D.P. Breen, C.Nombela, R.Vuono, P.S.Jones, K.Fisher, D.J.Burn, D.J. Brooks, A.B.Reddy, J.B.Rowe, R.A.Barker)

SENSORY SYSTEM

OLFACTORY SYSTEM

Overall, the left and the right olfactory bulb volumes are significantly reduced in people with Parkinson's Disease [1-5] but this did not always occur [6-9]. A difference in the lateralised olfactory bulb also occurs in Parkinson's Disease, indicating a larger right olfactory bulb than left olfactory bulb volume. This did not occur in those people assessed who did not have Parkinson's Disease [1, 10]. The reduced height of the left olfactory bulb is the most reliable indicator of the reduction in olfactory bulb volume [2]. The volume of the olfactory sulcus is also reduced in people with Parkinson's Disease in some [10], but not all cases [3]. There is a greater number of dopaminergic neurons when compared to people of a similar age, which might occur as a compensatory mechanism [9].

[1] PLoS One [2016] 11 (2) : e0149286 (J.Li, C.Z.Gu, J.B.Su, L.H. Zhu, Y.Zhou, H.Y.Huang, C.F.Liu)

[2] Movement Disorders [2012] 27 (8) : 1019-1025 (S.Brodoehl, C.Klingner, G.F.Volk, T.Bitter, O.W.Witte, C.Redecker)

[3] Zhonghua Er Bi Yan Hou Tou Jing Wai Ke Za Zhi [2015] 50 (1) : 20-24 (W.Hang, G.Liu, T.Han, P.Zhang, J.Zhang)

[4] Parkinsonism & Related Disorders [2015] 21 (7) : 771-777 (R. Sengoku, S.Matsushima, K.Bono, K.Sakuta, M.Yamazaki, S. Miyagawa, T.Komatsu, H.Mitsumura, Y.Kono, T.Kamiyama, et al)

[5] European Journal of Radiology [2014] 83 (3) : 564-570 (S.Chen, H.Y.Tan, Z.H.Wu, C.P.Sun, J.X.He, X.C.Li, M.Shao)

[6] European Journal of Neurology [2015] 22 (7) : 1068-1073 (L. Paschen, N.Schmidt, S.Wolff, C.Cnyrim, T.van Eimeren, K.E. Zeuner, G.Deuschl, K.Witt)

[7] European Review for Medical and Pharmacological Sciences [2014] 18 (23) : 3659-3664 (S.Altinayar, S.Oner, S.Can, A.Kizilay, S.Kamisli, K.Sarac)

[8] Journal of Clinical Neuroscience [2013] 20 (10) : 1469-1470 (H.A.Hakyemez, B.Veyseller, F.Ozer, S.Ozben, G.I.Bayraktar, D. Gurbuz, S.Cetin, Y.S.Yildirim)

[9] Acta Neuropathologica [2011] 122 (1) : 61-74 (I.C.Mundiñano, M.C.Caballero, C.Ordóñez, M.Hernandez, C.DiCaudo, I.Marcilla, M.E. Erro, M.T.Tuñon, M.R.Luquin)

[10] Neuroscience Letters [2016] 620 : 111-114 (N.Tanik, H.I.Serin, A.Celikbilek, L.E.Inan, F.Gundogdu)

VISUAL SYSTEM

The thickness of the retina is different in people with advanced Parkinson's Disease [1]. The inner retinal layer is significantly thinner in people with Parkinson's Disease [2-7], but not always [8]. The thickness of the outer retinal layer in Parkinson's Disease was no different [4]. There is reduced dopaminergic activity in the retina of people with Parkinson's Disease [2, 3, 9, 10, 11], which could lead to a reduction in the size of the retina.

[1] Retina [2014] 34 (5) : 971-980 (E.Garcia-Martin, M.Satue, S. Otin, I.Fuertes, R.Alarcia, J.M.Larrosa, V.Polo, L.E.Pablo)

[2] Journal of Neuro-Ophthalmology [2013] 33 (1) : 62-65 (S.Kirbas, K.Turkyilmaz, A.Tufekci, M.Durmus)

[3] Vision Research [2004] 44 (24) : 2793-2797 (R.Inzelberg, J.A. Ramirez, P.Nisipeanu, A.Ophir)

[4] Archives of Ophthalmology [2009] 127 (6) : 737-741 (M.E.Hajee, W.F.March, D.R.Lazzaro, A.H.Wolintz, E.M.Shrier, S.Glazman, I.G. Bodis-Wollner)

[5] European Journal of Ophthalmology [2014] 24 (1) : 114-119 (A. Sen, B.Tugcu, C.Coskun, C.Ekinci, S.A.Nacaroglu)

[6] European Journal of Neurology [2013] 20 (1) : 198-201 (C.La Morgia, P.Barboni, G.Rizzo, M.Carbonelli, G.Savini, C.Scaglione, S. Capellari, S.Bonazza, M.P.Giannoccaro, G.Calandra-Buonaura, et al)

[7] American Journal of Ophthalmology [2014] 157 (2) : 470-478 (E. Garcia-Martin, J.M.Larrosa, V.Polo, M.Satue, M.L.Marques), R. Alarcia, M.Seral, I.Fuertes, S.Otin, L.E.Pablo)

[8] Parkinsonism & Related Disorders [2011] 17 (6) : 431-436 (N.K. Archibald, M.P.Clarke, U.P.Mosimann, D.J.Burn)

[9] Journal of Parkinson's Disease [2014] 4 (2) : 197-204 (J.Y.Lee, J.Ahn, T.W.Kim, B.S.Jeon)

[10] Neurology Clinical Practice [2003] 21 (3) : 709-728 (G.R. Jackson, C.Owsley)

[11] Surgical and Radiologic Anatomy [1988] 10 (2) : 137-144 (J. Nguyen-Legros)

AUDITORY SYSTEM

Hearing is perceived in the Cochlea, in the Organ of Corti, which is the sensory organ of hearing. Dopamine helps to protect against noise exposure in the Cochlea [1-4]. Therefore, the insufficient dopamine that occurs in Parkinson's Disease can therefore lead to damage of the Cochlea.

[1] Neurochemical International [2011] 59 (2) : 150-158 (B.Lendvai, G.B.Halmos, G.Polony, J.Kapocsi, T.Horváth, M.Aller, E.Sylvester Vizi, T.Zelles)

[2] Advances in to Oto-Rhino-Laryngology [2002] 59 : 131-139 (E. Oestreicher, A.Wolfgang, D.Felix)

[3] European Journal of Neuroscience [2001] 14 (6) : 977-986 (J.Ruel, R.Nouvian, C.Gervais d'Aldin, R.Pujol, M.Eybalin, J.L.Puel)

[4] Progress in Neurobiology [1995] 47 (6) : 449-476 (J.L.Puel)

GUSTATORY SYSTEM

The fungiform papillae are innervated projections on the upper surface of the tongue. They have taste buds on their upper surface. In a number of neurological disorders there is a decrease in fungiform papillae. It is uncertain as to whether or not the decrease in taste that often occurs in Parkinson's Disease is accompanied by a reduction in fungiform papillae [1].

[1] The Neuroscientist [2008] 14 (3) : 240-250 (J.Gardiner, D.Barton, J.M.Vanslambrouck, F.Braet, D.Hall, J.Marc, R.Overall)

IMMUNE SYSTEM

The blood-brain barrier is a tightly regulated interface in the Central Nervous System that regulates the exchange of molecules in and out from the brain. It is mainly composed of endothelial cells, pericytes and astrocytes [1]. During the course of Parkinson's Disease there is dysfunction of the blood-brain barrier [1]. There is increased permeability of the blood-brain barrier [2, 3], which more specifically is in the postcommissural putamen in people who have Parkinson's Disease [3]. There are alterations in the tight junction, transport and endothelial cell surface proteins, and vascular density changes, all of which result in altered permeability of the blood-brain barrier [4].

[1] Journal of Cerebral Blood Flow and Metabolism [2015] 35 (5) : 747-750 (M.T.Gray, J.M.Woulfe)

[2] Neurodegenerative Disease [2015] 15 (2) : 63-69 (M.Fakhoury)

[3] Frontiers in Cellular Neuroscience [2014] 8 : 211 (R.Cabezas, M.Avila, J.Gonzalez, R.S.El-Bachá, E.Báez, L.M.García-Segura, J.C. Jurado Coronel, F.Capani, G.P.Cardona-Gomez, G.E.Barreto)

[4] Cell Transplantation [2007] 16 (3) : 285-99 (B.S.Desai, A.J. Monahan, P.M.Carvey, B.Hendey)

CHAPTER 16

PHYSIOLOGY OF PARKINSON'S DISEASE

DOPAMINERGIC PATHWAYS

DOPAMINERGIC PATHWAYS

Dopaminergic pathways, which are sometimes called dopaminergic projections, are neural pathways in the brain that transmit dopamine from one region of the brain to another. The neurons of the dopaminergic pathways have axons that run the entire length of the pathway. The major dopaminergic pathways in the brain are : the nigrostriatal pathway, the mesocortical pathway, the mesolimbic pathway, the tuberoinfundibular pathway, the diencephalospinal pathway, the incertohypothalamic pathway, neuroendocrine pathways, the olfactory pathway, and the visual pathway.

NIGROSTRIATAL PATHWAY

Pathway : In the substantia nigra, A9 dopaminergic neurons form the nigrostriatal pathway [1]. The functional activity of the nigrostriatal pathway is also modulated by A8 dopaminergic neurons [2]. The nigrostriatal pathway transmits dopamine from the substantia nigra pars compacta (SNc), which is located in the midbrain, to the caudate nucleus and putamen, which are located in the dorsal striatum [3].

Functions : The primary effect of the dopaminergic neurons via the nigrostriatal pathway is the maintenance of muscle tone in skeletal muscles by reducing muscle contraction [4, 5, 6]. The nigrostriatal pathway is necessary for efficient motor performance [6, 7]. Dopamine, via the nigrostriatal pathway, also acts on smooth muscle [8, 9].

[1] Proceedings, National Academy of Sciences, U.S.A. [2009] 106 (36) : 15454-15459 (M.Biagioli, M.Pinto, D.Cesselli, M.Zaninello, D. Lazarevic, P.Roncaglia, R.Simone, C.Vlachouli, C.Plessy, et al)

[2] Annals of the New York Academy of Sciences [1988] 537 : 27-50 (A.Y.Deutch, M.Goldstein, F.Baldino Jr, R.H.Roth)

[3] Movement Disorders [2015] 30 (9) : 1229-1236 (Y.Zhang, I.W. Wu, S.Buckley, C.S.Coffey, E.Foster, S.Mendick, J.Seibyl, N.Schuff)

[4] Clinical and Experimental Pharmacology and Physiology [1995] 22 (11) : 846-850 (A.D.Crocker)

[5] Journal of Neural Transmission [2010] 117 (12) : 1359-1369 (A. Korchounov, M.F.Meyer, M.Krasnianski)

[6] Reviews in the Neurosciences [1997] 8 (1) : 55-76 (A.D.Crocker)

[7] Biochemical Society Transactions [2007] 35 (Part 2) : 428-432 (E. Dowd, S.B.Dunnett)

[8] Journal of Pharmacology and Experimental Therapeutics [2016] 356 (2) : 434-444 (M.Fornai, C.Pellegrini, L.Antonioli, C.Segnani, C. Ippolito, E.Barocelli, V.Ballabeni, G.Vegezzi, Z.Al Harraq, et al)

[9] Neurourology and Urodynamics [2009] 28 (6) : 549-554 (T. Yamamoto, R.Sakakibara, K.Nakazawa, T.Uchiyama, E.Shimizu, T. Hattori)

Mesolimbic pathway

Pathway : In the ventral tegmental area (VTA), A10 dopaminergic neurons form the mesolimbic pathway [1, 2]. Functional activity of the mesolimbic pathway is also modulated by A8 dopaminergic neurons [3]. The mesolimbic pathway transmits dopamine form the ventral tegmental area (VTA), which is located in the midbrain, to the nucleus accumbens, which is located in the ventral striatum [4, 5].

Functions : The primary effect of dopamine in the nucleus accumbens is motivation. Dopamine release in the nucleus accumbens varies in accordance with reward rate and motivation. Changing dopamine immediately alters willingness to make effort and reinforces preceding action choices. Dopamine conveys the available reward for the investment of effort, which is employed for motivational functions [6].

[1] Proceedings, National Academy of Sciences, U.S.A. [2009] 106 (36) : 15454-15459 (M.Biagioli, M.Pinto, D.Cesselli, M.Zaninello, D. Lazarevic, P.Roncaglia, R.Simone, C.Vlachouli, C.Plessy, et al)

[2] Neuroscience Letters [1992] 139 (1) : 73-76 (M.Yoshida, H.Yokoo, K.Mizoguchi, H.Kawahara, A.Tsuda, T.Nishikawa, M.Tanaka)

[3] Annals of the New York Academy of Sciences [1988] 537 : 27-50 (A.Y.Deutch, M.Goldstein, F.Baldino Jr, R.H.Roth)

[4] Behavioural Brain Research [2015] 292 : 508-514 (M.Moradi, M.Yazdanian, A.Haghparast)

[5] Schizophrenia Bulletin [2015] 41 (1) : 291-299 (B.Rolland, A. Amad, E.Poulet, R.Bordet, A.Vignaud, R.Bation, C.Delmaire, P. Thomas, O.Cottencin, R.Jardri)

[6] Nature Neuroscience [2016] 19 (1) : 117-126 (A.A.Hamid, J.R. Pettibone, O.S.Mabrouk, V.L.Hetrick, R.Schmidt, C.M.Vander Weele, R.T.Kennedy, B.J.Aragona, J.D.Berke)

Mesocortical pathway

Pathway : The ventral tegmental area contains the A10 dopaminergic neurons [1]. The mesocortical pathway transmits dopamine from the ventral tegmental area (VTA), which is located in the midbrain, to the neurons of the prefrontal cortex (PFC). The prefrontal cortex is the part of the cerebral cortex that covers the front part of the frontal lobe [2, 3, 4].

Functions : The mesocortical pathway is associated with emotional responsiveness and the capacity for emotional arousal. The prefrontal cortex is known to play an important role in the regulation of emotion responses [5]. Emotion regulation enables the initiation of new emotional responses or the alteration of ongoing emotional responses. The emotional regulation can be voluntary or learned [6].

[1] Brain Research [1987] 434 (2) : 117-165 (R.D.Oades, G.M. Halliday)

[2] Psychopharmacology [2016] Apr 30 [Epub ahead of print] (G. Giannotti, L.Caffino, F.Mottarlini, G.Racagni, F.Fumagalli)

[3] Cerebral Cortex [2012] 22 (2) : 327-336 (N.Gorelova, P.J. Mulholland, L.J.Chandler, J.K.Seamans)

[4] Neuroreport [1996] 7 (8) : 1437-1441 (S.Pirot, J.Glowinski, A.M. Thierry)

[5] Stress [2004] 7 (2) : 131-143 (R.M.Sullivan)

[6] The effects of prefrontal cortex damage on the regulation of emotion [2009] (David Matthew Driscoll)

TUBEROINFUNDIBULAR PATHWAY

Pathway : A12 and A14 dopaminergic neurons [1, 2, 3] form the tuberoinfundibular pathway. The tuberoinfundibular pathway transmits dopamine from the dopaminergic neurons in the hypothalamus (in the arcuate nucleus and the periventricular mucleus), which forms the ventral part of the diencephalon, to the pituitary gland, which is one of the endocrine glands [1].

Functions : The hypothalamic control of prolactin secretion is different from other anterior pituitary hormones in that it is predominantly inhibitory. The function of dopamine that is transmitted from the dopaminergic neurons via the tuberoinfundibular pathway is to inhibit the secretion of prolactin from the pituitary gland. Prolactin has a broad range functions in the body [4].

[1] Neuroendocrinology [1986] 44 (1) : 95-101 (P.A.Rose, R.F.Weick)

[2] Journal of Endocrinology [2015] 226 (2) : T101-T122 (D.R. Grattan)

[3] Neuroendocrinology [1997] 65 (6) : 436-445 (A.Lerant, M.E. Freeman)

[4] Endocrinology [1996] 137 (9) : 3621-3628 (A.Lerant, M.E.Herman, M.E.Freeman)

Diencephalospinal pathway

Pathway : A11 dopaminergic neurons form the diencephalospinal pathway. The diencephalospinal pathway transmits dopamine from the dopaminergic neurons in the periventricular grey matter of the caudal thalamus and the posterior hypothalamic area to the spinal cord [1].

Functions : The A11 diencephalospinal pathway is essential for the modulation of the sensory and motor processes and pain control at the spinal cord level. Dopamine in the spinal cord contributes to spinal reflex excitability. Dopamine also activates spinal motor networks involved in locomotion [1].

[1] PLoS One [2010] 5 (10) : e13306 (Q.Barraud, I.Obeid, I.Aubert, G.Barrière, H.Contamin, S.McGuire, P.Ravenscroft, G.Porras, F. Tison, E.Bezard, I.Ghorayeb)

Incertohypothalamic pathway

Pathway : A13 dopaminergic neurons form the incertohypothalamic pathway. The incertohypothalamic pathway transmits dopamine from the dopaminergic neurons in the zona incerta, which is in the subthalamus, to the dorsolateral column of the periaqueductal gray, which is the grey matter located around the cerebral aqueduct within the tegmentum of the midbrain [1, 2].

Functions : The periaqueductal gray (PAG) (also known as the central gray) has enkephalin and endorphin producing cells. Consequently, the periaqueductal gray is the primary control centre for descending pain modulation, due to the ability of enkephalins and endorphins to suppress pain [3].

[1] Frontiers in Neuroanatomy [2013] 7 : 41 (F.Messanvi, E.Eggens-Meijer, B.Roozendaal, J.J.van der Want)

[2] Brain Research [1994] 659 (1-2) : 201-207 (M.J.Eaton, C.K. Wagner, K.E.Moore, K.J.Lookingland)

[3] Brain Research Bulletin [2006] 71 (1-3) : 193-199 (J.Yang, Y.Yang, H.T.Xu, J.M.Chen, W.Y.Liu, B.C.Lin)

NEUROENDOCRINE PATHWAYS

Pathway : Neuroendocrine pathways transmit dopamine from A15 dopaminergic neurons, which are located in the periventricular nucleus and adjacent parts of the anterior hypothalamic region [1, 2, 3], and A14 dopaminergic neurons, which are located in the periventricular nucleus of the hypothalamus [4], to the GnRH neurons in the hypothalamus.

Functions : The GnRH neurons produce Gonadotropin-releasing hormone (GnRH), which is also known as follicle-stimulating hormone releasing hormone (FSH-RH), and luteinizing hormone–releasing hormone (LHRH). GnRH is a releasing hormone responsible for the release of follicle-stimulating hormone (FSH) and luteinizing hormone (LH) from the anterior pituitary gland [5-8].

[1] European Journal of Neuroscience [2010] 32 (12) : 2152-2164 (M.N.Lehman, Z.Ladha, L.M.Coolen, S.M.Hileman, J.M.Connors, R.L. Goodman)

[2] Journal of Reproductivity and Fertility (Supplement) [1995] 49 : 285-296 (J.C.Thiéry, V.Gayrard, S.Le Corre, C.Viguié, G.B.Martin, P. Chemineau, B.Malpaux)

[3] Journal of Endocrinology [2010] 22 (7) : 674-681 (R.L.Goodman, H.T.Jansen, H.J.Billings, L.M.Coolen, M.N.Lehman)

[4] Journal of Endocrinology [1996] 148 (2) : 291-301 (S.K.Park, D.A. Strouse, M.Selmanoff)

[5] Bulletin of Mathematical Biology [2008] 70 (8) : 2211-2228 (R.Bertram, Y.X.Li)

[6] Proceedings, National Academy Sciences, U.S.A. [2005] 102 (5) : 1761-1766 (S.Messager, E.E.Chatzidaki, D.Ma, A.G.Hendrick, D. Zahn, J.Dixon, R.R.Thresher, I.Malinge, D.Lomet, et al)

[7] European Journal of Contraception and Reproductive Health Care [1998] 3 (1) : 21-28 (M.Stomati, A.D.Genazzani, F.Petraglia, A.R. Genazzani)

[8] Brain Research [1986] 399 (1) : 15-23. (K.Y.Pau, H.G.Spies)

OLFACTORY PATHWAY

Pathway : The olfactory bulb contains the A16 dopaminergic neurons [1]. The olfactory pathway transmits the stimulatory effects of olfaction. Stimulatory effects occur when odorant molecules bind to specific sites on the olfactory receptors to the olfactory bulb [2]. The olfactory receptors are in the cell membranes of olfactory receptor neurons.

Functions : The olfactory bulb has one source of sensory input, which are axons from olfactory receptor neurons of the olfactory epithelium. The olfactory bulb transmits information concerning odours to the brain, and is therefore necessary for a proper sense of smell. The olfactory bulb discriminates among odours, and enhances the sensitivity of odour detection [3].

[1] Brain Research [1999] 842 (2) : 491-495 (T.Hida, Y.Hasegawa, R. Arai)

[2] Neuroscience [1993] 52 (1) : 115-134 (H.Baker, A.I.Farbman)

[3] HNO [2014] 62 (12) : 846-852 (I.Manzini, J.Frasnelli, I.Croy)

VISUAL PATHWAY

Pathway : The retina contains the A17 dopaminergic neurons [1]. The visual pathway transmits the effects of dopamine from the retina, which is the inner coat of the eye. Light striking the retina initiates a cascade of chemical and electrical events that ultimately trigger nerve impulses. These are sent through the fibres of the optic nerve to the visual cortex [2, 3].

Functions : The visual cortex of the brain is the part of the cerebral cortex responsible for processing visual information. Dopamine mediates a wide variety of visual functions [4]. These functions include visual perception, colour perception, colour discrimination, contrast sensitivity, visual acuity, and darkness adaptation [5].

[1] Brain Research [2000] 885 (1) : 122-127 (L.W.Chen, L.C.Wei, H.L. Liu, L.Duan, G.Ju, Y.S.Chan)

[2] Fundamental and Clinical Pharmacology [1993] 7 (6) : 293-304 (P. Denis, J.P.Nordmann, P.P.Elena, M.Dussaillant, H.Saraux, P.Lapalus)

[3] Brain [2009] 132 : 1128-1145 (N.K.Archibald, M.P.Clarke, U.P. Mosimann, D.J.Burn)

[4] Neuroscience and Biobehavioral Review [2008] 32 (4) : 611-656 (R.Brandies, S.Yehuda)

[5] Frontiers in Psychology [2014] 5 : 1594 (A.J.Zele1, D.Cao)

CHAPTER 17

PHYSIOLOGY OF PARKINSON'S DISEASE

PHYSIOLOGICAL EFFECTS

Physiological effects

Most of the physiological effects in Parkinson's Disease are due to the insufficient formation of dopamine. When there is insufficient dopamine, there is a reduction in each of the physiological functions that dopamine normally stimulates via the various dopaminergic pathways.

Muscular system

The muscular system includes skeletal, smooth muscles and cardiac muscles. Skeletal muscles are attached to the skeleton. The skeletal muscles enable movement of the body and the maintenance of posture.

The primary dopaminergic effect via the nigrostriatal pathway is the reduction of muscle contraction in the skeletal and smooth muscles. Consequently, reduced dopaminergic stimulation, as occurs in Parkinson's Disease, causes excessive contraction of the skeletal and smooth muscles.

Acetylcholine affects muscle contraction via the five cholinergic receptors : m1, m2, m3, m4, and m5. The receptors m1, m3 and m5 are stimulatory. The receptors m2 and m4 are inhibitory. The combined stimulatory effect of m1, m3 and m5 is more powerful in total than the combined inhibitory effect of m2 and m4. So the overall effect of acetylcholine is to stimulate muscle contraction.

Dopamine affects muscle contraction via the five dopamine receptors : D1, D2, D3, D4, and D5. The receptors D2, D3 and D4 are inhibitory. The receptors D1 and D5 are stimulatory. The combined inhibitory effect of D2, D3 and D4 is more powerful in total than the combined stimulatory effect of D1 and D5. In the cholinergic neurons this causes an inhibition of the release of acetylcholine. So when there is insufficient formation of dopamine, as occurs in Parkinson's Disease, the cholinergic neurons are not inhibited. As acetylcholine stimulates muscle contraction this can lead to excessive muscle contraction.

In Parkinson's Disease there is increased muscle contraction : of the neck muscles, including the anterior neck muscles [1], of the leg muscles including those of gastrocnemius medialis and tibialis anterior [2], of the trunk, including the paravertebral muscles [3, 4], of the arm muscles, including those of brachioradialis and the biceps [5], of the hand muscles, including the dorsal interossei muscles [6], and of the facial muscles, including the orbicularis oris, mentalis muscles and labial muscles [7, 8].

[1] Journal of the Neurological Sciences [1999] 167 (1) : 22-25 (Y. Yoshiyama, J.Takama, T.Hattori)

[2] Functional Neurology [2003] 18 (3) : 165-170 (G.Albani, G. Sandrini, G.Künig, C.Martin-Soelch, A.Mauro, R.Pignatti, C.Pacchetti, V.Dietz, K.L.Leenders)

[3] Journal of Neurology [2007] 254 (2) : 202-209 (M.K.Mak, E.C. Wong, C.W.Hui-Chan)

[4] Journal of Neurology [2011] 258 (5) : 740-745 (A.Di Matteo, A.Fasano, G.Squintani, L.Ricciardi, T.Bovi, A.Fiaschi, P.Barone, M. Tinazzi)

[5] Journal of Neurology, Neurosurgery and Psychiatry [1987] 50 (10) : 1274-1283 (F.Viallet, J.Massion, R.Massarino, R.Khalil)

[6] Electroencephalography and Clinical Neurophysiology [1995] 97 (5) : 215-222 (R.Cantello, M.Gianelli, C.Civardi, R.Mutani)

[7] Neurology [1982] 32 (7) : 749-754 (C.J.Hunker, J.H.Abbs, S.M. Barlow)

[8] Journal of Neurology, Neurosurgery and Psychiatry [1971] 34 (6) : 679-681 (R.Leanderson, B.A.Meyerson, A.Persson)

NERVOUS SYSTEM

The nervous system is made up of the brain, the spinal cord, the nerves, and the sense organs, such as the eye and the ear. The nervous system receives, interprets, and responds to stimuli from inside and outside the body.

Reduced dopaminergic stimulation of the mesolimibic pathway is associated with bradyphrenia [1, 2], which is mental slowness and reduced motivation. Reduced dopaminergic stimulation of the mesocortical pathway is associated with emotional depression [3, 4]. Reduced dopaminergic stimulation of the incertohypothalamic pathway affects periaqueductal gray, which has both enkephalin and endorphin producing cells. Consequently, in Parkinson's Disease, there are reduced levels of enkephalins [5, 6] and endorphins [7], both of which suppress pain. Reduced stimulation of the diencephalospinal pathway contributes to insufficient pain control at the spinal cord level [8].

[1] Brain Nerve [2007] 59 (9) : 943-951 (M.Yokochi)

[2] Journal of Molecular Neuroscience [2007] 32 (1) : 72-79 (A. Friedman, I.Deri, Y.Friedman, E.Dremencov, S.Goutkin, E. Kravchinsky, M,Mintz, D.Levi, D.H.Overstreet, G.Yadid)

[3] Canadian Journal of Neurological Sciences [1984] 11 (1 Supplement) : 105-107 (H.C.Fibiger)

[4] American Journal of Psychiatry [1992] 149 (4) : 443-454 (J.L. Cummings)

[5] Neuropeptides [1991] 18 (4) : 201-207 (S.P.Sivam)

[6] Lancet [1981] 1 (8234) : 1367-1368 (H.Taquet, F.Javoy-Agid, F. Cesselin, Y.Agid)

[7] Neurology [1985] 35 (9) : 1371-1374 (G.Nappi, F.Petraglia, E. Martignoni, F.Facchinetti, G.Bono, A.R.Genazzani)

[8] PLoS One [2010] 5 (10) : e13306 (Q.Barraud, I.Obeid, I.Aubert, G.Barrière, H.Contamin, S.McGuire, P.Ravenscroft, G.Porras, F. Tison, E.Bezard, I.Ghorayeb)

ALIMENTARY SYSTEM

The Alimentary System includes the : oral cavity, pharynx, oesophagus, stomach, small intestine, large intestine (colon), rectum and anus. The muscles in the pharynx involved in swallowing are the superior, medial and inferior pharyngeal constrictors. There are muscles in the colon and the anal sphincter involved in waste elimination.

In people with Parkinson's Disease there is an increased contraction of the pharyngeal muscles [1], the anal sphincter [2, 3], and the colon [4]. There is prolonged passage through the small intestine [5]. More than 79% of people with Parkinson's Disease exhibit prolonged colonic transit time [6, 7]. About 66% of people with Parkinson's Disease had significantly increased colonic volume, with the transverse and rectosigmoid segments being particularly affected [7]. The most common effects on the esophagus are : a failure by the esophagus to contract properly (ineffective esophageal peristalsis) (55%), fragmented contraction in the esophagus (fragmented peristalsis) (48%), spasms in the esophagus (DES - diffuse esophageal spasm) (48%), and obstruction of the exit of the esophagus to the stomach (EGJ outflow obstruction) (39%) [8].

[1] Neurology [2007] 68 (8) : 583-589 (E.Alfonsi, M.Versino, I.M. Merlo, C.Pacchetti, E.Martignoni, G.Bertino, A.Moglia, C.Tassorelli, G.Nappi)

[2] Acta Neurologica Scandinavica [2012] 126 (4) : 248-255 (J.Linder, R.Libelius, E.Nordh, B.Holmberg, H.Stenlund, L.Forsgren)

[3] Acta Neurologica Scandinavica [2008] 117 (1) : 60-64 (K.Krogh, K.Ostergaard, S.Sabroe, S.Laurberg)

[4] Experimental Neurology [2007] 207 (1) : 4-12 (G.Anderson, A.R. Noorian, G.Taylor, M.Anitha, D.Bernhard, S.Srinivasan, J.G.Greene)

[5] Journal of Neural Transmission [2015] 122 (12) : 1659-1661 (J. Dutkiewicz, S.Szlufik, M.Nieciecki, I.Charzynska, L.Królicki, P. Smektala, A.Friedman)

[6] Movement Disorders [2016] Nov 22 [Epub ahead of print] (K. Knudsen, K.Krogh, K.Østergaard, P.Borghammer)

[7] Journal of Parkinsons Disease [2017] Jan 30 [Epub ahead of print] (K.Knudsen, T.D.Fedorova, A.C.Bekker, P.Iversen, K. Østergaard, K. Krogh, P.Borghammer)

[8] Diseases of the Esophagus [2017] 30 (4) : 1-6 (A.Su, R.Gandhy, C.Barlow, G.Triadafilopoulos)

Urinary system

The urethral sphincter is one of two muscles used to control the elimination of urine from the bladder through the urethra. The two muscles are the male or female external urethral sphincter and the internal urethral sphincter.

When the sphincter muscles contract, the urethra is sealed shut. In Parkinson's Disease there is normally overactivity of the urethral sphincter [1, 2, 3], or delayed relaxation of the sphincter [3, 4], that often results in urethral closure [1]. The detrusor muscle is smooth muscle found in the wall of the bladder. It remains relaxed to allow the bladder to store urine and contracts during urination to release urine. There is detrusor overactivity in most people with Parkinson's Disease [5, 6].

[1] Urological Research [1976] 4 (3) : 133-138 (S.Raz)

[2] International Urology and Nephrology [1985] 17 (1) : 35-41 (J.T.Andersen)

[3] British Journal of Urology [1983] 55 (6) : 691-693 (N.T.Galloway)

[4] Clinical Neuroscience [1998] 5 (2) : 78-86 (C.Singer)

[5] Journal of Neurological and Neurosurgical Psychiatry [2011] 82 (12) : 1382-1386 (T.Uchiyama, R.Sakakibara, T.Yamamoto, T.Ito, C. Yamaguchi, Y.Awa, M.Yanagisawa, Y.Higuchi, Y.Sato, et al)

[6] Urology [1989] 33 (6) : 486-489 (Z.Khan, P.Starer, A.Bhola)

Cardiovascular system

The cardiovascular system, also known as the circulatory system, is an organ system that encompasses the heart and blood vessels of the body. The cardiovascular system carries blood, oxygen, and nutrients to organs and tissues of the body, and carries waste and carbon dioxide from these tissues for removal from the body.

In Parkinson's Disease, symptoms can often occur in the cardiovascular system, and dopamine can contribute to those symptoms, but there are no direct dopaminergic effects on the cardiovascular system.

Respiratory system

The muscles of respiration are : the diaphragm, and the intercostal muscles, which includes the external intercostal muscles, internal intercostal muscles and innermost intercostal muscles. Accessory muscles are : the pectoralis major and minor, serratus anterior, the scalene group of muscles and the sternocleidomastoid muscle.

In people with Parkinson's Disease there is an increased contraction of the muscles involved in respiration [1, 2].

[1] Journal Electromyography and Kinesiology [2009] 19 (4) : 591-597 (L.U.Guedes, V.F.Parreira, A.C.Diório, F.Goulart, A.D.Andrade, R.R. Britto)

[2] Respiration Physiology [1999] 118 (2-3) : 163-172 (L.Vercueil, J.P. Linard, B.Wuyam, P.Pollak, G.Benchetrit)

Skeletal system

The skeletal system includes all of the bones and joints in the body. The skeleton provides support and protection for the soft tissues that make up the rest of the body. The skeletal system also provides attachment points for muscles to allow movements at the joints.

In Parkinson's Disease, although symptoms can occur in the skeletal system, there are no direct dopaminergic effects on the skeletal system. However, the excessive muscle contraction that occurs in Parkinson's Disease can cause the upper body to bend towards one side rather than the other, thereby affecting skeletal formation [1].

[1] Journal of Clinical Neurology [2009] 5 (2) : 91-94 (J.S.Baik, J.Y. Kim, J.H.Park, S.W.Han, J.H.Park, M.S.Lee)

Integumentary system

The integumentary system is the skin and its associated glands, including the sweat glands, as well as the hair and nails. The skin protects the body from various kinds of damage, such as loss of water or abrasion from outside.

In Parkinson's Disease there is increased secretion of sebum from the sebaceous glands [1]. The reduced dopamine levels in Parkinson's Disease enable higher levels of prolactin [2], which stimulates, via luteinizing hormone, the formation of testosterone [3]. Increased testosterone stimulates sebum formation [1].

[1] Dermatoendocrinology [2011] 3 (1) : 41-49 (E.Makrantonaki, R. Ganceviciene, C.Zouboulis)

[2] Endocrine Reviews [2001] 22 (6) : 724-763 (N.Ben-Jonathan, R. Hnasko)

[3] Journal of Andrology [1989] 10 (1) : 37-42 (Man-Cheong Fung, G.C.Wah, W.D.Odell)

Sensory system

Olfactory system

The olfactory system is the sensory system used for olfaction, which is the sense of smell. Odorants are inhaled through the nose where they contact the main olfactory epithelium. The olfactory epithelium contains olfactory receptors, which turns receptor activation for a variety of smells into electrical signals in neurons, which is where the stimulus is perceived.

The dopamine deficiency that occurs in Parkinson's Disease causes a reduction in the stimulation of the dopaminergic neurons in the olfactory bulb and in the olfactory tract through which smells are perceived [1].

[1] International Journal of Neuroscience [1999] 97 (3-4) : 225-233 (R.Sandyk)

VISUAL SYSTEM

The visual system is required for visual perception – processing and interpreting visual information to build a representation of the visual environment. The visual system consists of the eye, retina, fibres that conduct visual information, the superior colliculus and parts of the cerebral cortex. Its functions include visual perception, visual acuity, colour perception, colour discrimination, contrast sensitivity, and darkness adaptation [1].

There is reduced dopaminergic activity in the retina of people with Parkinson's Disease [2-6]. In people with Parkinson's Disease there is more sustained contraction of the muscles of the eye, including the orbicularis oculi, which controls eye closure and visual convergence [7].

[1] Frontiers in Psychology [2014] 5 : 1594 (A.J.Zele1, D.Cao)

[2] Journal of Parkinson's Disease [2014] 4 (2) : 197-204 (J.Y.Lee, J.Ahn, T.W.Kim, B.S.Jeon)

[3] Journal of Neuro-Ophthalmology [2013] 33 (1) : 62-65 (S.Kirbas, K.Turkyilmaz, A.Tufekci, M.Durmus)

[4] Neurology Clinical Practice [2003] 21 (3) : 709-728 (G.R. Jackson, C.Owsley)

[5] Surgical and Radiologic Anatomy [1988] 10 (2) : 137-144 (J. Nguyen-Legros)

[6] Vision Research [2004] 44 (24) : 2793-2797 (R.Inzelberg, J.A. Ramirez, P.Nisipeanu, A.Ophir)

[7] Neurology [1982] 32 (7) : 749-754 (C.J.Hunker, J.H.Abbs, S.M. Barlow)

ENDOCRINE SYSTEM

PITUITARY GLAND

The pituitary gland is a small endocrine gland in the brain. It is a protrusion off the bottom of the hypothalamus at the base of the brain. The function of dopamine that is transmitted from the dopaminergic neurons via the tuberoinfundibular pathway is to inhibit the secretion of prolactin from the pituitary gland.

In Parkinson's Disease there is low dopamine [1], which enables the increased secretion of prolactin from the pituitary gland.

[1] Endocrine Reviews [2001] 22 (6) : 724-763 (N.Ben-Jonathan, R. Hnasko)

PINEAL GLAND

The pineal gland is a small endocrine gland in the brain. It is located in the epithalamus, near the centre of the brain. The pineal gland produces melatonin, which regulates sleep in seasonal and circadian rhythms.

Dopamine regulates melatonin secretion [1]. Therefore, the reduced dopamine that occurs in Parkinson's Disease leads to altered melatonin levels.

[1] PLoS Biology [2012] 10 (6) : e1001347 (S.González, D.Moreno-Delgado, E.Moreno, K.Pérez-Capote, R.Franco, J.Mallol, A.Cortés, V. Casadó, C.Lluís, J.Ortiz, S.Ferré, E.Canela, P.J.McCormick)

Reproductive system

The male reproductive system consists of the penis, urethra, vas deferens, Cowper's gland, the testes, the scrotum, and the ejaculatory fluid producing glands, which include the seminal vesicles, prostate, and the vas deferens. The female reproductive system consists of the vagina, the labia, clitoris and urethra, which leads from the vulva, the vaginal opening, to the uterus, which holds the developing fetus. The vagina is attached to the uterus through the cervix. The uterus is attached to ovaries via the fallopian tubes.

Dopamine, via the neuroendocrine pathways, stimulates the secretion of GnRH (Gonadotropin-releasing hormone). In Parkinson's Disease there is low dopamine that reduces the secretion of GnRH. GnRH is a releasing hormone responsible for the release of follicle-stimulating hormone (FSH) and luteinizing hormone (LH) from the anterior pituitary gland [1-4]. Follicle-stimulating hormone (FSH) and luteinizing hormone (LH) have effects on the male reproductive system, including on testosterone secretion which is consequently lower in Parkinson's Disease [5, 6,]. Follicle-stimulating hormone (FSH), and luteinizing hormone (LH), which is low in women with Parkinson's Disease [7], have effects on the female reproductive system by lowering estrogen levels.

[1] Bulletin of Mathematical Biology [2008] 70 (8) : 2211-2228 (R.Bertram, Y.X.Li)

[2] Proceedings, National Academy Sciences, U.S.A. [2005] 102 (5) : 1761-1766 (S.Messager, E.E.Chatzidaki, D.Ma, A.G.Hendrick, D.Zahn, J.Dixon, R.R.Thresher, I.Malinge, D.Lomet, M.B.Carlton, et al)

[3] European Journal of Contraception and Reproductive Health Care [1998] 3 (1) : 21-28 (M.Stomati, A.D.Genazzani, F.Petraglia, A.R. Genazzani)

[4] Brain Research [1986] 399 (1) : 15-23. (K.Y.Pau, H.G.Spies)

[5] Journal of Neurology, Neurosurgery and Psychiatry [2004] 75 (9) : 1323-1326 (R.E.Ready, J.Friedman, J.Grace, H.Fernandez)

[6] Neurology [2004] 62 (3) : 411-413 (M.S.Okun, M.R.DeLong, J. Hanfelt, M.Gearing, A.Levey)

[7] Journal of Neural Transmission (Parkinson's Disease and Dementia Section) [1990] 2 (3) : 225-231 (U.Bonuccelli, P.Piccini, A.Napolitano, A.Cagnacci, A.M.Paoletti, G.B.Melis, A.Muratorio)

IMMUNE SYSTEM

The immune system is a diffuse network of interacting cells, cell products, and cell-forming tissues. The immune system includes the thymus, spleen, lymph nodes and lymph tissue, macrophages, lymphocytes, antibodies and lymphokines. The immune system protects the body from pathogens and other foreign substances, destroys infected and malignant cells, and removes cellular debris.

In Parkinson's Disease there is low dopamine. The low dopamine that occurs in Parkinson's Disease enables increased secretion of prolactin from the pituitary gland [1]. Prolactin prevents the action of glucocorticoids on the immune response [2]. Glucocorticoids regulate inflammation and the permeability of the blood brain barrier inflammation and normally reduce inflammation [3]. Consequently, prolactin promotes pro-inflammatory immune responses [4].

[1] Endocrine Reviews [2001] 22 (6) : 724-763 (N.Ben-Jonathan, R. Hnasko)

[2] Rossiiskii Fiziologicheskii Zhurnal Imeni I M Sechenova [2003] 89 (9) : 1117-1126 (E.E.Fomicheva, E.A.Nemirovich-Danchenko)

[3] Frontiers in Neuroanatomy [2015] 9 : 32 (M.T.Herrero, C.Estrada, L.Maatouk, S.Vyas)

[4] European Cytokine Network [2004] 15 (2) : 99-104 (J.M.Brand, C.Frohn, K.Cziupka, C.Brockmann, H.Kirchner, J.Luhm)

CHAPTER 18

SYMPTOMS OF PARKINSON'S DISEASE

PRIMARY SYMPTOMS

TYPES OF SYMPTOMS

The symptoms of Parkinson's Disease differ from person to person, over time, and in their severity. Muscular symptoms, such as rigidity, tremor, bradykinesia (slowness of movement) and walking difficulties are the most apparent and characteristic symptoms of Parkinson's Disease. However, Parkinson's Disease can eventually affect every system in the body : the muscular, nervous, alimentary, urinary, cardiovascular, respiratory, skeletal, integumentary, sensory, endocrine, reproductive, and immune systems.

Instead of being due to Parkinson's Disease, some of the symptoms commonly experienced in Parkinson's Disease, such as dyskinesia, can be caused by Parkinson's Disease drugs, especially when the Parkinson's Disease is more advanced.

There are other symptoms, such as dementia, that are not due to Parkinson's Disease but often coincide with Parkinson's Disease, especially when the Parkinson's Disease is more advanced.

MOST PREVALENT SYMPTOMS

EARLIER PARKINSON'S DISEASE

The most common symptoms in earlier Parkinson's Disease are rigidity (stiffness), tremor, bradkynesia (slowness of movement), freezing, falling, microphagia (reduced handwriting size), reduced arm swing, mirror movements, dysarthria (speech difficulties), hypomimia (reduced facial expression), depression, apathy, fatigue, anxiety, pain, sleep disturbance, constipation, dysphagia (swallowing difficulty), urinary symptoms, cardiovascular symptoms, respiratory muscle dysfunction, anosmia (reduced sense of smell), and sexual dysfunction.

The perception in patients of which symptoms are the most troublesome often differ from the clinicians view. In earlier Parkinson's Disease, the five most prevalent complaints ranked in descending order were : slowness, tremor, stiffness, pain, and then loss of smell or taste.

ADVANCED PARKINSON'S DISEASE

Some symptoms become far more common as Parkinson's Disease worsens. The most prevalent of these are hypokinesia, bradykinesia (slowness of movement), akinesia, dyskinesia, dementia, excessive daytime sleepiness, and siallhorea (drooling).

In advanced Parkinson's Disease the five most prevalent complaints ranked in descending order were : fluctuating response to medication (most commonly wearing off, followed by dyskinesia), mood changes, drooling, sleep problems (most commonly middle and late night insomnia followed by daytime sleepiness), and then tremor.

MUSCULAR SYSTEM

In Parkinson's Disease there are symptoms that can affect the muscles generally. These can include rigidity, tremor, hypokinesia (reduced movement), bradykinesia (slowness of movement), akinesia (loss of movement), dyskinesia (abnormal involuntary movements), akathisia (motor restlessness), and dystonia (abnormal involuntary postures) [CHAPTER 20].

Those muscular symptoms that can specifically affect the lower limbs are : shuffling (when walking), freezing (feeling unable to walk forwards), festination, falling, and restless legs syndrome. Those muscular symptoms that can specifically affect the upper limbs are : impaired finger dexterity, micrographia (small handwriting), reduced arm swing, mirror movement, and frozen shoulder syndrome. Those muscular symptoms that can specifically affect the head and neck are hypomimia (reduced facial expression), reduced blinking, dysarthria (difficulty speaking), and neck rigidity [CHAPTER 20].

The most common symptoms of these in Parkinson's Disease are rigidity (stiffness), tremor, bradkynesia (slowness of movement), freezing, falling, microphagia (reduced handwriting size), reduced arm swing, mirror movements, dysarthria (speech difficulties), and hypomimia (reduced facial expression) [CHAPTER 20].

Nervous system

In Parkinson's Disease there can be an increased likelihood of depression, dementia, pain, sleep disturbance, excessive daytime sleepiness, fatigue, apathy, anhedonia, bradyphrenia, alexithymia, anxiety, hallucinations, compulsions, neuropathy, and vertigo. The most prominent and prevalent of these symptoms are depression, apathy, fatigue, anxiety, pain, sleep disturbance and dementia (in more severe Parkinson's Disease) [CHAPTER 21].

Alimentary system

In Parkinson's Disease there can be an increased likelihood of constipation, dysphagia (swallowing difficulty), sialorrhea (excessive saliva and drooling), obesity, gastroparesis (slow gastric emptying), and intestinal bacterial overgrowth. The most common symptoms of these in Parkinson's Disease are constipation, which occurs in most people, followed by dysphagia, then sialorrhea, both of which occur in a large minority of people [CHAPTER 22].

Urinary system

In Parkinson's Disease there is often nocturia (frequent urinating at night), urinary incontinence (loss of urinary control), increased urinary frequency, and urinary retention (an inability to completely empty the bladder). Urinary symptoms occur in between 27% and 85% of people with Parkinson's Disease [CHAPTER 23].

CARDIOVASCULAR SYSTEM

Cardiovascular dystautonomia usually occurs in Parkinson's Disease and can include a variety of cardiovascular symptoms. Certain Parkinson's Disease drugs can increase the likelihood of heart failure, in which breathlessness, feeling very tired and ankle swelling are the main symptoms. Cardiovascular symptoms occur in 70% of people with Parkinson's Disease [CHAPTER 24].

RESPIRATORY SYSTEM

Respiratory muscle dysfunction usually, but not always, occurs in Parkinson's Disease. Respiratory muscle dysfunction makes respiratory diseases such as pneumonia more dangerous due to the reduced respiratory capacity it causes [CHAPTER 25].

SKELETAL SYSTEM

In Parkinson's Disease there can be an increased likelihood of osteoporosis and osteopenia. Postural deformities can be frequent and disabling complications of Parkinson's Disease. The postural deformities can include scoliosis, Pisa syndrome, and camptocormia. [CHAPTER 26].

INTEGUMENTARY SYSTEM

In Parkinson's Disease there is an increased likelihood of melanoma, which is a form of skin cancer; seborrhea, which is increased sebum secretion; and hyperhidrosis, which is increased sweat secretion. Increased sweat secretion is usually due to Parkinson's Disease drugs [CHAPTER 27].

SENSORY SYSTEM

In Parkinson's Disease there can be an increased likelihood of anosmia (which is a loss of the sense of smell), rhinorrhea (which is nasal discharge), visual disturbance, retinal thinning, hypogeusia (which is impaired sense of taste, and hearing loss. Visual disturbances and anosmia (loss of sense of smell) are particularly prominent in Parkinson's Disease. Most people with Parkinson's Disease have a loss of the sense of smell (anosmia) or reduction in the sense of smell (hyposmia) [CHAPTER 28].

ENDOCRINE SYSTEM

In Parkinson's Disease there is an increased likelihood of hyperprolactinemia in the pituitary gland, blunted circadian rhythms in the pineal gland, catecholamine deficiency in the adrenal gland, and hypothyroidism in the thyroid gland. Hypothyroidism is not a Parkinson's Disease symptom but can often coincide with Parkinson's Disease [CHAPTER 29].

REPRODUCTIVE SYSTEM

Parkinson's Disease can cause sexual dysfunction in men and women. Sexual dysfunction is common in Parkinson's Disease, with over 40% of people with Parkinson's Disease being affected in this way. Over two thirds of people with Parkinson's Disease had decreased sexual activity. Nearly two thirds of people with Parkinson's Disease had a loss of sex drive [CHAPTER 30].

IMMUNE SYSTEM

Neuroinflammation commonly, but not always, occurs in Parkinson's Disease. There is a greater likelihood of CNS infections occurring in Parkinson's Disease after diagnosis, and also before being diagnosed with Parkinson's Disease [CHAPTER 31].

CHAPTER 19

SYMPTOMS OF PARKINSON'S DISEASE

SYMPTOM PROGRESSION

EARLIEST SYMPTOMS

Many people have already had Parkinson's Disease for years by the time they are diagnosed with Parkinson's Disease or have had symptoms that were progressing towards it.

A comparison was made between those symptoms before diagnosis and their subsequent diagnosis. At 10 years before diagnosis the incidence of tremor was many times higher and constipation was higher in those who went on to develop Parkinson's Disease. At 5 years before diagnosis those who went on to develop Parkinson's Disease had a much higher incidence of tremor, a higher incidence of imbalance, constipation, hypotension, and a slightly higher incidence of erectile dysfunction, urinary dysfunction, dizziness, fatigue, depression, and anxiety. At 2 years before diagnosis the incidence of all studied features except neck pain and stiffness were higher in people who went on to develop Parkinson's Disease. A range of symptoms can therefore be detected years before diagnosis of Parkinson's Disease, with tremor being especially common prior to diagnosis [1].

Whether somebody is right handed or left handed can greatly affect on which side Parkinson's Disease symptoms initiate and which symptoms they initially have. Out of those people with Parkinson's Disease 92% were right handed. Nearly 62% of them had an initial onset of symptoms on the right hand side. Out of those people with Parkinson's Disease 8% were left handed. Around 75% of them had an initial onset of symptoms on the left hand side. Out of those people with Parkinson's Disease who were right handed 77% had Parkinson's Disease symptoms that were dominant on the right hand side. Out of those people with Parkinson's Disease who were left handed 58% of them had Parkinson's Disease symptoms that were dominant on the left hand side. In general, the dominant side of Parkinson's Disease symptoms was in accordance with which handed they were. In people who were right handed, rest tremor was the most common initial symptom. In people who were left handed, rest tremor and rigidity and bradykinesia were the most common initial symptoms [2].

Starting treatment

A lot of medical practitioners are reluctant to start L-dopa. Their main concern in starting Parkinson's Disease drugs is their temporary and limited benefits. Patients are more than twice as reluctant to start dopamine agonists compared with starting L-dopa. The most common reasons patients have for not starting Parkinson's Disease drugs are the fear of side effects, followed by the refusal to accept a diagnosis of Parkinson's Disease [3].

Most troubling symptoms

The perception in patients of which symptoms are the most troublesome often differ from the clinicians view. In typical Parkinson's Disease, the five most prevalent complaints ranked in descending order were : slowness, tremor, stiffness, pain, and then loss of smell or taste. In advanced Parkinson's Disease the five most prevalent complaints ranked in descending order were : fluctuating response to medication (most commonly wearing off, followed by dyskinesia), mood changes, drooling, sleep problems (most commonly middle and late night insomnia followed by daytime sleepiness), and then tremor. So as Parkinson's Disease progresses the most troublesome symptoms change considerably [4].

Worsening of symptoms

Episodes of sudden and transient worsening of symptoms commonly occur in Parkinson's Disease, especially when the Parkinson's Disease is more severe. A quarter of people with Parkinson's Disease were found to be affected in this way. Infection was the single most frequent cause, accounting for a quarter of cases. Other common causes were anxiety, medication errors, poor adherence to taking the required drugs, medication side effects, and postoperative decline. Overall, over 80% of reasons were attributable to reversible or treatable causes. Most people who experienced a sudden worsening of symptoms recovered fully but a third of people experienced recurrent episodes. One in six people suffered permanent decline. Those people most prone to sudden or transient worsening were those who had Parkinson's Disease for nearly eight years or more, had more severe symptoms, had greater use of dopaminergic drugs, and had a greater prevalence of motor complications [5].

People with Parkinson's Disease retired about 4 to 7 years earlier than average, with 23% to 75% reporting that they retired early because of Parkinson's Disease, with slowness and fatigue being the most debilitating symptoms in relation to working capacity [6].

Wearing off

Wearing off of the effect of drugs for Parkinson's Disease has been found to occur far earlier and in more people with Parkinson's Disease than previously assumed. Wearing off is very individual and there is no standard time frame for when this may occur or which symptoms are experienced. Neurologists found that there was wearing off in 57% of people with Parkinson's Disease. However, when this was assessed by the patients themselves, there was found to be wearing off in 67% of people with Parkinson's Disease. Even in people who had Parkinson's Disease for less than 2.5 years there was wearing off in 21% of people when assessed by neurologists and in 41% when patients assessed themselves. The most frequent wearing off symptoms were slowness of movements (55%) and reduced dexterity (48%). Those factors most associated with wearing off were : younger age, female gender, severer symptoms, and duration of treatment. Wearing off is already common in the early stages of Parkinson's Disease and is usually underestimated by routine neurological clinical evaluations. The effect of Parkinson's Disease drugs is therefore often relatively short lived [7].

Long term effects

After more than 5 years with Parkinson's Disease, the number of people who were dependent in activities of daily living went from 16% at the time of diagnosis up to 41%. Loss of independence was more likely when, at the time of diagnosis, the patient had been older, and had shorter symptom duration, increasing motor severity, and presence of mild cognitive impairment. Dependency was irreversible in most people [8].

After more than 10 years with Parkinson's Disease many people were minimally disabled (44%) or were experiencing postural instability (40%). Most (88%) were able to stand unaided but falls were common (55%). Almost all (93%) were living at home with a family member as a regular caregiver (84%). They had an average of two additional medical disorders, with arthritis (49%) and heart problems (32%) being the most common. Most of them (87%) took at least 2 medications, with L-dopa (96%), dopamine agonists (45%) and antidepressants (37%) being the most common. Most of them were not currently utilizing physical, occupational or speech therapy, but two-thirds of them reported engaging in physical activity. Deep brain stimulation was documented in 22% of people. Overall the mean health-related quality of life and caregiver burden was impaired in all domains [9].

After more than 20 years with Parkinson's Disease is associated with having fractures, or being confined to a wheelchair or bed, and major milestones of disease disability. Older age at onset and longer duration of Parkinson's Disease were both associated with a higher prevalence of major milestones of disease disability. Confinement to a wheelchair or bed had by then occurred in just over 1 in 5 people (21%). Those factors making confinement to a wheelchair or bed more likely were older age, postural instability and institutionalisation. Fractures occurred in 16% of people. Fractures were associated with postural instability. The most frequent outcome was death (28%). However, given the age of diagnosis and the duration of Parkinson's Disease this might have been no more than normal. Mortality was associated with male gender, older age, dysphagia, orthostatic hypotension, postural instability, fractures and institutionalisation [10].

Many people with Parkinson's Disease eventually require nursing to assist them with their symptoms. The average age of nursing home residents with Parkinson's Disease was nearly 80 years old with about half of them being male. Prevalence of dementia and depression in those in nursing homes was high [11, 12]. Over two thirds of people with Parkinson's Disease in nursing homes had to be helped with eating. Nearly all of them had to be helped with bathing [13].

MORTALITY

Parkinson's Disease usually nearly doubled or more than doubled the mortality rate [14-35, 52]. However, the mortality rates generally have been gradually declining [36]. The average survival time from diagnosis could be 9 years [37], over 10 years [38, 39], or even as much as 16 years or more [40].

Factors associated with early mortality are : male gender [40-43], older age [24, 42], older age at diagnosis [17, 40, 41], more severe symptoms [17, 40, 42, 43], duration of Parkinson's Disease [23], walking slowly [44], dementia [14, 19, 24, 28, 42, 45], cognitive impairment [40, 43], dysphagia [41], pneumonia [43], orthostatic hypotension [41], postural instability [41], institutionalisation [41], psychotic symptoms [42], depression [24], severe bradykinesia [40], and problems with vision [43].

Factors associated with increased survival after treatment initiation were : female gender [45, 46], people who were Hispanic [45], people who were Asian [45], people who were African American [43], and a younger age when Parkinson's Disease drugs were initiated [46].

The mortality rate increases with age. The age-adjusted relative risk of mortality was 1.1 during the first 5 years from diagnosis, 2.3 from 5 to 10 years, and 3.5 after 10 years [23]. The mortality rate gradually increased with the duration of Parkinson's Disease [16, 38]. When L-dopa was initiated after 1 to 3 years the mortality rate was 1.4. When L-dopa was initiated after 4 to 6 years the mortality rate was 2.4. When L-dopa was initiated after 7 to 9 years the mortality rate was 2.9 [47].

Life expectancy

The average age at death was 78 [31, 39], or 81 [21]. Life expectancy is another 38 years instead of the expected 49 years for those whose onset was 25 to 39 years old, another 21 years instead of the expected 31 years for those whose onset was 40 to 64 years old, and another 5 years instead of the expected 9 years for those whose onset was after they were 64 years old. The anticipated age of death is 71 instead of 82 for those whose onset was 25-39 years old, and was 88 instead of 91 for those whose onset was after they were 64 years old. So life expectancy is shorter in people with Parkinson's Disease regardless of the age of onset [48, 49].

Parkinson's Disease is not a fatal illness because even in those with early onset there was a life expectancy of decades [48]. Parkinson's Disease can reduce the ability to cope with certain medical disorders and thereby make fatality more likely. This is why some people are reported as having died of the complications of Parkinson's Disease. Less than two thirds of people with Parkinson's Disease had Parkinson's Disease recorded on their death certificate. The most common cause of death in people with Parkinson's Disease is pneumonia, which was the cause of death in 45% of people. However, people with Parkinson's Disease were actually less likely to die of cancer or heart disease than the rest of the population [50].

The place of death differs a lot according to the country the person is in. Of those countries assessed, the proportion of deaths in hospital ranged from 17% in the USA, which was the lowest, to 75% in South Korea, which was the highest. Hospital was the most prevalent place of death in South Korea (75%), Hungary (60%) and France (40%). Nursing homes were the most prevalent place of death in New Zealand (71%), Belgium (52%), USA (50%), Canada (48%) and the Czech Republic (44%). Home was the most prevalent place of death in Mexico (73%), Italy (51%) and Spain (46%). The chances of dying in hospital were consistently higher for men (Belgium, France, Italy, USA, Canada), for those younger than 80 years (Belgium, France, Italy, USA, Mexico), and for those living in areas with a higher provision of hospital beds (Italy, USA) [51].

[1] Lancet Neurology [2014] 14 (1) : 57-64 (A.Schrag, L.Horsfall, K.Walters, A.Noyce, I.Petersen)

[2] Medicina Clinica [2014] 142 (4) : 141-144 (J.Shi, J.Liu, Q.Qu)

[3] Parkinsonism & Related Disorders [2014] 20 (6) : 608-612 (T.A. Mestre, T.Teodoro, W.Reginold, J.Graf, M.Kasten, J.Sale, M. Zurowski, J.Miyasaki, J.J.Ferreira, C. Marras)

[4] Movement Disorders [2010] 25 (11) : 1646-1651 (M.Politis, K.Wu, S.Molloy, P.G.Bain, K.R.Chaudhuri, P.Piccini)

[5] Neurologist [2012] 18 (3) : 120-124 (K.S..Zheng, B.J.Dorfman, P.J. Christos, N.R.Khadem, C.Henchcliffe, P.Piboolnurak, M.J. Nirenberg)

[6] Parkinsonism & Related Disorders [2016] 27 : 9-24 (J.Koerts, M. König, L.Tucha, O.Tucha)

[7] Parkinsonism & Related Disorders [2014] 20 (2) : 204-211 (F. Stocchi, A.Antonini, P.Barone, M.Tinazzi, M.Zappia, M.Onofrj, S. Ruggieri, L.Morgante, U.Bonuccelli, L.Lopiano, P.Pramstaller, et al)

[8] Neurology [2016] Sep 2 [Epub ahead of print] (A.Bjornestad, O.B.Tysnes, J.P.Larsen, G.Alves)

[9] Parkinsonism & Related Disorders [2012] 18 (Supplement 3) : S10-S14 28 (3) : 380-383 (A.Hassan, S.S.Wu, P.Schmidt, I.A.Malaty, Y.F.Dai, J.M.Miyasaki, M.S.Okun)

[10] Journal of Neurology, Neurosurgery and Psychiatry [2015] 86 (8) : 849-855 (R.Cilia, E.Cereda, C.Klersy, M.Canesi, A.L.Zecchinelli, C.B. Mariani, S.Tesei, G.Sacilotto, N.Meucci, M.Zini, C.Ruffmann, et al)

[11] Parkinsonism & Related Disorders [2002] 8 (5) : 369-80 (R.J. Buchanan, S.Wang, C.Huang, P.Simpson, B.V.Manyam)

[12] Journal of American Geriatritic Society [2000] 48 (8) : 938-942 (D.Aarsland, J.P.Larsen, E.Tandberg, K.Laake)

[13] Journal of Parkinsons Disease [2016] Jun 2 [Epub ahead of print] (F.Chekani, V.Bali, R.R.Aparasu)

[14] Acta Neurologica Scandinavica [2013] 129 (2) : 71-79 (J.Xu, D.D.Gong, C.F.Man, Y.Fan)

[15] Movement Disorders [2011] 26 (14) : 2522-2529 (I.J.Posada, J. Benito-León, E.D.Louis, R.Trincado, A.Villarejo, M.J.Medrano, F. Bermejo-Pareja)

[16] Movement Disorders [2009] 24 (6) : 819-825 (A.Diem-Zangerl, K.Seppi, G.K.Wenning, E.Trinka, G.Ransmayr, W.Oberaigner, W. Poewe)

[17] Parkinsonism & Related Disorders [2014] 20 (8) : 894-897 (J.T. Järvelä, J.O.Rinne, O.Eskola, V.Kaasinen)

[18] Acta Neurologica Scandinavica [2014] 129 (2) : 71-79 (J.Xu, D.D. Gong, C.F.Man, Y.Fan)

[19] Parkinsonism & Related Disorders [2012] 18 (4) : 327-331 (C. Allyson Jones, W.R.Wayne Martin, M.Wieler, P.King-Jesso, D.C. Voaklander)

[20] Neurology [2008] 70 (16 Part 2) : 1423-1430 (J.A.Driver, T.Kurth, J.E.Buring, J.M.Gaziano, G.Logroscino)

[21] Journal of Epidemiology [2011] 21 (3) : 211-216 (Y.Doi, T. Yokoyama, Y.Nakamura, M.Nagai, K.Fujimoto, I.Nakano)

[22] African Journal of Medicine and Medical Sciences [2005] 34 (4) : 365-369 (N.U.Okubadejo, F.I.Ojini, M.A.Danesi)

[23] Movement Disorders [2006] 21 (7) : 1002-1007 (H.Chen, S.M. Zhang, M.A.Schwarzschild, M.A.Hernán, A.Ascherio)

[24] Acta Neurologica Scandinavica [2004] 110 (2) : 118-123 (T.A. Hughes, H.F.Ross, R.H.Mindham, E.G.Spokes)

[25] Neurology [2004] 62 (6) : 937-942 (K.Herlofson, S.A.Lie, D. Arsland, J.P.Larsen)

[26] Neurology [2001] 57 (12) : 2278-2282 (M.Guttman, P.M. Slaughter, M.E.Theriault, D.P.DeBoer, C.D.Naylor)

[27] Journal of Neurology [2000] 247 (6) : 429-434 (Y.Minami, R. Yamamoto, M.Nishikouri, A.Fukao, S.Hisamichi)

[28] Archives of Neurology [1997] 54 (3) : 260-264 (E.D.Louis, K. Marder, L.Cote, M.Tang, R.Mayeux)

[29] Acta Neurologica Scandinavica [1995] 92 (1) : 55-58 (L.Wermuth, E.N.Stenager, E.Stenager, J.Boldsen)

[30] Acta Neurologica Scandinavica [1995] 91 (5) : 311-316 (Y. Imaizumi)

[31] Mechanisms of Ageing and Development [1995] 85 (1) : 15-23 (Y.Imaizumi)

[32] Acta Neurologica Scandinavica [1992] 86 (1) : 55-59 (K.Kuroda, K.Tatara, T.Takatorige, F.Shinsho)

[33] New England Journal of Medicine [1996] 334 (2) : 71-76 (D. A. Bennett, L.A.Beckett, A.M.Murray, K.M.Shannon, C.G.Goetz, D.M. Pilgrim, D.A.Evans)

[34] Neurologia [1992] 7 (3) : 89-93 (J.A.Burguera, J.Catalá, P. Taberner, R.Muñoz)

[35] Journal of Neurology [1977] 216 (3) : 147-153 (R.J.Marttila, U.K. Rinne, T.Siirtola, V.Sonninen)

[36] European Journal of Neurology [2009] 16 (9) : 1010-1016 (A.Q. Mylne, C.Griffiths, C.Rooney, P.Doyle)

[37] Journal of Neurology, Neurosurgery, and Psychiatry [1999] 67 (3) : 300-307 (M.A.Hely, J.G.Morris, R.Traficante, W.G.Reid, D.J. O'Sullivan, P.M.Williamson)

[38] Movement Disorders [2014] 29 (13) : 1615-1622 (A.D.Macleod, K.S.Taylor, C.E.Counsell)

[39] Acta Neurologica Scandinavica [2013] 127 (5) : 295-300 (J. Duarte, L.M.García Olmos, A.Mendoza, L.E.Clavería)

[40] Parkinsonism & Related Disorders [2015] 21 (3) : 226-230 (L.P. Oosterveld, J.C.Allen Jr, G.Reinoso, S.H.Seah, K.Y.Tay, W.L.Au, L.C. Tan)

[41] Journal of Neurology, Neurosurgery, and Psychiatry [2015] 86 (8) : 849-845 (R.Cilia, E.Cereda, C.Klersy, M.Canesi, A.L.Zecchinelli, C.B.Mariani, S.Tesei, G.Sacilotto, N.Meucci, M.Zini, et al)

[42] Neurology [2010] 75 (14) : 1270-1276 (E.B.Forsaa, J.P.Larsen, T. Wentzel-Larsen, G.Alves)

[43] Medical Science Monitor [2002] 8 (4) : CR241-CR246 (H.H. Fernandez, K.L.Lapane)

[44] Archives of Neurology [2012] 69 (5) : 601-607 (A.W.Willis, M. Schootman, N.Kung, B.A.Evanoff, J.S.Perlmutter, B.A.Racette)

[45] Acta Neurologica Scandinavica [2011] 123 (3) : 193-200 (M. Matinolli, J.T.Korpelainen, K.A.Sotaniemi, V.V.Myllylä, R. Korpelainen)

[46] Journal of Neurology [2013] 260 (1) : 62-70 (O.Chillag-Talmor, N.Giladi, S.Linn, T.Gurevich, B.El-Ad, B.Silverman, N.Friedman, C. Peretz)

[47] Annals of Neurology [1987] 22 (1) : 8-12 (S.G.Diamond, C.H. Markham, M.M.Hoehn, F.H.McDowell, M.D.Muenter)

[48] Journal of Neurology, Neurosurgery and Psychiatry [2007] 78 (12) : 1304-1309 (L.S.Ishihara, A.Cheesbrough, C.Brayne, A.Schrag)

[49] Parkinsonism & Related Disorders [2016] Aug 12 [Epub ahead of print] (S.Fielding, A.D.Macleod, C.E.Counsell)

[50] Parkinsonism & Related Disorders [2010] 16 (7) : 434-437 (S. Pennington, K.Snell, M.Lee, R.Walker)

[51] BMC Palliative Care [2015] 14 (1) : 28 (K.Moens, D.Houttekier, L.Van den Block, R.Harding, L.Morin, S.Marchetti, A.Csikos, M. Loucka, W.A.Naylor, D.M.Wilson, J.Teno, et el)

[52] BMJ Open [2016] 6 (9) : e011888 (A.C.Winter, P.M.Rist, J.E.Buring, T.Kurth)

CHAPTER 20

SYMPTOMS OF PARKINSON'S DISEASE

MUSCULAR SYSTEM

Muscular system

The muscular system consists of skeletal, smooth and cardiac muscles. Skeletal muscles are attached to the skeleton. They are called voluntary muscles because the muscles can be controlled. The muscular system enables movement of the body and the maintenance of posture.

Primary symptoms

In Parkinson's Disease there are symptoms that can affect the muscles generally. These include rigidity [PAGE 233], tremor [PAGE 234], hypokinesia (reduced movement) [PAGE 237], bradykinesia (slowness of movement) [PAGE 238], akinesia (loss of movement) [PAGE 239], dyskinesia (abnormal involuntary movements) [PAGE 240], akathisia (motor restlessness) [PAGE 243], and dystonia (abnormal involuntary postures) [PAGE 244].

Those muscular symptoms that can specifically affect the lower limbs are : shuffling (when walking) [PAGE 245], freezing (feeling unable to walk forwards) [PAGE 246], festination [PAGE 250], falling [PAGE 251], and restless legs syndrome [PAGE 255].

Those muscular symptoms that can specifically affect the upper limbs are : impaired finger dexterity [PAGE 258], micrographia (small handwriting) [PAGE 259], reduced arm swing [PAGE 260], mirror movement [PAGE 261], and frozen shoulder syndrome [PAGE 263].

Those muscular symptoms that can specifically affect the head and neck are hypomimia (reduced facial expression) [PAGE 264], reduced blinking [PAGE 265], dysarthria (difficulty speaking) [PAGE 267], dysphonia [PAGE 268], and neck rigidity [PAGE 268].

MUSCULAR SYSTEM

PART 1 : GENERAL SYMPTOMS

In Parkinson's Disease there can be an increased likelihood of rigidity [PAGE 233], tremor [PAGE 234], hypokinesia (reduced movement) [PAGE 237], bradykinesia (slowness of movement) [PAGE 238], akinesia (loss of movement) [PAGE 239], dyskinesia (abnormal involuntary movements) [PAGE 240], akathisia (motor restlessness) [PAGE 243], and dystonia (abnormal involuntary postures) [PAGE 244].

RIGIDITY

Symptoms : Muscle rigidity is a cardinal symptom of Parkinson's Disease, which can cause limbs to resist passive movement [1-4]. Rigidity increases with the movement of a limb on the opposite side [3, 5]. Rigidity can include cogweel rigidity in which the muscles respond with cogwheel-like jerks to the use of force in bending the limbs [6].

Prevalence : Rigidity is a cardinal symptom of Parkinson's Disease [1-4] to such an extent that, if it is abolished by dopaminergic drugs, it is a reliable sign for the diagnosis of Parkinson's Disease [7]. It usually worsens in Parkinson's Disease at an annual rate of 2% to 3% [8].

Causes of symptoms : Rigidity occurs in the muscles, because in Parkinson's Disease there is excessive muscle contraction. Apart from neck rigidity [9], rigidity is only marginally related to the severity of Parkinson's Disease, the intake of Parkinson's Disease drugs [1, 10], or aging [11]. Rigidity is correlated with tremor [12].

[1] Quality of Life Research [2011] 20 (6) : 817-823 (R.Cano-de-la-Cuerda, L.Vela-Desojo, J.C.Miangolarra-Page, Y.Macías-Macías, E. Muñoz-Hellín)

[2] Functional Neurology [2001] 16 (2) : 147-156 (P.J.Delwaide)

[3] Movement Disorders [2007] 22 (8) : 1164-1168 (M.Hong, J.S. Perlmutter, G.M.Earhart)

[4] Disability and Rehabilitation [1998] 20 (4) : 142-150 (A. Nieuwboer, W.De Weerdt, R.Dom, E.Lesaffre)

[5] Canadian Journal of Neurological Sciences [2008] 35 (4) : 501-505 (D.A.Mendonça, M.S.Jog)

[6] Archives of Neurology [2005] 62 (5) : 828-830 (P.Ghiglione, R. Mutani, A.Chiò)

[7] Nihon Rinsho [1993] 51 (11) : 2823-2828 (S.Kuno)

[8] Archives of Neurology [1999] 56 (3) : 334-337 (E.D.Louis, M.X. Tang, L.Cote, B.Alfaro, H.Mejia, K.Marder)

[9] Rinsho Shinkeigaku [1996] 36 (10) : 1129-1135 (K.Nagumo, K. Hirayama)

[10] Journal of Neurology, Neurosurgery, and Psychiatry [2009] 80 (8) : 846-850 (S.M.van Rooden, M.Visser, D.Verbaan, J.Marinus, J.J.van Hilten)

[11] Gerontology [2000] 46 (3) : 129-132 (H.Nagayama, M.Hamamoto, C.Nito, S.Takagi, T.Miyazaki, Y.Katayama)

[12] Computers in Biology and Medicine [2008] 38 (11-12) : 1133-1139 (M.Mashhadi Malek, F.Towhidkhah, S.Gharibzadeh, V.Daeichin, M.Ali Ahmadi-Pajouh)

TREMOR

Symptoms : Tremor is defined as a rhythmic and involuntary movement of any part of the body [1]. There are three main types of tremor in Parkinson's Disease : resting tremor, action tremor, and intention tremor. Resting tremor is present at rest and disappears with movement. Action tremor (or kinetic tremor) occurs during any type of movement of an affected part of the body. Intention tremor is present during a purposeful movement toward a target [2]. Tremors most commonly occur in the hands [3, 4], because of the large size of the colony of pyramidal tract cells concerned with hand and finger movement, but can also occur in the fingers [5], arms [3], head [3, 6], posture [7], eyes [8-11], face [12], jaw [3], chin [3], tongue [13], legs [3, 14], and feet [15]. Tremor can cease during sleep only to return again on waking [16].

Prevalence : Rest tremor is one of the most frequent signs of Parkinson's Disease, occurring with various degrees of severity in about 75% (between 60% and 90%) of people with Parkinson's Disease [17, 18]. Action tremor occurs in about 46% of people with mild Parkinson's Disease [19] but can occur in over 90% of people with Parkinson's Disease generally [20]. Action tremor is not associated with age, age at onset, or the duration of Parkinson's Disease [20]. Nearly everybody with action tremor also had rest tremor [20, 21]. Essential Tremor is no more common in people who have Parkinson's Disease than it is in people who do not have Parkinson's Disease [22].

Causes of symptoms : It has been proposed that rest tremor is a result of increased muscle contraction and increased synchronisation of central oscillators. The increased variability of tremor frequency is attributed to poor synchronisation of the central oscillators. The recurrence of clinically visible rest tremor is accompanied by a reduction in tremor frequency variability. This reduction is attributed to increased synchronisation of central oscillators in the basal ganglia. If the number of active central oscillators is very low the muscle stimulating impulses are too weak to cause clinically evident tremor. If central oscillator synchronisation is poor the impulses originating from different central oscillators are not in phase and thus cancel out, again leading to reduced stimulation of muscles and reduced tremor amplitude. [23]. About 6% of people with Parkinson's Disease think that caffeine provokes and increases their tremor [24]. As rigidity becomes increasingly severe in Parkinson's Disease, tremor may diminish because the sustained discharges of motor units which cause rigidity inhibit their rhythmical interruptions, which are the physiological basis for tremor.

[1] JAMA [2014] 311 (9) : 948-954 (W.J.Elias, B.B.Shah)

[2] Postgraduate Medicine [1977] 61 (2) : 195-199 (A.S.McKinney)

[3] Acta Neurologica Taiwanica [2010] 19 (1) : 62-69 (Y.D.Hsu)

[4] Conference Procedings : IEEE Engineering in Medicine and Biology and Society [2011] : 470-473 (F.Rahimi, C.Bee, A.South, D. Debicki, M.Jog)

[5] Journal of Neurology, Neurosurgery and Psychiatry [1989] 52 (3) : 392-394 (M. Lakie, W.J.Mutch)

[6] Revue Neurologique [2010] 50 (11) : 676-684 (A.Gironell, B.Vives, J.Pagonabarraga)

[7] Clinical Neuropharmacology [1994] 17 (3) : 277-285 (J.M. Henderson, C.Yiannikas, J.G.Morris, R.Einstein, D.Jackson, K.Byth)

[8]. Parkinsonism & Related Disorders [2014] 20 (12) : 1449-1450 (M.S.Baron, G.T.Gitchel, P.A.Wetzel)

[9] Movement Disorders [2013] 28 (6) : 713-714 (C.Duval)

[10] Archives of Neurology [2012] 69 (8) : 1011-1017 (G.T.Gitchel, P.A.Wetzel, M.S.Baron)

[11] Movement Disorders [2013] 28 (4) : 534-537 (D.Kaski, T.A. Saifee, D.Buckwell, A.M.Bronstein)

[12] Movement Disorders [2009] 24 (10) : 1542-1545 (P. Schwingenschuh, C.Cordivari, J.Czerny, M.Esposito, K.P.Bhatia)

[13] Balkan Medical Journal [2015] 32 (1) : 127-128 (S.Delil, F. Bölükbasi, N.Yeni, G.Kiziltan)

[14] Journal of Movement Disorders [2009] 2 (1) : 29-32 (S.Y.Kang, S.K.Song, J.S. Kim, Y.H.Sohn)

[15] Journal of Physiology [2000] 529 (Part 1) : 273-281 (G.P.Moore, L.Ding, H.M.Bronte-Stewart)

[16] Neurophysiologie Clinique [1994] 24 (3) : 218-226 (A.Autret, B.Lucas, F.Henry, D.Saudeau, B.de Toffol)

[17] Neurologia i Neurochirurgia Polska [2008] 42 (1) : 12-21 (A. Budzianowska, K.Honczarenko)

[18] Neurology [1991] 41 (8) : 1298-1299 (A.H.Rajput, B.Rozdilsky, L.Ang)

[19] European Journal of Neurology [2015] 22 (2) : 223-228 (A.F. Gigante, G.Bruno, G.Iliceto, M.Guido, D.Liuzzi, P.V.Mancino, M.F.De Caro, P.Livrea, G.Defazio)

[20] Archives of Neurology [2001] 58 (10) : 1630-1634 (E.D.Louis, G. Levy, L.J.Côte, H.Mejia, S.Fahn, K.Marder)

[21] Neurological Research [2014] 36 (2) : 107-111 (A.Q.Rana, I. Siddiqui, A.A.Mosabbir, A.R.Qureshi, A.Fattah, N.Awan)

[22] International Journal of Neuroscience [2015] 125 (4) : 253-255 (A.Q.Rana, B.N.Böke, A.R.Qureshi, M.A.Rana, M.Rahman)

[23] Medical Hypotheses [2010] 74 (2) : 362-365 (A.Bartolic, Z. Pirtosek, J.Rozman, S.Ribaric)

[23] Neurology [1987] 37 (1) : 169-172 (W.Koller, S.Cone, G. Herbster)

HYPOKINESIA

Symptoms : Hypokinesia is a low level of physical movement. With bradykinesia, it is one of the two components of akinesia [1]. Prior to bradykinesia developing, there is impaired movement without any obvious disturbance of power or coordination. Movement tends to be interrupted by pauses. There can also be difficulty with small movements. Hypokinesia can affect functions such as gait hypokinesia, which is related to the severity of Parkinson's Disease [2], nocturnal hypokinesia, which includes difficulty turning over on bed [3], and laryngeal hypokinesia, which is common in Parkinson's Disease [4].

Prevalence : Hypokinesia is prominent only in those people who are more affected by Parkinson's Disease [5]. Men are more affected than women. However, over time, trunk and arm movements occurred more frequently in women than in men [6]. People who have rigidity and hypokinesia as the first symptom take a shorter time to develop severer Parkinson's Disease than do people who start with tremor alone [7]. Hypokinesia is more prevalent than bradykinesia but dopaminergic drugs predominantly improve bradykinesia rather than hypokinesia [8].

Causes of symptoms : Hypokinesia can be due to the excessive muscle contraction that occurs in Parkinson's Disease reducing the capacity for movement.

[1] Brain and Nerve [2007] 59 (9) : 943-951 (M.Yokochi)

[2] Parkinsonism & Related Disorders [2012] 18 (2) : 117-124 (D.Tan, M.Danoudis, J.McGinley, M.E.Morris)

[3] Journal of the American Geriatrics Society [2012] 60 (6) : 1104-1108 (M.Louter, M.Munneke, B.R.Bloem, S.Overeem)

[4] Parkinsonism & Related Disorders [2012] 18 (7) : 824-827 (F. Karlsson, P.Blomstedt, K.Olofsson, J.Linder, E.Nordh, J.van Doorn)

[5] Journal of Neural Transmission [1998] 105 (2-3) : 229-237 (J.J.van Hilten, A.A.van Eerd, E.A.Wagemans, H.A.Middelkoop, R.A.Roos)

[6] Journal of Clinical Neurophysiology [1998] 15 (3) : 235-242 (R.J. Dunnewold, J.I.Hoff, H.C.van Pelt, P.Q.Fredrikze, E.A.Wagemans, B. J.van Hilten)

[7] Movement Disorders [1996] 11 (3) : 236-242 (R.A.Roos, J.C. Jongen, E.A.van der Velde)

[8] Movement Disorders [2011] 26 (14) : 2504-2508 (A.J.Espay, J.P. Giuffrida, R.Chen, M.Payne, F.Mazzella, E.Dunn, J.E.Vaughan, A.P. Duker, A.Sahay, S.J.Kim, F.J.Revilla, D.A.Heldman)

Bradykinesia

Symptoms : Bradykinesia means slowness of movement and is one of the cardinal manifestations of Parkinson's Disease [1].

Prevalence : Bradykinesia occurs in around 28% of people with Parkinson's Disease when they are diagnosed, which is far less than the number of people who have rest tremor when they are diagnosed with Parkinson's Disease [2]. Bradykinesia was clearly present in the less affected patients with Parkinson's Disease and worsened as the Parkinson's Disease severity increased [3]. The objective measures of bradykinesia had only a modest or no relation to the semi-quantitative subjective Unified Parkinson's Disease Rating Scale (UPDRS) motor scores, which most likely was due to differences between the methods used [4].

Causes of symptoms : Bradykinesia can be due to the excessive muscle contraction that occurs in Parkinson's Disease reducing the capacity for movement. Bradykinesia may reflect a defective internal cue that disrupts and impairs the outflow of motor responses [5]. Bradykinesia may also partly be due to the failure of the corticomuscular system to engage in high frequency oscillatory activity [6]. The major cause of bradykinesia is depression in the rate of rise of electromyographic activity. The amplitude of the peak of this activity did not change significantly. There was no change either in the sequential activation of muscles, in the amount of co-contraction activity, in the accuracy of aim toward the visual target, or in the movement trajectory [7].

[1] Brain [2001] 124 (Part 11) : 2131-2146 (A.Berardelli, J.C.Rothwell, P.D.Thompson, M.Hallett)

[2] Clinical Neurology and Neurosurgery [2009] 111 (10) : 812-815 (A. Alrefai, M.Habahbih, M.Alkhawajah, M.Darwish, W.Batayha, Y. Khader, K.El-Salem)

[3] Journal of Neural Transmission [1998] 105 (2-3) : 229-237 (J.J.van Hilten, A.A.van Eerd, E.A.Wagemans, H.A.Middelkoop, R.A.Roos)

[4] Journal of Clinical Neurophysiology [1998] 15 (3) : 235-242 (R.J. Dunnewold, J.I.Hoff, H.C.van Pelt, P.Q.Fredrikze, E.A.Wagemans, B. J.van Hilten)

[5] Journal of Neurology [1994] 241 (7) : 439-447 (J.G.Phillips, K.E. Martin, J.L.Bradshaw, R.Iansek)

[6] Neuroreport [2001] 12 (11) : 2577-2581 (P.Brown, J.Marsden, L. Defebvre, F.Cassim, P.Mazzone, A.Oliviero, M.G.Altibrandi, V.Di Lazzaro, P.Limousin-Dowsey, V.Fraix, P.Odin, P.Pollak)

[7] Annals of Neurology [1992] 31 (1) : 93-100 (E.Godaux, D. Koulischer, J.Jacquy)

Akinesia

Symptoms : Akinesia refers to a failure of willed movement to occur. Akinesia is classified into three groups. The first is that secondary to the existence of marked rigidity of muscles and the second is that due to striatal dopamine deficiency, which can simply be interpreted as "lack of movement". The third is freezing or festination in quick repetitive movement especially in gait, speech and handwriting, for which L-dopa therapy has no influence. In most of the parkinsonian patients, it is considered that all three groups of akinesia are mixed together with a variety of grades [1].

Prevalence : Akinesia in Parkinson's Disease usually only occurs when Parkinson's Disease is chronic and severe [2, 3].

Causes of symptoms : Akinesia can be due to the excessive muscle contraction that occurs in Parkinson's Disease reducing the capacity for movement. Akinesia may also occur for two other possible reasons. One is that the movement is so slow and so small that it cannot be seen. A second is that the time needed to initiate the movement becomes excessively long. Reaction time studies in patients with Parkinson's Disease demonstrate that simple reaction time is delayed [4].

[1] Journal of Neural Transmission (Supplementum) [1980] (16) : 129-136 (H.Narabayashi)

[2] Neurology [2005] 64 (7) : 1162-1169 (M.Onofrj, A.Thomas)

[3] European Journal of Neurology [2003] 10 (4) : 391-398 (J.D. Schaafsma, Y.Balash, T.Gurevich, A.L.Bartels, J.M.Hausdorff, N. Giladi)

[4] Revue Neurologique [1990] 146 (10) : 585-590 (M.Hallett)

Dyskinesia

Symptoms : Dyskinesia commonly occurs as the rapid, jerky, irregular and involuntary movements of chorea [1]. There can be excessive and abnormal movements of the head, face, trunk, upper limbs. lower limbs [1, 2, 3], feet [3], eyes [4], and sometimes respiratory muscles [1]. People tended to suffer dyskinesia on the side of the body first affected by Parkinson's Disease [5]. When dyskinesia is unilateral it is more likely to occur on the side on which Parkinson's Disease is more severe [6].

Prevalence : Around 24% to 64% of people with Parkinson's Disease have dyskinesia. The rate varies according to geographical location [7-13, 24]. Around 50% of people with Parkinson's Disease develop dyskinesia within 5 years of diagnosis [24]. Around 60% of people with advanced Parkinson's Disease have dyskinesia [11, 14]. Those factors that make dyskinesia more likely are : the severity of Parkinson's Disease [6, 15], being younger when Parkinson's Disease first developed [15, 16, 17], younger age [17], a longer time from diagnosis to first being treated [16], and sometimes [15], but not always [16], the duration of Parkinson's Disease. The average time before dyskinesia developed was 4 years for women and 6 years for men [6, 16]. About 40% to 62% of people with Parkinson's Disease have dyskinesias after about 5 years [5, 15] or even less [18]. The likelihood of developing dyskinesias increased every year [5]. The majority of people with Parkinson's Disease have dyskinesias after 10 years of treatment [15].

Causes of symptoms : Dyskinesia in people with Parkinson's Disease is not a Parkinson's Disease symptom. It is usually caused by the use of dopaminergic drugs, including L-dopa and dopamine agonists [6, 13, 15, 19-22]. The reduction or withdrawal of those drugs can rid or reduce the dsykinesia [19]. The symptoms can be worsened by mental and physical activities such as speaking aloud, mental calculations, and movements of the fingers and neck [23].

[1] Postgraduate Medical Journal [2007] 83 (980) : 384-388 (B. Thanvi, N.Lo, T.Robinson)

[2] Fortschritte der Neurologie Psychiatrie [2007] 75 (7) : 387-396 (G. Ellrichmann, H.Russ, T.Müller)

[3] Movement Disorders [1994] 9 (1) : 2-12 (R.Marconi, D. Lefebvre-Caparros, A.M.Bonnet, M.Vidailhet, B.Dubois, Y.Agid)

[4] European Journal of Neurology [2007] 14 (10) : 1124-1128 (H. Grötzsch, R.Sztajzel, P.R.Burkhard)

[5] Journal of Neurology [1999] 246 (12) : 1127-1133 (F.Grandas, M.L.Galiano, C.Tabernero)

[6] Arquivos de Neuropsiquiatria [1995] 53 (4) : 737-742 (M.S. Rocha, L.A.Andrade, H.B.Ferraz, V.Borges)

[7] Neuroepidemiology [2007] 29 (3-4) : 163-169 (D.Woitalla, T. Mueller, H.Russ, K.Hock, D.A.Haeger)

[8] European Journal of Neurology [2016] 23 (2) : 304-312 (N.W. Scott, A.D.Macleod, C.E.Counsell)

[9] Current Treatments and Options in Neurology [2007] 9 (3) : 205-209 (J.Rao)

[10] Journal of the Medical Association Thailand [2006] 89 (5) : 632-637 (K.Kulkantrakorn, S.Tiamkao, C.Pongchaiyakul, T.Pulkes)

[11] Archives of Neurology [2006] 63 (2) : 205-209 (J.A.Van Gerpen, N.Kumar, J.H.Bower, S.Weigand, J.E.Ahlskog)

[12] Brain [2000] 123 (Part 11) : 2297-2305 (A.Schrag, N.Quinn)

[13] Journal of Neurology [1985] 232 (1) : 29-31 (A.Friedman)

[14] Journal of Neural Transmission [2007] 114 (3) : 341-345 (S. Papapetropoulos, D.C.Mash)

[15] Journal of Parkinsons Disease [2012] 2 (3) : 189-198 (A.Manson, P.Stirpe, A.Schrag)

[16] Journal of Neurology [2011] 258 (11) : 2048-2053 (S.Hassin-Baer, I.Molchadski, O.S.Cohen, Z.Nitzan, L.Efrati, O.Tunkel, E. Kozlova, A.D.Korczyn)

[17] Parkinsonism & Related Disorders [2010] 16 (8) : 490-497 (J.C. Sharma, C.G.Bachmann, G.Linazasoro)

[18] Canadian Journal of Neurological Sciences [1996] 23 (3) : 189-193 (P.J.Blanchet, P.Allard, L.Grégoire, F.Tardif, P.J.Bédard)

[19] Drugs [2016] 76 (7) : 759-777 (D.Vijayakumar, J.Jankovic)

[20] Drug Discovery Today [2010] 15 (19-20) : 867-875 (K.Buck, B. Ferger)

[21] Movement Disorders [1992] 7 (2) : 117-124 (M.R.Luquin, O. Scipioni, J.Vaamonde, O.Gershanik, J.A.Obeso)

[22] Brain [1991] 114 (Part 1B) : 601-617 (J.Vaamonde, M.R. Luquin, J.A.Obeso)

[23] Movement Disorders [1999] 14 (2) : 242-245 (F.Durif, M. Vidailhet, B.Debilly, Y.Agid)

[24] Parkinsonism & Related Disorders [2016] 22 : 48-53 (A. Bjornestad, E.B.Forsaa, K.F. Pedersen, O.B.Tysnes, J.P.Larsen, G. Alves)

Akathisia

Symptoms : Akathisia, which is motor restlessness, can occur in Parkinson's Disease. It can include rocking while standing or sitting, lifting the feet, and crossing and uncrossing the legs while sitting [1-5].

Prevalence : Nearly half or more than half of people with Parkinson's Disease are affected by akathisia [3-5]. Akathisia can occur to a lesser extent at night [6-8].

Causes of symptoms : Akathisia is a common side effect of antipsychotic drugs [9, 10].

[1] Journal of the Neurological Sciences [2011] 310 (1-2) : 82-85 (K. Bayulkem, G.Lopez)

[2] Revue Neurologique [2005] 161 (4) : 407-418 (R.Giuffrida, F.J. Vingerhoets, J. Bogousslavsky, J.Ghika)

[3] Neurology [2002] 59 (3) : 408-413 (T.Witjas, E.Kaphan, J.P. Azulay, O.Blin, M. Ceccaldi, J.Pouget, M.Poncet, A.A.Chérif)

[4] Movement Disorders [1994] 9 (5) : 545-549 (C.L.Comella, C.G. Goetz)

[5] Neurology [1987] 37 (3) : 477-481 (A.E.Lang, K.Johnson)

[6] Zhurnal Nevrologii I Psikhiatrii imeni S.S.Korsakova [2011] 111 (9 Part 2) : 45-50 (T.K.Kulua, N.V.Fedorova, O.A.Popovkina)

[7] Journal of the Neurological Sciences [2010] 289 (1-2) : 89-92 (K. Bayulkem, G.Lopez)

[8] Neurology [2004] 63 (8 Supplement 3) : S8-S11 (F.Grandas, A. Iranzo)

[9] Journal of Nervous and Mental Disease [1991] 179 (7) : 381-391 (P.Sachdev, C.Longragan)

[10] Italian Journal of Neurological Sciences [1990] 11 (5) : 439-442 (R.Sandyk, S.R.Kay)

Dystonia

Symptoms : Dystonia is uncontrollable and sometimes painful muscle spasms and prolonged muscle contractions. This can cause twisting, repetitive, involuntary movements or abnormal postures. Sometimes there is also dystonic tremor. Limb symptoms tend to be unilateral [1].

Prevalence : Occasionally, dystonia can occur in Parkinson's Disease [2, 3]. However, it is uncommon in untreated patients [2]. A third of people with Parkinson's Disease have painful dystonic movements in the lower extremities [4]. Around 16% of people with Parkinson's Disease reported early morning dystonia [5].

Causes of symptoms : Dystonia can be caused by dopaminergic drugs [2, 6], especially L-dopa [1, 6], even more so in people taking higher amounts for longer [5]. Dopamine agonists are less liable to do this [1].

[1] Clinical Neuropharmacology [1986] 9 (3) : 298-302 (H.L.Klawans, N.Paleologos)

[2] Journal of Neurology [2006] 253 (Supplement 7) : VII 7-13 (E. Tolosa, YCompta)

[3] Clinical Neuropharmacology [1986] 9 (3) : 293-297 (P.A.LeWitt, R.S.Burns, R.P.Newman)

[4] Archives of Neurology [1980] 37 (3) : 132-136 (P.A.Nausieda, W.J. Weiner, H.L.Klawans)

[5] Neurology [1998] 51 (1) : 283-285 (L.J.Currie, M.B.Harrison, J.M. Trugman, J.P.Bennett Jr, G.F.Wooten)

[6] Annals of Neurology [1988] 23 (1) : 73-78 (W.H.Poewe, A.J.Lees, G.M.Stern)

MUSCULAR SYSTEM

PART 2 : LOWER LIMB SYMPTOMS

Those muscular symptoms that can specifically affect the lower limbs are : shuffling (when walking) [PAGE 245], freezing (feeling unable to walk forwards) [PAGE 246], festination [PAGE 250], falling [PAGE 251], and restless legs syndrome [PAGE 255].

SHUFFLING

Symptoms : Shuffling whilst walking (walking in a clumsy or dragging manner) can occur in Parkinson's Disease [1-6]. Shuffling is associated with a greater fear of falling [5], and has a negative effect on the quality of life [6]. At first walking is slower, steps become shorter, feet are often dragged. This can develop into shuffling, or a complete inability to walk or stand without assistance. Flexion can occur in the knees, toes, and also the ankles, which can become inverted. Walking is characterised by short steps, with the feet barely leaving the ground, which can cause a shuffling noise. Small obstacles tend to trip the patient.

Prevalence : Shuffling is not so commonly reported in Parkinson's Disease [7].

Causes of symptoms : The rigidity and loss of movement in the legs causes difficulty in walking and running. In Parkinson's Disease there is increased muscle contraction of the leg muscles including those of gastrocnemius medialis and tibialis anterior [8]. It has been postulated that the decreased walking speed, and small shuffling steps in people with Parkinson's Disease could stem from an inability to tilt the body forward enough to provide sufficient forward propulsion [9]. Shuffling can respond well to dopaminergic drugs [1].

[1] Current Treatment Options in Neurology [2001] 3 (6) : 495-506 (J. M.Bertoni, J.L.Prendes, P.Sprenkle)

[2] JAMA [2003] 289 (3) : 347-353 (G.Rao, L.Fisch, S.Srinivasan, F. D'Amico, T.Okada, C.Eaton, C.Robbins)

[3] Biomedical Sciences Instrumentation [2005] 41 : 329-334 (D.B. Keenan, F.H.Wilhelm)

[4] Journal of Neurology, Neurosurgery, and Psychiatry [2008] 79 (4) : 368-376 (J.Jankovic)

[5] Behavioural Neurology [2011] 24 (3) : 219-228 (S.Rahman, H.J. Griffin, N.P.Quinn, M.Jahanshahi)

[6] Movement Disorders [2008] 23 (10) : 1428-1434 (S.Rahman, H.J. Griffin, N.P.Quinn, M.Jahanshahi)

[7] Neuroepidemiology [1991] 10 (3) : 150-156 (W.J.Mutch, W.C. Smith, R.F.Scott)

[8] Functional Neurology [2003] 18 (3) : 165-170 (G.Albani, G. Sandrini, G.Künig, C.Martin-Soelch, A.Mauro, R.Pignatti, C.Pacchetti, V.Dietz, K.L.Leenders)

[9] Frontiers in Neurology [2012] 3 : 132 (J.H.Bultitude, R.D.Rafal, C. Tinker)

Freezing

Symptoms : Freezing of gait (FOG) is a frequent, disabling symptom of Parkinson's Disease. It is characterised by brief episodes of the inability to step, or is characterised by extremely short steps that typically occur on initiating gait or on turning while walking. It is sudden and transient and usually lasts only a few seconds [1]. Freezing is a common cause of falling [2], and more than doubled the risk of falling [3].

Prevalence : The prevalence of freezing of gait in Parkinson's Disease is between 33% and 60% [3-11]. Around 20% of people with Parkinson's Disease are frequent fallers [8]. Freezing of Gait typically appeared nearly five years after the onset of Parkinson's Disease [9]. In 16% of cases it was evident before starting L-Dopa. Freezing is more common in the later stages of Parkinson's Disease [7]. By the end of the first decade, around 68% to 87% of people with Parkinson's Disease had freezing of gait [12, 13]. Freezing of gait is actually more common in atypical parkinsonism [5, 14].

Causes of symptoms : In Parkinson's Disease there is increased muscle contraction of the leg muscles including those of gastrocnemius medialis and tibialis anterior [15]. Those factors associated with an increase in likelihood of freezing of Gait are : the severity of Parkinson's Disease [3, 4, 6, 10, 16, 17], duration of Parkinson's Disease [4, 9, 10, 17, 18], earlier onset [3], older age [4, 11, 19], previous falls [8, 20], earlier use of L-dopa [11], higher dose of L-dopa [11], not taking dopamine agonists [11], reduced levels of activity [21], a greater step length variability [22], asymmetry of gait [23], balance problems [18, 20], sleep disorders [11], speech problems [18], being akinetic-rigid [11], akinesia [9], to a lesser extent with bradykinesia [18], more non-tremor symptoms [24], a selective impairment on executive functions [24], cognitive impairment [11, 20], depression [11]. Turning 360° in combination with a dual-task is the most important trigger for freezing [16, 25, 26]. Consequently, the most efficient way to objectively ascertain freezing of gait is by asking patients to repeatedly make rapid 360° narrow turns on the spot, and in both directions [27]. L-dopa decreases the freezing of gait in Parkinson's Disease [6, 20, 28, 29, 30] in around 20% of people [28].

[1] Movement Disorders [2008] 23 (3) : 395-400 (M.Amboni, A. Cozzolino, K.Longo, M.Picillo, P.Barone)

[2] Neurologia i Neurochirurgia Polska [2013] 47 (5) : 423-430 (M. Rudzinska, S.Bukowczan, J.Stozek, K.Zajdel, E.Mirek, W.Chwala, M. Wójcik-Pedziwiatr, K.Banaszkiewicz, A.Szczudlik)

[3] Journal of the Neurological Sciences [2012] 320 (1-2) : 66-71 (A. Contreras, F.Grandas)

[4] Journal of Neurological Science [2014] 345 (1-2) : 56-60 (R.Ou, X. Guo, W.Song, B.Cao, J.Yang, Q.Wei, N.Shao, H.Shang)

[5] Movement Disorders [1997] 12 (3) : 302-305 (N.Giladi, R.Kao, S. Fahn)

[6] Journal of Neural Transmission [2001] 108 (1) : 53-61 (N.Giladi, T. A.Treves, E.S.Simon, H.Shabtai, Y.Orlov, B.Kandinov, D.Paleacu, A. D.Korczyn)

[7] Revista Medica de Chile [2013] 141 (6) : 758-764 (G.Gonçalves, J. Pereira)

[8] Neurologia i Neurochirurgia Polska [2013] 47 (5) : 431-437 (M. Rudzinska, S.Bukowczan, J.Stozek, K.Zajdel, E.Mirek, W.Chwala, M. Wójcik-Pedziwiatr, K.Banaszkiewicz, A.Szczudlik)

[9] European Neurology [1997] 38 (4) : 297-301 (P.Lamberti, S. Armenise, V.Castaldo, M.de Mari, G.Iliceto, P.Tronci, L.Serlenga)

[10] Parkinsonism & Related Disorders [2015] Apr 13 [Epub ahead of print] (M.Amboni, F.Stocchi, G.Abbruzzese, L.Morgante, M.Onofrj, S. Ruggieri, M.Tinazzi, M.Zappia, M.Attar, D.Colombo, L.Simoni, et al)

[11] Medicine (Baltimore) [2016] 95 (26) : e4056 (H.Zhang, X.Yin, Z.Ouyang, J.Chen, S.Zhou, C.Zhang, X.Pan, S.Wang, J.Yang, Y.Feng, P.Yu, Q.Zhang)

[12] Clinical Neuropharmacology [2012] 35 (1) : 1-5 (P.J.García-Ruiz, J. Del Val, I.M.Fernández, A.Herranz)

[13] Journal of Neurology, Neurosurgery, and Psychiatry [2012] 83 (6) : 607-611 (M.Auyeung, T.H.Tsoi, V.Mok, C.M.Cheung, C.N.Lee, R. Li, E.Yeung)

[14] Movement Disorders [2008] 23 (Supplement 2) : S431-S438 (S.A. Factor)

[15] Functional Neurology [2003] 18 (3) : 165-170 (G.Albani, G. Sandrini, G.Künig, C.Martin-Soelch, A.Mauro, R.Pignatti, C.Pacchetti, V.Dietz, K.L.Leenders)

[16] Journal of Neurology [2006] 253 (Supplement 7) : VII27-VII32 (Y. Okuma)

[17] JAMA Neurology [2014] 71 (7) : 884-890 (S.Perez-Lloret, L. Negre-Pages, P.Damier, A.Delval, P.Derkinderen, A.Destée, W.G. Meissner, L.Schelosky, F.Tison, O.Rascol)

[18] Neurology [2001] 56 (12) : 1712-1721 (N.Giladi, M.P.McDermott, S.Fahn, S.Przedborski, J.Jankovic, M.Stern, C.Tanner)

[19] Movement Disorders [2000] 15 (2) : 309-312 (K.Kompoliti, C.G. Goetz, S.Leurgans, M.Morrissey, I.M.Siegel)

[20] Movement Disorders [2012] 27 (13) : 1644-1651 (S.Vercruysse, H.Devos, L.Munks, J.Spildooren, J.Vandenbossche, W.Vandenberghe, A.Nieuwboer, E.Heremans)

[21] Archives of Physical Medicine and Rehabilitation [2011] 92 (7) : 1159-1165 (D.M.Tan, J.L.McGinley, M.E.Danoudis, R.Iansek, M.E. Morris)

[22] Journal of Neurology, Neurosurgery, and Psychiatry [2012] 83 (1) : 98-101 (P.Knobl, L.Kielstra, Q.Almeida)

[23] Journal of Neurology [2013] 260 (1) : 71-76 (G.Frazzitta, G. Pezzoli, G.Bertotti, R.Maestri)

[24] Parkinsonism & Related Disorders [2014] 20 (6) : 604-607 (J.M. Hall, J.M.Shine, C.C.Walton, M.Gilat, Y.P.Kamsma, S.L.Naismith, S.J. Lewis)

[25] Movement Disorders [2010] 25 (15) : 2563-2570 (J.Spildooren, S.Vercruysse, K.Desloovere, W.Vandenberghe, E.Kerckhofs, A. Nieuwboer)

[26] Brain [2011] 134 (Part 1) : 59-72 (A.H.Snijders, I.Leunissen, M. Bakker, S.Overeem, R.C.Helmich, B.R.Bloem, I.Toni)

[27] Parkinsonism & Related Disorders [2012] 18 (2) : 149-154 (A.H. Snijders, C.A.Haaxma, Y.J.Hagen, M.Munneke, B.R.Bloem)

[28] Parkinsonism & Related Disorders [2013] 19 (10) : 894-896 (U. M.Fietzek, J.Zwosta, F.E.Schroeteler, K.Ziegler, A.O.Ceballos-Baumann)

[29] Parkinsonism & Related Disorders [2014] 20 (7) : 779-781 (J.V. Jacobs, J.G.Nutt, P.Carlson-Kuhta, R.Allen, F.B.Horak)

[30] Journal of Clinical Neuroscience [2003] 10 (5) : 584-588 (A.L. Bartels, Y.Balash, T.Gurevich, J.D.Schaafsma, J.M.Hausdorff, et al)

FESTINATION

Symptoms : Festination is a combination of stooped posture, short steps and imbalance. It leads to a gait that gets progressively faster that often ends falling [1]. Most people with festination believe that it is a disabling symptom [2]. During festination the number of steps was excessively increased (68%) and stride length was decreased (69%) [3].

Prevalence : Festination occurs in around 29% to 32% of people with Parkinson's Disease [2, 4]. It occurs more frequently in patients with : lower limbs as the site of onset [4], longer duration of Parkinson's Disease [2, 4], and more severe Parkinson's Disease [4]. The mean age, L-dopa use, entacapone use, motor complications [4], falls, freezing of gait [2, 4], emotional distress [5], are higher in people with festination.

Causes of symptoms : Rigidity and bradykinesia reduce interlimb coordination in Parkinsonian gait [6].

[1] Presse Medicale [2001] 30 (9) : 452-459 (G.Kemoun, L.Defebvre)

[2] Parkinsonism & Related Disorders [2001] 7 (2) : 135-138 (N. Giladi, H.Shabtai, E.Rozenberg, E.Shabtai)

[3] Movement Disorders [2001] 16 (6) : 1066-1075 (A.Nieuwboer, R. Dom, W.De Weerdt, K.Desloovere, S.Fieuws, E.Broens-Kaucsik)

[4] Clinical Neurology and Neurosurgery [2015] 139 : 172-176 (R.Ou, X.Guo, Q.Wei, B.Cao, J.Yang, W.Song, N.Shao, B.Zhao, X.Chen, H. Shang)

[5] Journal of Neuropsychiatry and Clinical Neurosciences [2015] 27 (2) : 121-126 (S.Starkstein, M.Dragovic, S.Brockman, M.Wilson, V. Bruno, M.Merello)

[6] Archives of Physical Meditation and Rehabilitation [2005] 86 (2) : 183-189 (A.Winogrodzka, R.C.Wagenaar, J.Booij, E.C.Wolters)

FALLING

Symptoms : Falling over commonly occurs in Parkinson's Disease [1]. Around 34% to 40% of falls resulted in injury [2, 3]. Among them, bruises of body parts other than the head were most frequent [2]. So people with Parkinson's Disease increase their likelihood of accidental injuries, especially head injuries. These also include : bone fracture and dislocation, all injuries, injury to spinal cord, plexus and nerves, and superficial injuries. The risk of injury increases with age [4]. Serious injuries occurred in less than 16% of cases [5] or far fewer [3].

Prevalence : Low, moderate and high concerns about falling were reported by 29%, 24% and 47% of people with Parkinson's Disease [1]. Falling actually occurs in anywhere between 19% and 64% of people with Parkinson's Disease [2, 3, 6-25, 39]. Women fell more often than men [25]. Falling occurs at least twice as often as it does in people who do not have Parkinson's Disease [26]. Recurrent fallers reported an average of 20 falls (between 4 and 67) per year [21]. Over a year, and even more over longer periods of time the likelihood of falling almost doubles [27, 28, 29]. Falling is uncommon in people who are newly diagnosed with Parkinson's Disease [22], and in people with tremor dominant Parkinson's Disease [22]. Most falls happened at home [29], and during parts of the day when mobility was at its highest [30].

Causes of symptoms : Factors that were most commonly associated with an increased likelihood of falling are more severe Parkinson's Disease symptoms [3, 15, 19, 21, 22, 31, 32], freezing [2, 3, 14, 21, 28, 29, 33], and a history of falls [2, 17, 20, 21, 31, 33, 34]. Other factors associated with an increased likelihood of falling are : postural instability [2, 3, 10, 29], a fear of falling [8, 21, 35], dyskinesia [2, 3, 14], cognitive impairment [14, 21, 33], and less commonly : disturbance of gait [18], old age [17, 20], daytime sleepiness [36], tripping [29], cognitive impairment [16], urinary incontinence [19], a history of near falls [8], environmental factors [10], higher L-dopa doses [28], being female [37], less physical activity before onset of Parkinson's Disease [15], reduced activities of daily living [34], greater fatigue [32], more depressive [32], reduced leg muscle strength [14,

32], use of dopamine agonists [21], impaired mobility [21], reduced physical activity [21], loss of postural reflexes [31], alcohol intake [3], abnormal posture [3, 33], vertigo [2], orthostatic hypotension [2]. People with Parkinson's Disease prone to falling took shorter strides, walked slower, had poorer gait stability and did not project their centre of mass as far forward of their base of support [38].

[1] Journal of Parkinson's Disease [2015] 5 (2) : 341-349 (S.B. Jonasson, S.Ullén, S.Iwarsson, J.Lexell, M.H.Nilsson)

[2] Neurologia i Neurochirurgia Polska [2013] 47 (5) : 423-430 (M. Rudzinska, S.Bukowczan, J.Stozek, K.Zajdel, E.Mirek, W.Chwala, M. Wójcik-Pedziwiatr, K.Banaszkiewicz, A.Szczudlik)

[3] Journal of Neuroscience Nursing [2000] 32 (4) : 222-228 (P. Gray, K.Hildebrand)

[4] European Journal of Neurology [2014] Mar 17 [Epub ahead of print] (H.C.Wang, C.C.Lin, C.I.Lau, A,Chang, F.C.Sung, C.H.Kao)

[5] Drugs & Aging [2009] 26 (10) : 847-852 (M.Rhalimi, R.Helou, P. Jaecker)

[6] BMJ Open [2013] 3 (11) : e003367 (B.Homann, A.Plaschg, M. Grundner, A.Haubenhofer, T.Griedl, G.Ivanic, E.Hofer, F.Fazekas, C. N.Homann)

[7] Nihon Ronen Igakkai Zasshi [2003] 40 (3) : 231-233 (T.Tsuchida, Y.Mano)

[8] PLoS One [2015] 10 (1) : e0117018 (B.Lindholm, P.Hagell, O. Hansson, M.H.Nilsson)

[9] Journal of Neurologic Physical Therapy [2006] 30 (2) : 60-67 (L.E. Dibble, M.Lange)

[10] Neurologia i Neurochirurgia Polska [2008] 42 (3) : 216-222 (M. Rudzinska, S.Bukowczan, K.Banaszkiewicz, J.Stozek, K.Zajdel, A. Szczudlik)

[11] Parkinsonism & Related Disorders [2009] 15 (2) : 110-115 (L.M. Allcock, E.M.Rowan, I.N.Steen, K.Wesnes, R.A.Kenny, D.J.Burn)

[12] Taehan Kanho Hakhoe Chi [2004] 34 (6) : 1081-1091 (K.Y. Sohng, J.S.Moon, K.S.Lee)

[13] Neurology [2009] 73 (20) : 1670-1676 (N.I.Bohnen, M.L.Müller, R.A.Koeppe, S.A.Studenski, M.A.Kilbourn, K.A.Frey, R.L.Albin)

[14] Neurorehabilitation and Neural Repair [2014] 28 (3) : 282-290 (S.S.Paul, C.Sherrington, C.G.Canning, V.S.Fung, J.C.Close, S.R.Lord)

[15] Geriatrics & Gerontology International [2015] 15 (4) : 472-480 (T.Gazibara, T.Pekmezovic, D.Kisic Tepavcevic, A.Tomic, I. Stankovic, V.S.Kostic, M.Svetel)

[16] Archives of Clinical Neuropsychology [2014] 29 (6) : 513 (D. Denney, D.Brown, J.Galusha, C.Lobue, R.Dewey, L.Lacritz)

[17] Annals of the Academy of Medicine, Singapore [2005] 34 (1) : 60-72 (L.W.Chu, I.Chi, A.Y.Chiu)

[18] Journal of Neurology [2004] 251 (1) : 79-84 (H.Stolze, S.Klebe, C.Zechlin, C.Baecker, L.Friege, G.Deuschl)

[19] Journal of Neurology [2005] 252 (11) : 1310-1315 (Y.Balash, C. Peretz, G.Leibovich, T.Herman, J.M.Hausdorff, N.Giladi)

[20] Parkinsonism & Related Disorders [2012] 18 (7) : 837-841 (T.S. Voss, J.J.Elm, C.L.Wielinski, M.J.Aminoff, D.Bandyopadhyay, K.L. Chou, L.R.Sudarsky, B.C.Tilley)

[21] Parkinson's Disease [2013] : 906274 (N.E.Allen, A.K. Schwarzel, C.G.Canning)

[22] European Journal of Neurology [2013] 20 (1) : 160-166 (Y.H. Hiorth, K.Lode, J.P.Larsen)

[23] Journals of Gerontology. Biological Sciences and Medical Sciences [2002] 57 (8) : M504-M510 (P.C.Fletcher, J.P. Hirdes)

[24] Journal of the American Geriatrics Society [2016] 64 (1) : 96-101 (T.B.Weaver, S.N.Robinovitch, A.C.Laing, Y.Yang)

[25] International Journal of Neuroscience [2016] Jun 29 : 1-18 [Epub ahead of print] (C.Tassorelli, M.Berlangieri, S.Buscone, M.Bolla, R.De Icco, A.Baricich, C.Pacchetti, C.Cisari, G.Sandrini)

[26] PLoS One [2016] 11 (9) : e0161689 (L.Kalilani, M.Asgharnejad, T.Palokangas, T.Durgin)

[27] Parkinsonism & Related Disorders [2015] 21 (3) : 236-242 (K. Mactier, S.Lord, A.Godfrey, D.Burn, L.Rochester)

[28] Parkinsonism & Related Disorders [2014] 20 (10) : 1059-1064 (Y.H.Hiorth, J.P.Larsen, K.Lode, K.F.Pedersen)

[29] Disability and Rehabilitation [2008] 30 (16) : 1205-1212 (A. Ashburn, E.Stack, C.Ballinger, L.Fazakarley, C.Fitton)

[30] Revista de Neurología [2004] 38 (12) : 1128-1132 (R.Cano-de la Cuerda, A.I.Macías-Jiménez, M.L.Cuadrado-Pérez, J.C.Miangolarra-Page, M.Morales-Cabezas)

[31] Movement Disorders [2007] 22 (13) : 1892-1900 (R.M.Pickering, Y.A.Grimbergen, U.Rigney, A.Ashburn, G.Mazibrada, B.Wood, P. Gray, G.Kerr, B.R.Bloem)

[32] European Neurology [2012] 67 (6) : 326-330 (M.S.Bryant, D.H. Rintala, J.G.Hou, S.P.Rivas, A.L.Fernandez, E.C.Lai, E.J.Protas)

[33] Movement Disorders [2009] 24 (9) : 1280-1289 (M.D.Latt, S.R. Lord, J.G.Morris, V.S.Fung)

[34] Acta Neurologica Scandinavica [2011] 123 (3) : 193-200 (M. Matinolli, J.T.Korpelainen, K.A.Sotaniemi, V.V.Myllylä, R. Korpelainen)

[35] Journal of Aging and Physical Activity [2015] 23 (2) : 187-193 (M. S.Bryant, D.H.Rintala, J.G.Hou, E.J.Protas)

[36] Journal of Parkinson's Disease [2013] 3 (3) : 387-391 (M.Spindler, N.S.Gooneratne, A.Siderowf, J.E.Duda, C.Cantor, N.Dahodwala)

[37] Parkinsonism & Related Disorders [2014] 20 (1) : 88-92 (K.Y. Cheng, W.C.Lin, W.N.Chang, T.K.Lin, N.W.Tsai, C.C.Huang, H.C. Wang, Y.C.Huang, H.W.Chang, Y.J.Lin, L.H.Lee, et al)

[38] Movement Disorders [2010] 25 (14) : 2369-2378 (M.H.Cole, P.A. Silburn, J.M.Wood, C.J.Worringham, G.K.Kerr)

[39] Journal of Neurology [2016] Dec 20 [Epub ahead of print] (Y.H. Hiorth, G.Alves, J.P.Larsen, J.Schulz, O.B.Tysnes, K.F.Pedersen)

Restless legs syndrome

Symptoms : Restless legs syndrome (RLS) is characterised by an irresistible urge for somebody to move their legs in order to stop uncomfortable sensations. It most commonly affects the legs, but can affect elsewhere in the body. Moving the affected body part reduces the sensations, thereby providing temporary relief.

Prevalence : Restless Leg Syndrome commonly occurs in people with Parkinson's Disease [1, 2, 3], with a prevalence of between 6% and 40% [1-20]. The prevalence increases with the duration of Parkinson's Disease [20]. People with Restless Legs Syndrome were more prone to developing Parkinson's Disease [21, 22]. In around 68% of people, Parkinson's Disease symptoms preceded RLS symptoms [19]. All the Restless Legs Syndrome symptoms did not appear in people with RLS until the Parkinson's Disease symptoms became apparent [23]. RLS symptoms usually developed within 5 years of developing Parkinson's Disease [24]. Many people with Parkinson's Disease suffer from motor restlessness due to Parkinsonism and this may also mimic Restless Legs Syndrome [25].

Causes of symptoms : In Parkinson's Disease there is increased muscle contraction of the leg muscles including those of gastrocnemius medialis and tibialis anterior [26]. Restless Legs Syndrome is a neurological disorder that responds to dopaminergic drugs, indicating a common pathophysiology with Parkinson's Disease [4]. However, presently there is not enough evidence to suggest that the actual pathophysiologic mechanism in both disorders is identical [27]. People with Parkinson's Disease who had RLS had : more anxiety [7], greater depression [17], worse nutritional status [7], worse Quality of Life [7], reported more pain [9], worse sleep [10, 28], worse Parkinson's Disease [11], were more commonly female [13], had earlier onset of Parkinson's Disease [14], had a lower L-dopa dose [14], and had been taking Parkinson's Disease drugs for longer [15].

[1] International Journal of Neuroscience [2016] 126 (2) : 116-120 (A.Q.Rana, A.R.Qureshi, L.Rahman, A.Jesudasan, K.K. Hafez, M.A. Rana)

[2] Journal of Parkinson's Disease [2014] 4 (2) : 211-221 (W.Schrempf, M.D.Brandt, A.Storch, H.Reichmann)

[3] Parkinsonism & Related Disorders [2014] 20 (Supplement 1) : S5-S9 (R.M.Rijsman, L.F.Schoolderman, R.S.Rundervoort, M.Louter)

[4] Arquivos de Neuro-Psiquiatria [2010] 68 (6) : 869-872 (T.M. Guerreiro, D.R.Nishikawa, L.C.Ferreira, H.A.Melo, R.C.Prado)

[5] European Neurology [2015] 73 (3-4) : 212-219 (A.Ylikoski, K. Martikainen, M.Partinen)

[6] International Journal of Neuroscience [2014] Dec 18 [Epub ahead of print] (E.M.Dragan, Z.Chen, W.G.Ondo)

[7] Acta Neurologica Scandinavica [2015] 131 (4) : 211-218 (S.M. Fereshtehnejad, M.Shafieesabet, G.A.Shahidi, A.Delbari, J.Lökk)

[8] Journal of the Neurological Sciences (2014) 344 (1-2) : 186-189 (Y. S.Oh, J.S.Kim, I.S.Park, I.U.Song, Y.M.Son, J.W.Park, D.W.Yang, H. T.Kim, K.S.Lee)

[9] Journal of the Neurological Sciences [2013] 327 (1-2) : 32-34 (A.Q.Rana, I.Siddiqui, A.Mosabbir, A.Athar, O.Syed, M.Jesudasan, K. Hafez)

[10] Parkinsonism & Related Disorders [2013] 19 (4) : 426-430 (K. Bhalsing, K.Suresh, U.B.Muthane, P.K.Pal)

[11] Parkinsonism & Related Disorders [2013] 19 (3) : 355-358 (H.Y. Shin, J.Youn, W.T.Yoon, J.S.Kim, J.W.Cho)

[12] Neurology [2011] 77 (22) : 1941-1946 (M.D.Gjerstad, O.B. Tysnes, J.P.Larsen)

[13] Movement Disorders [2010] 25 (13) : 2142-2147 (D.Verbaan, S. M.van Rooden, J.J.van Hilten, R.M.Rijsman)

[14] Movement Disorders [2009] 24 (14) : 2076-2080 (C.M.Peralta, B. Frauscher, K.Seppi, E.Wolf, G.K.Wenning, B.Högl, W.Poewe)

[15] Movement Disorders [2009] 24 (4) : 579-582 (J.E.Lee, H.W. Shin, K.S.Kim, Y.H.Sohn)

[16] Movement Disorders [2007] 22 (13) : 1912-1916 (J.C.Gómez-Esteban, J.J.Zarranz, B.Tijero, F.Velasco, J.Barcena, I.Rouco, E. Lezcano, M.C.Lachen, A.Jauregui, A.Ugarte)

[17] Movement Disorders [2003] 18 (2) : 181-185 (P.R.Krishnan, M. Bhatia, M.Behari)

[18] Journal of the Neurological Sciences [2002] 196 (1-2) : 33-36 (E. K.Tan, S.Y.Lum, M.C.Wong)

[19] Archives of Neurology [2002] 59 (3) : 421-424 (W.G.Ondo, K.D. Vuong, J.Jankovic)

[20] Sleep [2016] 39 (2) : 405-412 (M.Moccia, R.Erro, M.Picillo, G. Santangelo, E.Spina, R.Allocca, K.Longo, M.Amboni, R.Palladino, R. Assante, S.Pappatà, M.T.Pellecchia, P.Barone, C.Vitale)

[21] Sleep [2014] 37 (2) : 369-372 (J.C.Wong, Y.Li, M.A. Schwarzschild, A.Ascherio, X.Gao)

[22] Movement Disorders [2010] 25 (15) : 2654-2657 (X.Gao, M.A. Schwarzschild, E.J.O'Reilly, H.Wang, A.Ascherio)

[23] Zhonghua Nei Ke Za Zhi [2010] 49 (11) : 947-950 (L.Q.Zhao, L. N.Wang, F.Y.Hu)

[24] Journal of the Neurological Sciences [2006] 250 (1-2) : 39-44 (T. Nomura, Y.Inoue, K.Nakashima)

[25] Journal of the Neurological Sciences [2010] 289 (1-2) : 135-137 (J.C.Möller, M.Unger, K.Stiasny-Kolster, W.H.Oertel)

[26] Functional Neurology [2003] 18 (3) : 165-170 (G.Albani, G. Sandrini, G.Künig, C.Martin-Soelch, A.Mauro, R.Pignatti, C.Pacchetti, V.Dietz, K.L.Leenders)

[27] Journal of Neurology [2006] 253 (Supplement 7) : VII33-VII37 (E.K. Tan)

[28] BMC Neurology [2012] 12 : 71 (E.Svensson, A.G.Beiske, J.H. Loge, K.K.Beiske, B.Sivertsen)

MUSCULAR SYSTEM
PART 3 : UPPER LIMB SYMPTOMS

Those muscular symptoms that can specifically affect the upper limbs are : impaired finger dexterity [PAGE 258], micrographia (small handwriting) [PAGE 259], reduced arm swing [PAGE 260], mirror movement (intentional movements of one side of the body are mirrored by involuntary movements of the other side) [PAGE 261], and frozen shoulder syndrome [PAGE 263].

IMPAIRED FINGER DEXTERITY

Symptoms : Impaired finger dexterity [1], including dysco-ordination of the wrist and fingers [2].

Prevalence : The finger dexterity of people with Parkinson's Disease is usually more impaired than people without Parkinson's Disease [1, 3].

Causes of symptoms : In Parkinson's Disease there is increased muscle contraction of the hand muscles, including the dorsal interossei muscles [4]. Previously, bradykinesia was regarded as the major cause. However, it is claimed that it is related to praxis function [5], an intrinsic dysfunction of the primary somatosensory cortex [6], or limb kinetic apraxia [3].

[1] Movement Disorders [2010] 25 (15) : 2531-2555 (M.S.Lee, C.H. Lyoo, M.J.Lee, J.Sim, H.Cho, Y.H.Choi)

[2] Neuropsychologia [2009] 47 (12) : 2504-2514 (N.Dounskaia, A.W. Van Gemmert, B.C.Leis, G.E.Stelmach)

[3] Movement Disorders [2008] 23 (12) : 1701-1706 (A.Gebhardt, T. Vanbellingen, F.Baronti, B.Kersten, S.Bohlhalter)

[4] Electroencephalography and Clinical Neurophysiology [1995] 97 (5) : 215-222 (R.Cantello, M.Gianelli, C.Civardi, R.Mutani)

[5] Brain and Cognition [2011] 77 (1) : 48-52 (T.Vanbellingen, B. Kersten, M.Bellion, P.Temperli, F.Baronti, R.Müri, S.Bohlhalter)

[6] Parkinsonism & Related Disorders [2015] 21 (3) : 259-265 (T. Foki, W.Pirker, A.Geißler, D.Haubenberger, M.Hilbert, I.Hoellinger, M. Wurnig, J.Rath, J.Lehrner, E.Matt, F.Fischmeister, S.Trattnig, et al)

MICROGRAPHIA

Symptoms : Micrographia, which is an abnormal reduction in writing size, is a specific deficit associated with Parkinson's Disease [1-4]. It is more characteristic of people with Parkinson's Disease who have rigidity and akinesia than in people with prominent tremor [4]. People with Parkinson's Disease also exhibit impaired handwriting, which is described as dysgraphia [1, 2]. It can be used to distinguish people with Parkinson's Disease [1, 5]. People with Parkinson's Disease had a linear decrease in overall character size and horizontal strokes along the writing sequence in the horizontal direction, but not in the vertical direction [6]. The decrease of handwriting size in the horizontal direction suggests that micrographia may be associated with wrist extension [6]. There is also a reduced capability to maintain a given force when writing [7]. Handwriting usually changed over time [8].

Prevalence : Microphagia occurs in nearly half of people with Parkinson's Disease [9].

Causes of symptoms : In Parkinson's Disease there is increased muscle contraction of the hand muscles, including the dorsal interossei muscles [10]. Handwriting improved in response to the use of dopaminergic drugs and deteriorated in response to their withdrawal [11]. Long term deterioration in Parkinson's Disease did not worsen handwriting [12].

[1] Computer Methods and Programs in Biomedicine [2014] 117 (3) : 405-411 (P.Drotár, J.Mekyska, I.Rektorová, L.Masarová, Z.Smékal, M. Faundez-Zanuy)

[2] Movement Disorders [2014] 29 (12) : 1467-1475 (A.Letanneux, J. Danna, J.L.Velay, F.Viallet, S.Pinto)

[3] Parkinsonism & Related Disorders [2005] 11 (1) : 57-63 (E.J.Kim, B.H.Lee, K.C.Park, W.Y.Lee, D.L.Na)

[4] Journal of Neurology [2012] 259 (11) : 2335-2340 (N.P.Bajaj, L. Wang, V.Gontu, D.G.Grosset, P.G.Bain)

[5] Journal of Neurology [2013] 260 (9) : 2357-2361 (S.Rosenblum, M. Samuel, S.Zlotnik, I.Erikh, I.Schlesinger)

[6] Behavioural Neurology [2013] 27 (2) : 169-174 (H.I.Ma, W.J. Hwang, S.H.Chang,T.Y. Wang)

[7] Neuropsychologia [1999] 37 (6) : 685-694 (A.W.Van Gemmert, H.L.Teulings, J.L.Contreras-Vidal, G.E.Stelmach)

[8] Forensic Science International [1997] 88 (3) : 197-214 (J.Walton)

[9] BMJ Open [2012] 2 (3) pii : e000628 (A.Wagle Shukla, S. Ounpraseuth, M.S.Okun, V.Gray, J.Schwankhaus, W.S.Metzer)

[10] Electroencephalography and Clinical Neurophysiology [1995] 97 (5) : 215-222 (R.Cantello, M.Gianelli, C.Civardi, R.Mutani)

[11] Journal of Neural Transmission [2006] 113 (5) : 609-623 (O. Tucha, L.Mecklinger, J.Thome, A.Reiter, G.L.Alders, H.Sartor, M. Naumann, K.W.Lange)

[12] Movement Disorders [1986] 1 (3) : 187-192 (H.L.Klawans)

Reduced arm swing

Symptoms : People with Parkinson's Disease commonly have reduced arm swing while walking, which can initially occur in one arm [1-4] before progressing to both arms. Asymmetric arm swing and accompanying tremor are indicators of early Parkinson's Disease [5, 6].

Prevalence : Reduced arm swing occurred in as many as 75% of people with Parkinson's Disease [4].

Causes of symptoms : In Parkinson's Disease there is increased muscle contraction of the arm muscles, including those of brachioradialis and the biceps [7]. Reduction in arm swing is associated with rigidity [8]. Asymmetric arm swing is related to Parkinson's Disease severity [9, 10]. It can be reduced using dopaminergic drugs [11].

[1] Conference proceedings : Annual International Conference of the IEEE Engineering in Medicine and Biology Society [2007] : 6665-6668 (I.Carpinella, P.Crenna, A.Marzegan, M.Rabuffetti, et al)

[2] Movement Disorders [2010] 25 (14) : 2369-2378 (M.H.Cole, P.A. Silburn, J.M.Wood, C.J.Worringham, G.K.Kerr)

[3] Movement Disorders [2012] 27 (12) : 1563-1566 (S.A.Schneider, L. Drude, M.Kasten, C.Klein, J.Hagenah)

[4] Disability and Rehabilitation [1998] 20 (4) : 142-150 (A. Nieuwboer, W.De Weerdt, R.Dom, E.Lesaffre)

[5] Gait & Posture [2014] 39 (4) : 1138-1141 (S.M.Lee, M.Kim, H.M. Lee, K.Y.Kwon, H.T.Kim, S.B.Koh)

[6] Gait & Posture [2010] 31 (2) : 256-260 (M.D.Lewek, R.Poole, J. Johnson, O.Halawa, X.Huang)

[7] Journal of Neurology, Neurosurgery and Psychiatry [1987] 50 (10) : 1274-1283 (F.Viallet, J.Massion, R.Massarino, R.Khalil)

[8] Journal of the Neurological Sciences [2014] 341 (1-2) : 32-35 (K.Y. Kwon, M.Kim, S.M.Lee, S.H.Kang, H.M.Lee, S.B.Koh)

[9] Gait & Posture [2012] 35 (3) : 373-377 (X.Huang, J.M.Mahoney, M.M.Lewis, D.U.Guangwei, S.J.Piazza, J.P.Cusumano)

[10] IEEE Transactions on Neural Systems and Rehabilitation Engineering [2010] 18 (3) : 303-310 (A.Salarian, F.B.Horak, C. Zampieri, P.Carlson-Kuhta, J.G.Nutt, K.Aminian)

[11] Journal of Parkinson's Disease [2015] 5 (1) : 141-150 (N.W. Sterling, J.P.Cusumano, N.Shaham, S.J.Piazza, G.Liu, L.Kong, G.Du, M.M.Lewis, X.Huang)

Mirror movement

Symptoms : Mirror movement is a condition in which intentional movements of one side of the body are mirrored by involuntary movements of the other side of the body. For example, when an affected individual makes a fist with the right hand, the left hand makes a similar movement. The mirror movements primarily involve the upper limbs, especially the hands and fingers [1, 2].

Prevalence : Over 90% of people who have Parkinson's Disease exhibit mirror movements [3, 4]. Mirror movements are often reported in people with early Parkinson's Disease [5, 6], and when the symptoms of Parkinson's Disease are less severe [3]. However, one study found that mirror movements were actually less common in Parkinson's Disease [7].

Causes of symptoms : Mirror movements reflect an abnormal enhancement of the mirroring that can be observed in normal circumstances during complex and effortful tasks. It was hypothesized that, in Parkinson's Disease, enhanced mirroring is caused by a failure of basal ganglia output to support the cortical network that is responsible for the execution of strictly unimanual movements [8]. Overt mirror movement may be due to the combination of enhanced motor cortex excitability [5, 6] and an earlier onset of activation in the mirror hand [6]. Mirror movements are usually a clinical feature of the less affected side in people who have mild Parkinson's Disease [4, 7].

[1] PLoS One [2013] 8 (6) : e66910 (A.Poisson, B.Ballanger, E. Metereau, J.Redouté, D.Ibarolla, J.C.Comte, H.G.Bernard, M. Vidailhet, E.Broussolle, S.Thobois)

[2] Tremor and other Hyperkinetic Movements [2012] 2 pii : tre-02-59-398-1 (B.C.Cox, M.Cincotta, A.J.Espay)

[3] Journal of Neurological Science [2016] 366 : 171-176 (P. Chatterjee, R.Banerjee, S.Choudhury, B.Mondal, M.U.Kulsum, K. Chatterjee, H.Kumar)

[4] Journal of Neurology, Neurosurgery and Psychiatry [2005] 76 (10) : 1355-1358 (A.J.Espay, J.Y.Li, L.Johnston, R.Chen, A.E.Lang)

[5] Movement Disorders [2007] 22 (6) : 813-821 (J.Y.Li, A.J.Espay, C.A.Gunraj, P.K.Pal, D.I.Cunic, A.E.Lang, R.Chen)

[6] Journal of Parkinsons Disease [2014] 4 (3) : 437-452 (S.A. Sharples, Q.J.Almeida, J.M.Kalmar)

[7] Movement Disorders [2008] 23 (2) : 253-258 (D.Ottaviani, D.Tiple, A.Suppa, C.Colosimo, G.Fabbrini, M.Cincotta, G.Defazio, A. Berardelli)

[8] Movement Disorders [2006] 21 (9) : 1461-1465 (M.Cincotta, F.Giovannelli, A.Borgheresi, F.Balestrieri, P.Vanni, A.Ragazzoni, G. Zaccara, U.Ziemann)

Frozen Shoulder Syndrome

Symptoms : In Frozen Shoulder Syndrome the shoulder becomes stiff and so greatly restricts movement of the shoulder. It can thereby cause chronic pain and physical disability [1]. The symptoms of Frozen Shoulder Syndrome tend to get gradually worse over a number of months or years.

Prevalence : Frozen Shoulder Syndrome can more commonly affect people with Parkinson's Disease [1-4], with from 12% to 46% of people with Parkinson's Disease being affected by it [1, 3, 4]. Those people prone to Frozen Shoulder Syndrome had initial symptoms of akinesia twice as frequently as they had tremor [4]. In at least 8% of people with Parkinson's Disease who have Frozen Shoulder Syndrome it was the first symptom they had, occurring up to 2 years before other common symptoms [4].

Causes of symptoms : In Parkinson's Disease there is increased muscle contraction of the arm muscles, including those of brachioradialis and the biceps [5]. Shoulder muscles can also be affected by excessive muscle contraction. "Frozen shoulders" and pain can respond to the use of L-dopa [6].

[1] Parkinson's Disease [2015] Jun 9 [Epub 2015] (Y.T.Chang, W.N. Chang, N.W.Tsai, K.Y.Cheng, C.C.Huang, C.T.Kung, Y.J.Su, W.C. Lin, B.C.Cheng, C.M.Su, Y.F.Chiang, C.H.Lu)

[2] Journal of Neurology, Neurosurgery and Psychiatry [1989] 52 (6) : 813-814 (L.Cleeves, L.Findley)

[3] Parkinsonism & Related Disorders [2013] 19 (7) : 666-669 (Y.E.Kim, W.W.Lee, J.Y.Yun, H.J.Yang, H.J.Kim, B.S.Jeon)

[4] Journal of Neurology, Neurosurgery and Psychiatry [1989] 52 (1) : 63-66 (D.Riley, A.E. Lang, R.D.Blair, A.Birnbaum, B.Reid)

[5] Journal of Neurology, Neurosurgery and Psychiatry [1987] 50 (10) : 1274-1283 (F.Viallet, J.Massion, R.Massarino, R.Khalil)

[6] Southern Medical Journal [2004] 97 (8) : 776-777 (G.J.Gilbert)

Muscular system

Part 4 : Head and neck symptoms

Those muscular symptoms that can specifically affect the head and neck are hypomimia (reduced facial expression) [PAGE 264], reduced blinking [PAGE 265], dysarthria (difficulty speaking), [PAGE 267], dysphonia [PAGE 268], and neck rigidity [PAGE 268].

Hypomimia

Symptoms : Hypomimia is a reduction and slowness of facial expression. This gives the appearance of a mask like face. Some individuals may appear uninterested when speaking, while others stare fixedly with unblinking eyes. Impaired facial expression, including spontaneous and emotional movements such as smiling, have been often reported in Parkinson's Disease [1, 2, 3]. Intentional facial expressions are slowed (bradykinetic) and involve less movement in much the same way that other intentional movements are affected by Parkinson's Disease [4].

Prevalence : There is a general consensus that spontaneous smiling is uncommon in people with Parkinson's Disease [1]. Posed smiling and voluntary grinning are related to the severity of Parkinson's Disease [1, 3].

Causes of symptoms : In Parkinson's Disease there is increased muscle contraction of the facial muscles, including the orbicularis oris, mentalis muscles and labial muscles [5, 6]. Hypomimia is not improved by taking L-dopa [1]. A reduction in eye movement caused by muscle rigidity leads to the staring appearance of the eyes.

[1] Parkinsonism & Related Disorders [2014] 20 (4) : 370-375 (L. Marsili, R.Agostino, M. Bologna, D.Belvisi, A.Palma, G.Fabbrini, A. Berardelli)

[2] Frontiers of Neurology and Neuroscience [2013] 31 : 178-187 (J. Haan)

[3] Journal of Neurological Science [2014] 347 (1-2) : 332-336 (M. Marneweck, G.Hammond)

[4] Journal of the International Neuropsychological Society [2006] 12 (6) : 765-773 (D.Bowers, K.Miller, W.Bosch, D.Gokcay, O.Pedraza, U. Springer, M.Okun)

[5] Neurology [1982] 32 (7) : 749-754 (C.J.Hunker, J.H.Abbs, S.M. Barlow)

[6] Journal of Neurology, Neurosurgery and Psychiatry [1971] 34 (6) : 679-681 (R.Leanderson, B.A.Meyerson, A.Persson)

Reduced blinking

Symptoms : Blinking, which consists of a closing and an opening eyelid movement, can be performed voluntarily, spontaneously, and reflexly [1]. Parkinson's Disease is characterised by a reduction in spontaneous blinking [1, 2], especially in the "off" period [1, 3]. The amplitudes of voluntary and reflex blinking also tended to be smaller than normal in people with Parkinson's Disease [1, 4]. The longer pauses between the closing and opening phase in comparison to normal subjects suggests bradykinesia of voluntary blinking [1]. In some people with Parkinson's Disease the blink rate is high and returns to normal after the administration of L-dopa [3]. In these cases it is suggested that the increased blink rate represents a form of dystonia [3]. In those with dyskinesia the blink rate becomes more extended [5].

Prevalence : In people with Parkinson's Disease the decline in blink rate increases with age [6, 7]. Blinking was reduced more in women than men younger than 50 years of age but did not differ from men older than 60 years of age [7]. There was no increased effect on blinking according to the duration, treatment or severity of Parkinson's Disease [6]. Blink rate is also correlated with corneal sensitivity [8]. Blink rates were highest when people were being interviewed and were lowest whilst reading a passage [6].

Causes of symptoms : In Parkinson's Disease there is increased muscle contraction of the orbicularis oris [9, 10]. The blink rate increased after the administration of L-dopa [3]. A reduction in eye movement caused by muscle rigidity leads to a poverty of blinking.

[1] Movement Disorders [2008] 23 (5) : 669-675 (R.Agostino, M. Bologna, L.Dinapoli, B.Gregori, G.Fabbrini, N.Accornero, A. Berardelli)

[2] Journal of Neurology, Neurosurgery, and Psychiatry [2013] 84 (6) : 681-685 (M.Bologna, G.Fabbrini, L.Marsili, G.Defazio, P.D. Thompson, A.Berardelli)

[3] Movement Disorders [2000] 15 (5) : 982-985 (T.E.Kimber, P.D. Thompson)

[4] Movement Disorders [2006] 21 (8) : 1248-1251 (M.Korosec, I. Zidar, D.Reits, C.Evinger, F.Vanderwerf)

[5] Functional Neurology [1989] 4 (3) : 257-261 (L.M.Iriarte, J. Chacon, J.Madrazo, P.Chaparro)

[6] Journal of Neurology [2012] 259 (4) : 739-744 (E.Fitzpatrick, N. Hohl, P.Silburn, C.O'Gorman, S.A.Broadley)

[7] Clinical Neurology and Neurosurgery [2003] 105 (2) : 90-92 (W.H. Chen, T.J.Chiang, M.C.Hsu, J.S.Liu)

[8] Cornea [2013] 32 (5) : 631-635 (V.C.Reddy, S.V.Patel, D.O.Hodge, J.A.Leavitt)

[9] Neurology [1982] 32 (7) : 749-754 (C.J.Hunker, J.H.Abbs, S.M. Barlow)

[10] Journal of Neurology, Neurosurgery and Psychiatry [1971] 34 (6) : 679-681 (R.Leanderson, B.A.Meyerson, A.Persson)

Dysarthria

Symptoms : Dysarthria is speech difficulties, such as unclear, softened or slurred speech. The voice becomes softer and loses volume (hypophonia). A loss of voice inflections makes the voice sound monotonous. People with Parkinson's Disease spoke more quietly than other people and yet overestimated the volume of their speech during both reading and conversation [1]. There is a reduced ability to express stress, even in the early stages of Parkinson's Disease [2]. Impaired vowel articulation is a possible early marker of Parkinson's Disease [3]. Vowel articulation is significantly reduced in people with Parkinson's Disease but this was not related to the severity of Parkinson's Disease [4].

Prevalence : The speech of around 70% of people with Parkinson's Disease was found to be affected in this way, making it one of the most common problems [5]. The average time taken to fully develop dysarthria is seven years [6].

Causes of symptoms : Dysarthria is caused by problems with the muscles used in speech, which includes the larynx and pharynx. The intelligibility of speech in people with Parkinson's Disease was not related to age or the duration of Parkinson's Disease. Dysarthria was only weakly related to the stage and the severity of Parkinson's Disease [5].

[1] Movement Disorders [2000] 15 (6) : 1125-1131 (A.K.Ho, J..L. Bradshaw, T.Iansek)

[2] Journal of Voice [2014] 28 (1) : 129.e1-129.e8 (T.Tykalova, J. Rusz, R.Cmejla, H.Ruzickova, E.Ruzicka)

[3] Journal of the Acoustical Society of America [2013] 134 (3) : 2171-2181 (J.Rusz, R.Cmejla, T.Tykalova, H.Ruzickova, J.Klempir, V. Majerova, J.Picmausova, J.Roth, E.Ruzicka)

[4] Journal of Voice [2011] 25 (4) : 467-472 (S.Skodda, W.Visser, U. Schlegel)

[5] Journal of Neurology, Neurosurgery and Psychiatry [2007] 78 (11) : 1188-1190 (N.Miller, L.Allcock, D.Jones, E.Noble, A.J.Hildreth, D.J. Burn)

[6] Archives of Neurology [2001] 58 (2) : 259-264 (J.Müller, G.K. Wenning, M.Verny, A.McKee, K.R.Chaudhuri, K.Jellinger, W.Poewe, I.Litvan)

Dysphonia

Symptoms : Dysphonia is an impairment in the ability to produce voice sounds using the vocal organs. It is distinct from dysarthria which signifies dysfunction in the muscles needed to produce speech. Thus, dysphonia is a phonation disorder. The voice can be hoarse, breathy, harsh, or rough, but some kind of phonation is still possible [1].

Prevalence : The prevalence of dysphonia is about 35% in Parkinson's Disease [1, 2].

Causes of symptoms : Dysphonia is related to the severity of Parkinson's Disease. However, dysphonia is more closely related to depression than to the severity of Parksinson's Disease [2].

[1] Laryngoscope [2006] 116 (10) : 1740-1744 (G.K.Sewall, J.Jiang, C.N.Ford)

[2] Journal of the Neurological Sciences [2014] 346 (1-2) : 112-115 (M.K.Sunwoo, J.Y.Hong, J.E.Lee, H.S.Lee, P.H.Lee, Y.H.Sohn)

Neck rigidity

Symptoms : Neck rigidity can cause a loss of movement and flexion of the neck. It can also cause antecollis, retrocollis or torticollis. In antecollis the neck bends forward and the head drops down. In retrocollis the head is drawn backwards. In torticollis the head becomes persistently turned to one side. Neck rigidity is significantly higher in patients with retrocollis and antecollis than in those with normal neck posture [1]. There is also anterior neck rigidity in Dropped Head Syndrome [2], in which the neck and also the trunk are bent forward [3, 4]. Dropped Head Syndrome can also cause a bending forward of the spine [5].

Prevalence : Neck rigidity is related to the duration and severity of Parkinson's Disease. There was neck rigidity in 27% of people with Parkinson's Disease who had unilateral involvement of the limbs. There was rigidity in the neck rigidity in all people with Parkinson's Disease who had bilateral involvement of the limbs [6]. In more advanced Parkinson's Disease (Hoehn and Yahr stage 5) 28% had retrocollis, 4% had antecollis, and 1% had antecollis and torticollis. However, in an earlier stage of Parkinson's Disease (Hoehn and Yahr stage 4) hardly anybody with Parkinson's Disease had retrocollis [1]. It took an average of 10 years to develop antecollis, but the time taken varies greatly [7]. Dropped Head Syndrome occurs in about 6% of people with Parkinson's Disease, and more commonly in women. It took an average of 5 years to develop Dropped Head Syndrome but the time taken varies greatly [4].

Causes of symptoms : In Parkinson's Disease there is increased muscle contraction of the neck muscles, including the anterior neck muscles [8]. Parkinson's Disease drugs lessened Dropped Head Syndrome in most but not all patients, but dopamine agonists can worsen it [3, 4].

[1] Journal of Neurological Science [2013] 324 (1-2) : 106-108 (K. Kashihara, T.Imamura)

[2] Journal of Neurological Science [1999] 167 (1) : 22-25 (Y. Yoshiyama, J.Takama, T.Hattori)

[3] Journal of Neurology [2006] 253 (Supplement 7) : VII21-VII26 (K. Fujimoto)

[4] Movement Disorders [2006] 21 (8) : 1213-1216 (K.Kashihara, M. Ohno, S.Tomita)

[5] Evidence Based Spine Care Journal [2011] 2 (2) : 41-47 (A.R. Martin, R.Reddy, M.G.Fehlings)

[6] Rinsho Shinkeigaku [1996] 36 (10) : 1129-1135 (K.Nagumo, K. Hirayama)

[7] Movement Disorders [2007] 22 (16) : 2325-2331 (B.P. van de Warrenburg, C.Cordivari, A.M.Ryan, R.Phadke, J.L.Holton, K.P. Bhatia, M.G.Hanna, N.P.Quinn)

[8] Journal of the Neurological Sciences [1999] 167 (1) : 22-25 (Y. Yoshiyama, J.Takama, T.Hattori)

CHAPTER 21

SYMPTOMS OF PARKINSON'S DISEASE

NERVOUS SYSTEM

Nervous system

The nervous system is made up of the brain, the spinal cord, the nerves, and the sense organs, such as the eye and the ear. The nervous system receives, interprets, and responds to stimuli from inside and outside the body.

Primary symptoms

In Parkinson's Disease there can be an increased likelihood of depression [PAGE 271], dementia [PAGE 277], pain [PAGE 283], sleep disturbance [PAGE 288], excessive daytime sleepiness [PAGE 291], fatigue [PAGE 296], apathy [PAGE 298], anhedonia [PAGE 302], bradyphrenia [PAGE 304], alexithymia [PAGE 305], neuropathy [PAGE 306], anxiety [PAGE 308], hallucinations [PAGE 310], compulsions [PAGE 314], vertigo [PAGE 317], and brain tumor [PAGE 317]. The most prominent, prevalent or troubling of these symptoms are depression, dementia, pain, fatigue and sleep disturbance.

Depression

Symptoms : Dopamine is involved in the control of behaviour. So its deficiency can cause emotional depression and slowness of thinking. Symptoms of depression can be evident in people with Parkinson's Disease at the time of diagnosis and might develop in the pre-motor stage of the disease [1, 2]. Depression made Parkinson's Disease as much as four times more likely to develop [3-9]. Depressive features did not differ according to whether or not people also had Parkinson's Disease [10]. Depression has been shown to contribute to an increased rate of decline of both cognitive and motor function, profoundly impacting on the patient's quality of life [11-13].

Prevalence : The average prevalence of depression in Parkinson's Disease is around 40%. The majority of studies put the prevalence of depression in Parkinson's Disease at between 20% and 50% [2, 11, 12, 14-46]. In some studies the prevalence is claimed to be between 10% and 60% [3, 46-56]. However, according to a few other studies the prevalence is claimed to be anywhere between 2% and 90% [56-59]. The prevalence can differ a lot according to the diagnostic criteria used [47]. The degree of depression varied from minimal, mild, and moderate to severe [22, 24, 49, 55, 60, 61]. Around 22% of home dwellers who had Parkinson's Disease, and 50% of people with Parkinson's Disease who were institutionalized, used antidepressants [72]. Prevalence increases according to : the duration of Parkinson's Disease [22, 51, 60, 62], more severe Parkinson's Disease [44, 54, 62, 63], more cognitive impairment [52], being female [3, 41, 54, 64], and being single [65]. There is an association between depression and the severity of bradykinesia [37], rigidity [37], and anxiety [66]. About half of the people who have Parkinson's Disease developed depression within 8 years of the onset of Parkinson's Disease. Around 72% of people with Parkinson's Disease developed depression within 10 years of the onset of Parkinson's Disease. The estimates of the likelihood of people who have Parkinson's Disease committing suicide differ enormously, from anywhere between twice as likely to far more likely to being far more unlikely [67, 68, 69].

Causes of symptoms : Depressive state, not major depression, is an essential feature of Parkinson's Disease derived from impairment of the mesocortical dopaminergic pathway [27]. Reduced dopaminergic stimulation of the mesocortical pathway is associated with emotional depression [70, 71].

[1] Movement Disorders [2003] 18 (4) : 414-418 (A.F.Leentjens, M. Van den Akker, J.F.Metsemakers, R.Lousberg, F.R.Verhey)

[2] Nature Reviews Neurology [2011] 8 (1) : 35-47 (D.Aarsland, S. Påhlhagen, C.G.Ballard, U.Ehrt, P.Svenningsson)

[3] Revista de Neurologia [1999] 28 (7) : 694-698 (J.M.Errea, J.R.Ara)

[4] Neurology [2002] 58 (10) : 1501-1504 (A.G.Schuurman, M.van den Akker, K.T.Ensinck, J.F.Metsemakers, J.A.Knottnerus, A.F.Leentjens, F.Buntinx)

[5] American Journal of Geriatric Psychiatry [2015] 23 (9) : 934-940 (Y.T.Hsu, C.C.Liao, S.N.Chang, Y.W.Yang, C.H.Tsai, T.L.Chen, F.C. Sung)

[6] Neurology [2013] 81 (17) : 1538-1544 (C.C.Shen, S.J.Tsai, C.L. Perng, B.I.Kuo, A.C.Yang)

[7] European Journal of Neurology [2011] 18 (3) : 448-453 (C.Becker, G.P.Brobert, S.Johansson, S.S.Jick, C.R.Meier)

[8] Movement Disorders [2010] 25 (9) : 1157-1162 (F.Fang, Q.Xu, Y. Park, X.Huang, A.Hollenbeck, A.Blair, A.Schatzkin, F.Kamel, H. Chen)

[9] Neurology [2015] 84 (24) : 2422-2429 (H.Gustafsson, A. Nordström, P.Nordström)

[10] Psychopathology [2003] 36 (5) : 221-225 (U.Merschdorf, D.Berg, I.Csoti, F.Fornadi, B.Merz, M.Naumann, G.Becker, T.Supprian)

[11] Expert Review of Neurotherapeutics [2005] 5 (6) : 803-810 (J. Lagopoulos, G.S.Malhi, B.Ivanovski, C.M.Cahill, J.G.Morris)

[12] Nihon Ronen Igakkai Zasshi [2013] 50 (6) : 752-754 (M.Murata, T.Okamoto)

[13] Arquivos de Neuro-Psiquiatria [2012] 70 (8) : 617-620 (F.H.Costa, A.L.Rosso, H.Maultasch, D.H.Nicaretta, M.B.Vincent)

[14] Fortschritte der Neurologie-Psychiatrie [2013] 81 (2) : 81-87 (O. Riedel, C.Schneider, J.Klotsche, H.Reichmann, A.Storch, H.U. Wittchen)

[15] Neurology [2007] 69 (4) : 342-347 (B.Ravina, R.Camicioli, P.G. Como, L.Marsh, J.Jankovic, D.Weintraub, J.Elm)

[16] Ideggyogyaszati Szemle [2014] 67 (7-8) : 229-236 (Z.Rihmer, X. Gonda, P.Döme)

[17] Journal of Neuropsychiatry and Clinical Neurosciences [2001] 13 (2) : 187-196 (J.R.Slaughter, K.A.Slaughter, D.Nichols, S.E.Holmes, M.P.Martens)

[18] Journal of Geriatric Psychiatry and Neurology [2003] 16 (3) : 178-183 (D.Weintraub, P.J.Moberg, J.E.Duda, I.R.Katz, M.B.Stern)

[19] American Journal of Psychiatry [1994] 151 (7) : 1010-1014 (P.Hantz, G.Caradoc-Davies, T.Caradoc-Davies, M.Weatherall, G. Dixon)

[20] Journal of Neural Transmission [2000] 107 (1) : 59-71 (N.Giladi, T.A.Treves, D.Paleacu, H.Shabtai, Y.Orlov, B.Kandinov, E.S.Simon, A.D.Korczyn)

[21] Parkinsonism & Related Disorders [2009] 15 (2) : 144-148 (P.G. Frisina, V.Haroutunian, L.S.Libow)

[22] BMC Psychiatry [2014] 14 : 278 (T.Ketharanathan, R.Hanwella, R.Weerasundera, V.A.de Silva)

[23] Journal of Neurology [2004] 251 (Supplement 6) : VI/24-VI/27 (M.R.Lemke, G.Fuchs, I.Gemende, B.Herting, C.Oehlwein, H. Reichmann, J.Rieke, J.Volkmann)

[24] Acta Clinica Croatica [2015] 54 (1) : 73-76 (O.Sinanovic, J.Hudic, S.Zukic, A.Kapidžic, L.Zonic, M.Vidovic)

[25] Arquivos de Neuro-Psiquiatria [2005] 63 (3B) : 766-771 (R.C. Prado, E.R.Barbosa)

[26] American Journal of Psychiatry [1992] 149 (4) : 443-454 (J.L. Cummings)

[27] Nihon Rinsho [2004] 62 (9) : 1661-1666 (M.Yamamoto)

[28] Archives of Neurology [1992] 49 (3) : 305-307 (G.Dooneief, E. Mirabello, K.Bell, K.Marder, Y.Stern, R.Mayeux)

[29] American Journal of Geriatric Psychiatry [1999] 7 (2) : 110-118 (T.A.Zesiewicz, M.Gold, G.Chari, R.A.Hauser)

[30] Journal of Psychology [1996] 130 (6) : 659-667 (J.B.Murray)

[31] Arquivos de Neuro-Psiquiatria [2008] 66 (2A) : 152-156 (V. Tumas, G.G.Rodrigues, T.L.Farias, J.A.Crippa)

[32] Journal of Neuroscience Nursing [1991] 23 (3) : 158-164 (L.K. Bunting, B.Fitzsimmons)

[33] Behavioural Neurology [1993] 6 (3) : 151-154 (S.E.Starkstein, R.G.Robinson, R.Leiguarda, T.J.Preziosi)

[34] American Journal of Psychiatry [1986] 143 (6) : 756-759 (R. Mayeux, Y.Stern, J.B.Williams, L.Cote, A.Frantz, I.Dyrenfurth)

[35] Neuropsychopharmacologia Hungarica [2004] 6 (2) : 82-85 (Z. Rihmer, K.Seregi, A.Rihmer)

[36] Nihon Rinsho [2000] 58 (10) : 2120-2124 (K.Kurokawa, T.Yuasa)

[37] Clinical Neurology and Neurosurgery [2006] 108 (5) : 465-469 (S.Papapetropoulos, J.Ellul, A.A.Argyriou, E.Chroni, N.P.Lekka)

[38] Neurology [2002] 58 (4 Supplement 1) : S63-S70 (M.S.Okun, R.L. Watts)

[39] Journal of Nervous and Mental Disease [1990] 178 (1) : 27-31 (S.E.Starkstein, T.J.Preziosi, P.L.Bolduc, R.G.Robinson)

[40] Journal of Neurology [2001] 248 (Supplement 3) : III5-III11 (M. Yamamoto)

[41] Journal of Clinical and Experimental Neuropsychology [2016] 38 (1) : 51-58 (A.I.Ghaddar, M.I.Fawaz, G.Khazen, J.Abdallah, A.Milane)

[42] Acta Neurologica Scandinavica [2006] 113 (1) : 1-8 (A. Lieberman)

[43] Movement Disorders [2009] 24 (9) : 1306-1311 (B.Ravina, J.Elm, R.Camicioli, P.G.Como, L.Marsh, J.Jankovic, D.Weintraub)

[44] Journal of Neurology, Neurosurgery, and Psychiatry [1994] 57 (10) : 1265-1267 (V.S.Kostíc, S.R.Filipovic, D.Lecic, D.Momcilovic, D.Sokic, N.Sternic)

[45] International Journal of Geriatric Psychiatry [2009] 24 (9) : 937-943 (D.A.Nation, H.L.Katzen, S.Papapetropoulos, B.K.Scanlon, B.E.Levin)

[46] Neurology [2016] Jun 29 [Epub ahead of print] (Z.Goodarzi, K.J.Mrklas, D.J.Roberts, N.Jette, T.Pringsheim, J.Holroyd-Leduc)

[47] Seishin Shinkeigaku Zasshi [2013] 115 (11) : 1135-1141 (S.Kitamura, H.Nagayama)

[48] Internal Medicine [2013] 52 (5) : 539-545 (T.Yamanishi, H. Tachibana, M.Oguru, K.Matsui, K.Toda, B.Okuda, N.Oka)

[49] Zhonghua Yi Xue Za Zhi [2013] 93 (1) : 26-29 (C.J.Mao, J.P. Chen, W.D.Hu, C.F.Liu)

[50] Journal of Geriatric Psychiatry and Neurology [2010] 23 (1) : 35-41 (M.Oguru, H.Tachibana, K.Toda, B.Okuda, N.Oka)

[51] Annals of Clinical Psychiatry [2011] 23 (3) : 171-177 (A.H. Farabaugh, J.J.Locascio, L.Yap, M.Fava, S.Bitran, J.L.Sousa, J.H. Growdon)

[52] Arquivos de Neuro-Psiquiatria [2014] 72 (6) : 426-429 (M.H. Chagas, T.S.Moriyama, A.C.Felício, A.L.Sosa, R.A.Bressan, C.P.Ferri)

[53] Canadian Journal of Neurological Sciences [2002] 29 (2) : 139-146 (A.Anguenot, P.Y.Loll, J.P.Neau, P.Ingrand, R.Gil)

[54] Parkinsonism & Related Disorders [2003] 10 (1) : 23-28 (A.Rojo, M.Aguilar, M.T.Garolera, E.Cubo, I.Navas, S.Quintana)

[55] Neurologia i Neurochirurgia Polska [2003] 37 (Supplement 5) : 165-173 (M.Golab, K.Honczarenko)

[56] Parkinsonism & Related Disorders [2016] S1353-S8020 (16) : 30119-30115 [Epub ahead of print] (Y.Haasum, J.Fastbom, K.Johnell)

[57] Movement Disorders [2008] 23 (2) : 183-189 (J.S.Reijnders, U. Ehrt, W.E.Weber, D.Aarsland, A.F.Leentjens)

[58] Brain and Nerve [2007] 59 (9) : 935-942 (M.Mimura)

[59] Journal of Neuropsychiatry and Clinical Neurosciences [2005] 17 (3) : 310-323 (C.Veazey, S.O.Aki, K.F.Cook, E.C.Lai, M.E.Kunik)

[60] Journal of the Neurological Sciences [2011] 310 (1-2) : 220-224 (T.C.van der Hoek, B.A.Bus, P.Matui, M.A.van der Marck, R.A. Esselink, I.Tendolkar)

[61] Neurologia i Neurochirurgia Polska [2003] 37 (2) : 351-364 (J. Slawek, M.Derejko, P.Lass)

[62] Canadian Journal of Neurological Sciences [2010] 37 (1) : 61-66 (B.Jasinska-Myga, J.D.Putzke, C.Wider, Z.K.Wszolek, R.J.Uitti)

[63] Journal of the Neurological Sciences [2008] 272 (1-2) : 158-163 (F.Stella, C.E.Banzato, E.M.Barasnevicius Quagliato, M.A.Viana)

[64] International Journal of Geriatric Psychiatry [2016] 31 (5) : 458-456 (G.M.Pontone, C.C.Bakker, S.Chen, Z.Mari, L.Marsh, P.V.Rabins, J.R.Williams, S.S.Bassett)

[65] Acta Neurologica Scandinavica [2016] 133 (4) : 276-280 (A.Q. Rana, A.R.Qureshi, A.Mumtaz, I.Abdullah, A.Jesudasan, K.K.Hafez, M.A.Rana)

[66] Biological Psychiatry [1993] 34 (7) : 465-470 (M.A.Menza, D.E. Robertson-Hoffman, A.S.Bonapace)

[67] Journal of the Neurological Sciences [2010] 289 (1-2) : 40-43 (V.S.Kostic, T.Pekmezovic, A.Tomic, M.Jecmenica-Lukic, T. Stojkovic, V.Spica. M.Svetel, E.Stefanova, I.Petrovic, E.Dzoljic)

[68] Parkinsonism & Related Disorders [2016] 32 : 102-107 (T.Lee, H.B.Lee, M.H.Ahn, J.Kim, M.S.Kim, S.J.Chung, J.P.Hong)

[69] Journal of Geriatric Psychiatry and Neurology [2001] 14 (3) : 120-124 (M.Myslobodsky, F.M.Lalonde, L.Hicks)

[70] Canadian Journal of Neurological Sciences [1984] 11 (1 Supplement) : 105-107 (H.C.Fibiger)

[71] American Journal of Psychiatry [1992] 149 (4) : 443-454 (J.L. Cummings)

[72] Parkinsonism and Related Disorders [2016] 27 : 85-88 (Y. Haasum, J.Fastbom, K.Johnell)

Dementia

Symptoms : Dementia can begin as mild cognitive impairment and then gradually develop in to Parkinson's Disease dementia (PDD) [1]. The symptoms of dementia can include memory loss [2, 3], cognitive impairment, disorientation, communication difficulties [2, 3], and confusion [2, 3, 4]. Dementia can consequently make normal tasks and interactions difficult.

Prevalence : Mild cognitive impairment can be identified in 15% to 20% of people with Parkinson's Disease at the time of diagnosis [5, 62], and 26% to 49% after that [1, 6-9, 61, 62]. After 5 years, 47% to 64% of people with Parkinson's Disease had cognitive impairment [1, 10, 59, 60]. People with mild Parkinson's Disease were twice as likely to develop dementia [11]. Over 27% of those people with mild cognitive impairment at the outset actually rid their cognitive impairment after 5 years, as did 24% of people who had developed mild cognitive impairment during the first 5 years [62]. Approximately 13% to 38% of people with Parkinson's Disease also have dementia [7, 12-45, 61]. Dementia in Parkinson's Disease is more common as people get older [24, 46]. So during the course of the disease approximately 40% of people with Parkinson's Disease develop dementia [19, 46, 47]. That is about 6 times more likely than those people that do not get Parkinson's Disease [46]. Approximately 50% or more of people who have had Parkinson's for ten years also have dementia [23, 48-52]. Approximately 80% or more of those people who have had Parkinson's Disease for twenty years or more also have dementia [48, 51, 53]. Those people who had Parkinson's Disease who developed dementia were more likely to be older [16, 43, 51, 54, 55], to have an older age of onset [42, 56, 57], to be male [16, 51, 55, 57], and to have more severe Parkinson's Disease symptoms [42, 43, 53, 55, 56, 58].

Causes of symptoms : Parkinson’s Disease and dementia are biochemically distinct. Parkinson’s Disease is primarily due to insufficient dopamine. Dementia is due to insufficient acetylcholine. The prevalence of dementia in Parkinson’s Disease is therefore probably due to Parkinson’s Disease and dementia both occurring more commonly as people get older rather than having a common cause.

[1] Neurology [2013] 81 (4) : 346-352 (M.Broeders, R.M.de Bie, D.C. Velseboer, J.D.Speelman, D.Muslimovic, B.Schmand)

[2] Nihon Koshu Eisei Zasshi [2016] 63 (4) : 202-208 (T.Miyamura)

[3] Zhurnal Nevrologii i Psikhiatrii Imeni S.S.Korsakova [2013] 113 (7 Part 2) : 25-31 (I.V.Kolykhanov, IaB.Fedorova, S.I.Gavrilova)

[4] Tijdschrift voor Gerontologie en Geriatrie [2003] 34 (5) : 222-226 (G.S.Spronk, C.J.Schölzel-Dorenbos, M.J.Jellesma-Eggenkamp)

[5] Parkinsonism & Related Disorders [2016] 22 (Supplement 1) : S144-S148 (D.Aarsland)

[6] Acta Neurologica Scandinavica [2014] 129 (5) : 307-318 (H.C. Pfeiffer, A.Løkkegaard, M.Zoetmulder, L.Friberg, L.Werdelin)

[7] Neuroepidemiology [2011] 37 (3-4) : 168-176 (M.Balzer-Geldsetzer, A.S.Costa, M.Kronenbürger, J.B.Schulz, S.Röske, A. Spottke, U.Wüllner, T.Klockgether, A.Storch, C.Schneider, et al)

[8] Movement Disorders [2011] 26 (10) : 1814-1824 (I.Litvan, D. Aarsland, C.H.Adler, J.G.Goldman, J.Kulisevsky, B.Mollenhauer, M.C.Rodriguez-Oroz, A.I.Tröster, D.Weintraub)

[9] Gaceta Medica de Mexico [2016] 152 (3) : 357-363 (S.Isais-Millán, D.Piña-Fuentes, C.Guzmán-Astorga, A.Cervantes-Arriaga, M. Rodríguez-Violante)

[10] Neurology [2015] 85 (15) : 1276-1282 (K.Pigott, J.Rick, S.X.Xie, H.Hurtig, A.Chen-Plotkin, J.E.Duda, J.F.Morley, LM.Chahine, N. Dahodwala, R.S.Akhtar, A.Siderowf, J.Q.Trojanowski, D.Weintraub)

[11] Movement Disorders [2010] 25 (2) : 172-178 (E.D.Louis, M.X. Tang, N.Schupf)

[12] Movement Disorders [2005] 20 (10) : 1255-1266 (D.Aarsland, J. Zaccai, C.Brayne)

[13] International Journal of Geriatric Psychiatry [2016] 31 (8) : 938-943 (O.Riedel, D.Bitters, U.Amann, E.Garbe, I.Langner)

[14] Geriatrics and Gerontology International [2016] 16 (2) : 230-236 (Y.S.Oh, J.S.Kim, I.S.Park, Y.S.Shim, I.U.Song, J.W.Park, P.H.Lee, C.H.Lyoo, T.B.Ahn, H.I.Ma, Y.D.Kim, S.B.Koh, S.J.Lee, K.S.Lee)

[15] American Journal of Alzheimers Disease and Other Dementias [2014] 29 (7) : 630-636 (J.Sanyal, T.K.Banerjee, V.R.Rao)

[16] Neurology [2014] 83 (14) : 1253-1260 (J.B.Anang, J.F.Gagnon, J.A.Bertrand, S.R.Romenets, V.Latreille, M.Panisset, J.Montplaisir, R.B.Postuma)

[17] Seishin Shinkeigaku Zasshi [2013] 115 (11) : 1142-1149 (H. Tachibana)

[18] Neurology [2014] 82 (3) : 263-270 (K.T.Olde Dubbelink, A. Hillebrand, J.W.Twisk, J.B.Deijen, D.Stoffers, B.A.Schmand, C.J. Stam, H.W.Berendse)

[19] Fortschritte der Neurologie-Psychiatrie [2013] 81 (2) : 81-87 (C. Schneider, J.Klotsche, H.Reichmann, A.Storch, H.U.Wittchen)

[20] Brain and Nerve [2012] 64 (12) : 1365-1375 (K.Wada, K. Nakashima)

[21] Clinical Neurology and Neurosurgery [2013] 115 (6) : 673-677 (E.M.Khedr, N.A.El Fetoh, H.Khalifa, M.A.Ahmed, K.M.El Beh)

[22] Neurodegenerative Diseases [2013] 12 (1) : 1-12 (J.Slawek, A.Roszmann, P.Robowski, M.Dubaniewicz, E.J.Sitek, K.Honczarenko, A.Gorzkowska, S.Budrewicz, M.Mak, M.Golab-Janowska, et al)

[23] Alzheimers and Dementia [2012] 8 (6) : 463-469 (F.Perez, C. Helmer, A.Foubert-Samier, S.Auriacombe, J.F.Dartigues,F. Tison)

[24] Psychiatry and Clinical Neurosciences [2012] 66 (1) : 64-68 (A.Q. Rana, M.S.Yousuf, S.Naz, N.Qa'aty)

[25] Parkinsonism & Related Disorders [2012] 18 (5) : 598-601 (O. Riedel, R.Dodel, G.Deuschl, J.Klotsche, H.Förstl, I.Heuser, W.Oertel, H.Reichmann, P.Riederer, C.Trenkwalder, H.U.Wittchen)

[26] Arquivos de Neuropsiquiatria [2011] 69 (5) : 733-738 (B.Baldivia, S.M.Brucki, S.Batistela, J.C.Esper, C.D.Augusto, M.S.Rocha)

[27] Journal of Neurology [2011] 258 (8) : 1513-1517 (M.Hu, J. Cooper, R.Beamish, E.Jones, R.Butterworth, L.Catterall, Y.Ben-Shlomo)

[28] MMW Fortschritte der Medizin [2010] 152 (Supplement 1) : 1-6 (H.Von Reichmann, G.Deuschl, O.Riedel, A.Spottke, H.Förstl, F.Henn, I.Heuser, W.Oertel, P.Riederer, C.Trenkwalder, R.Dodel, et al)

[29] Journal of Neurology [2010] 257 (7) : 1073-1082 (O.Riedel, J. Klotsche, A.Spottke, G.Deuschl, H.Förstl, F.Henn, I.Heuser, W. Oertel, H.Reichmann, P.Riederer, C.Trenkwalder, R.Dodel, H.U. Wittchen)

[30] Revista de Neurologia [2009] 49 (8) : 393-398 (P.Martínez-Martín, C.Prieto-Jurczynska, B.Frades-Payo0

[31] Journal of Neurological Science [2010] 289 (1-2) : 18-22 (D. Aarsland, M.W.Kurz)

[32] Parkinsonism & Related Disorders [1997] 3 (3) : 151-158 (A.N. Lieberman)

[33] Acta Neurologica Scandinavica [2007] 116 (3) : 190-195 (M. Kitayama, K.Wada-Isoe, K.Nakaso, Y.Irizawa, K.Nakashima)

[34] Journal of Neurology, Neurosurgery and Psychiatry [2007] 78 (11) : 1182-1187 (D.Verbaan, J.Marinus, M.Visser, S.M.van Rooden, A.M. Stiggelbout, H.A.Middelkoop, J.J.van Hilten)

[35] Journal of Neurological Science [2006] 248 (1-2) : 138-142 (A. Lieberman)

[36] Movement Disorders [2004] 19 (9) : 1043-1049 (P.Hobson, J. Meara)

[37] Neurologia i Neurochirurgia Polska [2003] 37 (Supplement 5) : 103-115 (J.Slawek, M.Derejko)

[38] Neurologia i Neurochirurgia Polska [2001] 35 (4) : 569-581 (J. Slawek, E.Bojko, J.Szady)

[39] Neurologia [1999] 14 (Supplement 1) : 72-81 (J.Kulisevsky, B. Pascual-Sedano)

[40] Archives of Neurology [1996] 53 (6) : 538-542 (D.Aarsland, E.Tandberg, J.P.Larsen, J.L.Cummings)

[41] Archives of Neurology [1995] 52 (7) : 695-701 (K.Marder, M.X. Tang, L.Cote, Y.Stern, R.Mayeux)

[42] Journal of Neural Transmission [2000] 107 (1) : 59-71 (N.Giladi, T.A.Treves, D.Paleacu, H.Shabtai, Y.Orlov, B.Kandinov, E.S.Simon, A.D.Korczyn)

[43] Neurology [1995] 45 (4) : 705-708 (F.Tison, J.F.Dartigues, S. Auriacombe, L.Letenneur, F.Boller, A.Alpérovitch)

[44] Journal of Neurology, Neurosurgery and Psychiatry [1988] 51 (12) : 1498-1502 (F.Girotti, P.Soliveri, F.Carella, I.Piccolo, P.Caffarra, M. Musicco, T.Caraceni)

[45] Annals of Neurology [1979] 6 (4) : 355-359 (A.Lieberman, M. Dziatolowski, M.Kupersmith, M.Serby, A.Goodgold, J.Korein, M. Goldstein)

[46] Neurological Sciences [2006] 27 (Supplement 1) : S40-S43 (A. Padovani, C.Costanzi, N.Gilberti, B.Borroni)

[47] Journal of the Medical Association of Thailand [2013] 96 (4) : 440-445 (P.Mekawichai, L.Choeikamhaeng)

[48] Postgraduate Medical Journal [2015] 91 (1074) : 212-220 (J. Cosgrove, J.E.Alty, S.Jamieson)

[49] Journal of Neurology, Neurosurgery and Psychiatry [2013] 84 (11) : 1258-1264 (C.H.Williams-Gray, S.L.Mason, J.R.Evans, T.Foltynie, C.Brayne, T.W.Robbins, R.A.Barker)

[50] Journal of Neurology [2010] 257 (9) : 1524-1532 (M.Coelho, M.J. Marti, E.Tolosa, J.J.Ferreira, F.Valldeoriola, M.Rosa, C.Sampaio)

[51] Neurology [2008] 70 (13) : 1017-1022 (T.C.Buter, A.van den Hout, F.E.Matthews, J.P.Larsen, C.Brayne, D.Aarsland)

[52] Archives of Neurology [2003] 60 (3) : 387-392 (D.Aarsland, K. Andersen, J.P.Larsen, A.Lolk, P.Kragh-Sørensen)

[53] Movement Disorders [2008] 23 (6) : 837-844 (M.A.Hely, W.G. Reid, M.A.Adena, G.M.Halliday, J.G.Morris)

[54] Movement Disorders [2007] 22 (12) : 1689-1707 (M.Emre, D. Aarsland, R.Brown, D.J.Burn, C.Duyckaerts, Y.Mizuno, G.A.Broe, J. Cummings, D.W.Dickson, S.Gauthier, J.Goldman, C.Goetz, et al)

[55] Neurology [2000] 54 (8) : 1596-1602 (T.A.Hughes, H.F.Ross, S.Musa, S.Bhattacherjee, R.N.Nathan, R.H.Mindham, E.G.Spokes)

[56] Neuroepidemiology [1996] 15 (1) : 20-25 (S.L.Glatt, J.P.Hubble, K.Lyons, A.Paolo, A.I.Tröster, R.E.Hassanein, W.C.Koller)

[57] Archives of Neurology [1992] 49 (5) : 492-497 (R.Mayeux, J. Denaro, N.Hemenegildo, K.Marder, M.X.Tang, L.J.Cote, Y.Stern)

[58] Journal of Neurology [2008] 255 (2) : 255-264 (O.Riedel, J. Klotsche, A.Spottke, G.Deuschl, H.Förstl, F.Henn, I.Heuser, W.Oertel, H.Reichmann, P.Riederer, C.Trenkwalder, R.Dodel, H.U.Wittchen)

[59] Journal of Clinical and Experimental Neuropsychology [2016] 38 (1) : 40-50 (I.Galtier,, A.Nieto, J.N.Lorenzo, J.Barroso)

[60] Scientific Reports [2016] 6 : 33929 (B.J.Lawrence, N.Gasson, A.M.Loftus)

[61] Geriatrics and Gerontology International [2016] 16 (2) : 230-236 (Y.S.Oh, J.S.Kim, I.S.Park, Y.S.Shim, I.U.Song, J.W.Park, P.H.Lee, C.H.Lyoo, T.B.Ahn, H.I.Ma, Y.D.Kim, S.B.Koh, S.J.Lee, K.S.Lee)

[62] Neurology [2017] Jan 20 [Epub ahead of print] (K.F.Pedersen, J.P. Larsen, O.B.Tysnes, G.Alves)

PAIN

Symptoms : Pain commonly occurs in Parkinson's Disease [1-11]. In most people with Parkinson's Disease the pain is chronic [7, 12]. In a minority of people with Parkinson's Disease the pain is so severe that it overshadows the motor symptoms [13]. As Parkinson's Disease progresses pain threshold and pain tolerance tend to decrease, which can predispose to pain development [14]. Overall, analgesic use is low [6], but only 48% to 52% of people with Parkinson's Disease used analgesics to deal with pain [15, 45]. The pain fluctuates with on-off periods [15]. The off period resulted in an increased frequency of pain, which was related to stiffness [16].

Prevalence : Pain occurs in 30% to 95% of people with Parkinson's Disease depending on the definition of pain [9, 11, 13, 15, 17-36, 45, 46, 47]. People with symptoms of pain are more likely to develop Parkinson's Disease. The likelihood is nearly doubled in those with mild pain and nearly tripled in those with moderate or severe pain [37]. Only 3% of them resolved during the development of the disease [20].

Of those people with Parkinson's Disease who went on to develop motor features of Parkinson's Disease, one third manifested musculoskeletal pain as the initial symptom [38]. Pain preceded the motor disorders in 39% of people with Parkinson's Disease [18]. Over half of people with Parkinson's Disease reported pain prior to diagnosis [11], or at clinical onset [10]. The number of types of pain reported was one in 53% of people with Parkinson's Disease, two in 24%, three in 5% [25], and two or more in 27% of people [11]. Musculoskeletal pains occurred in 28% to 74% of people with Parkinson's Disease [11, 15, 21, 25, 31-34, 46]. The primary musculoskeletal pains were : back (71% to 74%) [21, 39, 46], upper limbs (72%) [18, 21], lower limbs (68%) [15, 18], legs (38%) [21, 40], neck (15%) [18]. Other pains included : joints (52% to 54%) [18, 46], rheumatologic pain (51%) [20], paravertebral (45%) [18], due to dystonia (19% to 48%) [21, 25, 31, 32, 33], radicular or neuropathic (11% to 36%) [11, 25, 31, 32, 33, 46], and central pain (10% to 12%) [25, 31]. People with Parkinson’s Disease described their experience of pain as aching (46%), a feeling of tension (18%), sharp pain (12%), deep pain (12%) and dull pain (11%) [32]. In 75% of people with Parkinson's Disease pain was on the side of more severe motor symptoms [5, 12]. Factors associated with pain are : being younger at onset [7], severer depression [7, 11, 18, 33], more motor complications [7, 19], female gender [14, 25], severity of disease [14, 33], akathisia [31]. About a third of pains were linked to motor fluctuations, mostly in the off phase [20].

Causes of symptoms : Reduced dopaminergic stimulation of the incertohypothalamic pathway affects periaqueductal gray, which has enkephalin and endorphin producing cells. Consequently, there is a reduction in enkephalins [41, 42] and endorphins [43], both of which can suppress pain. Reduced stimulation of the diencephalospinal pathway contributes to insufficient pain control at the spinal cord level [44].

[1] International Journal of Geriatric Psychiatry [2010] 25 (5) : 519-524 (P.McNamara, K. Stavitsky, E.Harris, O.Szent-Imrey, R.Durso)

[2] Journal of Neural Transmission [2013] 120 (4) : 583-586 (G. Defazio, A.Gigante, P.Mancino, M.Tinazzi)

[3] Revista de Neurologia [2010] 50 (Supplement 2) : S65-S74 (D.Santos García, A.Aneiros Díaz, M.Macias Arribi, M.A.Llaneza González, J. Abella Corral, H.Santos Canelles)

[4] Revue Neurologique [2012] 168 (8-9) : 576-584 (S.Thobois, B. Ballanger, A.Poisson, E.Broussolle)

[5] Brain and Nerve [2012] 64 (4) : 364-372 (F.Yoshii)

[6] Journal of Pain and Symptom Management [2006] 32 (5) : 462-469 (M.A.Lee, R.W.Walker, T.J.Hildreth, W.M.Prentice)

[7] Movement Disorders [2008] 23 (10) : 1361-1369 (L.Nègre Pagès, W.Regragui, D.Bouhassira, H.Grandjean, O.Rascol)

[8] Tidsskrift for den Norske Laegeforening [1989] 109 (5) : 561-563 (S.I.Bekkelund, B.Selseth, S.I.Mellgren)

[9] Movement Disorders [1986] 1 (1) : 45-49 (C.G.Goetz, C.M.Tanner, M.Levy, R.S.Wilson, D.C.Garron)

[10] Archives of Neurology [2008] 65 (9) : 1191-1194 (G.Defazio, A.Berardelli, G.Fabbrini, D.Martino, E.Fincati, A.Fiaschi, G.Moretto, G.Abbruzzese, R.Marchese, U.Bonuccelli, P.Del Dotto, et al)

[11] Revista de Neurologia [2011] 52 (7) : 385-393 (D.Santos-García, J.Abella-Corral, A.Aneiros-Díaz, H.Santos-Canelles, M.A.Llaneza-González, M.Macías-Arribi)

[12] Zhurnal Nevrologii i Psikhiatrii Imeni S.S.Korsakova [2013] 113 (7 Part 2) : 39-44 (S.O.Makhnev, O.S.Levin)

[13] Movement Disorders [2010] 25 (Supplement 1) : S98-S103 (B. Ford)

[14] Journal of Neurology [2011] 258 (4) : 627-633 (S.Zambito Marsala, M.Tinazzi, R.Vitaliani, S.Recchia, F.Fabris, C.Marchini, A. Fiaschi, G.Moretto, B.Giometto, A.Macerollo, G.Defazio)

[15] Movement Disorders [2012] 27 (4) : 480-484 (M.P.Broen, M.M. Braaksma, J.Patijn, W.E.Weber)

[16] Arquivos de Neuro-Psiquiatria [2009] 67 (3A) : 591-594 (G.H. Letro, E.M.Quagliato, M.A.Viana)

[17] Clinical Neuroscience [1998] 5 (2) : 63-72 (B.Ford)

[18] Srpski Arhiv za Celokupno Lekarstvo [1990] 118 (11-12) : 463-466 (Z.Marinkovic, V.Kostic, N.Covikovic-Sternic, S.Marinkovic)

[19] Journal of Neurology, Neurosurgery and Psychiatry [2006] 77 (7) : 822-825 (M.Tinazzi, C.Del Vesco, E.Fincati, S.Ottaviani, N.Smania, G.Moretto, A.Fiaschi, D.Martino, G.Defazio)

[20] Revue Neurologique [2005] 161 (4) : 407-418 (R.Giuffrida, F.J. Vingerhoets, J.Bogousslavsky, J.Ghika)

[21] Clinical Neurology and Neurosurgery [2013] 115 (11) : 2313-2317 (A.Q.Rana, A.Kabir, M.Jesudasan, I.Siddiqui, S.Khondker)

[22] Parkinsonism & Related Disorders [2013] 19 (3) : 285-294 (A. Fil, R.Cano de la Cuerda, E.Muñoz Hellín, L.Vela, M.Ramiro González, C.Fernández de Las Peñas)

[23] CNS Drugs [2012] 26 (11) : 937-948 (M.Sophie, B.Ford)

[24] American Journal of Geriatric Psychiatry [2009] 17 (4) : 269-275 (U.Ehrt, J.P.Larsen, D.Aarsland)

[25] Pain [2009] 141 (1-2) : 173-177 (A.G.Beiske, J.H.Loge, A. Rønningen, E.Svensson)

[26] Parkinsonism & Related Disorders [2012] 18 (7) : 828-832 (D.L. Terriff, J.V.Williams, S.B.Patten, D.H.Lavorato, A.G.Bulloch)

[27] Nature Reviews Neurology [2012] 8 (5) : 284-294 (G.Wasner, G.Deuschl)

[28] Parkinsonism & Related Disorders [2012] 18 (Supplement 1) : S222-S225 (H.B.Wen, A.X.Zhang, H.Wang, L.Li, H.Chen, Y.Liu, B. Zhang B, Q.Xu)

[29] Parkinsonism & Related Disorders [2007] 13 (5) : 312-314 (K. Toda, T.Harada, F.Ishizaki, N.Horie, T.Yamada)

[30] Joint Bone Spine [2006] 73 (3) : 298-302 (F.Etchepare, S. Rozenberg, T.Mirault, A.M.Bonnet, C.Lecorre, Y.Agid, P.Bourgeois, B.Fautrel)

[31] Clinical Neurology and Neurosurgery [2011] 113 (1) : 11-13 (H.A. Hanagasi, S.Akat, H.Gurvit, J.Yazici, M.Emre)

[32] Functional Neurology [2013] 28 (4) : 297-304 (A.Rana, U.Saeed, M.S.Masroor, M.S.Yousuf, I.Siddiqui)

[33] PLoS One [2015] 10 (8) : e0136541 (P.Valkovic, M.Minar, H. Singliarova, J.Harsany, M.Hanakova, J.Martinkova, J.Benetin)

[34] International Psychogeriatrics [2016] 28 (2) : 283-289 (X.J.Lin, N.Yu, X.G.Lin, Y.F.Zhang, Y.Chen, K.Zhang, X.S. Wang, W.G.Liu)

[35] Journal of Neurological Science [2016] 365 : 162-166 (S.Kubo, S.Hamada, T.Maeda, T.Uchiyama, M.Hashimoto, N.Nomoto, O.Kano, T.Takahashi, H.Terashi, T.Takahashi, T.Hatano, T.Hasegawa, et al)

[36] Journal of Back and Musculoskeletal Rehabilitation [2016] Jun 3 [Epub ahead of print] (E.A.Ozturk, I.Gundogdu, B.Kocer, S.Comoglu, A.Cakci)

[37] European Journal of Neurology [2013] 20 (10) : 1398-1404 (C.H. Lin, R.M.Wu, H.Y.Chang, Y.T.Chiang, H.H.Lin)

[38] Journal of the Neurological Sciences [2012] 319 (1-2) : 102-104 (K.Farnikova, A.Krobot, P.Kanovsky)

[39] Movement Disorders [2007] 22 (6) : 853-856 (D.Broetz, M. Eichner, T.Gasser, M.Weller, J.P.Steinbach)

[40] Movement Disorders [2009] 24 (11) : 1641-1649 (P.Barone, A. Antonini, C.Colosimo, R.Marconi, L.Morgante, T.P.Avarello, E. Bottacchi, A.Cannas, G.Ceravolo, R.Ceravolo, G.Cicarelli, et al)

[41] Neuropeptides [1991] 18 (4) : 201-207 (S.P.Sivam)

[42] Lancet [1981] 1 (8234) : 1367-1368 (H.Taquet, F.Javoy-Agid, F. Cesselin, Y.Agid)

[43] Neurology [1985] 35 (9) : 1371-1374 (G.Nappi, F.Petraglia, E. Martignoni, F.Facchinetti, G.Bono, A.R.Genazzani)

[44] PLoS One [2010] 5 (10) : e13306 (Q.Barraud, I.Obeid, I.Aubert, G.Barrière, H.Contamin, S.McGuire, P.Ravenscroft, G.Porras, F. Tison, E.Bezard, I.Ghorayeb)

[45] Clinical Journal of Pain [2016] Sep 10 [Epub ahead of print] (S.Yust Katz, R.Hershkovitz, T.Gurevich, R.Djaldetti)

[46] Journal of Neurology [2017] Feb 27 [Epub ahead of print] (C. Buhmann, N.Wrobel, W.Grashorn, O.Fruendt, K.Wesemann, S. Diedrich, U.Bingel)

[47] Pain Practice [2017] Mar 30 [Epub ahead of print] (Y.T.Fu, C.J. Mao, L.J.Ma, H.J.Zhang, Y.Wang, J.Li, J.Y.Huang, J.Y.Liu, C.F.Liu)

Sleep Disturbance

Symptoms : Sleep disorders in Parkinson's Disease are common and have a negative impact on the quality of life [1, 2]. They include : insomnia [1, 3-11], impaired bed mobility [12], sleep-disordered breathing [4, 5, 6], sleep fragmentation [2, 3, 4, 8, 13], restless legs syndrome (RLS) [1, 3, 6, 10], REM-sleep behaviour disorder (RBD) [1, 6, 14-17], periodic limb movements [4], vivid dreams [7, 8, 10], nightmares [18, 19], enuresis (loss of urine control during sleep) [19], night terrors [19], snoring [10], and sleepwalking [19].

Prevalence : Sleep disturbances are one of the most common non-motor symptoms in Parkinson's Disease [3, 20, 21]. Sleep disorders occur in 42% to 94% of people with Parkinson's Disease [4, 5, 13, 22, 23, 29]. Younger people with Parkinson's Disease are affected more in this way [18]. The most prevalent sleep disorders in people with Parkinson's Disease are : poor sleep quality (77%) [29], insomnia (27% to 60%) [4, 5, 9, 10, 24, 28, 30], impaired bed mobility (54%) [12], sleep-disordered breathing (54%) [4], sleep fragmentation (52%) [4], restless legs syndrome (50%) [10], REM- sleep behaviour disorder (RBD) (34% to 42%) [14, 16, 17], periodic limb movements (32%) [4], vivid dreams (71%) [10], nightmares (17% to 32%) [18, 19], enuresis (21%) [19], night terrors (4%) [19], snoring (31%) [10], sleepwalking (2%) [19], disrupted sleep 81% [24], awakenings during night 31% [24], early morning awakenings 40% [24], and non-restorative sleep 38% [24].

Causes of symptoms : In Parkinson's Disease the main causes of having sleep disturbances generally are having movement disturbances during sleep, disturbances of neurotransmission, certain drugs and having concomitant diseases [25]. Insomnia is usually associated with having more progressed Parkinson's Disease [5], having Parkinson's Disease for a longer duration [9], having a higher dosage of L-dopa [5, 11, 26], a higher dosage of dopamine agonists [27], and being female gender [9].

[1] Journal of Parkinson's Disease [2014] 4 (2) : 211-221 (W. Schrempf, M.D.Brandt, A. Storch, H.Reichmann)

[2] Parkinsonism & Related Disorders [2009] 15 (1) : 15-19 (K. Suzuki, M.Miyamoto, T.Miyamoto, Y.Okuma, N.Hattori, S.Kamei, F. Yoshii, H.Utsumi, Y.Iwasaki, M.Iijima, K.Hirata)

[3] Nature and Science of Sleep [2011] 3 : 125-133 (D.O.Claassen, S.J. Kutscher)

[4] Parkinsonism & Related Disorders [2009] 15 (9) : 670-674 (M.I. Norlinah, K.N.Afidah, A.T.Noradina, A.S.Shamsul, B.B.Hamidon, R. Sahathevan, A.A.Raymond)

[5] Movement Disorders [2002] 17 (4) : 775-781 (S.Kumar, M.Bhatia, M.Behari)

[6] International Journal of Neuroscience [2012] 122 (8) : 407- 412 (A.Barber, K.Dashtipour)

[7] Clinical Neurology and Neurosurgery [2013] 115 (10) : 2103-2107 (M.Z.Zhou, J.Gan, Y.R.Wei, X.Y.Ren, W.Chen, Z.G.Liu)

[8] Biomedicine and Pharmacotherapy [1999] 53 (3) : 149-153 (F. Valldeoriola, J. Molinuevo)

[9] Journal of Neurology, Neurosurgery and Psychiatry [2007] 78 (5) : 476-479 (M.D.Gjerstad, T.Wentzel-Larsen, D.Aarsland, J.P.Larsen)

[10] Journal of the Neurological Sciences [2004] 217 (1) : 41-45 (P. Braga-Neto, F.P.da Silva-Júnior, F.Sueli Monte, P.F.de Bruin, V.M.de Bruin)

[11] PLoS One [2011] 6 (7) : e22511 (M.H.Yong, S.Fook-Chong, R. Pavanni, L.L.Lim, E.K. Tan)

[12] Sleep Medicine [2013] 14 (7) : 668-674 (M.Louter, R.J.van Sloun, D.A.Pevernagie, J.B. Arends, P.J.Cluitmans, B.R.Bloem, S.Overeem)

[13] Journal of Clinical and Diagnostic Research [2016] 10 (2) : OC09-OC12 (V.K.Selvaraj, B.Keshavamurthy)

[14] Journal of Clinical Sleep Medicine [2013] 9 (1) : 55A-59A (R. Poryazova, M.Oberholzer, C.R.Baumann, C.L.Bassetti)

[15] Clinical Neurology and Neurosurgery [2011] 113 (6) : 472-476 (D. Vibha, G.Shukla, V. Goyal, S.Singh, A.K.Srivastava, M.Behari)

[16] Parkinsonism & Related Disorders [2009] 15 (Supplement 3) : S101- S104 (I.Arnulf, S.Leu-Semenescu)

[17] Clinical Neurology and Neurosurgery [2014] 124C : 37-43 (K.A. Bjørnarå, E.Dietrichs, M.Toft)

[18] Annals of Clinical and Laboratory Science [1996] 26 (5) : 389-395 (M.L.Wagner, M.N. Fedak, J.I.Sage, M.H.Mark)

[19] Journal of Neurological Science [2014] 346 (1-2) : 204-208 (A.Ylikoski, K.Martikainen, M.Partinen)

[20] Movement Disorders [2009] 24 (11) : 1641-1649 (P.Barone, A. Antonini, C.Colosimo, R.Marconi, L.Morgante, T.P.Avarello, E. Bottacchi, A.Cannas, G.Ceravolo, R.Ceravolo, G.Cicarelli, et al)

[21] Movement Disorders [2010] 25 (11) : 1646-1651 (M.Politis, K.Wu, S.Molloy, P.G Bain, K.R.Chaudhuri, P.Piccini)

[22] Minerva Medica [2005] 96 (3) : 155-173 (E.C.Lauterbach)

[23] Journal of the International Neuropsychological Society [2012] (1) : 108-117 (K.Stavitsky, S.Neargarder, Y.Bogdanova, P.McNamara, A. Cronin-Golomb)

[24] Neurological Sciences [2015] 36 (11) : 2003-2010 (A.Ylikoski, K.Martikainen, M.Sieminski, M.Partinen)

[25] Neurologia i Neurochirurgia Polska [2005] 39 (5) : 380-388 (M. Boczarska-Jedynak, G. Opala)

[26] Journal of Clinical Sleep Medicine [2013] 9 (11) : 1131-1137 (S. Chung, N.I.Bohnen, R.L.Albin, K.A.Frey, M.L.Müller, R.D.Chervin)

[27] Parkinsonism and Related Disorders [2016] Sep 9 [Epub ahead of print] (K.Zhu, J.J.van Hilten, J.Marinus)

[28] Parkinsonism & Related Disorders [2016] Sep 9 [Epub ahead of print] (K.Zhu, J.J.van Hilten, J.Marinus)

[29] Journal of Huazhong University of Science and Technology - Medical Sciences [2017] 37 (1) : 100-104 (Z.J.Mao, C.C.Liu, S.Q.Ji, Q.M.Yang, H.X.Ye, H.Y.Han, Z.Xue)

[30] Annals of the American Thoracic Society [2017] Feb 23 [Epub ahead of print] (S.Shafazand, D.M.Wallace, K.L.Arheart, S.Vargas, C.C.Luca, H.Moore, H.Katzen, B.Levin, C.Singer)

Excessive daytime sleepiness

Symptoms : Excessive daytime sleepiness (EDS) is described as inappropriate and undesirable sleepiness during waking hours [1]. Excessive daytime sleepiness can greatly increase the time spent napping [2]. Excessive daytime sleepiness is more likely to make people with Parkinson's Disease fall [3], and to cause fatigue [4]. Excessive daytime sleepiness could cause blunted circadian rhythms of melatonin secretion [5]. In the advanced stages of Parkinson's Disease the mean level of sleepiness is quite high [6]. Excessive daytime sleepiness is an early sign of Parkinson's Disease [7, 8], and may precede Parkinson's Disease [8, 9]. However, excessive daytime sleepiness can emerge during the course of Parkinson's Disease [10]. Sleep attacks can also occur [11-15].

Prevalence : Excessive daytime sleepiness is common in Parkinson's Disease [14, 16-31]. The prevalence of excessive daytime sleepiness in Parkinson's Disease is between 9% and 51% [1, 7, 14, 23, 26, 30-47, 60]. However, a lot of people with Parkinson's Disease who have excessive daytime sleepiness are unaware that they have it [48]. The prevalence rate increases over the course of Parkinson's Disease [40]. Sleep attacks can occur in at least 15% of people [49].

Causes of symptoms : Dopamine agonists contribute to excessive daytime sleepiness [5, 7, 19, 36, 43, 44, 50-53], but not in all cases [54]. However, total dopaminergic drug dose rather than the dopamine agonists used is a better predictor of excessive daytime sleepiness [54]. Excessive daytime sleepiness is also related to : the duration of Parkinson's Disease [19, 23, 42, 55, 56], cognitive impairment [9, 42, 43, 47], male gender [56, 57], poor sleep quality [43, 44, 50, 58], autonomic dysfunction [43], hallucinations [43], depression [47], anxiety [59], and use of anti-hypertensives [43].

[1] CNS Drugs [2011] 25 (3) : 203-212 (B.Knie, M.T.Mitra, K. Logishetty, K.R.Chaudhuri)

[2] PLoS One [2013] 8 (11) : e81233 (S.J.Bolitho, S.L.Naismith, P. Salahuddin, Z.Terpening, R.R.Grunstein, S.J.Lewis)

[3] Journal of Parkinson's Disease [2013] 3 (3) : 387-391 (M.Spindler, N.S.Gooneratne, A.Siderowf, J.E.Duda, C.Cantor, N.Dahodwala)

[4] Journal of Clinical Sleep Medicine [2013] 9 (11) : 1131-1137 (S. Chung, N.I.Bohnen, R.L.Albin, K.A.Frey, M.L.Müller, R.D.Chervin)

[5] JAMA Neurology [2014] 71 (4) : 463-469 (A.Videnovic, C.Noble, K.J.Reid, J.Peng, F.W.Turek, A.Marconi, A.W.Rademaker, T.Simuni, C.Zadikoff, P.C.Zee)

[6] Journal of Sleep Research [2013] 22 (2) : 197-200 (F.Giganti, S. Ramat, I.Zilli, S.Guidi, L.M.Raglione, S.Sorbi, P.Salzarulo)

[7] Oman Medical Journal [2015] 30 (1) : 3-10 (F.Salawu, A.Olokoba)

[8] American Journal of Epidemiology [2011] 173 (9) : 1032-1038 (J. Gao, X.Huang, Y.Park, A.Hollenbeck, A.Blair, A.Schatzkin, H.Chen)

[9] Parkinsonism & Related Disorders [2013] 19 (9) : 806-811 (J.G. Goldman, R.A.Ghode, B.Ouyang, B.Bernard, C.G.Goetz, G.T. Stebbins)

[10] Neurological Sciences [2003] 24 (3) : 178-179 (G.Fabbrini, P. Barbanti, C.Aurilia, C.Pauletti, N.Vanacore, G.Meco)

[11] Journal of Parkinson’s Disease [2014] 4 (2) : 211-221 (W. Schrempf, M.D.Brandt, A. Storch, H.Reichmann)

[12] Minerva Medica [2005] 96 (3) : 155-173 (E.C.Lauterbach)

[13] International Journal of Neuroscience [2012] 122 (8) : 407-412 (A.Barber, K.Dashtipour)

[14] Clinical Neurology and Neurosurgery [2014] 124C : 37-43 (K.A. Bjørnarå, E.Dietrichs, M.Toft)

[15] Parkinsonism & Related Disorders [2013] 19 (12) : 1152-1155 (M.M.Kurtis, C. Rodriguez-Blazquez, P.Martinez-Martin)

[16] Parkinsonism & Related Disorders [2014] 20 (6) : 578-583 (K. Kotschet, W.Johnson, S.McGregor, J.Kettlewell, A.Kyoong, D.M. O'Driscoll, A.R.Turton, R.I.Griffiths, M.K.Horne)

[17] Sleep Medicine [2003] 4 (4) : 339-342 (S.Kumar, M.Bhatia, M. Behari)

[18] Journal of Neural Transmission - Parkinson's Disease and Dementia section [1993] 5 (3) : 235-244 (J.J.van Hilten, M.Weggeman, E.A.van der Velde, G.A.Kerkhof, J.G.van Dijk, R.A.Roos)

[19] European Neurology [2010] 63 (3) : 129-135 (R.Poryazova, D. Benninger, D.Waldvogel, C.L.Bassetti)

[20] Neurology [2005] 65 (9) : 1442-1446 (R.D.Abbott, G.W.Ross, L. R.White, C.M.Tanner, K.H.Masaki, J.S.Nelson, J.D.Curb, H. Petrovitch)

[21] Journal of the Neurological Sciences [2008] 271 (1-2) : 47-52 (K. Suzuki, T.Miyamoto, M.Miyamoto, Y.Okuma, N.Hattori, S.Kamei, F. Yoshii, H.Utsumi, Y.Iwasaki, M.Iijima, K.Hirata)

[22] Movement Disorders [2014] 29 (2) : 259-262 (B.Prudon, G.W. Duncan, T.K.Khoo, A.J.Yarnall, K.N.Anderson)

[23] Neurology [2015] 85 (2) : 162-168 (L.K.Tholfsen, J.P.Larsen, J. Schulz, O.B.Tysnes, M.D.Gjerstad)

[24] Parkinsonism & Related Disorders [2009] 15 (1) : 15-19 (K. Suzuki, M.Miyamoto, T.Miyamoto, Y.Okuma, N.Hattori, S.Kamei, F. Yoshii, H.Utsumi, Y.Iwasaki, M.Iijima, K. Hirata)

[25] Nature and Science of Sleep [2011] 3 : 125-133 (D.O.Claassen, S.J. Kutscher)

[26] Parkinsonism & Related Disorders [2009] 15 (9) : 670-674 (M.I. Norlinah, K.N.Afidah, A.T.Noradina, A.S.Shamsul, B.B.Hamidon, R. Sahathevan, A.A.Raymond)

[27] PLoS One [2014] 9 (9) : e107278 (V.Cochen De Cock, S.Bayard, I.Jaussent, M.Charif, M.Grini, M.C.Langenier, H.Yu, R.Lopez, C. Geny, B.Carlander, Y.Dauvilliers)

[28] Parkinsonism & Related Disorders [2009] 15 (Supplement 3) : S101- S104 (I.Arnulf, S.Leu-Semenescu)

[29] Journal of Clinical and Diagnostic Research [2016] 10 (2) : OC09-OC12 (V.K.Selvaraj, B.Keshavamurthy)

[30] JAMA [2002] 287 (4) : 455-463 (D.E.Hobson, A.E.Lang, W.R. Martin, A.Razmy, J.Rivest, J.Fleming)

[31] Sleep Medicine Reviews [2005] 9 (3) : 185-200 (I.Arnulf)

[32] Translational Neurodegeneration [2015] 4 (1) : 1 (H.Chen, E.J. Zhao, W.Zhang, Y.Lu, R.Liu, X.Huang, A.J.Ciesielski-Jones, M.A. Justice, D.S.Cousins, S.Peddada)

[33] European Journal of Neurology [2010] 17 (12) : 1428-1436 (P.O. Valko, D.Waldvogel, M.Weller, C.L.Bassetti, U.Held, C.R. Baumann)

[34] Movement Disorders [2008] 23 (1) : 35-41 (D.Verbaan, S.M.van Rooden, M.Visser, J.Marinus, J.J.van Hilten)

[35] Movement Disorders [2007] 22 (11) : 1567-1572 (I.Ghorayeb, A. Loundou, P.Auquier, Y.Dauvilliers, B.Bioulac, F.Tison)

[36] CNS Drugs [2001] 15 (4) : 267-275 (J.P.Larsen, E.Tandberg)

[37] Neurology [2002] 58 (10) : 1544-1546 (M.D.Gjerstad, D.Aarsland, J.P.Larsen)

[38] Movement Disorders [2006] 21 (9) : 1432-1438 (I.Shpirer, A. Miniovitz, C.Klein, R.Goldstein, T.Prokhorov, J.Theitler, L.Pollak, J. M.Rabey)

[39] Neurology [2006] 67 (5) : 853-858 (M.D.Gjerstad, G.Alves, T. Wentzel-Larsen, D.Aarsland, J.P.Larsen)

[40] Neurology [2015] 85 (2) : 162-168 (L.K.Tholfsen, J.P.Larsen, J.I. Schulz, O.B.Tysnes, M.D.Gjerstad)

[41] PLoS One [2014] 9 (9) : e107278 (V.Cochen De Cock, S.Bayard, I.Jaussent, N.Charif, M.Grini, M.C.Langenier, H.Yu, R.Lopez, C.Geny, B.Carlander, Y.Dauvilliers)

[42] Movement Disorders [1999] 14 (6) : 922-927 (E.Tandberg, J.P. Larsen, K.Karlsen)

[43] Parkinsonism & Related Disorders [2016] Jan 22 [Epub ahead of print] (K.Zhu, J.J.van Hilten, J.Marinus)

[44] Neurologic Clinics [2005] 23 (4) : 1187-1208 (M.J.Thorpy, C.H. Adler)

[45] Annals of Clinical and Laboratory Science [1996] 26 (5) : 389-395 (M.L.Wagner, M.N. Fedak, J.I.Sage, M.H.Mark)

[46] Journal of the Medical Association of Thailand [2014] 97 (10) : 1022-1027 (S.Setthawatcharawanich, K.Limapichat, P.Sathirapanya, K. Phabphal)

[47] Zhonghua Nei Ke Za Zhi [2016] 55 (7) : 515-519 (Y.Gong, C.F.Liu)

[48] Sleep Disorders [2014] 2014 : 767181 (M.Ataide, C.M.Franco, O. G.Lins)

[49] Neurologia i Neurochirurgia Polska [2005] 39 (5) : 380-388 (M. Boczarska-Jedynak, G.Opala)

[50] Journal of Neural Transmission (Supplementum) [2006] (70) : 349-355 (C.L.Comella)

[51] Journal of Neural Transmission (Supplementum) [2006] (70) : 357-360 (I.Arnulf)

[52] European Neurology [2003] 49 (1) : 30-33 (I.Schlesinger, P.D. Ravin)

[53] Parkinsonism & Related Disorders [2001] 7 (4) : 283-286 (C.C. Sanjiv, M.Schulzer, E.Mak, J.Fleming, W.R.Martin, T.Brown, S.M. Calne, J.Tsui, A.J.Stoessl, C.S.Lee, D.B.Calne)

[54] Archives of Neurology [2004] 61 (1) : 97-102 (A.Razmy, A.E. Lang, C.M.Shapiro)

[55] Clinical Neurology and Neurosurgery [2014] 124 : 37-43 (K.A. Bjørnarå, E.Dietrichs, M.Toft)

[56] Neurology [2001] 57 (8) : 1392-1396 (W.G.Ondo, K.Dat Vuong, H.Khan, F.Atassi, C.Kwak, J.Jankovic)

[57] Sleep Medicine [2003] 4 (4) : 275-280 (T.Roth, D.B.Rye, L.D. Borchert, C.Bartlett, D.L.Bliwise, C.Cantor, J.M.Gorell, J.P.Hubble, B.Musch, C.W.Olanow, C.Pollak, M.B.Stern, R.L.Watts)

[58] Sleep [2004] 27 (5) : 967-972 (S.Stevens, C.L.Cormella, E.J. Stepanski)

[59] Clinical Neurology and Neurosurgery [2016] 148 : 29-34 (S. Pandey, B.K.Bajaj, A.Wadhwa, K.S.Anand)

[60] Journal of Huazhong University of Science and Technology - Medical Sciences [2017] 37 (1) : 100-104 (Z.J.Mao, C.C.Liu, S.Q.Ji, Q.M.Yang, H.X.Ye, H.Y.Han, Z.Xue)

FATIGUE

Symptoms : People with Parkinson's Disease are more prone to fatigue [1-14].

Prevalence : The prevalence of fatigue in people who have Parkinson's Disease was found to be anywhere between 35% and 70% [15-24].

Causes of symptoms : Fatigue Parkinson's Disease is most associated with depression [11, 12, 19, 24-27]. Fatigue is also associated with the severity of Parkinson's Disease [1, 11, 25], female gender [12, 27, 28], daytime sleepiness [11, 12, 27], older age [1], and anxiety [11].

[1] Neurology [2014] 83 (3) : 215-220 (F.Stocchi, G.Abbruzzese, R. Ceravolo, P.Cortelli, M.D'Amelio, M.F.De Pandis, G.Fabbrini, C. Pacchetti, G.Pezzoli, A.Tessitore, M.Canesi, C.Iannacone, M.Zappia)

[2] Neurology [1993] 43 (10) : 2016-2018 (J.Friedman, H.Friedman)

[3] American Family Physician [2013] 87 (4) : 267-273 (J.D. Gazewood, D.R.Richards, K.Clebak)

[4] Journal of Neural Transmission [2013] 120 (4) : 577-581 (C.Falup-Pecurariu)

[5] Expert Opinion on Pharmacotherapy [2011] 12 (13) : 1999-2007 (J. H.Friedman, A,Abrantes, L.H.Sweet)

[6] Movement Disorders [2007] 22 (3) : 297-308 (J.H.Friedman, R.G. Brown, C.Comella, C.E.Garber, L.B.Krupp, J.S.Lou, L.Marsh, L.Nail, L.Shulman, C.B.Taylor)

[7] Praxis [2002] 91 (10) : 407-410 (H.P.Ludin)

[8] Journal of Neurology [2006] 253 (Supplement 7) : VII48-VII53 (F. Yoshii, H.Takahashi, R.Kumazawa, S.Kobori)

[9] Neurological Sciences [2003] 24 (3) : 225-226 (A.Zenzola, G.Masi, M.De Mari, G.Defazio, P.Livrea, P.Lamberti)

[10] Parkinsonism & Related Disorders [2013] 19 (2) : 148-152 (G. Fabbrini, A.Latorre, A.Suppa, M.Bloise, M.Frontoni, A.Berardelli)

[11] Parkinson's Disease [2011] : 125271 (V.Metta, K.Logishetty, P. Martinez-Martin, H.M.Gage, P.E.Schartau, A.Martin, T.K. Kaluarachchi, P.Odin, P.Barone, F.Stocchi, A.Antonini, et al)

[12] Movement Disorders [2010] 25 (14) : 2456-2460 (A.G.Beiske, J. H.Loge, M.J.Hjermstad, E.Svensson)

[13] Neurology [2008] 71 (7) : 481-485 (G.Schifitto, J.H.Friedman, D. Oakes, L.Shulman, C.L.Comella, K.Marek, S.Fahn)

[14] Movement Disorders [2001] 16 (2) : 190-196 (J.S.Lou, G.Kearns, B.Oken, G.Sexton, J.Nutt)

[15] Acta Neurologica Scandinavica [2010] (Supplementum) (190) : 78- 81 (A.G.Beiske, E.Svensson)

[16] Internal Medicine [2011] 50 (15) : 1553-1558 (H.Miwa, T.Miwa)

[17] Journal of Neurology [2012] 259 (8) : 1639-1647 (P.Martinez-Martin, C.Falup Pecurariu, P.Odin, J.J.van Hilten, A.Antonini, J.M. Rojo-Abuin, V.Borges, C.Trenkwalder, D.Aarsland, D.J.Brooks, et al)

[18] Movement Disorders [2009] 24 (13) : 1977-1983 (Y.Okuma, S. Kamei, A.Morita, F.Yoshii, T.Yamamoto, S.Hashimoto, H.Utsumi, T. Hatano, N.Hattori, M.Matsumura, K.Takahashi, S.Nogawa, et al)

[19] Brazilian Journal of Medical and Biological Research [2009] 42 (8) : 771-775 (F.O.Goulart, B.A.Godke, V.Borges, S.M.Azevedo-Silva, M.F.Mendes, M.S.Cendoroglo, H.B.Ferraz)

[20] Movement Disorders [2001] 16 (6) : 1120-1122 (J.H.Friedman, H. Friedman)

[21] Movement Disorders [1999] 14 (2) : 237-241 (K.Karlsen, J.P. Larsen, E.Tandberg, K.Jørgensen)

[22] Parkinsonism & Related Disorders [2012] 18 (Supplement 1) : S222-S225 (H.B.Wen, Z.X.Zhang, H.Wang, L.Li, H.Chen, Y.Liu, B. Zhang, Q.Xu)

[23] European Journal of Neurology [2012] 19 (7) : 963-968 (K. Herlofson, S.O.Ongre, L.K.Enger, O.B.Tysnes, J.P.Larsen)

[24] Parkinsons Disease [2016] : 2835945 (M.Golab-Janowska, D. Kotlega, K.Safranow, A.Meller, A.Budzianowska, K.Honczarenko)

[25] Journal of Neurological Sciences [2008] 270 (1-2) : 107-113 (E. Havlikova, J.P.van Dijk, J.Rosenberger, I.Nagyova, B.Middel, T. Dubayova, Z.Gdovinova, J.W.Groothoff)

[26] European Neurology [2013] 70 (1-2) : 59-64 (S.Y.Kang, H.I.Ma, Y.M.Lim, S.H.Hwang, Y.J.Kim)

[27] Acta Neurologica Scandinavica [2011] 123 (2) : 130-136 (A. Kummer, P.Scalzo, F.Cardoso, A.L.Teixeira).

[28] Neurological Sciences [2014] 35 (12) : 1991-1996 (Y.Song, Z.Gu, J.An, P.Chan)

Apathy

Symptoms : Apathy is characterised by lack of interest, loss of initiative, diminished motivation, and a flattening of affect [1, 2].

Prevalence : Apathy occurs more commonly in Parkinson's Disease [3, 4, 5], especially when there is also depression [6]. Apathy is also one of the most common neuropsychiatric symptoms in Parkinson's Disease [7, 8]. Estimates of the prevalence of apathy in Parkinson's Disease varies according to the study, from 16% to 70%, with an average of around 40% [8-24]. The extent of agreement concerning the degree of apathy between self reporting and caregiver reports is low at only 45% [25]. When people that also have depression and dementia are excluded, the prevalence of apathy decreases to between 5% and 10% [26].

Causes of symptoms : Apathy is associated with depression [19, 21, 23], but not in all studies [27]. Researchers have suggested links between apathy and dopamine depletion in Parkinson's Disease [28]. Consistent with this, apathy in Parkinson's Disease is significantly improved by an acute intake of L-dopa [29], and apathy is associated with the severity of Parkinson's Disease [17, 19, 21, 23, 30]. Apathy in Parkinson's Disease is also associated with postural instability [31], right-onset disease by as much as four times more [27], male gender [19], older age [23], and cognitive impairment [21, 29, 32], but not in all studies [19]. These findings suggest that in non-demented, non-depressed PD patients, apathy may be a predictive factor for dementia and cognitive decline over time [33].

[1] Movement Disorders [2014] 29 (7) : 897-903 (N.Carriere, P. Besson, K.Dujardin, A.Duhamel, L.Defebvre, C.Delmaire, D.Devos)

[2] Journal of Neuroscience [2014] 34 (17) : 5918-5926 (S.Martínez-Horta, J.Riba, R.F.de Bobadilla, J.Pagonabarraga, B.Pascual- Sedano, R.M.Antonijoan, S.Romero, M.A.Mañanas, et al)

[3] Movement Disorders [2015] 30 (7) : 919-927 (D.Weintraub, T. Simuni, C.Caspell-Garcia, C.Coffey, S.Lasch, A.Siderowf, D. Aarsland, P.Barone, D.Burn, L.M.Chahine, J.Eberling, et al)

[4] Neurology [2014] 83 (12) : 1096-1103 (P.de la Riva, K.Smith, S.X. Xie, D.Weintraub)

[5] Movement Disorders [2012] 27 (3) : 432-434 (L.D.Louis, E.D. Huey, M.Gerbin, A.S.Viner)

[6] Acta Neurologica Scandinavica [2015] 131 (2) : 80-87 (M. Skorvanek, Z.Gdovinova, J.Rosenberger, R.Ghorbani Saeedian, I. Nagyova, J.W.Groothoff, J.P.van Dijk)

[7] Dementia and Geriatric Cognitive Disorders [2013] 35 (5-6) : 249-255 (S.Laatu, M.Karrasch, K.Martikainen, R.Marttila)

[8] Movement Disorders [2008] 23 (13) : 1889-1896 (J.Kulisevsky, J. Pagonabarraga, B.Pascual-Sedano, C.García-Sánchez, A.Gironell)

[9] Behavioural Neurology [2013] 27 (4) : 501-513 (G.Santangelo, L. Trojano, P.Barone, D.Errico, D.Grossi, C.Vitale)

[10] Neurological Sciences [2014] 35 (5) : 729-734 (M.Rodríguez-Violante, P.González-Latapi, A.Cervantes-Arriaga, D.Martínez-Ramírez, S.Velázquez-Osuna, A.Camacho-Ordoñez)

[11] Journal of Geriatric Psychiatry and Neurology [2013] 26 (4) : 237-243 (M.Skorvanek, J.Rosenberger, Z.Gdovinova, I.Nagyova, R.G. Saeedian, J.W.Groothoff, J.P.Dijk)

[12] Parkinsonism & Related Disorders [2012] 18 (4) : 339-342 (L. Ziropadja, E.Stefanova, M.Petrovic, T.Stojkovic, V.S. Kostic)

[13] Geriatrie et Psychologie Neuropsychiatrie du Vieillissement [2013] 11 (2) : 197-207 (D.Delgadillo-Iniguez, C.Derouesné, L. Lacomblez, M. C.Gély-Nargeot)

[14] Movement Disorders [2015] Jan 20 [Epub ahead of print] (H.C. Baggio, B.Segura, J.L.Garrido-Millan, M.J.Marti, Y.Compta, F. Valldeoriola, E.Tolosa, C.Junque)

[15] Clinical Neurology and Neurosurgery [2010] 112 (10) : 883-885 (M.Rodríguez-Violante, A.Cervantes-Arriaga, A.Villar-Velarde, T. Corona)

[16] Neurologia [2010] 25 (1) : 40-50 (R.García-Ramos, C.Villanueva, J.del Val, J.Matías-Guíu)

[17] Journal of Geriatric Psychiatry and Neurology [2010] 23 (1) : 35-41 (M.Oguru, H.Tachibana, K.Toda, B.Okuda, N.Oka)

[18] Journal of Neurology, Neurosurgery, and Psychiatry [2009] 80 (11) : 1279-1282 (K.F.Pedersen, G.Alves, D.Aarsland, J.P.Larsen)

[19] Journal of Neurology [2010] 257 (2) : 217-223 (K.F.Pedersen, G. Alves, K.Brønnick, D.Aarsland, O.B.Tysnes, J.P.Larsen)

[20] Medicina [2009] 69 (2) : 253-258 (A.Bottini Bonfanti, J.L. Etcheverry, G.G.Persi, H.Zezza, S.Starkstein, E.M.Gatto)

[21] Parkinsonism & Related Disorders [2009] 15 (4) : 295-299 (K.F. Pedersen, J.P.Larsen, G.Alves, D.Aarsland)

[22] Neurology [2006] 67 (1) : 33-38 (L.Kirsch-Darrow, H.H. Fernandez, M.Marsiske, M.S.Okun, D.Bowers)

[23] Movement Disorders [2015] 30 (6) : 759-769 (M.G.den Brok, J.W.Dalen, W.A.van Gool, E.P.Moll van Charante, R.M.de Bie, E. Richard)

[24] Journal of Neurologial Science [2016] 367 : 342-346 (M.Petrovic, E.Stefanova, L.Ziropadja, T.Stojkovic, V.S.Kostic)

[25] Aging and Mental Health [2008] 12 (5) : 647-653 (A.McKinlay, R.C.Grace, J.C.Dalrymple-Alford, T.J.Anderson, J.Fink, G.Roger)

[26] Movement Disorders [2012] 27 (2) : 174-178 (S.E.Starkstein)
[27] Journal of Geriatric Psychiatry and Neurology [2013] 26 (2) : 95-104 (E.Harris, P.McNamara, R.Durso)

[28] Health Psychology [2011] 30 (4) : 386-400 (K.R.Bogart)

[29] Frontiers in Aging Neuroscience [2014] 6 : 164 (V.Fleury, E. Cousin, V.Czernecki, E.Schmitt, E.Lhommée, A.Poncet, V.Fraix, I. Troprès, P.Pollak, A.Krainik, P.Krack)

[30] Movement Disorders [2014] 29 (14) : 1796-1801 (K.Dujardin, C. Langlois, L.Plomhause, A.S.Carette, M.Delliaux, A.Duhamel, L. Defebvre)

[31] Journal of the Neurological Sciences [2014] 338 (1-2) : 162-165 (A.Hassan, S.Vallabhajosula, L.B.Zahodne, D.Bowers, M.S.Okun, H. H.Fernandez, C.J.Hass)

[32] Journal of Neuropsychiatry and Clinical Neurosciences [1998] 10 (3) : 314-319 (M.L.Levy, J.L.Cummings, L.A.Fairbanks, D. Masterman, B.L.Miller, A.H.Craig, J.S.Paulsen, I.Litvan)

[33] Movement Disorders [2009] 24 (16) : 2391-2397 (K.Dujardin, P.Sockeel, M.Delliaux, A.Destée, L.Defebvre)

ANHEDONIA

Symptoms : Anhedonia is the inability to gain pleasure from normally pleasurable experiences. This can include what somebody used to find pleasurable such as their interests, and social interactions. Anhedonia often occurs in Parkinson's Disease [1-14].

Prevalence : Anhedonia occurs in up to 45% of people with Parkinson's Disease [12, 15], and in up to 80% of people who also had depression [12].

Causes of symptoms : Anhedonia is related to the severity of depression [9, 16, 17, 18], but some people with Parkinson's Disease do not have depression [18]. It is also related to apathy [9, 13, 17, 19, 20], cognitive impairment [1, 9, 17, 19], neuropsychiatric symptoms [21], and more severe Parkinson's Disease [22].

[1] Seishin Shinkeigaku Zasshi [2013] 115 (11) : 1135-1141 (S. Kitamura, H.Nagayama)

[2] Movement Disorders [2015] 30 (2) : 229-237 (C.Pont-Sunyer, A. Hotter, C.Gaig, K.Seppi, Y.Compta, R.Katzenschlager, N.Mas, D. Hofeneder,T.Brücke, A.Bayés, K.Wenzel, J.Infante, H.Zach, et al)

[3] Journal of Neurology [2014] 261 (2) : 382-391 (P.Solla, A.Cannas, C.S.Mulas, S.Perra, A.Corona, P.P.Bassareo, F. Marrosu)

[4] Psychiatry Research [2014] 215 (2) : 448-452 (M.Pettorruso, G. Martinotti, A.Fasano, G.Loria, M.Di Nicola, L.De Risio, L.Ricciardi, G.Conte, L.Janiri, A.R.Bentivoglio)

[5] Zhonghua Yi Xue Za Zhi [2013] 93 (1) : 26-29 (C.J.Mao, J.P.Chen, W.D.Hu, C.F.Liu)

[6] Journal of Neuropsychiatry and Clinical Neurosciences [2012] 24 (4) : 444-451 (G.Loas, P.Krystkowiak, O.Godefroy)

[7] Clinical Neurology and Neurosurgery [2012] 114 (4) : 352-355 (S. Miura, H.Kida, J.Nakajima, K.Noda, K.Nagasato, M.Ayabe, H. Aizawa, M.Hauser, T.Taniwaki)

[8] Journal of Huazhong University of Science and Technology [2009] 29 (6) : 725-728 (J.Zheng, S.Sun, X.Qiao, Y.Liu)

[9] Parkinsonism & Related Disorders [2009] 15 (8) : 576-581 (G. Santangelo, L.Morgante, R.Savica, R.Marconi, L.Grasso, A.Antonini, D.De Gaspari, D.Ottaviani, D.Tiple, L.Simoni, P.Barone)

[10] Movement Disorders [2007] 22 (5) : 666-672 (K.M.Miller, M.S. Okun, H.F.Fernandez, C.E.4th Jacobson, R.L.Rodriguez, D. Bowers)

[11] Journal of Neuropsychiatry and Clinical Neurosciences [2006] 8 (3) : 397-401 (K.Witt, C.Daniels, J.Herzog, D.Lorenz, J.Volkmann, J.Reiff, M.Mehdorn, G.Deuschl, P.Krack)

[12] Journal of Neuropsychiatry and Clinical Neurosciences [2005] 17 (2) : 214-220 (M.R.Lemke, H.M.Brecht, J.Koester, P.H.Kraus, H. Reichmann)

[13] International Journal of Psychiatry in Clinical Practice [2003] 7 (Supplement 1) : 25-27 (T.Maruyama)

[14] Journal of Neurology, Neurosurgery, and Psychiatry [2003] 74 (9) : 1308-1311 (V.Isella, S.Iurlaro, R.Piolti, C.Ferrarese, L.Frattola, I. Appollonio, P.Melzi, M.Grimaldi)

[15] Clinical Neurology and Neurosurgery [2013] 115 (12) : 2524-2527 (K.Matsui, H.Tachibana, T.Yamanishi, M.Oguru, K.Toda, B.Okuda, N.Oka)

[16] Depression and Anxiety [2013] 30 (1) : 85-91 (G.Spalletta, S. Fagioli, G.Meco, M.Pierantozzi, A.Stefani, V.Pisani, C.Caltagirone, F. E.Pontieri, F.Assogna)

[17] Movement Disorders [2011] 26 (10) : 1825-1834 (F.Assogna, L. Cravello, C.Caltagirone, G.Spalletta)

[18] Geriatrics & Gerontology International [2011] 11 (3) : 275-281 (S.Fujiwara, F.Kimura, T.Hosokawa, S.Ishida, M.Sugino, T.Hanafusa)

[19] Journal of Neurology [2009] 256 (4) : 632-638 (G.Santangelo, C. Vitale, L.Trojano, K.Longo, A.Cozzolino, D.Grossi, P.Barone)

[20] Movement Disorders [2014] 29 (14) : 1796-1801 (K.Dujardin, C. Langlois, L.Plomhause, A.S.Carette, M.Delliaux, A.Duhamel, L. Defebvre)

[21] Clinical Neurology and Neurosurgery [2009] 111 (8) : 665-669 (J.C.Gómez-Esteban, B.Tijero, J.Somme, I.Bilbao, J.Fernández, S. Boyero, F.Velasco, E.Lezcano, J.J.Zarranz)

[22] Journal of Neurological Science [2016] Nov 3 [Epub ahead of print] (H.Nagayama, T.Maeda, T.Uchiyama, M.Hashimoto, N.Nomoto, O.Kano, T.Takahashi, H.Terashi, S.Hamada, T.Hasegawa, et al)

Bradyphrenia

Symptoms : Bradyphrenia is mental slowness [1]. Bradyphrenia can consist of slowness of thought, impaired attention and motivation, lack of spontaneity, and inflexibility [2].

Prevalence : Bradyphrenia often occurs in Parkinson's Disease [1, 3-7]. Between 11% and 51% of people with Parkinson's Disease were found to exhibit mental slowness by performing significantly worse on neuropsychological tests including tests of attention and executive function [1]. However, bradyphrenia is uncommon in people with Parkinson's Disease who do not have dementia or depression [8, 9, 10].

Causes of symptoms : Bradyphrenia is associated with reduced dopaminergic stimulation of the mesolimibic pathway [11, 12]. Bradyphrenia in Parkinson's Disease may reflect advancing age because the effects of age may be greater in some cases than the effects of basal ganglia disease once motor dysfunction has been allowed for [13].

[1] Journal of Clinical and Experimental Neuropsychology [2016] May 1 : 1-9 [Epub ahead of print] (T.T.Vlagsma, J.Koerts, O.Tucha, H.T.Dijkstra, A.A.Duits, T.van Laar, J.M.Spikman)

[2] Revue Neurologique [1994] 150 (12) : 823-826 (A.J.Lees)

[3] Neuropsychologia [2002] 40 (8) : 1488-1493 (B.A.Shipley, I.J. Deary, J.Tan, G.Christie, J.M.Starr)

[4] Electromyography and Clinical Neurophysiology [1996] 36 (4) : 215-220 (A.Aotsuka, S.J.Weate, M.E.Drake Jr, G.W.Paulson)

[5] Neuropsychologia [1995] 33 (5) : 561-575 (M.O.Russ, L.Seger)

[6] Acta Neurologica Scandinavica [1993] 87 (4) : 255-261 (R.J. Dobbs, S.G.Bowes, A.Charlett, M.Henley, C.Frith, J.Dickins, S.M. Dobbs)

[7] Neurology [1987] 37 (7) : 1130-1134 (R.Mayeux, Y.Stern, M. Sano, L.Cote, J.B.Williams)

[8] Neuropsychologia [1994] 32 (11) : 1383-1396 (M.E.Duncombe, J.L.Bradshaw, R.Iansek, J.G.Phillips)

[9] Journal of Clinical and Experimental Neuropsychology [1994] 16 (3) : 457-471 (K.B.Spicer, G.G.Brown, J.M.Gorell)

[10] Brain and Cognition [1993] 21 (1) : 87-110 (A.Revonsuo, R.Portin, L.Koivikko, J.O.Rinne, U.K.Rinne)

[11] Journal of Molecular Neuroscience [2007] 32 (1) : 72-79 (A. Friedman, I.Deri, Y.Friedman, E.Dremencov, S.Goutkin, E. Kravchinsky, M,Mintz, D.Levi, D.H.Overstreet, G.Yadid)

[12] Brain Nerve [2007] 59 (9) : 943-951 (M.Yokochi)

[13] The Journals of Gerontology, Series A [1999] 54 (8) : M404-M409 (J.G.Phillips, T.Schiffter, M.E.Nicholls, J.L.Bradshaw, R.Iansek, L.L.Saling)

Alexithymia

Symptoms : Alexithymia is a personality trait characterised by difficulties identifying and describing feelings and a reduced tendency to think about emotions [1, 2].

Prevalence : About 20% to 50% of people with Parkinson's Disease have alexithymia [2-5], which is about 2 to 4 times normal [2-5].

Causes of symptoms : There is a strong association between alexithymia and the severity of depression [6, 7].

[1] Movement Disorders [2014] 29 (2) : 214-220 (K.S.Goerlich-Dobre, C.Probst, L.Winter, K.Witt, G.Deuschl, B.Möller, T.van Eimeren)

[2] Psychosomatics [2010] 51 (1) : 22-28 (A.Costa, A.Peppe, G.A. Carlesimo, G.Salamone, C.Caltagirone)

[3] Parkinsonism & Related Disorders [2016] 28 : 1-11 (F.Assogna, L.Cravello, M.D.Orfei, N.Cellupica, C.Caltagirone, G.Spalletta)

[4] Frontiers in Psychology [2014] 5 : 1168 (L.Castelli, D.Tonello, L. Rizzi, M.Zibetti, M.Lanotte, L.Lopiano)

[5] American Journal of Geriatric Psychiatry [2012] 20 (2) : 133-141 (F.Assogna, K.Palmer, F.E.Pontieri, M.Pierantozzi, A.Stefani, W. Gianni, C.Caltagirone, G.Spalletta)

[6] Psychotherapy and Psychosomatics [2011] 80 (4) : 251-253 (M. Poletti, D.Frosini, C.Pagni, C.Lucetti, P.Del Dotto, R.Ceravolo, U. Bonuccelli)

[7] European Journal of Neurology [2006] 13 (8) : 836-841 (A.Costa, A.Peppe, G.A. Carlesimo, P.Pasqualetti, C.Caltagirone)

Neuropathy

Symptoms : Neuropathy is damage or disease of the nerves. Peripheral neuropathy develops when nerves in the body's extremities, such as the hands, feet and arms are damaged. The main symptoms of peripheral neuropathy can include : numbness and tingling in the feet or hands; burning, stabbing or shooting pain in affected areas; loss of balance and co-ordination; muscle weakness, especially in the feet. The symptoms are usually constant but may come and go.

Prevalence : Neuropathy is far more common in people who have

Parkinson's Disease [1]. Around 37% to 57% of people who have Parkinson's Disease can be affected [2, 3, 4], which means that it is about twenty times more likely to occur in people with Parkinson's Disease. It occurs more commonly than in people with a Parkinsonism [4].

Causes of symptoms : Neuropathy is related to age [1, 5], vitamin B12 deficiency [2], serum folate levels [1], and L-dopa use [1, 2, 5, 6, 7]. Neuropathy is more than twice as likely in people who have Parkinson's Disease who have been taking L-dopa for a long time [5]. However, one study could not relate neuropathy to the long term use of L-dopa, the duration of Parkinson's Disease, or the age of the people affected [3]. Another study proposed multifactorial causes of neuropathy [4].

[1] Journal of Neurology [2013] 260 (11) : 2844-2848 (Y.A.Rajabally, J.Martey)

[2] Neurology [2011] 77 (22) : 1947-1950 (Y.A.Rajabally, J.Martey)

[3] Neuro Endocrinology Letters [2015] 36 (4) : 363-367 (Z. Grambalova, M.Kaiserova, M.Vastik, K.Mensíkova, P.Otruba, J. Zapletalova, J. Dufek, P.Kanovsky)

[4] BMC Neurology [2016] 16 : 139 (D.F.de Araújo, A.P.de Melo Neto, I.S. Oliveira, B.S.Brito, I.T.de Araújo, I.S.Barros, J.W.Lima, W.G.Horta, FdeA.Gondim)

[5] Movement Disorders [2013] 28 (10) : 1391-1397 (R.Ceravolo, G. Cossu, M.Bandettini di Poggio, L.Santoro, P.Barone, M.Zibetti, D. Frosini, V.Nicoletti, F.Manganelli, R.Iodice, M. Picillo, et al)

[6] Parkinsonism & Related Disorders [2014] 20 (1) : 27-31 (F. Mancini, C.Comi, G.D.Oggioni, C.Pacchetti, D.Calandrella, M.Coletti Moja, G.Riboldazzi, S.Tunesi, M.Dal Fante, L.Manfredi, et al)

[7] Journal of Neurology [2012] 259 (8) : 1668-1672 (D.Santos-García, R.de la Fuente-Fernández, F.Valldeoriola, A.Palasí, F.Carrillo, M. Grande, P.Mir, O.De Fabregues, J. Casanova)

Anxiety

Symptoms : Anxiety can precede the onset of Parkinson's Disease or can develop after diagnosis [1]. Anxiety commonly occurred in combination with depression [2, 3, 19]. An anxious personality was associated with an increased risk of developing Parkinson's Disease [4, 5].

Prevalence : Anxiety is more than twice as common in Parkinson's Disease [6]. Anxiety disorders, especially anxiety, panic, and social phobia, occur in up to 40% of people with Parkinson's Disease [7, 8]. Anxiety occurs in 37% to 73% of people with Parkinson's Disease [9-13]. Around 30% of people with Parkinson's Disease had a general anxiety diagnosis [3, 14]. Social phobia was diagnosed in 42% of people with Parkinson's Disease [15]. Panic disorder occurs in around 30% of people with Parkinson's Disease [16].

Causes of symptoms : Anxiety is greater during "off" periods than during "on" periods. The change in anxiety is related to the changes in Parkinson's Disease symptom scores [17]. Anxiety is not significantly associated with the severity of motor symptoms or cognitive functioning [18]. Panic disorder is associated with the earlier onset of Parkinson's Disease, motor fluctuations (77%), and morning dystonia (38%) [12].

[1] Movement Disorders [2014] 29 (8) : 967-975 (N.N.Dissanayaka, E. White, J.D.O'Sullivan, R.Marsh, N.A.Pachana, G.J.Byrne)

[2] Internal Medicine [2013] 52 (5) : 539-545 (T.Yamanishi, H. Tachibana, M.Oguru, K.Matsui, K.Toda, B.Okuda, N.Oka)

[3] Biological Psychiatry [1993] 34 (7) : 465-470 (M.A.Menza, D.E. Robertson-Hoffman, A.S.Bonapace)

[4] Parkinsonism & Related Disorders [2010] 16 (9) : 576-581 (E.L. Jacob, N.M.Gatto, A.Thompson, Y.Bordelon, B.Ritz)

[5] Movement Disorders [2010] 25 (13) : 2105-2113 (J.H.Bower, B.R. Grossardt, D.M.Maraganore, J.E.Ahlskog, R.C.Colligan, Y.E.Geda, T. M.Therneau, W.A.Rocca)

[6] Movement Disorders [2000] 15 (4) : 669-677 (M.Shiba, J.H. Bower, D.M.Maraganore, S.K.McDonnell, B.J.Peterson, J.E.Ahlskog, D.J.Schaid, W.A.Rocca)

[7] Journal of Neuropsychiatry and Clinical Neurosciences [1996] 8 (4) : 383-392 (I.H.Richard, R.B.Schiffer, R.Kurlan)

[8] Journal of Neuropsychiatry and Clinical Neurosciences [2010] 22 (4) : 390-394 (B.Bolluk, E.T.Ozel-Kizil, M.C.Akbostanci, E.C. Atbasoglu)

[10] Parkinsonism & Related Disorders [2015] 21 (3) : 189-193 (S. Rutten, I.Ghielen, C.Vriend, A.W.Hoogendoorn, H.W.Berendse, A.F. Leentjens, Y.D.van der Werf, J.H.Smit, O.A.van den Heuvel)

[11] Journal of Geriatric Psychiatry and Neurology [2013] 26 (1) : 34-40 (E.Stefanova, L.Ziropadja, M.Petrovic, T.Stojkovic, V.Kostic)

[12] Movement Disorders [2009] 24 (9) : 1333-1338 (G.M.Pontone, J.R.Williams, K.E.Anderson, G.Chase, S.A.Goldstein, S.Grill, E.S. Hirsch, S.Lehmann, J.T.Little, R.L.Margolis, P.V.Rabins, et al)

[13] Journal of Neurologial Science [2016] 367 : 342-346 (M.Petrovic, E.Stefanova, L.Ziropadja, T.Stojkovic, V.S.Kostic)

[14] Movement Disorders [2016] Apr 29 [Epub ahead of print] (M.P. Broen, N.E.Narayen, M.L.Kuijf, N.N.Dissanayaka, A.F.Leentjens)

[15] Movement Disorders [2008] 23 (14) : 2015-2025 (A.F.Leentjens, K.Dujardin, L.Marsh, P.Martinez-Martin, I.H.Richard, S.E.Starkstein, D.Weintraub, C.Sampaio, W.Poewe, O.Rascol, G.T.Stebbins, et al)

[16] Neuropsychiatric Disease and Treatment [2014] 10 : 829-834 (B.K.Gultekin, B.Ozdilek, E.E. Bestepe)

[17] Movement Disorders [1993] 8 (4) : 501-506 (E.R.Siemers, A. Shekhar, K.Quaid, H.Dickson)

[18] Journal of Psychosomatic Research [2015] 78 (2) : 143-148 (R.G. Brown, B.A.Fernie)

[19] European Journal of Neurology [2016] [Epub ahead of print] (K. Zhu, J.J.van Hilten, J.Marinus)

HALLUCINATIONS

Symptoms : Hallucinations in Parkinson's Disease are initially almost exclusively visual [1-4]. Pareidolia, which is a form of visual illusion, is also more common in Parkinson's Disease [5]. Some people also have auditory hallucinations [6, 7], including verbal hallucinations [8, 9], but not commonly in isolation [4, 10]. Fewer people still experience olfactory hallucinations [11]. Although visual hallucinations in isolation are typical, non-visual hallucinations emerge over time, so that a combination of visual with non-visual hallucinations pre dominates in later Parkinson's Disease [4, 12].

Prevalence : The number of people with Parkinson's Disease who have hallucinations varies from 10% to 50% with the average figure being around 30% [1-7, 13-41, 52]. Around 60% of people with Parkinson's Disease eventually develop hallucinations [42].

Causes of symptoms : The likelihood of hallucinations in Parkinson's Disease increases with the use of dopaminergic drugs [7, 13, 43, 44, 45], duration of Parkinson's Disease [12, 43, 46, 47, 48], Parkinson's Disease severity [43, 48], impaired visual acuity [49], and is associated with cognitive impairment [48], depression [48], vivid dreams and nightmares [50], sleep disorders [43, 51], and ocular disorders [51].

[1] Acta Neurologica Belgica [2012] 112 (1) : 33-37 (M.Svetel, T. Smiljkovic, T.Pekmezovic, V.Kostic)

[2] Journal of Neurology [2010] 257 (9) : 1524-1532 (M.Coelho, M.J. Marti, E.Tolosa, J.J.Ferreira, F.Valldeoriola, M.Rosa, C.Sampaio)

[3] Archives of Neurology [1996] 53 (12) : 1265-1268 (J.R. Sanchez-Ramos, R.Ortoll, G.W.Paulson)

[4] Journal of Neurology, Neurosurgery, and Psychiatry [1998] 64 (4) : 533-535 (R.Inzelberg, S.Kipervasser, A.D.Korczyn)

[5] Parkinsonism & Related Disorders [2015] 21 (6) : 603-609 (M.Uchiyama, Y.Nishio, K.Yokoi, Y.Hosokai, A.Takeda, E.Mori)

[6] Brain [2000] 123 (Part 4) : 733-745 (G.Fénelon, F.Mahieux, R. Huon, M.Ziégler)

[7] Journal of the Association of Physicians of India [2004] 52 : 703-706 (M.Gupta, G.Singh, G.A.Khwaja, M.M.Mehndiratta)

[8] Journal of Neural Transmission [2010] 117 (10) : 1183-1188 (R. Debs, V.Cochen De Cock, L.Nègre-Pagès, M.Aristin, A.Senard, O. Rascol)

[9] European Neurology [1996] 36 (Supplement 1) : 49-58 (K.Miyoshi, A.Ueki, O.Nagano)

[10] BMC Neurology [2008] 8 : 21 (S.Papapetropoulos, H.Katzen, A. Schrag, C.Singer, B.K.Scanlon, D.Nation, A.Guevara, B.Levin)

[11] Journal of Parkinsons Disease [2012] 2 (3) : 199-205 (J.H. McAuley, S.Gregory)

[12] Movement Disorders [2011] 26 (12) : 2196-2200 (C.G.Goetz, G.T. Stebbins, B.Ouyang)

[13] Geriatrie et Psychologie Neuropsychiatrie du Vieillissement [2013] 11 (3) : 295-304 (A.M.Bonnet, V.Czernecki)

[14] Parkinsonism & Related Disorders [2014] 20 (1) : 17-21 (M. Giorelli, J.Bagnoli, L.Consiglio, M.Lopane, G.B.Zimatore, D.Zizza, P. Difazio)

[15] Psychiatry and Clinical Neurosciences [2013] 67 (7) : 509-516 (A. Q.Rana, I.Siddiqui, M.Zangeneh, A.Fattah, N.Awan, M.S.Yousuf)

[16] BMJ Case Reports [2013] May 22 (O.Vaou, M.Saint-Hilaire, J. Friedman)

[17] American Journal of Geriatric Pharmacotherapy [2010] 8 (4) : 316-330 (M.L.Eng, T.E.Welty)

[18] Clinical Neurology and Neurosurgery [2013] 115 (10) : 2103-2107 (M.Z.Zhou, J.Gan, Y.R.Wei, X.Y.Ren, W.Chen, Z.G.Liu)

[19] Annals of Internal Medicine [1989] 111 (3) : 218-222 (W.E. Golden, R.C.Lavender, W.S.Metzer)

[20] Geriatrics [1986] 41 (8) : 59-62, 67 (G.W.Paulson, K. Schafer, B. Hallum)

[21] Italian Journal of Neurological Sciences [1990] 11 (4) : 373-379 (G.Meco, V.Bonifati, G.Cusimano, E.Fabrizio, N.Vanacore)

[22] Movement Disorders [2011] 26 (13) : 2387-2395 (N.K.Archibald, M.P.Clarke, U.P.Mosimann, D.J.Burn)

[23] Clinical Neurology and Neurosurgery [2010] 112 (10) : 883-885 (M.Rodríguez-Violante, A.Cervantes-Arriaga, A.Villar-Velarde, T. Corona)

[24] Southern Medical Journal [2010] 103 (8) : 837-841 (M.Mittal, L. T.Jr.Giron)

[25] Archives of Neurology [2010] 67 (6) : 670-676 (M.Kasten, L. Kertelge, N.Brüggemann, J.van der Vegt, A.Schmidt, V.Tadic, C. Buhmann, S.Steinlechner, M.I.Behrens, A.Ramirez, F.Binkofski, et al)

[26] Movement Disorders [2005] 20 (11) : 1439-1448 (C.Pacchetti, R.Manni, R.Zangaglia, F.Mancini, E.Marchioni, C.Tassorelli, M. Terzaghi, M.Ossola, E.Martignoni, A.Moglia, G.Nappi)

[27] Neurology [2005] 64 (10) : 1712-1715 (D.Paleacu, E.Schechtman, R.Inzelberg)

[28] International Journal of Geriatric Psychiatry [2005] 20 (7) : 668-673 (D.Grossi, L.Trojano, M.T.Pellecchia, M.Amboni, N.A.Fragassi, P.Barone)

[29] Zeitschrift für Gerontologie [1994] 27 (4) : 260-269 (P.Vieregge, D.Körtke, C.Meyer-Bornsen)

[30] Revue Neurologique [2002] 158 (2) : 203-210 (M.Bailbé, S. Karolewicz, J.P.Neau, P.Dumas, R.Gil)

[31] Archives of Neurology [1999] 56 (5) : 595-601 (D.Aarsland, J.P. Larsen, J.L.Cummins, K.Laake)

[32] Neurology [2007] 69 (2) : 187-195 (K.M.Biglan, R.G.Jr Holloway, M.P.McDermott, I.H.Richard)

[33] Journal of Neurology, Neurosurgery, and Psychiatry [1999] 67 (4) : 492-496 (D.Aarsland, J.P.Larsen, N.G.Lim, C.Janvin, K.Karlsen, E. Tandberg, J.L.Cummings)

[34] Movement Disorders [2013] 28 (6) : 755-762 (K.Zhu, J.J.van Hilten, H.Putter, J.Marinus)

[35] Journal of Neurology, Neurosurgery and Psychiatry [2008] 79 (6) : 652-655 (D.R.Williams, J.D.Warren, A.J.Lees)

[36] Journal of Neurology [2002] 249 (12) : 1699-1703 (G.Fénelon, S. Thobois, A.M.Bonnet, E.Broussolle, F.Tison)

[37] Fortschritte der Neurologie-Psychiatrie [2000] 68 (3) : 129-136 (N.J.Diederich, V.Pieri, C.G.Goetz)

[38] Journal of Neurology, Neurosurgery and Psychiatry [2001] 70 (6) : 734-738 (S.Holroyd, L.Currie, G.F.Wooten)

[39] Lancet Neurology [2005] 4 (10) : 605-610 (D.R.Williams, A. J.Lees)

[40] Neurology [2004] 63 (2) : 293-300 (L.Marsh, J.R.Williams, M. Rocco, S.Grill, C.Munro, T.M.Dawson)

[41] Parkinsonism & Related Disorders [2014] 20 (3) : 318-322 (P. Urwyler, T.Nef, A.Killen, D.Collerton, A.Thomas, D.Burn, I.McKeith, U.P.Mosimann)

[42] Archives of Neurology [2010] 67 (8) : 996-1001 (E.B.Forsaa, J.P.Larsen, T.Wentzel-Larsen, C.G.Goetz, G.T.Stebbins, D.Aarsland, G.Alves)

[43] Neurologia [2006] 21 (1) : 12-18 (E.Cubo, M.González, A. Aguilar, S.Quintana)

[44] Tidsskrift for den Norske Laegeforening [1998] 118 (25) : 3959-3963 (D.Arsland, J.P.Larsen)

[45] Movement Disorders [2010] 25 (Supplement 1) : S104-S109 (C.G. Goetz)

[46] Neurology [2001] 57 (11) : 2078-2082 (C.G.Goetz, S.Leurgans, E. J.Pappert, R.Raman, A.B.Stemer)

[47] Neurology [2005] 64 (1) : 81-86 (C.G.Goetz, J.Wuu, L.M.Curgian, S.Leurgans)

[48] Journal of Neurology, Neurosurgery and Psychiatry [2001] 70 (6) : 727-733 (J.Barnes, A.S.David)

[49] Journal of Geriatric Psychiatry and Neurology [2006] 19 (1) : 36-40 (H.Matsui, F.Udaka, A.Tamura, M.Oda, T.Kubori, K.Nishinaka, M.Kameyama)

[50] Neurology [2010] 75 (20) : 1773-1779 (C.G.Goetz, B.Ouyang, A. Negron, G.T.Stebbins)

[51] Movement Disorders [2005] 20 (2) : 212-217 (A.D.de Maindreville, G.Fénelon, F.Mahieux)

[52] Journal of the Neurological Sciences [2016] Oct 27 [Epub ahead of print] (J.Zhu, B.Shen, L.Lu, W.Lan, Y.Pan, L.Zhang, J.Dong, M.Wang, L.Zhang)

Compulsions

Symptoms : Compulsions and impulse control disorders occur in Parkinson's Disease [1-6]. These can take the form of compulsive eating [3, 4, 7-10, 11], pathological gambling [3, 4, 7-11], punding (in which there is an intense fascination with repetitive handling and examining of mechanical objects or arranging common objects, such as lining up pebbles, rocks, or small objects) [7, 8, 10, 12], compulsive shopping [3, 4, 7, 8, 11], hypersexuality [3, 4, 7, 8, 10, 11], medication hoarding [8], an irrepressible need to drum and beat percussion instruments [13].

Prevalence : Compulsions and impulse control disorders (ICDs) occur in 8% to 30% of people with Parkinson's Disease [1-6, 24, 25]. The most prevalent compulsions in people with Parkinson's Disease are : compulsive eating (3% to 7%) [2, 14, 15, 25], pathological gambling (1% to 7%) [2, 14-19], punding (0.3% to 6.5%) [11, 14, 19], compulsive shopping (3% to 6%) [2, 15], hypersexuality (3% to 4%) [2, 14, 15, 19, 20], medication hoarding [8], an irrepressible need to drum and beat percussion instruments [13].

Causes of symptoms : The main risk factors for compulsions are especially, the use of dopamine agonists [1, 2, 6, 7, 21, 22, 24] and L-dopa [6, 13, 14]. Compulsions are also associated with younger age [2, 6, 14, 22, 23], male gender [23], earlier age at the onset of Parkinson's Disease [6, 13], longer duration of Parkinson's Disease [6, 14], a history of impulse-compulsive disorders [23], insomnia, anxiety, and depression [22].

[1] Journal of Clinical Psychopharmacology [2013] 33 (5) : 691-694 (M.Poletti, C.Logi, C. Lucetti, P.Del Dotto, F.Baldacci, A.Vergallo, M.Ulivi, S.Del Sarto, G.Rossi, R.Ceravolo, U.Bonuccelli)

[2] Archives of Neurology [2010] 67 (5) : 589-595 (D.Weintraub, J. Koester, M.N.Potenza, A.D.Siderowf, M.Stacy, V.Voon, J. Whetteckey, G.R.Wunderlich, A.E.Lang)

[3] Parkinsonism & Related Disorders [2012] 18 (Supplement 1) : S80-S84 (D.Vilas, C.Pont-Sunyer, E.Tolosa)

[4] Der Nervenarzt [2012] 83 (12) : 1582-1589 (R.Katzenschlager, K. S.Goerlich, T.van Eimeren)

[5] Movement Disorders [2012] 27 (2) : 242-247 (D.Weintraub, E. Mamikonyan, K.Papay, J. A.Shea, S.X.Xie, A.Siderowf)

[6] Parkinsonism & Related Disorders [2014] 20 (1) : 22-26 (M.B. Callesen, D.Weintraub, M.F.Damholdt, A.Møller)

[7] Journal of the Neurological Sciences [2011] 310 (1-2) : 197-201 (A. Ávila, X.Cardona, M. Martín-Baranera, J.Bello, F.Sastre)

[8] CNS Spectrums [2008] 13 (8) : 690-698 (J.M.Ferrara, M.Stacy)

[9] Neurocase [2008] 14 (6) : 480-484 (H.Miwa, T.Kondo)

[10] Parkinsonism & Related Disorders [2011] 17 (10) : 761-764 (S.Y.Lim, Z.K.Tan, P.I. Ngam, T.L.Lor, H.Mohamed, J.P.Schee, A.K. Tan, J. Y.Goh, E.Ooi, P.C.Soh)

[11] Translational Neurodegeneration [2016] 5 : 4 (X.P.Wang, M.Wei, Q.Xiao)

[12] Movement Disorders [2006] 21 (8) : 1217-1218 (A.Fasano, A.E. Elia, F.Soleti, A. Guidubaldi, A.R.Bentivogli)

[13] Behavioural Neurology [2013] 27 (4) : 559-562 (C.Vitale, L. Trojano, P.Barone, D.Errico, V.Agosti, G.Sorrentino, D.Grossi, G. Santangelo)

[14] Journal of the Neurological Sciences [2013] 331 (1-2) : 76-80 (K. Tanaka, K.Wada-Isoe, S.Nakashita, M.Yamamoto, K.Nakashima)

[15] Neurology [2013] 80 (2) : 176-180 (D.Weintraub, K.Papay, A. Siderowf)

[16] Parkinsonism & Related Disorders [2013] 19 (7) : 645-653 (G. Santangelo, P.Barone, L.Trojano, C.Vitale)

[17] Brain and Nerve [2008] 60 (9) : 1039-1046 (K.Fujimoto)

[18] Movement Disorders [2011] 26 (11) : 1976-1984 (A.Djamshidian, F.Cardoso, D. Grosset, H.Bowden-Jones, A.J.Lees)

[19] European Journal of Neurology [2012] 19 (3) : 494-500 (H.L. Chiang, Y.S.Huang, S.T. Chen, Y.R.Wu)

[20] International Journal of General Medicine [2009] 2 : 57-61 (C.A. Cooper, A.Jadidian, M. Paggi, J.Romrell, M.S.Okun, R.L.Rodriguez, H.H.Fernandez)

[21] Fortschritte der Neurologie-Psychiatrie [2013] 81 (9) : 503-510 (K.Rohde, O.Riedel, U.Lueken, S.Rietzel, M.Fauser, C.Ossig, H. Reichmann, A.Storch)

[22] Journal of Neurology, Neurosurgery, and Psychiatry [2011] 82 (6) : 620-622 (S.S. O'Sullivan, C.M.Loane, A.D.Lawrence, A.H.Evans, P. Piccini, A.J.Lees)

[23] Annals of Neurology [2008] 64 (Supplenent 2) : S93-S100 (D. Weintraub)

[24] Clinical Neuropharmacology [2017] 40 (2) : 51-55 (C.C.Ramírez Gómez, M.Serrano Dueñas, O.Bernal, N.Araoz, M.Sáenz Farret, V. Aldinio, V.Montilla, F.Micheli)

[25] Journal of Neurology, Neurosurgery and Psychiatry [2017] 88 (4) : 317-324 (A.Antonini, P.Barone, U.Bonuccelli, K.Annoni, M. Asgharnejad, P.Stanzione)

Vertigo

Symptoms : Vertigo is when a person feels as if they or what is around them are moving when they are not. This may be associated with nausea, vomiting, sweating, or walking difficulties. Vertigo is the most common type of dizziness, which can cause a tendency to fall.

Prevalence : Dizziness is a frequent complaint of people who have Parkinson's Disease. Nearly half of people with Parkinson's Disease have dizziness. Many of them appear to have orthostatic hypotension, but about 8% of them have benign paroxysmal positional vertigo, which can be rid in the vast majority of cases. About 3% of people with Parkinson's Disease have a more atypical presentation of benign paroxysmal positional vertigo. So in total about 11% of people with Parkinson's Disease have paroxysmal positional vertigo, which can be treated easily and successfully [1].

Causes of symptoms : Orthostatic hypotension (OH) is often thought to be the cause. However, benign paroxysmal positional vertigo (BPPV) can also be an explanation [1].

[1] Parkinsonism & Related Disorders [2013] 19 (12) : 1110-1112 (E. Van Wensen, R.B.van Leeuwen, H.J.van der Zaag-Loonen, S.Masius-Olthof, B.R.Bloem)

Brain tumor

Symptoms : A brain tumour is a growth of cells that multiplies in an uncontrollable way. It can be cancerous (malignant) or non-cancerous (benign). The symptoms can include : severe headaches [1, 2], seizures [1, 2], nausea [1, 2], vomiting [1, 2], drowsiness [2], progressive weakness on one side of the body [1], confusion [2], mental or behavioural changes [1], vision or speech problems.

Prevalence : The risk of developing a brain tumor in people with Parkinson's Disease is 1.5 to 2.1 times more likely [3, 4, 5]. Benign brain tumor exhibited a slightly higher risk than that. The risk of developing a benign brain tumor was even higher in females. Mostly only those between 50 and 64 years old had a higher risk of developing a brain tumor [3].

Causes of symptoms : The cause of the increased risk of brain tumor is unknown [3].

[1] Neurological Sciences [2011] 32 (Supplement 2) : S207-S208 (A. Silvani, P.Gaviani, E.Lamperti, A.Botturi, D.Ferrari, G.Simonetti, A. Salmaggi)

[2] Seminars in Diagnostic Pathology [2010] 27 (2) : 97-104 (S.A. Alomar)

[3] Acta Neurologica Scandinavia [2016] 134 (2) : 148-153 (C.F.Tang, M.K.Lu, C.H.Muo, C.H.Tsai, C.H.Kao)

[4] PLoS One [2016] 11 (10) : e0164388 (R.Ye, T.Shen, Y.Jiang, L.Xu, X.Si, B.Zhang)

[5] Practical Radiation Oncology [2015] 5 (4) : e327-e335 (A. Engelman, K.Perumal, M.Mehta)

CHAPTER 22

SYMPTOMS OF PARKINSON'S DISEASE

ALIMENTARY SYSTEM

ALIMENTARY SYSTEM

The Alimentary System includes all the body structures involved in eating food, preparing food for absorption, digesting food and the excretion of waste products. This includes the : oral cavity, pharynx, oesophagus, stomach, small intestine, large intestine (colon), rectum and anus.

PRIMARY SYMPTOMS

In Parkinson's Disease there can be an increased likelihood of constipation [PAGE 319], dysphagia (swallowing difficulty) [PAGE 321], sialorrhea (excessive saliva and drooling) [PAGE 323], xerostomia [PAGE 324], intestinal bacterial overgrowth [PAGE 325], gastroparesis (slow gastric emptying) [PAGE 326], and obesity [PAGE 327]. The most common symptoms of these in Parkinson's Disease are constipation, which occurs in most people, followed by dysphagia, then sialorrhea, both of which occur in a large minority of people.

CONSTIPATION

Symptoms : Constipation refers to bowel movements that are infrequent or hard to pass. Constipation is a common cause of painful defecation. Severe constipation can progress to bowel obstruction.

Prevalence : Most people with Parkinson's Disease suffer from constipation [1-10]. Severe constipation is associated with the time since diagnosis and the severity of Parkinson's Disease [6]. Severity of constipation is associated with a future diagnosis of Parkinson's Disease [11, 12]. Constipation is more common when Parkinson's

Disease is more advanced [13]. Constipation usually precedes the motor manifestations of Parkinson's Disease [14].

Cause of symptoms : In people with Parkinson's Disease there is an increased contraction of the anal sphincter [8, 15], and the colon [16]. Constipation can be due to slow transit through the intestine [17] and the colon [7, 8], and excessive contraction of the anal sphincter [8]. Bowel dysfunction in Parkinson's Disease may be the result of both delayed colon transit and impaired anorectal muscle coordination [18].

[1] Movement Disorders [2000] 15 (1) : 71-76 (F.Stocchi, D.Badiali, L. Vacca, L.D'Alba, F.Bracci, S.Ruggieri, M.Torti, A.Berardelli, E. Corazziari)

[2] Journal of Neurology [2004] 251 (Supplement 7) : vII 18-23 (A. Ueki. M.Otsuka)

[3] American Journal of Gastroenterology [1994] 89 (1) : 15-25 (L.L. Edwards, E.M.Quigley, R.K.Harned, R.Hofman, R.F.Pfeiffer)

[4] Movement Disorders [1993] 8 (1) : 83-86 (L.Edwards, E.M. Quigley, R.Hofman, R.F.Pfeiffer)

[5] European Neurology [1992] 32 (3) : 134-140 (C.Singer, W.J. Weiner, J.R.Sanchez-Ramos)

[6] Wiener Klinische Wochenschrift [1998] 110 (15) : 535-537 (W.H. Jost, B.Schrank)

[7] Wiener Klinische Wochenschrift [1991] 69 (20) : 906-909 (W.H. Jost, B.Schimrigk)

[8] Acta Neurologica Scandinavica [2008] 117 (1) : 60-64 (K.Krogh, K.Ostergaard, S.Sabroe, S.Laurberg)

[9] British Journal of Nutrition [2013] 110 (2) : 347-353 (M. Barichella, E.Cereda, C.Madio, L.Iorio, C.Pusani, R.Cancello, R. Caccialanza, G.Pezzoli, E.Cassani)

[10] Journal of Neurology [2013] 260 (5) : 1332-1338 (M.G. Cersosimo, G.B.Raina, C.Pecci, A.Pellene, C.R.Calandra, C.Gutiérrez, F.E.Micheli, E.E.Benarroch)

[11] Parkinsonism & Related Disorders [2014] 20 (12) : 1371-1375 (C.H.Lin, J.W.Lin, Y.C.Liu, C.H.Chang, R.M.Wu)

[12] Journal of Neurology, Neurosurgery and Psychiatry [2016] 87 (7) : 710-716 (K.L.Adams-Carr, J.P.Bestwick, S.Shribman, A. Lees, A. Schrag, A.J.Noyce)

[13] Parkinsonism & Related Disorders [2015] 21 (5) : 455-460 (H. Park, J.Y.Lee, C.M.Shin, J.M.Kim, T.J.Kim, J.W.Kim)

[14] Journal of Neurology [2013] 260 (5) : 1332-1338 (M.G. Cersosimo, G.B.Raina, C.Pecci, A.Pellene, C.R.Calandra, C.Gutiérrez, F.E.Micheli, E.E.Benarroch)

[15] Acta Neurologica Scandinavica [2012] 126 (4) : 248-255 (J. Linder, R.Libelius, E.Nordh, B.Holmberg, H.Stenlund, L.Forsgren)

[16] Experimental Neurology [2007] 207 (1) : 4-12 (G.Anderson, A.R. Noorian, G.Taylor, M.Anitha, D.Bernhard, S.Srinivasan, J.G.Greene)

[18] Clinical Neuroscience [1998] 5 (2) : 136-146 (R.F.Pfeiffer)

Dysphagia

Symptoms : Dysphagia is the impaired ability to swallow. Some people with dysphagia have problems swallowing certain foods or liquids, while others cannot swallow at all. Dysphagia can cause coughing or choking when eating or drinking [1].

Prevalence : Anywhere from 10% to more than 90% of people with Parkinson's Disease have dysphagia [2-10, 15, 16]. That is several times more common than in people that do not have Parkinson's Disease [9]. Some people (around 6%) also suffer from odynophagia (painful swallowing) (6%) [15]. Dysphagia probably contributed to weight loss in around 40% of people with Parkinson's Disease because they were unable to eat as much [15]. Although most people with Parkinson's Disease had swallowing problems in the oral phase, nearly all of them had swallowing problems in the pharangeal phase [10]. About half of them had swallowing problems in the esophageal phase [10]. Major esophageal disorders regarding movement through the esophagus were detected in nearly one third of people with Parkinson's Disease [11]. Minor impairment in this respect was present in 95% of people with Parkinson's Disease throughout all stages of Parkinson's Disease [11]. There is a moderate correlation between the rate of swallowing and the severity of Parkinson's Disease [12, 13].

Cause of symptoms : In people with Parkinson's Disease there is an increased contraction of the pharyngeal muscles [1], which are the muscles involved in swallowing. Parkinson's Disease can cause dysphagia because of the effect that Parkinson's Disease can have on the muscles involved in swallowing [13].

[1] The Essential Dysphagia Handbook : Real Life Decisions, Mind Mapping and More [2013] (Claire Langdon, Karen Jardine)

[2] Movement Disorders [2010] 25 (14) : 2361-2368 (H.Y.Sung, J.S. Kim, K.S.Lee, Y.I.Kim, I.U.Song, S.W.Chung, D.W.Yang, Y.K.Cho, J.M.Park, I.S.Lee, S.W.Kim, I.S.Chung, M.G.Choi)

[3] Clinical Neurology and Neurosurgery [1997] 99 (2) : 106-112 (J. L.Fuh, R.C.Lee, S.J.Wang, C.H.Lin, P.N.Wang, J.H.Chiang, H. C.Liu)

[4] European Neurology [1997] 38 (1) : 49-52 (C.Coates, A.M. Bakheit)

[5] British Journal of Nutrition [2013] 110 (2) : 347-353 (M. Barichella, E.Cereda, C.Madio, L.Iorio, C.Pusani, R.Cancello, R. Caccialanza, G.Pezzoli, E.Cassani)

[6] Journal of Neurology [2013] 260 (5) : 1332-1338 (M.G.Cersosimo, G.B.Raina, C.Pecci, A.Pellene, C.R.Calandra, C. Gutiérrez, F.E. Micheli, E.E.Benarroch)

[7] Clinical Neuroscience [1998] 5 (2) : 136-146 (R.F.Pfeiffer)

[8] Acta Otorrinolaringologica Espanola [2016] Jun 3 [Epub ahead of print] (S.Mamolar Andrés, M.L.Santamarina Rabanal, C.M.Granda Membiela, M.J.Fernández Gutiérrez, P.Sirgo Rodríguez, et al)

[9] Parkinsonism & Related Disorders [2012] 18 (4) : 311-315 (J.G. Kalf, B.J.de Swart, B.R.Bloem, M.Munneke)

[10] Rinsho Shinkeigaku [2016] Jul 29 [Epub ahead of print] (S. Hisashi, R.Fukumitsu, M.Ishida, A.Nodera, T.Otani, T.Maruoka, K. Nakamura, Y.Izumi, R.Kaji, Y.Nishida)

[11] Neurogastroenterology and Motility [2016] Jul 31 [Epub ahead of print] (I.Suttrup, J.Suttrup, S.Suntrup-Krueger, M.L.Siemer, J.Bauer, C.Hamacher, S.Oelenberg, D.Domagk, R.Dziewas, T.Warnecke)

[12] Journal of Neurology, Neurosurgery and Psychiatry [2009] 80 (9) : 1047-1049 (N.Miller, L.Allcock, A.J.Hildreth, D.Jones, E.Noble, D.J. Burn)

[13] Parkinsonism & Related Disorders [2015] 21 (5) : 455-460 (H. Park, J.Y.Lee, C.M.Shin, J.M.Kim, T.J.Kim, J.W.Kim)

[14] Neurology [2007] 68 (8) : 583-589 (E.Alfonsi, M.Versino, I.M. Merlo, C.Pacchetti, E.Martignoni, G.Bertino, A.Moglia, C.Tassorelli, G.Nappi)

[15] Diseases of the Esophagus [2017] 30 (4) : 1-6 (A.Su, R.Gandhy, C.Barlow, G.Triadafilopoulos)

[16] European Journal of Clinical Nutrition [2017] Jul 12 [Epub ahead of print] (X.Ding, J.Gao, C.Xie, B.Xiong, S.Wu, Z.Cen, Y.Lou, D.Lou, F.Xie, W.Luo)

Sialorrhea

Symptoms : Sialorrhea is drooling, due to either excessive salivation or a failure to swallow saliva.

Prevalence : Sialorrhea occurs in more than a third of people with Parkinson's Disease [1, 2, 3]. About a quarter of people with Parkinson’s Disease have drooling that occurs day and night [1, 4, 5]. Sialorrhea is more common in advanced Parkinson's Disease [6].

Cause of symptoms : Sialorrhea in Parkinson's Disease is thought to be caused by dysphagia (impaired or infrequent swallowing) rather than hypersecretion of saliva [7, 8], because people with the worst dysphagia had the worst drooling [9]. The immobility of the mouth, tongue, palatal and pharyngeal musculature causes excessive salivation, which leads to drooling, as there is no intermittent spontaneous and subconscious swallowing movements that can dispose of saliva. Oropharyngeal bradykinesia may be responsible for drooling [10].

[1] Parkinsonism & Related Disorders [2014] Dec 16 [Epub ahead of print] (R.Ou, X.Guo, Q.Wei, B.Cao, J.Yang, W.Song, N.Shao, B.Zhao, X.Chen, H.Shang)

[2] European Journal of Neurology [2012] 19 (1) : 28-37 (S.Perez-Lloret, L.Nègre-Pagès, A.Ojero-Senard, P.Damier, A.Destée, F. Tison, M.Merello, O.Rascol)

[3] British Journal of Nutrition [2013] 110 (2) : 347-353 (M. Barichella, E.Cereda, C.Madio, L.Iorio, C.Pusani, R.Cancello, R. Caccialanza, G.Pezzoli, E.Cassani)

[4] Journal of Neurology [2009] 256 (9) : 1391-1396 (J.G.Kalf , B.J.de Swart, G.F.Borm, B.R.Bloem, M.Munneke)

[5] Journal of Neurological Science [2015] 353 (1-2) : 74-78 (R.Ou, X.Guo, Q.Wei, B.Cao, J.Yang, W.Song, K.Chen, B.Zhao, X.Chen, H. Shang)

[6] Parkinsonism & Related Disorders [2015] Feb 14 [Epub ahead of print] (H.Park, J.Y.Lee, C.M.Shin, J.M.Kim, T.J.Kim, J.W.Kim)

[7] Movement Disorders [2007] 22 (16) : 2306-2313 (K.L.Chou, M. Evatt, V.Hinson, K.Kompoliti)

[8] Clinical Neuroscience [1998] 5 (2) : 136-146 (R.F.Pfeiffer)

[9] Parkinsonism & Related Disorders [2008] 14 (3) : 243-245 (A.C. Nóbrega, B.Rodrigues, A.C.Torres, R.D.Scarpel, C.A.Neves, A. Melo)

[10] Neurological Sciences [2016] 37 (12) : 1987-1991 (M.Karakoc, M.I.Yon, G.Y.Cakmakli, E.K.Ulusoy, A.Gulunay, N.Oztekin, F.Ak)

Xerostomia

Symptoms : Xerostomia is dryness in the mouth, which can be associated with reduced salivary flow (hyposalivation) [1].

Prevalence : Around 87% of people with Parkinson's Disease have hyposalivation [1]. Around 50% of people with Parkinson's Disease reported xerostomia [1, 2].

Cause of symptoms : L-dopa influences the production of saliva [3].

[1] Oral Disease [2016] Dec 14 [Epub ahead of print] (A.G.Barbe, A.Heinzler, S.H.Derman, M.Hellmich, L.Timmermann, M.J.Noack)

[2] Gerodontology [2016] May 27 [Epub ahead of print] (A.G.Barbe, N.Bock, S.H.Derman, M.Felsch, L.Timmermann, M.J.Noack)

[3] Movement Disorders [2005] 20 (2) : 204-207 (M.Proulx, F.P.de Courval, M.A.Wiseman, M.Panisset)

Intestinal bacterial overgrowth

Symptoms : Parkinson's Disease is associated with gastrointestinal motility abnormalities that can favour the occurrence of small intestinal bacterial overgrowth. Small intestinal bacterial overgrowth can lead to the following symptoms : abdominal bloating and distension, excess gas, abdominal pain, diarrhea or sometimes chronic constipation [1].

Prevalence : Small intestinal bacterial overgrowth occurs in somewhere between 30% and over half of all people with Parkinson's Disease in contrast to only 8% to 10% of people that do not have Parkinson's Disease. It is very significantly related to the severity of Parkinson's Disease [1, 2].

Causes of symptoms : In Parkinson's Disease there is an increased contraction of the colon [3], and prolonged passage through the small intestine [4]. The occurrence of small intestinal bacterial overgrowth in Parkinson's Disease could therefore be due to gastrointestinal motility abnormalities leaving bacteria for longer in the intestines [1].

[1] Movement Disorders [2011] 26 (5) : 889-892 (M.Gabrielli, P. Bonazzi, E.Scarpellini, E.Bendia, E.C.Lauritano, A.Fasano, M.G. Ceravolo, M.Capecci, A.Rita Bentivoglio, L.Provinciali, et al)

[2] Journal of Neural Transmission [2016] Sep 2 [Epub ahead of print] (X.L.Niu, L.Liu, Z.X.Song, Q.Li, Z.H.Wang, J.L.Zhang, H.H.Li)

[3] Experimental Neurology [2007] 207 (1) : 4-12 (G.Anderson, A.R. Noorian, G.Taylor, M.Anitha, D.Bernhard, S.Srinivasan, J.G.Greene)

[4] Journal of Neural Transmission [2015] 122 (12) : 1659-1661 (J. Dutkiewicz, S.Szlufik, M.Nieciecki, I.Charzynska, L.Królicki, P. Smektala, A.Friedman)

Gastroparesis

Symptoms : Gastroparesis is delayed gastric emptying [1]. It can lead to Early Morning Off (EMO), which is lengthy delay in the therapeutic effect of the initial dose of oral medication in the morning [2].

Prevalence : Gastric emptying time is delayed in 60% to 70% of people with Parkinson's Disease [3, 4]. EMO is a symptom experienced by people at every stage of Parkinson's Disease. People with Parkinson's Disease who felt they had EMO amounted to around 80%, with 37% of them stating that EMO was a daily occurrence. Even 52% of people with early Parkinson's Disease had EMO. The prevalence of EMO increased as Parkinson's Disease worsened [2].

Cause of symptoms : In people with Parkinson's Disease there is an increased contraction of the colon [5], and prolonged passage through the small intestine [6]. Most of the gastrointestinal abnormalities associated with Parkinson's Disease are attributable to impaired motility [1]. The delayed gastric emptying this causes can cause Early Morning Off (EMO) [2]. The muscles around the stomach, small gut and oesophagus are also affected so that there is reduced motility of them, and spasms in the oesophagus.

[1] Movement Disorders [2014] 29 (1) : 23-32 (S.Marrinan, A.V. Emmanuel, D.J.Burn)

[2] Journal of Neurological Science [2016] 364 : 1-5 (R.Onozawa, J. Tsugawa, Y.Tsuboi, J.Fukae, T.Mishima, S.Fujioka)

[3] Parkinsonism & Related Disorders [2009] 15 (9) : 692-696 (A. Krygowska-Wajs, W.P.Cheshire Jr, Z.K.Wszolek, A.Hubalewska-Dydejczyk, B.Jasinska-Myga, M.J.Farrer, M.Moskala, et al)

[4] Neurology [1996] 46 (4) : 1051-1054 (R.Djaldetti, J.Baron, I.Ziv, E.Melamed)

[5] Experimental Neurology [2007] 207 (1) : 4-12 (G.Anderson, A.R. Noorian, G.Taylor, M.Anitha, D.Bernhard, S.Srinivasan, J.G.Greene)

[6] Journal of Neural Transmission [2015] 122 (12) : 1659-1661 (J. Dutkiewicz, S.Szlufik, M.Nieciecki, I.Charzynska, L.Królicki, P. Smektala, A.Friedman)

Obesity

Symptoms : Obesity is when excess body fat has accumulated to the extent that it may have a negative effect on health. Obesity is often measured according to the body mass index (BMI).

Prevalence : In people with Parkinson's Disease, 1% to 4% were underweight, 33% to 46% were within the normal range, 33% to 47% were overweight, and 15% to 19% were obese [1, 2]. Obesity and a higher BMI (body mass index) is not related to the risk of developing Parkinson's Disease [3]. However, in early Parkinson's Disease people tend to increase their weight [4], and subsequently become overweight. Parkinson's Disease was found to be associated with an increased BMI (body mass index) [5, 6], but to a lesser extent in other studies [7, 8]. The BMI tended to decline with a lengthier duration of Parkinson's Disease [9, 10] but it was accompanied by increased adiposity [10]. Fat distribution is altered in people who have Parkinson's Disease. In people with Parkinson's Disease there is an increased ratio of visceral fat to subcutaneous fat [11].

Causes of symptoms : A higher daily dosage per kilogramme of L-dopa and dopaminergic drugs was correlated with a lower BMI (body mass index) [8]. Obesity could be due to a reduction in the physical activity that often occurs in people with Parkinson's Disease.

[1] Clinical Nutrition [2014] 33 (6) : 1132-1139 (M.Vikdahl, M. Carlsson, J.Linder, L.Forsgren, L.Håglin)

[2] Movement Disorders [2011] 26 (12) : 2253-2259 (N.Palacios, X.Gao, M.L.McCullough, E.J.Jacobs, A.V.Patel, T.Mayo, M.A. Schwarzschild, A.Ascherio)

[3] Arquivos de Neuropsiquiatra [2012] 70 (11) : 843-846 (H.Morales-Briceño, A.Cervantes-Arriaga, M.Rodríguez-Violante, J.Calleja-Castillo, T.Corona)

[4] European Journal of Neurology [2009] 16 (8) : 895-901 (C.G. Bachmann, A.Zapf, E.Brunner, C.Trenkwalder)

[5] Neurology [2006] 67 (11) : 1955-1959 (G.Hu, P.Jousilahti, A. Nissinen, R.Antikainen, M.Kivipelto, J.Tuomilehto)

[6] American Journal of Epidemiology [2004] 159 (6) : 547-555 (H. Chen, S.M.Zhang, M.A.Schwarzschild, M.A.Hernán, W.C.Willett, A. Ascherio)

[7] European Journal of Clinical Nutrition [2003] 57 (4) : 543-547 (M. Barichella, A.Marczewska, A.Vairo, M.Canesi, G.Pezzoli)

[8] European Journal of Epidemiology [2014] 29 (4) : 285-292 (K. Sääksjärvi, P.Knekt, S.Männistö, J.Lyytinen, T.Jääskeläinen, N. Kanerva, M.Heliövaara)

[9] European Journal of Neurology [2008] 15 (9) : 965-968 (P. Ragonese, M.D'Amelio, G.Callari, N.Di Benedetto, B.Palmeri, M.A. Mazzola, V.Terruso, G.Salemi, G.Savettieri, P.Aridon)

[10] Acta Diabetologica [2003] 40 (Supplement 1) : S187-S190 (M.L. Petroni, G.Albani, V.Bicchiega, S.Baudo, C.Vinci, A.Montesano, G.Izzo, P.Bertocco, S.Mazzotta, E.Zorzetto, F.Balzola, A.Mauro)

[11] Parkinsonism & Related Disorders [2016] Sep 16 [Epub ahead of print] (D.Bernhardt, H.P.Müller, A.C.Ludolph, L.Dupuis, J.Kassubek)

CHAPTER 23

SYMPTOMS OF PARKINSON'S DISEASE

URINARY SYSTEM

URINARY SYSTEM

The urinary system consists of the two kidneys, ureters, the bladder, and the urethra. The urinary system is the primary means of eliminating liquid from the body.

PRIMARY SYMPTOMS

In Parkinson's Disease there is often nocturia (frequent urinating at night) [PAGE 329], urinary incontinence (loss of urinary control) and increased urinary frequency [PAGE 330], and urinary retention [PAGE 330]. Urinary symptoms occur in between 27% and 85% of people with Parkinson's Disease [1-8].

NOCTURIA

Symptoms : Nocturia is the need to often urinate at night. Most people with Parkinson's Disease have nocturia, which is the most common urinary symptom that people with Parkinson's Disease experience [2, 4, 7, 8, 9, 10, 11].

Prevalence : More than a third of people with Parkinson’s Disease are diagnosed with nocturia [8, 12]. Those people who had Parkinson's Disease who were 70 years old and older were more likely to have both nocturia and nocturnal polyuria, which is the passing of an excessive quantity of urine - 72% instead of 55% for those younger than 70. Men had nocturia more frequently - 33% for men and 20% for women [7]. However, in another study, only 15% of men had nocturia [13]. Asian and Indian males were especially at a significantly greater risk of nocturia than other ethnicities [12]. Symptoms of nocturia were not related to gender in some studies [5, 6] but were in others [7, 12, 14]. Symptoms of nocturia were related to age in some studies [4, 7, 9] but not in another study [2].

Causes of symptoms : The prevalence of nocturnal polyuria and nocturia are not higher than in the general population of the same age. This suggests that they occur, not because of Parkinson's Disease, but because of the older age that is associated with Parkinson's Disease and nocturia [7].

Urinary incontinence

Symptoms : Urinary incontinence, which is urinary leakage, and also increased urinary frequency also commonly occur in Parkinson's Disease [1, 2, 4, 5, 8-11, 13, 15].

Prevalence : Most women with Parkinson's Disease who have urinary symptoms have urinary urgency with or without urinary incontinence [16]. Urinary incontinence occurred in 25% of men [13]. Symptoms were not related to gender in some studies [5, 6] but were in others [12, 15]. Symptoms were related to age in some studies [4, 9] but not in another [2].

Causes of symptoms : Urodynamic tests revealed neurogenic detrusor overactivity in most people with Parkinson's Disease [5, 17], with over 67% having detrusor overactivity, 12% having detrusor underactivity, and with 20% having normal detrusor function [10].

Urinary retention

Symptoms : Urinary retention, also known as ischuria, is an inability to completely empty the bladder that results in urine being retained in the bladder.

Prevalence : More than 25% of people with Parkinson's Disease have obstructive urinary symptoms, the most frequent of which is incomplete emptying of the bladder [4, 18]. Symptoms of urinary retention are not related to gender in some studies [5, 6] but were in others [8, 12, 14], with men being 2 to 3 times more likely than women to have urinary retention [8]. Symptoms were related to age in some studies [4, 9] but not in another [2].

Causes of symptoms : Whilst urinating, detrusor underactivity rather than detrusor overactivity occurred in half of people [5]. The detrusor muscle contracts when urinating to squeeze out urine [5].

[1] Neurourology and Urodynamics [2012] 31 (8) : 1279-1283 (K. Winge, K.K.Nielsen)

[2] Neurourology and Urodynamics [2006] 25 (2) : 116-122 (K.Winge, A.M.Skau, H.Stimpel, K.K.Nielsen, L.Werdelin)

[3] Clinical Neurology and Neurosurgery [2010] 112 (10) : 883-885 (M.Rodríguez-Violante, A.Cervantes-Arriaga, A.Villar-Velarde, T. Corona)

[4] Arquivos de Neuro-Psiquiatria [2003] 61 (2B) : 359-363 (R.N. Campos-Sousa, E.Quagliato, B.B.da Silva, R.M.deCarvalho Jr, S.C. Ribeiro, D.F.de Carvalho)

[5] Journal of Neurological and Neurosurgical Psychiatry [2011] 82 (12) : 1382-1386 (T.Uchiyama, R.Sakakibara, T.Yamamoto, T.Ito, C. Yamaguchi, Y.Awa, M.Yanagisawa, Y.Higuchi, Y.Sato, et al)

[6] Japanese Journal of Psychiatry and Neurology [1992] 46 (1) : 181-186 (T.Hattori, K.Yasuda, K.Kita, K.Hirayama)

[7] Progres en Urologie [2015] 25 (6) : 312-317 (J. Romain, F.Torny, J.P. Dumas, X.Gamé, A.Descazeaud)

[8] Chinese Medical Journal [2015] 128 (21) : 2906-2912 (L.M. Zhang, X.P.Zhang)

[9] Clinical Neurology and Neurosurgery [2013] 115 (10) : 2103- 2107 (M.Z.Zhou, J.Gan, Y.R.Wei, X.Y.Ren, W.Chen, Z.G.Liu)

[10] Neurourology and Urodynamics [2011] 30 (7) : 1258-1261 (M. M. Ragab, E.S.Mohammed)

[11] International Urology and Nephrology [2012] 44 (2) : 415-424 (L. Yeo, R.Singh, M.Gundeti, J.M.Barua, J.Masood)

[12] Neurology Research [2014] 36 (3) : 234-238 (A.Q.Rana, H.Vaid, M.R.Akhter, N.Y.Awan, A.Fattah, M. H. Cader, K.Hafez, M.A. Rana, M.S.Yousuf)

[13] Journal of Neuroscience Nursing [2013] 45 (6) : 382-392 (J.P. Robinson, C.W.Bradway, L.Bunting-Perry, T.Avi-Itzhak, M.Mangino, J.Chittams, J.E.Duda)

[14] Journal of Neurology, Neurosurgery and Psychiatry [2000] 68 (4) : 429-433 (I.Araki, S.Kuno)

[15] Wiener Klinische Wochenschrift [1996] 108 (10) : 296-302 (W. H. Jost, K.Schimrigk)

[16] International Urogynecology Journal and Pelvic Floor Dysfunction [1999] 10 (2) : 144-151 (R.R.Dmochowski)

[17] Urology [1989] 33 (6) : 486-489 (Z.Khan, P.Starer, A.Bhola)

[18] Der Urologe [1990] 29 (4) : 170-175 (K.P.Jünemann, H. Melchior)

CHAPTER 24

SYMPTOMS OF PARKINSON'S DISEASE

CARDIOVASCULAR SYSTEM

CARDIOVASCULAR SYSTEM

The cardiovascular system, also known as the circulatory system, is an organ system that encompasses the heart and blood vessels of the body. The cardiovascular system carries blood, oxygen, and nutrients to organs and tissues of the body, and carries waste and carbon dioxide from these tissues for removal from the body.

PRIMARY SYMPTOMS

Cardiovascular dystautonomia usually occurs in Parkinson's Disease and can include a variety of cardiovascular symptoms [PAGE 333]. Certain Parkinson's Disease drugs can increase the likelihood of heart failure, in which breathlessness, feeling very tired and ankle swelling are the main symptoms [PAGE 335]. Supine hypotension can also occur [PAGE 337].

CARDIOVASCULAR DYSAUTONOMIA

Symptoms : Cardiovascular dystautonomia includes signs or symptoms of impaired autonomic regulation of circulation and are often affected in Parkinson's Disease [1]. Over a period of three years there is progression of an impairment of sympathetic and parasympathetic control of the cardiovascular functions in people with Parkinson's Disease [2]. Cardiovascular autonomic function, especially orthostatic hypotension, is often affected in Parkinson's Disease [1, 3, 4, 5]. Mild impairment of autonomic cardiovascular control occurred early in the course of Parkinson's Disease [6]. Latent cardiac and vasomotor sympathetic dysfunction but not parasympathetic dysfunction is already present early in Parkinson's Disease, even without orthostatic hypotension [7]. There is a cardiovascular dysfunction, which occurs solely in people with Parkinson's Disease, that the researchers describe as "Parkinsonian Heart". Parkinsonian Heart is characterized by a severe loss of the physiological noradrenergic innervation and a slight impairment of central autonomic control. Both of these prevent the heart's proper functioning [8]. Heart rate variability is a marker of cardiovascular dysautonomia [9, 10] and tends to be reduced in Parkinson's Disease [11, 12, 13].

Prevalence : Cardiovascular symptoms occur in 70% of people with Parkinson's Disease. There is a higher percentage in those people with Parkinson's Disease who predominantly had rigidity or akinesia [14]. The prevalence of Orthostatic hypotension in Parkinson's disease is 51% [17]. Cardiovascular Diseases are one of the most common comorbid events in Parkinson's Disease [15]. Those most affected by impairment of autonomic cardiovascular control tend to be older [16].

Causes of symptoms : The catecholamines that regulate autonomic function, adrenaline and noradrenaline, are biosynthesized from dopamine. So the insufficient dopamine that occurs in people with Parkinson's Disease will also lead to low levels of adrenaline and noradrenaline.

[1] Neurobiology of Disease [2012] 46 (3) : 572-580 (S.Jain, D.S. Goldstein)

[2] Acta Neurologica Scandinavica [1999] 100 (5) : 296-299 (A. Mesec, S.Sega, M.Trost, T.Pogacnik)

[3] Movement Disorders [2010] 25 (15) : 2493-2500 (D.A.Gallagher, A.J.Lees, A.Schrag)

[4] Cleveland Clinic Journal of Medicine [2008] 75 (Supplement 2) : S54-S58 (B.L.Walter)

[5] Journal of Movement Disorders [2016] 9 (2) : 97-103 (J.S.Kim, S.H.Lee, Y.S.Oh, J.W.Park, J.Y.An, S.K.Park, S.R.Han, K.S.Lee)

[6] Autonomic Neuroscience [2004] 116 (1-2) : 30-38 (M.Bouhaddi, F. Vuillier, J.O.Fortrat, S.Cappelle, M.T.Henriet, L.Rumbach, J. Regnard)

[7] European Journal of Neurology [2011] 18 (2) : 286-292 (H.Oka, C.Toyoda, M.Yogo, S.Mochio)

[8] Current Medicinal Chemistry [2007] 14 (23) : 2421-2428 (F. Fornai, R.Ruffoli, P.Soldani, S.Ruggieri, A.Paparelli)

[9] Journal of Neural Transmission [2003] 110 (9) : 997-1011 (D. Devos, M.Kroumova, R.Bordet, H.Vodougnon, J.D.Guieu, C.Libersa, A.Destee)

[10] Journal of Neurology [2002] 249 (11) : 1535-1540 (V.Pursiainen, T.H.Haapaniemi, J.T.Korpelainen, H.V.Huikuri, K.A.Sotaniemi, V. Myllylä)

[11] European Journal of Neurology [2000] 7 (6) : 667-672 (M.Kallio, T.Haapaniemi, J.Turkka, K.Suominen, U.Tolonen, K.Sotaniemi, V.P. Heikkilä, V.Myllylä)

[12] Annals of Neurology [2015] 77 (5) : 877-883 (A.Alonso, X. Huang, T.H.Mosley, G.Heiss, H.Chen)

[13] Arquivos de Neuropsiquiatria [2014] 72 (10) : 762-767 G. Delgado, B.Estañol, M.Rodríguez-Violante, R.Martínez-Memije, Ó. Infante-Vázquez, N.Bertado-Ramírez)

[14] Clinical Neurology and Neurosurgery [2013] 115 (6) : 673-677 (E. M.Khedr, N.A.El Fetoh, H.Khalifa, M.A.Ahmed, K.M.El Beh)

[15] Neurological Sciences [2004] 25 (2) : 66-71 (E.Martignoni, L. Godi, A.Citterio, R.Zangaglia, G.Riboldazzi, D.Calandrella, C. Pacchetti, G.Nappi)

[16] Italian Journal of Neurological Science [1993] 14 (6) : 437-442 (R. Martín, R.Manzanares, J.M.Moltó, T.Canet, C.Ruiz, J.Matías-Guiu)

[17] Journal of Parkinson's Disease [2016] Sep 20 [Epub ahead of print] (A.Hommel, M.J.Faber, N.J.Weerkamp, J.G.van Dijk, B.R. Bloem, R.T.Koopmans)

Heart failure

Symptoms : Heart failure is a condition caused by the heart failing to pump enough blood around the body at the right pressure. It usually occurs because the heart muscle has become too weak or stiff to work properly. Breathlessness, feeling very tired and ankle swelling are the main symptoms. These symptoms can have other causes only some of which are serious. Symptoms of heart failure can develop quickly (acute heart failure) or develop gradually (chronic heart failure).

Prevalence : The likelihood of heart failure in elderly people with Parkinson's Disease is more than doubled [1].

Causes of symptoms : The primary cause of an increased likelihood of heart failure in Parkinson's Disease is the use of dopamine agonists [2], especially pramipexole [3, 4, 5], pergolide [6, 7, 8], and cabergoline [4, 9].

[1] Parkinsonism & Related Disorders [2004] 10 (7) : 417-420 (T.A. Zesiewicz, J.A.Strom, A.R.Borenstein, R.A.Hauser, C.R.Cimino, H.L. Fontanet, G.B.Cintron, J.F.Staffetti, P.B.Dunne, K.L.Sullivan)

[2] ISRN Neurology [2014] : 956353 (K.Abou Farha, C.Baljé-Volkers, W.Tamminga, I.den Daas, S.van Os)

[3] The Consultant Pharmacist [2015] 30 (3) : 136-140 (K.Lockett, D. De Backer, K.A.Cauthon)

[4] Expert Opinions on Drug Safety [2014] 13 (3) : 351-360 (S.Perez-Lloret, M.V.Rey, J.Crispo, D.Krewski, M.Lapeyre-Mestre, J.L. Montastruc, O.Rascol)

[5] Pharmacological Research [2012] 65 (3) : 358-364 (M.M.Mokhles, G.Trifirò, J.P.Dieleman, M.D.Haag, E.M.van Soest, K.M.Verhamme, G.Mazzaglia, R.Herings, C.Luise, D.Ross, G.Brusselle, A.Colao, et al)

[6] Canadian Journal of Neurological Sciences [2008] 35 (2) : 173-178 (C.Zadikoff, M.Duong-Hua, K.Sykora, C.Marras, A.Lang, P.Rochon)

[7] Canadian Journal of Neurological Sciences [2006] 33 (1) : 111-113 (J.Scozzafava, J.Takahashi, W.Johnston, L.Puttagunta, W.R. Martin)

[8] Neurology [2003] 61 (6) : 859-861 (G.Van Camp, A.Flamez, B. Cosyns, J.Goldstein, C.Perdaens, D.Schoors)

[9] Neurology [1993] 43 (12) : 2587-2590 (G.Lera, J.Vaamonde, M. Rodriguez, J.A.Obeso)

Supine hypertension

Symptoms : Supine hypertension is a feature of cardiovascular autonomic failure [1]. Supine hypertension is defined as a diastolic blood pressure of greater than 140/90 mmHg [2].

Prevalence : Supine hypertension occurs in 34 % of people with Parkinson's Disease (mildly in 71 % of them, moderate in 27 % of them, and severe in 2 %) [1]. Supine hypertension is more common in older age [2], and when there is preexisting hypertension [2].

Causes of symptoms : Supine blood pressure positively correlates with the degree of orthostatic hypotension [2]. Cardiovascular comorbidities significantly contribute to the development of supine hypertension [1]. Supine blood pressure positively correlates with the degree of orthostatic hypotension [2].

[1] Clinical Autonomic Research [2016] 26 (2) : 97-105 (A.Fanciulli, G.Göbel, J.P.Ndayisaba, R.Granata, S.Duerr, S.Strano, C.Colosimo, W. Poewe, F.E.Pontieri, G.K.Wenning)

[2] Clinical Autonomic Research [2016] 26 (1) : 15-21 (T.Umehara, H.Matsuno, C.Toyoda, H.Oka)

CHAPTER 25

SYMPTOMS OF PARKINSON'S DISEASE

RESPIRATORY SYSTEM

RESPIRATORY SYSTEM

The respiratory system includes the nasal passages, larynx, trachea, bronchial tubes, diaphragm and the lungs. Muscles are involved in facilitating the function of the respiratory system. The respiratory system enables a person to breathe and exchange oxygen and carbon dioxide throughout the body.

PRIMARY SYMPTOMS

Respiratory muscle dysfunction usually, but not always, occurs in Parkinson's Disease. Respiratory muscle dysfunction makes respiratory diseases such as pneumonia more dangerous due to the reduced respiratory capacity it causes.

RESPIRATORY MUSCLE DYSFUNCTION

Symptoms : Repetitive ventilatory tasks can be limited and contribute to respiratory muscle fatigue. Consequently, the breathing rate can not be sustained as well and breathing efficiency is reduced [1]. There is often abnormal ventilatory control despite normal lung volumes and flows [2]. Respiratory muscle strength and endurance are also decreased [3]. Due to the reduced respiratory capacity, people with Parkinson's Disease are more prone to the effects of pneumonia, which occurs more commonly than expected in Parkinson's Disease, but not because of Parkinson's Disease [4, 5, 6]. Consequently, pneumonia is the most common cause of death associated with Parkinson's Disease [7-13]. However, death certificates indicated that pneumonia was a substantial contributor to the cause of death in only 20% of people with Parkinson's Disease [13]. Asthmatics, especially those people with severe asthma are far more likely to develop Parkinson's Disease. However, asthma does not occur far more commonly in Parkinson's Disease [14].

Prevalence : Most, but not all, people with Parkinson's Disease have respiratory muscle dysfunction [1, 2, 3].

Causes of symptoms : In people with Parkinson's Disease there is an increased contraction of the muscles involved in respiration [15, 16]. Excessive muscle contraction of the respiratory muscles hinders the ability of people with Parkinson's Disease to increase respiration in order to cope with respiratory infections.

[1] The American Review of Respiratory Disease [1988] 138 (2) : 266-271 (G.E.Tzelepis, F.D.McCool, J.H.Friedman, F.G.Hoppin Jr.)

[2] Respiratory Physiology and Neurobiology [2011] 179 (2-3) : 300-304 (L.M.Seccombe, H.L.Giddings, P.G.Rogers, A.J.Corbett, M.W. Hayes, M.J.Peters, E.M.Veitch)

[3] Canadian Journal of Neurological Sciences [2002] 29 (1) : 68-72 (P.Weiner, R.Inzelberg, A.Davidovich, P.Nisipeanu, R.Magadle, N. Berar-Yanay, R.L.Carasso)

[4] Progress in Palliative Care [2013] 21 (3) : 140-145 (L.Lethbridge, G.M.Johnston, G.Turnbull)

[5] Parkinsonism & Related Disorders [2015] 21 (9) : 1082-1086 (U.Akbar, B.Dham, Y.He, N.Hack, S.Wu, M.Troche, P.Tighe, E. Nelson, J.H.Friedman, M.S.Okun)

[6] Neuropsychiatric Disease and Treatment [2016] 12 : 1037-1046 (Y.P.Chang, C.J.Yang, K.F.Hu, A.C.Chao, Y.H.Chang, K.P.Hsieh, J.H. Tsai, P.S.Ho, S.Y.Lim)

[7] Parkinsonism & Related Disorders [2010] 16 (7) : 434-437 (S. Pennington, K.Snell, M.Lee, R.Walker)

[8] Archives of Neurology [2000] 57 (4) : 507-512 (L.Morgante, G. Salemi, F.Meneghini, A.E.Di Rosa, A.Epifanio, F.Grigoletto, P. Ragonese, F.Patti, A.Reggio, R.Di Perri, G.Savettieri)

[9] Medical Science Monitor [2002] 8 (4) : CR241-CR246 (H.H. Fernandez, K.L.Lapane)

[10] Neurology, Neurosurgery and Psychiatry [1999] 67 (3) : 300-307 (M.A.Hely, J.G.Morris, R.Traficante, W.G.Reid, D.J.O'Sullivan, P.M. Williamson)

[11] European Neurology [1997] 38 (Supplement 2) : 60-63 (K. Nakashima, M.Maeda, M.Tabata, Y.Adachi, M.Kusumi, H.Ohshiro)

[12] Movement Disorders [1994] 9 (3) : 350-352 (R.K.Mosewich, A.H. Rajput, A.Shuaib, B.Rozdilsky, L.Ang)

[13] Journal of Neurology, Neurosurgery and Psychiatry [2013] 84 (11) : 1258-1264 (C.H.Williams-Gray, S.L.Mason, J.R.Evans, T.Foltynie, C.Brayne, T.W.Robbins, R.A.Barker)

[14] Allergy [2015] 70 (12) : 1605-1612 (C.M.Cheng, Y.H.Wu, S.J. Tsai, Y.M.Bai, J.W.Hsu, K.L.Huang, T.P.Su, C.T.Li, C.F.Tsai, A.C. Yang, W.C.Lin, T.L.Pan, W.H.Chang, T.J.Chen, M.H.Chen)

[15] Journal Electromyography and Kinesiology [2009] 19 (4) : 591-597 (L.U.Guedes, V.F.Parreira, A.C.Diório, F.Goulart, A.D. Andrade, R.R. Britto)

[16] Respiration Physiology [1999] 118 (2-3) : 163-172 (L.Vercueil, J.P.Linard, B.Wuyam, P.Pollak, G.Benchetrit)

CHAPTER 26

SYMPTOMS OF PARKINSON'S DISEASE

SKELETAL SYSTEM

Skeletal system

The skeletal system includes all of the bones and joints in the body. The skeleton acts as a scaffold by providing support and protection for the soft tissues that make up the rest of the body. The skeletal system also provides attachment points for muscles to allow movements at the joints.

Primary symptoms

In Parkinson's Disease there can be an increased likelihood of osteoporosis [PAGE 342] and osteopenia [PAGE 342]. The postural deformities can include camptocormia [PAGE 344], scoliosis [PAGE 345], and Pisa syndrome [PAGE 345].

Postural deformities can be frequent and disabling complications of Parkinson's Disease [1]. The prevalence of skeletal problems is higher in people with Parkinson's Disease. Up to two thirds of people with Parkinson's Disease have them [2, 3]. Only just over a quarter of people with Parkinson's Disease answered that their musculoskeletal problems were recovering. Musculoskeletal problems tended to receive less treatment when people had Parkinson's Disease. The most common sites of musculoskeletal problems are the lower back, in nearly half of people, and the shoulder and knee, which were affected far less [2]. Striatal foot deformities are the most common deformity observed (25%). Camptocormia is the second most common deformity (20%). Striatal and postural deformities were seen in more advanced Parkinson's Disease. Striatal deformities almost always (94%) occurred more on the same side of the body as the onset of Parkinson's Disease symptoms. Pisa and scoliosis occurred more (66%) on the opposite side to the onset of Parkinson's Disease symptoms [3].

[1] Lancet Neurology [2011] 10 (6) : 538-549 (K.M.Doherty, B.P.van de Warrenburg, M.C.Peralta, L.Silveira-Moriyama, J.P.Azulay, O.S. Gershanik, B.R.Bloem)

[2] Parkinsonism & Related Disorders [2013] 19 (7) : 666-669 (Y.E. Kim, W.W.Lee, J.Y.Yun, H.J.Yang, H.J.Kim, B.S.Jeon)

[3] Indian Journal of Medical Research [2016] 144 (5) : 682-688 (S. Pandey, H.Kumar)

Osteoporosis and Osteopenia

Symptoms : Osteoporosis is a decrease in bone mass and density which can lead to an increased risk of fracture. Osteopenia is low bone mineral density. Osteopenia often develops in to osteoporosis. Due to the proneness to falling that some people with Parkinson's Disease have, the risk of fractures becomes even greater in those people that also have Osteoporosis.

Prevalence : Osteoporosis and fractures are more common in Parkinson's Disease [1-7]. One in six people with Parkinson's Disease were found to have already developed Osteoporosis [1]. However, the prevalence of osteoporosis in Parkinson's Disease does not exceed that of other people of a similar age [8]. Osteoporosis is related to the severity of Parkinson's Disease [1], and is far more likely to occur in Parkinson's Disease in those people prone to falls [9]. Osteopenia is more common in people with Parkinson's Disease [10]. Over half of people with Parkinson's Disease have been found to have osteopenia [1]. Osteopenia is about four times more likely than osteoporosis [11, 12]. As many as 91% of women [8, 13] and 61% of men who have Parkinson's Disease have osteoporosis or osteopenia [13]. Ostepenia is more common with a longer duration of Parkinson's Disease [14].

Causes of symptoms : Although the biochemistry of Parkinson's Disease and osteoporosis do not coincide, osteoporosis is very common in Parkinson's Disease and is related to the severity of Parkinson's Disease. This is largely due to them both being more common with age [1].

[1] Rheumatology International [2008] 28 (12) : 1205-1209 (A. Bezza, Z.Ouzzif, H.Naji, L.Achemlal, A.Mounach, M.Nouijai, A. Bourazza, R.Mossadeq, A.El Maghraoui)

[2] Parkinsonism & Related Disorders [2013] 19 (7) : 666-669 (Y.E. Kim, W.W.Lee, J.Y.Yun, H.J.Yang, H.J.Kim, B.S.Jeon)

[3] Bone [2013] 52 (1) : 498-505 (Y.Zhao, L.Shen, H.F.Ji)

[4] Nihon Ronen Igakkai Zasshi [1995] 32 (10) : 637-640 (T. Yamada, T.Kachi, K.Ando)

[5] Journal of Neurology, Neurosurgery and Psychiatry [2014] 85 (10) : 1159-1166 (K.M.Torsney, A.J.Noyce, K.M.Doherty, J.P.Bestwick, R. Dobson, A.J.Lees)

[6] Parkinsonism & Related Disorders [2016] May 26 [Epub ahead of print] (I.Sleeman, Z.C.Che, C.Counsell)

[7] International Journal of Neuroscience [2016] Jun 29 : 1-18 [Epub ahead of print] (C.Tassorelli, M.Berlangieri, S.Buscone, M.Bolla, R.De Icco, A.Baricich, C.Pacchetti, C.Cisari, G.Sandrini)

[8] Movement Disorders [2005] 20 (12) : 1636-1640 (B.Wood, R. Walker)

[9] Parkinsonism & Related Disorders [2014] 20 (1) : 88-92 (K.Y. Cheng, W.C.Lin, W.N.Chang, T.K.Lin, N.W.Tsai, C.C.Huang, H.C. Wang, Y.C.Huang, H.W.Chang, Y.J.Lin, L.H.Lee, B.C.Cheng, et al)

[10] Age and Ageing [2013] 42 (2) : 156-162 (F.Van den Bos, A.D. Speelman, M.Samson, M.Munneke, B.R.Bloem, H.J.Verhaar)

[11] Journal of Neurology [2013] 260 (3) : 754-760 (F.van den Bos, A.D. Speelman, M.van Nimwegen, Y.T.van der Schouw, F.J.Backx, B.R. Bloem, M.Munneke, H.J.Verhaar)

[12] Rheumatology International [2008] 28 (12) : 1205-1209 (A. Bezza, Z.Ouzzif, H.Naji, L.Achemlal, A.Mounach, M.Nouijai, A. Bourazza, R.Mossadeq, A.El Maghraoui)

[13] Parkinsonism & Related Disorders [2009] 15 (5) : 339-346 (M. Invernizzi, S.Carda, G.S.Viscontini, C.Cisari)

[14] International Journal of Neuroscience [2012] 122 (9) : 523-527 (S.K.Daniel, M.C.Lansang, M.S.Okun)

CAMPTOCORMIA

Symptoms : Camptocormia is characterised as an extreme bent-forward posture of the trunk that disappears in the recumbent position [1].

Prevalence : Less than 10% of people with Parkinson's Disease have Camptocornia [2-5]. Camptocormia is more common : in females [2], in people with late onset Parkinson's Disease [2], in people with more severe Parkinson's Disease [3, 4], in people who had a longer duration of Parkinson's Disease [4], in people with Parkinson's Disease who are older and had more severe motor symptoms and had a higher L-dopa dose [5], but there was not a clear correlation with L-dopa use. Camptocornia in people with Parkinson's Disease is associated with more severe symptoms of Parkinson's Disease [6]. In some people the posture improved, and in others it was unchanged or even aggravated following L-dopa use [7, 8]. Camptocormia that developed a long time after Parkinson's Disease developed responded poorly to L-dopa [9].

Causes of symptoms : Camptocornia can be caused by the muscle rigidity that occurs in Parkinson's Disease. Parkinson's Disease induces functional changes in the organisation of the corticospinal and reticulospinal tracts, where dysfunction could contribute to axial rigidity. Rigidity of the spinal flexion muscles could lead to the under use of the spinal extension muscles, which become progressively atrophic. Rigidity may also induce spinal deformations, leading to a neurogenic syndrome via compression of the spinal nerves [10].

[1] Annales de Readaptation et de Medecine Physique [2007] 50 (1) : 55-59 (E.Bouzgarou, A.Dupeyron, G.Castelnovo, V.Boudousq, L. Collombier, P.Labauge, J.Pélissier)

[2] Parkinsonism & Related Disorders [2013] 19 (8) : 725-731 (A. Yoritaka, Y.Shimo, M.Takanashi, J.Fukae, T.Hatano, T.Nakahara, N. Miyamato, T.Urabe, H.Mori, N.Hattori)

[3] Journal of Neurology, Neurosurgery and Psychiatry [2009] 80 (2) : 145-148 (D.Tiple, G.Fabbrini, C.Colosimo, D.Ottaviani, F.Camerota, G.Defazio, A.Berardelli)

[4] Journal of Neurological Science [2014] 337 (1-2) : 173-175 (W. Song, X.Guo, K.Chen, R.Huang, B.Zhao, B.Cao, Y.Chen, H.F.Shang)

[5] Movement Disorders [2011] 26 (14) : 2567-2571 (M.Seki, K. Takahashi, A.Koto, B.Mihara, Y.Morita, K.Isozumi, K.Ohta, K. Muramatsu, J.Gotoh, K.Yamaguchi, Y.Tomita, H.Sato, Y.Nihei, et al)

[6] Journal of Neurological Science [2015] Sep 8 [Epub ahead of print] (S.Nakane, M.Yoshioka, N.Oda, T.Tani, K.Chida, M.Suzuki, I. Funakawa, A.Inukai, K.Hasegawa, K.Kuroda, K.Mizoguchi, et al)

[7] Movement Disorders [1999] 14 (3) : 443-447 (R.Djaldetti, R. Mosberg-Galili, H.Sroka, D.Merims, E.Melamed)

[8] Gait Posture [2015] 42 (3) : 263-268 (F.Benninger, A.Khlebtovsky, Y.Roditi, O.Keret, I.Steiner, E.Melamed, R.Djaldetti)

[9] Journal of Neurology, Neurosurgery and Psychiatry [2006] 77 (11) : 1223-1228 (F.Bloch, J.L.Houeto, S.Tezenas du Montcel, F. Bonneville, F.Etchepare, M.L.Welter, S.Rivaud-Pechoux, V.Hahn-Barma, et al)

[10] Journal of Neurology, Neurosurgery and Psychiatry [2006] 77 (11) : 1229-1234 (A-C.Lepoutre, D.Devos, A.Blanchard-Dauphin, V. Pardessus, C-A.Maurage, D.Ferriby, J-F.Hurtevent, A.Cotten, et al)

Scoliosis

Symptoms : Scoliosis and Pisa Syndrome are often referred to interchangeably. Pisa syndrome describes a person who lists to the side whereas scoliosis is defined by spinal curvature and rotation and may not be associated with lateral flexion [1]. Scoliosis is often a painful medical condition in which a person's spine is curved from side to side. Scoliosis was defined as a deviation of the spine of ten degrees or more.

Prevalence : Scoliosis was found in a third of people with Parkinson's

Disease. Scoliosis was found to be seven times more likely in women than it is in men. The likelihood also increased with age [2]. Pisa Syndrome occurs in around 8% of people with Parkinson's Disease. Those with Pisa Syndrome tended to be older, have had Parkinson's Disease for longer, and take more L-dopa [3].

Causes of symptoms : The use of dopaminergic drugs did not appear to have any effect on the degree of scoliosis. However, the excessive muscle contraction that occurs in Parkinson's Disease can cause the upper body to bend towards one side rather than the other [2].

[1] Journal of Neurology, Neurosurgery and Psychiatry [2013] 84 (12) : 1400-1403 (K.M.Doherty, I.Davagnanam, S.Molloy, L.Silveira-Moriyama, A.J.Lees)

[2] Journal of Clinical Neurology [2009] 5 (2) : 91-94 (J.S.Baik, J.Y. Kim, J.H.Park, S.W.Han, J.H.Park, M.S.Lee)

[3] Neurology [2015] 85 (20) : 1769-1779 (M.Tinazzi, A.Fasano, C. Geroin, F.Morgante, R.Ceravolo, S.Rossi, A.Thomas, G.Fabbrini, A. Bentivoglio, F.Tamma, G.Cossu, N.Modugno, M.Zappia, et al)

CHAPTER 27

SYMPTOMS OF PARKINSON'S DISEASE

INTEGUMENTARY SYSTEM

INTEGUMENTARY SYSTEM

The integumentary system is the skin and its associated glands, including the sweat glands, as well as the hair and nails. The skin protects the body from various kinds of damage such as loss of water or abrasion from outside.

PRIMARY SYMPTOMS

In Parkinson's Disease there is an increased likelihood of melanoma [PAGE 347], which is a form of skin cancer; hyperhidrosis [PAGE 349], which is increased sweat secretion; and seborrhea [PAGE 350], which is increased sebum secretion.

MELANOMA

Symptoms : Melanoma is a type of skin cancer that forms from the melanocytes. Most melanomas present as a dark, mole-like spot that spreads and, unlike a mole, has an irregular border.

Prevalence : There is a higher than expected frequency of melanoma in people with Parkinson's Disease [1-8], which is not due to L-dopa [5, 9, 10, 11]. Melanoma was over three times more likely in people with Parkinson's Disease after they have been diagnosed but was not more likely before diagnosis. The risk of melanoma could sometimes be as much as four to nine times higher in Parkinson's Disease [12, 13]. There was no relationship between Parkinson's Disease and other skin cancers [14].

Causes of symptoms : The melanocytes in the skin produce melanin, which is made from L-tyrosine via L-dopa [15-18]. This is the same means as dopamine in the dopaminergic neurons. In the dopaminergic neurons L-dopa forms dopamine [19-23]. The reduced ability in Parkinson's Disease to produce L-dopa reduces the capacity to produce melanin. Melanin helps to protect skin cells from Ultra Violet induced damage. So melanoma is probably increased in Parkinson's Disease because of the reduced capacity to produce L-dopa in the melanocytes.

[1] British Journal of Dermatology [2014] 170 (1) : 11-19 (V. Nikolaou, A.J.Stratigos)

[2] Movement Disorders [2010] 25 (2) : 139-148 (J.J.Ferreira, D. Neutel, T.Mestre, M.Coelho, M.M.Rosa, O.Rascol, C.Sampaio)

[3] Movement Disorders [2007] 22 (10) : 1471-1475 (J.Ferreira, J. M.Silva, R.Freire, J.Pignatelli, L.C.Guedes, A.Feijó, M.M.Rosa, M. Coelho, J.Costa, A.Noronha, R.Hewett, A.M.Gomes, et al)

[4] Epidemiology [2006] 17 (5) : 582-587 (J.H.Olsen, S.Friis, K. Frederiksen)

[5] Melanoma Research [2006] 16 (3) : 201-206 (R.Zanetti, D.Loria, S. Rosso)

[6] American Journal of Epidemiology [2014] 179 (1) : 85-94 (K. Wirdefeldt, C.E.Weibull, H.Chen, F.Kamel, C.Lundholm, F.Fang, W. Ye)

[7] JAMA Oncology [2015] 1 (5) : 633-640 (P.Y.Lin, S.N.Chang, T.H. Hsiao, B.T.Huang, C.H.Lin, P.C.Yang)

[8] Parkinsonism & Related Disorders [2016] Jun 20 [Epub ahead of print] (P.Tacik, S.Curry, S.Fujioka, A.Strongosky, R.J.Uitti, J.A.van Gerpen, N.N.Diehl, M.G.Heckman, Z.K.Wszolek)

[9] Journal of Neural Transmission [2009] 116 (11) : 1503-1507 (R. Inzelberg, S.D.Israeli-Korn)

[10] Movement Disorders [2007] 22 (5) : 720-722 (R.Constantinescu, M.Romer, K.Kieburtz)

[11] Parkinsonism & Related Disorders [2003] 9 (6) : 321-327 (K.H. Fiala, J.Whetteckey, B.V.Manyam)

[12] Movement Disorders [2007] 22 (9) : 1252-1257 (J.H.Olsen, K. Tangerud, L.Wermuth, K.Frederiksen, S.Friis)

[13] Neuroepidemiology [2016] 46 (2) : 128-136 (S.Y.Shalaby, E.D. Louis)

[14] Neurology [2011] 76 (23) : 2002-2009 (R.Liu, X.Gao, Y.Lu, H. Chen)

[15] Journal of Biological Chemistry [1964] 239 : 2910 (T.Nagatsu, M.Levitt, S.Udenfriend)

[16] Archives of Biochemistry and Biophysics [1967] 120 : 420 (M. Ikeda, M.Levitt, S.Udenfriend)

[17] Nature [1983] 302 : 830 (S.El Mestikawy, J.Glowinski, M.Hamon)

[18] Comptes Rendus Academie des Sciences [1986] 302 : 435 (D. Pigeon, R.Drissi-Daoudi, F. Gros, J.Thibault)

[19] Journal of Biological Chemistry [1948] 174 : 813 (R.W.Mc Gilvery, P.P.Cohen)

[20] Journal of Biological Chemistry [1957] 227 : 617 (H.Weissbach, D.F.Bogdanski, B.G.Redfield, S.Udenfriend)

[21] Journal of Biological Chemistry [1962] 237 : 89 (W.Lovenberg, H.Weissbach, S. Udenfriend)

[22] Proceedings, National Academy of Science USA [1972] 69 : 343 (J.G.Christenson, W.Dairman, S.Udenfriend)

[23] Hoppe-Seyler's Zeitschrift fuer Physiologische Chemie [1963] 332 : 70 (C.E. Sekeris)

Hyperhidrosis

Symptoms : Hyperhidrosis is due to the overactivity of the sweat glands that can result in the excessive secretion of sweat.

Prevalence : There is an increased likelihood of hyperhidrosis in Parkinson's Disease [1, 2, 3].

Causes of symptoms : Instead of being due to Parkinson's Disease, the increased sweat secretion that can occur in Parkinson’s Disease is usually due to Parkinson's Disease drugs. As an unintended side effect, L-dopa can produce adrenaline [4], which in turn stimulates the sweat glands [5].

[1] European Journal of Neurology [1987] 26 (1) : 1-7 (J.T.Turkka, V.V.Myllylä)

[2] Journal of Neurology [1994] 241 (10) : 573-576 (Y.Mano, T. Nakamuro, T.Takayanagi, R.F.Mayer)

[3] Journal of Neural Transmission [2001] 108 (2) : 205-213 (M. Fischer, I.Gemende, W.C.Marsch, P.A.Fischer)

[4] Journal of Neural Transmission [2009] 116 (11) : 1355-1362 (A. Nakashima, N.Hayashi, Y.S.Kaneko, K.Mori, E.L.Sabban, T.Nagatsu, A.Ota)

[5] International Journal of Cosmetic Science [2007] 29 (3) : 169 -179 (K.Wilke, A.Martin, L.Terstegen, S.S.Biel)

Seborrhea

Symptoms : Seborrhea is overactive sebaceous glands. The sebaceous glands are glands in the skin that secrete sebum in order to lubricate the skin and hair of mammals. Seborrhea can result in the excessive secretion of sebum by the sebaceous glands on to the surface of the skin [1, 2, 3].

Prevalence : There is an increased likelihood of seborrhea occurring in Parkinson's Disease [1, 2, 3].

Causes of symptoms : In Parkinson's Disease there is low dopamine. Dopamine inhibits the formation of prolactin [4]. So in Parkinson's Disease the reduced dopamine levels enable higher levels of prolactin. Prolactin stimulates, via luteinizing hormone, the formation of testosterone [5]. Increased testosterone stimulates sebum formation thereby causing seborrhea [6].

[1] Primary Care [1977] 4 (3) : 475-480 (A.Flint)

[2] Journal of Neural Transmission [1997] 104 (11-12) : 1295-1304 (E.Martignoni, L.Godi, C.Pacchetti, E.Berardesca, G.P.Vignoli, G. Albani, F.Mancini, G.Nappi)

[3] Journal of Neural Transmission [2001] 108 (2) : 205-213 (M. Fischer, I.Gemende, W.C.Marsch, P.A.Fischer)

[4] Endocrine Reviews [2001] 22 (6) : 724-763 (N.Ben-Jonathan, R. Hnasko)

[5] Journal of Andrology [1989] 10 (1) : 37-42 (Man-Cheong Fung, G.C.Wah, W.D.Odell)

[6] Dermatoendocrinology [2011] 3 (1) : 41-49 (E.Makrantonaki, R. Ganceviciene, C.Zouboulis)

CHAPTER 28

SYMPTOMS OF PARKINSON'S DISEASE

SENSORY SYSTEM

SENSORY SYSTEM

The sensory system consists of the olfactory system (for olfaction, which is the sense of smell), the gustatory system (for the sense of taste), the visual system (for visual perception), and the auditory system (for the sense of hearing).

PRIMARY SYMPTOMS

In Parkinson's Disease there can be an increased likelihood of anosmia (which is a loss of the sense of smell) [PAGE 352], rhinorrhea (which is nasal discharge) [PAGE 354], visual disturbance [PAGE 355], retinal thinning [PAGE 356], hypogeusia (which is impaired sense of taste [PAGE 359], and hearing loss [PAGE 361]. Visual disturbances and anosmia are particularly prominent.

OLFACTORY SYSTEM

The olfactory system is the sensory system used for olfaction, which is the sense of smell. Odorants are inhaled through the nose where they contact the main olfactory epithelium. The olfactory epithelium contains olfactory receptors, which turns receptor activation for a variety of smells into electrical signals in neurons, which is where the stimulus is perceived.

ANOSMIA

Symptoms : A loss of the sense of smell (anosmia) and reduced sense of smell (hyposmia) often occur in Parkinson’s Disease [1-11]. Those people with mild cognitive impairment are often unaware of it [12].

Prevalence : Most people with Parkinson's Disease have a loss of the sense of smell (anosmia) or reduction (hyposmia) in the sense of smell [1-11, 13, 18]. Hyposmia was found in 73% of patients at diagnosis [19].

Causes of symptoms : The dopamine deficiency that occurs in Parkinson's Disease causes a reduction in the stimulation of the dopaminergic neurons in the olfactory bulb and in the olfactory tract through which smells are perceived [14]. However, the reduction in the sense of smell is not due entirely to the deficiency of dopamine [15, 16]. Excessive contraction of the nasal muscles can reduce the physical ability to inhale through the nose. Parkinson's Disease consequently impairs sniffing, reducing sniff airflow rate and volume [17].

[1] ORL Journal for Otorhinolaryngology Related Specialities [1991] 53 (3) : 143-146 (T.Murofushi, M.Mizuno, R.Osanai, T. Hayashida)

[2] Chemical Senses [1997] 22 (1) : 105-110 (J.P.Lehrner, T.Brucke, P. Dal-Bianco, G.Gatterer, I.Kryspin-Exner)

[3] Neurology [1988] 38 (8) : 1237-1244 (R.L.Doty, D.A.Deems, S. Stellar)

[4] Archives in Neurology [2003] 60 (4) : 545-549 (K.L.Double, D.B.Rowe, M.Hayes, D.K.Chan, J.Blackie, A.Corbett, R.Joffe, V.S. Fung, J.Morris, G.M.Halliday)

[5] Journal of Clinical Neuroscience [2002] 9 (5) : 521-524 (A.Muller, M.Mungersdorf, H.Reichmann, G.Strehle, T.Hummel)

[6] Journal of Neurology, Neurosurgery and Psychiatry [2003] 74 (7) : 956-958 (J.M.Henderson, Y.Lu, S.Wang, H.Cartwright, G.M.Halliday)

[7] Arquivos de Neuro-Psiquiatria [2007] 65 (3A) : 647-652 (L.B. Quagliato, M.A.Viana, E.M.Quagliato, S.Simis)

[8] Parkinsonism & Related Disorders [2009] 15 (7) : 490-494 (A. Haehner, S.Boesveldt, H.W.Berendse, A.Mackay-Sim, J.Fleischmann, P.A.Silburn, A.N.Johnston, G.D.Mellick, B.Herting, et al)

[9] Movement Disorders [2014] 29 (8) : 1069-1074 (E.B.Lucassen, N.W.Sterling, E.Y.Lee, H.Chen, M.M.Lewis, L.Kong, X.Huang)

[10] Zhonghua Er Bi Yan Hou Tou Jing Wai Ke Za Zhi [2015] 50 (1) : 20-24 (W.Hang, G.Liu, T.Han, P.Zhang, J.Zhang)

[11] Behavioural Neurology [2015] : 976589 (S.Cavaco, A.Gonçalves, A.Mendes, N.Vila-Chã, I.Moreira, J.Fernandes, J.Damásio, A.Teixeira-Pinto, A.Bastos Lima)

[12] Parkinsonism & Related Disorders [2016] 22 : 74-79 (I.Kawasaki, T.Baba, A.Takeda, E.Mori)

[13] Journal of Neural Transmission [2016] 123 (4) : 421-424 (J. Haugen, M.L.Müller, V.Kotagal, R.L.Albin, R.A.Koeppe, P.J.Scott, K.A.Frey, N.I.Bohnen)

[14] International Journal of Neuroscience [1999] 97 (3-4) : 225-233 (R.Sandyk)

[15] Functional Neurology [1998] 13 (2) : 99-103 (J.Roth, T.Radil, E.Ruzicka, R.Jech, J.Tichy)

[16] Journal of Neurology, Neurosurgery and Psychiatry [1987] 50 (1) : 88-89 (N.P.Quinn, M.N.Rosser, C.D.Marsden)

[17] Proceedings, National Academy Sciences U.S.A. [2001] 98 (7) : 4154-4159 (N.Sobel, M.E.Thomason, I.Stappen, C.M.Tanner, J.W. Tetrud, J.M.Bower, E.V.Sullivan, J.D.Gabrieli)

[18] Clinical Otolaryngology [2016] Dec 22 [Epub ahead of print] (G.C.Passali, F.Bove, L.Vargiu, A.R.Bentivoglio, R.Anzivino, E.De Corso, J.Galli, M.Rigante, M.Pandolfini, B.Sergi, M.Giuliani, et al)

[19] Parkinsonism and Related Disorders [2017] Feb 21 [Epub ahead of print] (M.E.Domellöf, K.F.Lundin, M.Edström, L.Forsgren)

Rhinorrhea

Symptoms : Rhinorrhea is nasal discharge, commonly referred to as a runny nose. It is an early feature of Parkinson's Disease, being present at the time of onset [1]. The nasal discharge of over half of those people with Parkinson's Disease is accompanied with lightheadedness. Lightheadedness is usually uncommon, occurring in less than one in ten people [2]. The increased frequency of nasal discharge can lead to a reduction in the sense of smell [1, 2].

Prevalence : Although, nasal discharge is usually assumed to occur for a variety of reasons such as colds, flu or allergies, it commonly occurs in Parkinson's Disease [1-5]. It is more common in men [4, 5].

Causes of symptoms : Nasal discharge occurring so frequently in Parkinson's Disease is not directly due to low dopamine [2]. A previous study found no relationship between rhinorrhea and dopamine agonists [2]. There was no relationship with age or severity of symptoms [2, 4].

[1] Movement Disorders [2008] 23 (3) : 452-454 (J.H.Friedman, M.M.Amick)

[2] Movement Disorders [2011] 26 (2) : 320-323 (K.L.Chou, R.A. Koeppe, N.I.Bohnen)

[3] International Journal of Neuroscience [2010] 120 (4) : 258-260 (L.Sedig, J.Leibner, A.L.Ramjit, S.S.Wu, Y.Dai, M.S.Okun, R.L. Rodriguez, I.A.Malaty, H.H.Fernandez)

[4] Journal of Neurological Science [2014] 343 (1-2) : 88-90 (O.Kano, M.Yoshioka, H.Nagayama, S.Hamada, T.Maeda, T.Hasegawa, T. Kadowaki, R.Sengoku, H.Terashi, T.Hatano, N.Nomoto, et al)

VISUAL SYSTEM

The visual system is required for visual perception – processing and interpreting visual information to build a representation of the visual environment. It consists of the eye, retina, fibres that conduct visual information, the superior colliculus and parts of the cerebral cortex.

VISUAL DISTURBANCE

Symptoms : In Parkinson's Disease there is a reduction in convergence ability [1], in visual acuity [2, 38], contrast sensitivity [3-8, 38], colour discrimination [7, 9-16], and impaired visual perception [17, 18]. There is increased double vision [19, 20], the need to turn the head to see objects in the periphery [19], misjudging objects when walking [20], words moving whilst reading [20], asthenopia, upgaze deficiency, and convergence insufficiency [21]. Ocular complaints suggesting ocular surface irritation, altered tear film, blepharospasm, decreased blink rate, and decreased convergence amplitudes occur more frequently [22]. There are also larger pupil diameters after the adaptation to light [23].

Prevalence : The prevalence of recurrent visual complaints (RVC) and recurrent visual hallucinations (RVH) in Parkinson's Disease and their effects are recurrent visual complaints (17%), recurrent visual hallucinations (29%), double vision (18%), misjudging objects when walking (12%), words moving whilst reading (17%), freezing in narrow spaces (30%) [20].

Causes of symptoms : Reduced dopamine could give rise to many of the visual abnormalities observed in Parkinson's Disease [24]. There is reduced dopaminergic activity in the retina of people with Parkinson's Disease [25-29]. Retinal dopamine loss in Parkinson's Disease is reflected by visual neurophysiological dysfunction [29]. In people with Parkinson's Disease there is also more sustained contraction of the muscles of the eye, including the orbicularis oculi, which controls eye closure and visual convergence [30].

Retinal thinning

Symptoms : The thickness of the retina is different in people with advanced Parkinson's Disease [31]. The inner retinal layer is thinner in people with Parkinson's Disease [26, 29, 32-35]. However, this is not always true [36]. Parkinson's Disease treatment made no difference to the degree of thinness of the retina [33]. The thickness of the outer retinal layer in Parkinson's Disease was no different [32].

Prevalence : Lengthier duration of Parkinson's Disease was associated with greater thinning of the retina [34]. In those people taking L-dopa, Age-related Macular Degeneration (AMD) occurred significantly later than in those people who did not take L-dopa. The likelihood of developing AMD at all is reduced in those people taking L-dopa [37].

Causes of symptoms : There is reduced dopaminergic activity in the retina of people with Parkinson's Disease [25-29], which could lead to a reduction in size of the retina.

[1] Ophthalmology [2012] 119 (1) : 178-182 (Z.Almer, K.S.Klein, L. Marsh, M.Gerstenhaber, M.X.Repka)

[2] Movement Disorders [1992] 7 (3) : 232-238 (R.D.Jones, I.M. Donaldson, P.L.Timmings)

[3] Neurology [1988] 38 (1) : 76-81 (C.Bulens, J.D.Meerwaldt, G.J. Van der Wildt)

[4] Brain [1987] 110 (Part 2) : 415-432 (D.Regan, C.Maxner)

[5] Movement Disorders [2011] 26 (13) : 2387-2395 (N.K.Archibald, M.P.Clarke, U.P. Mosimann, D.J.Burn)

[6] Neurology [1992] 42 (4) : 887-890 (M.J.Price, R.G.Feldman, D. Adelberg, H.Kayne)

[7] Journal of the Neurological Sciences [2000] 172 (1) : 7-11 (V.Pieri, N.J.Diederich, R.Raman, C.G.Goetz)

[8] Journal of Neuroophthalmology [2015] 35 (3) : 254-258 (M.Kaur, R.Saxena, D.Singh, M.Behari, P.Sharma, V.Menon)

[9] Movement Disorders [2012] 27 (14) : 1781-1788 (J.A.Bertrand, C.Bedetti, R.B.Postuma, O.Monchi, D.Génier Marchand, T.Jubault, J.F.Gagnon)

[10] European Journal of Neurology [2011] 18 (4) : 577-583 (Y.S.Oh, J.S.Kim, S.W.Chung, I.U.Song, Y.D.Kim, Y.I.Kim, K.S.Lee)

[11] Acta Neurologica Scandinavica [2002] 105 (4) : 256-260 (T. Müller, D.Woitalla, S.Peters, K.Kohla, H.Przuntek)

[12] Vision Research [1998] 38 (21) : 3427-3431 (B.C.Regan, N. Freudenthaler, R.Kolle, J.D.Mollon, W.Paulus)

[13] Neurology [1995] 45 (2) : 386-387 (T.Büttner, W.Kuhn, T.Müller, T.Patzold, K.Heidbrink, H.Przuntek)

[14] Journal of Neurology [1998] 245 (10) : 659-664 (T.Müller, W. Kuhn, T.Büttner, E.Eising, H.Coenen, M.Haas, H.Przuntek)

[15] Neurologica Scandinavica Acta [1997] 96 (5) : 293-296 (T. Müller, W.Kuhn, T. Büttner, H.Przuntek)

[16] Vision Research [1998] 38 (21) : 3421-3426 (J.Birch, R.U.Kolle, M.Kunkel, W.Paulus, P.Upadhyay)

[17] Neurology [2005] 65 (12) : 1907-1913 (E.Y.Uc, M.Rizzo, S.W. Anderson, S.Qian, R.L.Rodnitzky, J.D.Dawson)

[18] Neurology [2004] 63 (11) : 2091-2096 (U.P.Mosimann, G.Mather, K.A.Wesnes, J.T.O'Brien, D.J.Burn, I.G.McKeith)

[19] Behavioural Neurology [1997] 10 (2) : 77-81 (S.A.McDowell, J.P. Harris)

[20] Parkinsonism & Related Disorders [2014] 20 (3) : 318-322 (P. Urwyler, T.Nef, A.Killen, D.Collerton, A.Thomas, D.Burn, I. McKeith, U.P.Mosimann)

[21] Journal of Pediatric Ophthalmology and Strabismus [1996] 33 (3) : 144-147 (M.X.Repka, M.C.Claro, D.N.Loupe, S.G.Reich)

[22] Neurology [2004] 62 (2) : 177-180 (V.Biousse, B.C.Skibell, R.L.Watts, D.N.Loupe, C.Drews-Botsch, N.J.Newman)

[23] Clinical Autonomic Research [1991] 1 (1) : 55-58 (G.Micieli, C. Tassorelli, E.Martignoni, C.Pacchetti, P.Bruggi, M.Magri, G.Nappi)

[24] Vision Research [1997] 37 (24) : 3509-3529 (M.B.Djamgoz, M.W.Hankins, J.Hirano, S.N.Archer)

[25] Journal of Parkinson's Disease [2014] 4 (2) : 197-204 (J.Y.Lee, J.Ahn, T.W.Kim, B.S.Jeon)

[26] Journal of Neuro-Ophthalmology [2013] 33 (1) : 62-65 (S.Kirbas, K.Turkyilmaz, A.Tufekci, M.Durmus)

[27] Neurology Clinical Practice [2003] 21 (3) : 709-728 (G.R. Jackson, C.Owsley)

[28] Surgical and Radiologic Anatomy [1988] 10 (2) : 137-144 (J. Nguyen-Legros)

[29] Vision Research [2004] 44 (24) : 2793-2797 (R.Inzelberg, J.A. Ramirez, P.Nisipeanu, A.Ophir)

[30] Neurology [1982] 32 (7) : 749-754 (C.J.Hunker, J.H.Abbs, S.M. Barlow)

[31] Retina [2014] 34 (5) : 971-980 (E.Garcia-Martin, M.Satue, S. Otin, I.Fuertes, R.Alarcia, J.M.Larrosa, V.Polo, L.E.Pablo)

[32] Archives of Ophthalmology [2009] 127 (6) : 737-741 (M.E.Hajee, W.F.March, D.R.Lazzaro, A.H.Wolintz, E.M.Shrier, S.Glazman, I.G. Bodis-Wollner)

[33] European Journal of Ophthalmology [2014] 24 (1) : 114-119 (A. Sen, B.Tugcu, C.Coskun, C.Ekinci, S.A.Nacaroglu)

[34] European Journal of Neurology [2013] 20 (1) : 198-201 (C.La Morgia, P.Barboni, G.Rizzo, M.Carbonelli, G.Savini, C.Scaglione, S. Capellari, S.Bonazza, M.P.Giannoccaro, G.Calandra-Buonaura, et al)

[35] American Journal of Ophthalmology [2014] 157 (2) : 470-478 (E. Garcia-Martin, J.M.Larrosa, V.Polo, M.Satue, M.L.Marques, R. Alarcia, M.Seral, I.Fuertes, S.Otin, L.E.Pablo)

[36] Parkinsonism & Related Disorders [2011] 17 (6) : 431-436 (N.K. Archibald, M.P.Clarke, U.P.Mosimann, D.J.Burn)

[37] American Journal of Medicine [2016] 129 (3) : 292-298 (M.H. Brilliant, K.Vaziri, T.B.Connor Jr, S.G.Schwartz, J.J.Carroll, C.A. McCarty, S.J. Schrodi, S.J.Hebbring, K.S.Kishor, et al)

[38] Investigative Ophthalmology and Visual Science [2017] 58 (2) : 1151-1157 (M.Satue, M.J.Rodrigo, J.Obis, E.Vilades, H.Gracia, S.Otin, M.I.Fuertes, R.Alarcia, J.A.Crespo, V.Polo, J.M.Larrosa, et al)

Gustatory system

The gustatory system is the sensory system for the sense of taste. Taste reception occurs in specialised receptors in the mouth known as taste cells. They are contained in bundles called taste buds, which are contained in raised areas known as papillae. Papillae are found across the tongue. There are different types of taste receptor for each type of taste.

HYPOGEUSIA

Symptoms : There is often an impaired sense of taste (hypogeusia) in people with Parkinson's Disease [1-9]. The sense of taste is least impaired at the front of the tongue [10].

Prevalence : More than 25% of people with Parkinson's Disease have a diminished sense of taste [7]. Diminished sense of taste is more prevalent in late onset Parkinson's Disease [9], and in women more than men [11].

Causes of symptoms : Diminished sense of taste in Parkinson's Disease is not correlated with age, the duration of Parkinson's Disease, the severity of Parkinson's Disease or the strength of the sense of smell [7, 8]. In a number of neurological disorders there is a decrease in fungiform papillae. It is uncertain as to whether or not the decrease in taste that often occurs in people who have Parkinson's Disease is accompanied by a reduction in fungiform papillae or is caused by it [12].

[1] Clinical Neurology and Neurosurgery [2013] 115 (10) : 2103- 2107 (M.Z.Zhou, J.Gan, Y.R.Wei, X.Y.Ren, W.Chen, Z.G.Liu)

[2] Canadian Journal of Neurological Science [2013] 40 (1) : 36-41 (J.S.Kim, J.Youn, H.Shin, J.W.Cho)

[3] Journal of Neural Transmission [2013] 120 (4) : 531-535 (K.C. Breen, G.Drutyte)

[4] PLoS One [2013] 8 (2) : e49596 (M.H.Yong, J.C.Allen Jr, K.M. Prakash, E.K.Tan)

[5] Movement Disorders [2010] 25 (11) : 1646-1651 (M.Politis, K. Wu, S.Molloy, P.Bain, K.R.Chaudhuri, P.Piccini)

[6] Internal Medicine [2011] 50 (20) : 2311-2315 (K.Kashihara, A. Hanaoka, T.Imamura)

[7] Parkinsonism & Related Disorders [2009] 15 (3) : 232-237 (M. Shah, J.Deeb, M.Fernando, A.Noyce, E.Visentin, L.J.Findley, C.H. Hawkes)

[8] Journal of Neurology [2011] 258 (6) : 1076-1079 (H.J.Kim, B.S.Jeon, J.Y.Lee, Y.J.Cho, K.S.Hong, J.Y.Cho)

[9] Journal of Neurology [2013] 260 (1) : 131-137 (V.Spica, T. Pekmezovic, M.Svetel, V.S.Kostic)

[10] Journal of Neurology [2015] 262 (3) : 547-557 (R.L.Doty, M.T. Nsoesie, I.Chung, A.Osman, I.Pawasarat, J.Caulfield, H.Hurtig, J.Silas, J.Dubroff, J.E.Duda, G.S.Ying, H.Tekeli, F.E.Leon-Sarmiento)

[11] Journal of Neurology [2012] 259 (8) : 1639-1647 (P.Martinez-Martin, C.Falup Pecurariu, P.Odin, J.J.van Hilten, A.Antonini, J.M. Rojo-Abuin, V.Borges, C.Trenkwalder, D.Aarsland, D.J.Brooks, et al)

[12] The Neuroscientist [2008] 14 (3) : 240-250 (J.Gardiner, D.Barton, J.M.Vanslambrouck, F.Braet, D.Hall, J.Marc, R.Overall)

AUDITORY SYSTEM

The auditory system is the sensory system for the sense of hearing. It includes both the sensory organs, the ears, and the auditory parts of the sensory system. The key structure in the auditory system is the hair cell. Hair cells in the Organ of Corti in the cochlea can respond to sound.

HEARING LOSS

Symptoms : Hearing loss, which is also known as hearing impairment is a partial or total inability to hear. An affected person may be described as hard of hearing. A deaf person has little to no hearing. Hearing loss may occur in one or both ears. Hearing loss can be temporary or permanent.

Prevalence : Hearing loss is three times more likely in elderly people who have Parkinson's Disease. However, hearing loss is still 1.77 times more likely in elderly people with Parkinson's Disease than it is in elderly people who do not have Parkinson's Disease [1]. Impaired

speech recognition was more affected in people with Parkinson's Disease who had hearing impairment [2].
Causes of symptoms : Hearing is perceived in the Cochlea, in the Organ of Corti, which is the sensory organ of hearing. Dopamine helps to protect against noise exposure in the Cochlea [3-6]. Insufficient dopamine can therefore lead to damage that can result in loss or reduction of hearing.

[1] European Journal of Neurology [2014] 21 (5) : 752-757 (S.W.Lai, K.F.Liao, C.L.Lin, C.C.Lin, F.C.Sung)

[2] Parkinsonism & Related Disorders [2016] 22 (Supplement 1) : S138-S143 (C.Vitale, V.Marcelli, T.Abate, A.Pianese, R.Allocca, M.Moccia, E.Spina, P,Barone, G.Santangelo, M.Cavaliere)

[3] Neurochemical International [2011] 59 (2) : 150-158 (B.Lendvai, G.B.Halmos, G.Polony, J.Kapocsi, T.Horváth, M.Aller, E.Sylvester Vizi, T.Zelles)

[4] Advances in to Oto-rhino-laryngology [2002] 59 : 131-139 (E. Oestreicher, A.Wolfgang, D.Felix)

[5] European Journal of Neuroscience [2001] 14 (6) : 977-986 (J.Ruel, R.Nouvian, C.Gervais d'Aldin, R.Pujol, M.Eybalin, J.L.Puel)

[6] Progress in Neurobiology [1995] 47 (6) : 449-476 (J.L.Puel)

CHAPTER 29

SYMPTOMS OF PARKINSON'S DISEASE

ENDOCRINE SYSTEM

ENDOCRINE SYSTEM

The endocrine glands include the pineal gland, pituitary gland, thyroid gland, thymus, adrenal gland, pancreas, parathyroid gland, ovaries, testes, and hypothalamus. The endocrine system refers to glands that secrete hormones directly into the circulatory system to be carried towards target organs.

PRIMARY SYMPTOMS

In Parkinson's Disease there is an increased likelihood of hyperprolactinemia [PAGE 363] in the pituitary gland, blunted circadian rhythms [PAGE 364] in the pineal gland, hypothyroidism [PAGE 365] in the thyroid gland, and catecholamine deficiency [PAGE 367] in the adrenal gland.

PITUITARY GLAND

The pituitary gland (hypophysis) is a small endocrine gland in the brain. It is a protrusion off the bottom of the hypothalamus at the base of the brain. The pituitary gland produces a number of hormones including prolactin.

HYPERPROLACTINEMIA

Symptoms : Hyperprolactinemia is the increased secretion of prolactin from the pituitary gland. It affects the reproductive functions.

Prevalence : In most people with Parkinson's Disease the levels of prolactin are raised [1, 2, 3], but in some people with Parkinson's

Disease the prolactin levels are normal [4, 5]. In those people with normal levels of prolactin, the normal levels appear to be due to the effects of Parkinson's Disease drugs [3, 5].

Causes of symptoms : In Parkinson's Disease there is low dopamine. Dopamine inhibits the formation of prolactin [6]. So in Parkinson's Disease the reduced dopamine levels enable higher levels of prolactin.

[1] Acta Neurologica Scandinavica [2015] 131 (6) : 411-416 (M. Nitkowska, R.Tomasiuk, M.Czyzyk, A.Friedman)

[2] Journal of Neurology [1991] 238 (1) : 19-22 (G.Bellomo, L. Santambrogio, M.Fiacconi, A.M.Scarponi, G.Ciuffetti)

[3] Acta Medica Hungarica [1994] 50 (1-2) : 3-13 (K.Otake, Y.Oiso, T.Mitsuma, Y.Hirooka, K.Adachi)

[4] Journal of Neuroendocrinology [2011] 23 (6) : 519-524 (N.A.Aziz, H.Pijl, M.Frölich, F.Roelfsema, R.A.Roos)

[5] Neurology [1986] 36 (3) : 393-395 (A.Laihinen, U.K.Rinne)

[6] Endocrine Reviews [2001] 22 (6) : 724-763 (N.Ben-Jonathan, R. Hnasko)

Pineal gland

The pineal gland is a small endocrine gland in the brain. It is located in the epithalamus, near the centre of the brain. The pineal gland produces melatonin, which regulates sleep patterns in seasonal and circadian rhythms.

Blunted circadian rhythms

Symptoms : Most people with Parkinson's Disease have been found to have blunted circadian rhythms. The pineal gland produces melatonin, which is a hormone that regulates the circadian rhythms. Circadian rhythms are the alterations of endocrine functions that take place in a regulated manner over a roughly 24 hour period [1].

Prevalence : The differences and the range of secretion of melatonin from the pineal gland were found to be lower in Parkinson's Disease than in people that do not have Parkinson's Disease. Overall Parkinson's Disease symptoms and duration of symptoms were not significantly related to the circadian rhythm. So it was only daytime sleepiness and not Parkinson's Disease symptoms generally that can be affected by the blunted circadian rhythm that can occur in Parkinson's Disease [1].

Cause of symptoms : Dopamine regulates melatonin secretion [2]. Therefore, the reduced dopamine that occurs in Parkinson's Disease will lead to an altered circadian rhythm.

[1] JAMA Neurology [2014] 71 (4) : 463-469 (A.Videnovic, C.Noble, K.J.Reid, J.Peng, F.W.Turek, A.Marconi, A.W. Rademaker, T.Simuni, C.Zadikoff, P.C.Zee)

[2] PLoS Biology [2012] 10 (6) : e1001347 (S.González, D.Moreno-Delgado, E.Moreno, K.Pérez-Capote, R.Franco, J.Mallol, A.Cortés, V. Casadó, C.Lluís, J.Ortiz, S.Ferré, E.Canela, P.J.McCormick)

Thyroid gland

The thyroid gland is an endocrine gland that produces thyroid hormones, the main ones being thyroxine (T4) and triiodothyronine (T3), which is more active. These hormones regulate the growth and rate of function of many other systems in the body.

Hypothyroidism

Symptoms : Common symptoms of hypothyroidism are fatigue, feeling cold, poor memory and concentration, depression, reduced sex drive, constipation, weight gain, muscle cramps, shortness of breath, poor hearing, hair loss [1]. There is a similarity between some of the symptoms of hypothyroidism and Parkinson’s Disease [2-5]. Consequently hypothyroidism can remain undiagnosed [2-4] or Parkinson’s Disease can at first appear to be hypothyroidism [6].

Prevalence : The prevalence of hypothyroidism was found to be marginally greater in Parkinson's Disease in some studies [7, 8], more so when there was akinesia and rigidity [9]. However, in some other studies the prevalence of hypothyroidism was found to be no greater than normal [5, 10].

Causes of symptoms : Hypothyroidism is not a symptom of Parkinson's Disease. However, the symptoms of hypothyroidism and Parkinson's Disease can sometimes occur together to some degree because L-tyrosine is required for the formation of dopamine and the thyroid hormones.

[1] Harrison's Principles of Internal Medicine [2011] : 341 (Disorders of the thyroid gland) (D.L.Longo, A.S.Fauci, D.L.Kasper, S.L.Hauser, J.L.Jameson, J.Loscalzo)

[2] Movement Disorders [2003] 18 (9) : 1058-1059 (J.M. García-Moreno, J.Chacón-Peña)

[3] Revista de Neurologia [2002] 35 (8) : 741-742 (J.M.García-Moreno, J.Chacón)

[4] Postgraduate Medicine [1993] 94 (5) : 187-190 (H.B.Tandeter, P. Shvartzman)

[5] Acta Neurologica Scandinavica [1987] 75 (5) : 364-365 (A.C. Johannessen, A.Boye, H.Pakkenberg)

[6] Diseases of the Nervous System [1968] 29 (6) : 396-398 (R.R. Strang)

[7] Parkinsonism & Related Disorders [2004] 10 (6) : 381-383 (R.P. Munhoz, H.A.Teive, A.R.Troiano, P.R.Hauck, M.H.Herdoiza M.H. Leiva, H.Graff, L.C.Werneck)

[8] Neurology [1981] 31 (1) : 93-95 (J.R.Berger, R.E.Kelley)

[9] Canadian Journal of Neurological Sciences [1983] 10 (1) : 37-42 (M.Roy, L.Boyer, A.Barbeau)

[10] Archives of Gerontology and Geriatrics [2001] 33 (3) : 295-300 (H.Tandeter, A.Levy, G.Gutman, P.Shvartzman)

Adrenal gland

The adrenal glands are endocrine glands that produce several hormones including adrenaline and the steroids aldosterone and cortisol. The adrenal glands are above the kidneys. The adrenal medulla is part of the adrenal gland. It is located at the centre of the adrenal gland and is surrounded by the adrenal cortex. It secretes the hormones adrenaline and noradrenaline.

Catecholamine deficiency

Symptoms : In Parkinson's Disease there is a reduction in the levels of the catecholamines (adrenaline and noradrenaline) in the adrenal medulla [1-4].

Prevalence : There have not been any assessments of the prevalence of catecholamine deficiency in Parkinson's Disease. However, Parkinson's Disease is frequently accompanied by a variety of autonomic symptoms.

Causes of symptoms : The catecholamines adrenaline and noradrenaline are biosynthesized from dopamine. So the insufficient dopamine that occurs in Parkinson's Disease will lead to low levels of catecholamines in the adrenal medulla. The catecholamine deficiency is not due to Parkinson's Disease drugs [4].

[1] New England Journal of Medicine [1988] 318 (4) : 254 (S.W. Carmichael, R.J.Wilson, W.S.Brimijoin, L.J.Melton, H.Okazaki, T.L. Yaksh, J.E.Ahlskog, S.L.Stoddard, G.M.Tyce)

[2] Experimental Neurology [1989] 104 (1) : 22-27 (S.L.Stoddard, G.M.Tyce, J.E.Ahlskog, A.R.Zinsmeister, S.W.Carmichael)

[3] Reviews in the Neurosciences [1994] 5 (4) : 293-307 (S.L. Stoddard)

[4] Microscopy Research and Technique [1994] 29 (2) : 151-154 (S.L. Stoddard, G.J.Merkel, J.A.Cook, A.R.Zinsmeister, S.W. Carmichael)

CHAPTER 30

SYMPTOMS OF PARKINSON'S DISEASE

REPRODUCTIVE SYSTEM

Reproductive system

The reproductive system is a system of sex organs which work together for the purpose of sexual activity and sexual reproduction. Many non-living substances such as fluids, hormones, and pheromones are important accessories for the proper functioning of the reproductive system.

Primary symptoms

Parkinson's Disease can cause sexual dysfunction in men and women. Sexual dysfunction is common in Parkinson's Disease, with over 40% of people with Parkinson's Disease being affected in this way [1]. Over two thirds of people with Parkinson's Disease had decreased sexual activity [2]. Nearly two thirds of people with Parkinson's Disease had a loss of sex drive [3, 4]. Sexual dissatisfaction is experienced by 37% of people [5]. Associated illnesses, use of medications, and advanced stage of Parkinson's Disease contributed to sexual dysfunction [6]. Sexual dysfunction was not otherwise related to age or age of onset [1] or duration [7] of Parkinson's Disease. Perception of sexual functioning is also considerably influenced by depression [8]. The neurological features that were most associated with a greater loss of sex drive and sexual activity were autonomic dysfunction, aging, depression, female gender and severer Parkinson's Disease [4, 9].

Male reproductive system

The male reproductive system can be grouped into three categories. The first category is the production and storage of sperm. This takes place in the testes, which are inside the scrotum. Immature sperm travel to the epididymis for development and storage. The second category are the ejaculatory fluid producing glands, which include the seminal vesicles, prostate, and the vas deferens. The third category are those organs and glands used for copulation, and deposition of the spermatozoa within the male. These include the penis, urethra, vas deferens, and Cowper's gland.

Male sexual dysfunction

Symptoms : There can be a profound impairment in sexual arousal, behaviour, orgasm, and sex drive [10]. Men with Parkinson's Disease report erectile dysfunction [2-6], premature ejaculation [6], difficulty ejaculating [6], sexual dissatisfaction [6, 8], and cessation of sexual activity during the course of the disease [6].

Prevalence : Men with Parkinson's Disease reported erectile dysfunction (38% to 68%) [2-6] (which was more frequent over 61 years of age [2]), sexual dissatisfaction (65%) [6], premature ejaculation (40%) [6], difficulty ejaculating (39%) [6], and cessation of sexual activity during the course of the disease (23%) [6]. In younger people with Parkinson's Disease 40% of men reported altered sex drive, while 33% of men experienced altered sexual activity [9].

Causes of symptoms : In Parkinson's Disease there is low dopamine that reduces the secretion of Gonadotropin-releasing hormone. Gonadotropin-releasing hormone is a releasing hormone responsible for the release of follicle-stimulating hormone (FSH) and luteinizing hormone (LH) [11-14]. Follicle-stimulating hormone (FSH) and luteinizing hormone (LH) have effects on the male reproductive system, including on testosterone secretion which is consequently lower in Parkinson's Disease [15, 16].

Female reproductive system

The female reproductive system contains three main parts. The vagina, which also includes the labia, clitoris and urethra, leads from the vulva, the vaginal opening, to the uterus. The uterus holds the developing fetus. The ovaries produce the female's ova. The vagina is attached to the uterus through the cervix. The uterus is attached to the ovaries via the fallopian tubes.

Female sexual dysfunction

Symptoms : There can be a profound impairment in sexual arousal, behaviour, orgasm, and sex drive [10]. Women with Parkinson's Disease report difficulties with arousal [6], reaching orgasm [6], sexual dissatisfaction [6, 7, 8, 17], cessation of sexual activity during the course of the disease [6], and reduced sexual desire [6, 7].

Prevalence : Sexual dysfunction is more prevalent in women with Parkinson's Disease, with as many as 87% experiencing sexual dysfunction [18]. Women reported difficulties with arousal (87%), reaching orgasm (75%), low sexual desire (46%), sexual dissatisfaction (37%), and cessation of sexual activity during the course of the disease (21%) [6]. The age of women was associated with significant changes in satisfaction and activity [17]. The severity and duration of Parkinson's Disease were not associated with sexual dysfunction in women [19]. In younger people with Parkinson's Disease 70% of women reported altered sex drive, while 80% of women experienced altered sexual activity [9].

Causes of symptoms : In Parkinson's Disease there is low dopamine that reduces the secretion of Gonadotropin-releasing hormone. Gonadotropin-releasing hormone is a releasing hormone responsible for the release of follicle-stimulating hormone (FSH) and luteinizing hormone (LH) [11-14]. Follicle- stimulating hormone (FSH), and luteinizing hormone (LH), which is low in women with Parkinson's Disease [20], have effects on the female reproductive system by lowering estrogen levels.

[1] Zhonghua Nan Ke Xue [2013] 19 (6) : 518-521 (X.Hu, W.G.Liu, F.L.Yan)

[2] Neurologia [1994] 9 (5) : 178-181 (J.A.Burguera, L.García Reboll, E.Martínez Agulló)

[3] Journal of Sexual Medicine [2009] 6 (4) : 1024-1031 (A. Kummer, F.Cardoso, A.L.Teixeira)

[4] Journal of Sexual Medicine [2009] 6 (4) : 1024-1031 (A. Kummer, F.Cardoso, A.L.Teixeira)

[5] Journal of Sexual Medicine [2010] 7 (4 Part 1) : 1438-1444 (C.L.Wielinski, S.C.Varpness, C.Erickson-Davis, A.J.Paraschos, S.A. Parashos)

[6] Journal of Sex and Marital Therapy [2004] 30 (2) : 95-105 (G.Bronner, V.Royter, A.D.Korczyn, N.Giladi)

[7] European Journal of Neurology [2008] 15 (11) : 1168-1172 (E.Celikel, E.T.Ozel-Kizil, M.C.Akbostanci, A.Cevik)

[8] Journal of Neurology, Neurosurgery and Psychiatry [2000] 69 (4) : 550-552 (H. Jacobs, A. Vieregge, P.Vieregge)

[9] Acta Neurologica Scandinavica [1995] 91 (6) : 453-455 (L.Wermuth, E.Stenager)

[10] American Journal of Geriatric Psychiatry [2004] 12 (2) : 221-226 (M.Yu, D.M.Roane, C.R.Miner, M.Fleming, J.D.Rogers)

[11] Bulletin of Mathematical Biology [2008] 70 (8) : 2211-2228 (R.Bertram, Y.X.Li)

[12] Proceedings, National Academy Sciences, U.S.A. [2005] 102 (5) : 1761-1766 (S.Messager, E.E.Chatzidaki, D.Ma, A.G.Hendrick, D. Zahn, J.Dixon, R.R.Thresher, I.Malinge, D.Lomet, M.B.Carlton, et al)

[13] European Journal of Contraception and Reproductive Health Care [1998] 3 (1) : 21-28 (M.Stomati, A.D.Genazzani, F.Petraglia, A.R. Genazzani)

[14] Brain Research [1986] 399 (1) : 15-23. (K.Y.Pau, H.G.Spies)

[15] Journal of Neurology, Neurosurgery and Psychiatry [2004] 75 (9) : 1323-1326 (R.E.Ready, J.Friedman, J.Grace, H.Fernandez)

[16] Neurology [2004] 62 (3) : 411-413 (M.S.Okun, M.R.DeLong, J. Hanfelt, M.Gearing, A.Levey)

[17] Movement Disorders [1997] 12 (6) : 923-927 (M.Welsh, L.Hung, C.H.Waters)

[18] Movement Disorders [2016] Aug 8 [Epub ahead of print] (S. Varanda, J.Ribeiro da Silva, A.S.Costa, C.Amorim de Carvalho, J.N. Alves, M.Rodrigues, G.Carneiro)

[19] European Journal of Neurology [2008] 15 (11) : 1168-1167 (E.Celikel, E.T.Ozel-Kizil, M.C.Akbostanci, A.Cevik)

[20] Journal of Neural Transmission (Parkinson's Disease and Dementia Section) [1990] 2 (3) : 225-231 (U.Bonuccelli, P.Piccini, A.Napolitano, A.Cagnacci, A.M.Paoletti, G.B.Melis, A.Muratorio)

CHAPTER 31

SYMPTOMS OF PARKINSON'S DISEASE

IMMUNE SYSTEM

Immune system

The immune system is a diffuse network of interacting cells, cell products, and cell-forming tissues. The immune system includes the thymus, spleen, lymph nodes and lymph tissue, macrophages, lymphocytes, antibodies and lymphokines. The immune system protects the body from pathogens and other foreign substances, destroys infected and malignant cells, and removes cellular debris.

Primary symptoms

Neuroinflammation commonly, but not always, occurs in Parkinson's Disease [PAGE 373]. There is a greater likelihood of CNS infections occurring in Parkinson's Disease after diagnosis, and also before being diagnosed with Parkinson's Disease [PAGE 375].

Neuroinflammation

Symptoms : Neuroinflammation is a defence mechanism associated with the restoration of the normal structure and function of the brain [1]. People with Parkinson's Disease who have neuroinflammation present with all of the classical features of inflammation including phagocyte activation, complement activation, increased synthesis and release of proinflammatory cytokines [2]. In people with Parkinson's Disease activated microglial cells and T lymphocytes have been detected in the substantia nigra concomitantly with an increased expression of pro-inflammatory mediators [3]. Under conditions of increased glucocorticoids, the elevated prolactin that occurs in Parkinson's Disease functions physiologically to maintain the survival and function of T-lymphocytes [4].

Prevalence : In people with Parkinson's Disease neuroinflammation appears to be a ubiquitous finding [2]. Neuroinflammatory changes have been repeatedly demonstrated in people with Parkinson's Disease [1, 5, 6]. Increases in pro-inflammatory factor levels are common features of Parkinson's Disease [7, 8].

Causes of symptoms : In Parkinson's Disease there is low dopamine. The low dopamine that occurs in Parkinson's Disease enables the increased secretion of prolactin from the pituitary gland [9]. Prolactin prevents the action of glucocorticoids on the immune response [10]. Glucocorticoids normally reduce inflammation and the permeability of the blood brain barrier [11]. Consequently, the increased prolactin promotes pro-inflammatory immune responses [12].

[1] Mediators of Inflammation [2013] : 952375 (S.V.More, H.Kumar, I.S.Kim, S.Y.Song, D.K.Choi)

[2] British Journal of Pharmacology [2007] 150 (8) : 963-976 (P.S. Whitton)

[3] Parkinsonism & Related Disorders [2012] 18 (Supplement 1) : S210-S212 (E.C.Hirsch, S.Vyas, S.Hunot)

[4] Endocrinology [2003] 144 (5) : 2102-2110 (N.Krishnan, O.Thellin, D.J.Buckley, N.D.Horseman, A.R.Buckley)

[5] Journal of Neuroimmune Pharmacology [2013] 8 (1) : 189-201 (F. Blandini)

[6] Histology and Histopathology [2006] 21 (6) : 673-678 (H.Arai, T.Furuya, Y.Mizuno, H.Mochizuki)

[7] Translational Neurodegeneration [2015] 4 : 19 (Q.Wang, Y.Liu, J.Zhou)

[8] Brain Pathology [2014] 24 (6) : 584-598 (P.Garcia-Esparcia, F.Llorens, M.Carmona, I.Ferrer)

[9] Endocrine Reviews [2001] 22 (6) : 724-763 (N.Ben-Jonathan, R. Hnasko)

[10] Rossiiskii Fiziologicheskii Zhurnal Imeni I M Sechenova [2003] 89 (9) : 1117-1126 (E.E.Fomicheva, E.A.Nemirovich-Danchenko)

[11] Frontiers in Neuroanatomy [2015] 9 : 32 (M.T.Herrero, C.Estrada, L.Maatouk, S.Vyas)

[12] European Cytokine Network [2004] 15 (2) : 99-104 (J.M.Brand, C.Frohn, K.Cziupka, C.Brockmann, H.Kirchner, J.Luhm)

CNS INFECTIONS

Symptoms : Infections in the central nervous system (CNS) are caused by a wide range of microorganisms resulting in distinct clinical syndromes including meningitis, encephalitis, and pyogenic infections, such as empyema (accumulations of pus) and brain abscesses. As pus and other material from an infection accumulate, pressure is exerted on the brain or spinal cord. This pressure can damage the nervous system tissue, possibly permanently. Bacterial and viral infections in the central nervous system can be rapidly fatal and can result in severe disability in survivors [1].

Prevalence : People with Parkinson's Disease are 1.8 times more likely to be hospitalized for a CNS infection. People who had been hospitalized in the year preceding being diagnosed with Parkinson's Disease or who had multiple CNS infections at least five years before diagnosis were over 3 times more likely to develop Parkinson's Disease [2].

Causes of symptoms : The blood-brain barrier is a tightly regulated interface in the Central Nervous System that regulates the exchange of molecules in and out from the brain. It is mainly composed of endothelial cells, pericytes and astrocytes [3]. During the course of Parkinson's Disease there is dysfunction of the blood-brain barrier [3]. There is consequently increased permeability of the blood-brain barrier [4, 5], which more specifically is in the postcommissural putamen in people who have Parkinson's Disease [5].

[1] Neurotherapeutics [2012] 9 (1) : 124-138 (J.D.Beckham, K.L.Tyler)

[2] International Journal of Epidemiology [2012] 41 (4) : 1042-1049 (F.Fang, K.Wirdefeldt, A.Jacks, F.Kamel, W.Ye, H.Chen)

[3] Journal of Cerebral Blood Flow and Metabolism [2015] 35 (5) : 747-750 (M.T.Gray, J.M.Woulfe)

[4] Neurodegenerative Disease [2015] 15 (2) : 63-69 (M.Fakhoury)

[5] Frontiers in Cellular Neuroscience [2014] 8 : 211 (R.Cabezas, M.Avila, J.Gonzalez, R.S.El-Bachá, E.Báez, L.M.García-Segura, J.C. Jurado Coronel, F.Capani, G.P.Cardona-Gomez, G.E.Barreto)

CHAPTER 32

DIAGNOSIS OF PARKINSON'S DISEASE

OBSERVATIONAL METHODS

DIAGNOSIS

Diagnosis is usually based on physical observation and questioning of the patients. The most commonly used symptom questionnaire is the Unified Parkinson Disease Rating Scale (UPDRS). Assessments can also involve the SPECT or PET scans, which are the most accurate methods of diagnosing Parkinson's Disease.

MISDIAGNOSIS

Misdiagnosis in Parkinson's Disease is very common. The average accuracy of diagnosing Parkinson's Disease is only 80% [1]. For clinical diagnosis performed by non-experts the accuracy is even less, at 73% [1]. Accuracy of clinical diagnosis performed by movement disorders experts rose from 79% at the initial assessment to 84% after a follow-up assessment [1]. However, initial diagnoses of Parkinson's Disease made by general neurologists were only infrequently changed [2]. They were incorrect in 18% to 35% of cases [1, 2, 3]. This means that many people have been treated for Parkinson's Disease without ever having had Parkinson's Disease. In people taking Parkinson's Disease drugs Parkinsonism was confirmed in only 74% of cases and only 53% of them had probable Parkinson's Disease. Over a quarter of the people diagnosed with Parkinson's Disease did not benefit from Parkinson's Disease drugs [3, 4]. More than 1 in 3 people with tremor were misdiagnosed as having Essential Tremor when most of them actually had Parkinson's Disease [5]. From 17% to 26% of people with tremor disorders were wrongly diagnosed as having tremor dominant Parkinson's Disease [6]. From 6% to 20% of people with tremor dominant Parkinson's Disease were wrongly diagnosed as having other tremor disorders [6]. The accuracy of diagnosing Parkinson's Disease had not significantly improved in the previous 25 years [1].

[1] Neurology [2016] 86 (6) : 566-576 (G.Rizzo, M.Copetti, S.Arcuti, D.Martino, A.Fontana, G.Logroscino)

[2] Archives of Neurology [2000] 57 (3) : 369-372 (J.Jankovic, A.H. Rajput, M.P.McDermott, D.P.Perl)

[3] Lancet Neurology [2006] 5 (1) : 75-86 (E.Tolosa, G.Wenning, W. Poewe)

[4] Age and Ageing [1999] 28 (2) : 99-102 (J.Meara, B.K.Bhowmick, P.Hobson)

[5] Archives of Neurology [2006] 63 (8) : 1100-1104 (S.Jain, S.E.Lo, E.D.Louis)

[6] Journal of Neurology, Neurosurgery and Psychiatry [2010] 81 (11) : 1223-1228 (N.P.Bajaj, V.Gontu, J.Birchall, J.Patterson, D.G.Grosset, A.J.Lees)

Observational methods of diagnosis

Besides the Unified Parkinson Disease Rating Scale (UPDRS) [PAGE 378], less common means of assessment are : the Hoen and Yahr [PAGE 389], which grades patients according to five stages of severity; the MDS-UPDRS [PAGE 390], which is a revision of the UPDRS; the modified Rankin Scale (mRS) [PAGE 391], which assesses the level of disability; the PDQ-39 [PAGE 392] and the PDQL [PAGE 395], which assess the quality of life; the Schwab and England Activities of Daily Living [PAGE 397]; and the Webster disability rating scale [PAGE 398], Systematic Screening of Handwriting Difficulties (SOS-test) [PAGE 402].

Unified Parkinson Disease Rating Scale (UPDRS)

The most commonly used symptom questionnaire is the Unified Parkinson Disease Rating Scale (UPDRS). The UPDRS involves scoring by a clinician, based on motor examination, and a historical report of mental functioning and activities of daily living obtained by questioning the patient. It enables the assessment of the worsening or improvement of symptoms over time. It encompasses earlier rating scales : the Hoehn and Yahr staging scale, and the modified Schwab and England activities of daily living scale [1]. There are four parts : I Mentation, behavior and mood, II Activities of daily living (for both "on" and "off"), III Motor examination, IV Complications of therapy. Only one option is chosen. The numbers next to each option is the score for that option. In monotherapy, a "Total UPDRS" score is the combined sum of parts I, II, and III : with a total score of from 0 (not affected) to 176 (most severely affected). In adjunct therapy, part IV is included. Part IV contains 11 questions and the scale can range from 0 to 23 [1].

I Mentation, behavior and mood

1. Intellectual Impairment

0 = None.
1 = Mild. Consistent forgetfulness with partial recollection of events and no other difficulties.
2 = Moderate memory loss, with disorientation and moderate difficulty handling complex problems. Mild but definite impairment of function at home with need of occasional prompting.
3 = Severe memory loss with disorientation for time and often to place. Severe impairment in handling problems.
4 = Severe memory loss with orientation preserved to person only. Unable to make judgements or solve problems. Requires much help with personal care. Cannot be left alone at all.

2. Thought Disorder (Due to dementia or drug intoxication)

0 = None.
1 = Vivid dreaming.
2 = "Benign" hallucinations with insight retained.
3 = Occasional to frequent hallucinations or delusions; without insight; could interfere with daily activities.
4 = Persistent hallucinations, delusions, or florrid psychosis. Not able to care for self.

3. Depression

0 = None.
1 = Periods of sadness or guilt greater than normal, never sustained for days or weeks.
2 = Sustained depression (1 week or more).
3 = Sustained depression with vegetative symptoms (insomnia, anorexia, weight loss, loss of interest).
4 = Sustained depression with vegetative symptoms and suicidal thoughts or intent.

4. Motivation/Initiative

0 = Normal.
1 = Less assertive than usual; more passive.
2 = Loss of initiative or disinterest in elective (nonroutine) activities.
3 = Loss of initiative or disinterest in day to day (routine) activities.
4 = Withdrawn, complete loss of motivation.

II Activities of daily living (for both "on" and "off")

5. Speech

0 = Normal.
1 = Mildly affected. No difficulty being understood.
2 = Moderately affected. Sometimes asked to repeat statements.
3 = Severely affected. Frequently asked to repeat statements.
4 = Unintelligible most of the time.

6. Salivation

0 = Normal.
1 = Slight but definite excess of saliva in mouth; may have nighttime drooling.
2 = Moderately excessive saliva; may have minimal drooling.
3 = Marked excess of saliva with some drooling.
4 = Marked drooling, requires constant tissue or handkerchief.

7. Swallowing

0 = Normal.
1 = Rare choking.
2 = Occasional choking.
3 = Requires soft food.
4 = Requires NG tube or gastrotomy feeding.

8. Handwriting

0 = Normal.
1 = Slightly slow or small.
2 = Moderately slow or small; all words are legible.
3 = Severely affected; not all words are legible.
4 = The majority of words are not legible.

9. Cutting food and handling utensils

0 = Normal.
1 = Somewhat slow and clumsy, but no help needed.
2 = Can cut most foods, although clumsy and slow; some help needed.
3 = Food must be cut by someone, but can still feed slowly.
4 = Needs to be fed.

10. Dressing

0 = Normal.
1 = Somewhat slow, but no help needed.
2 = Occasional assistance with buttoning, getting arms in sleeves.
3 = Considerable help required, but can do some things alone.
4 = Helpless.

11. Hygiene

0 = Normal.
1 = Somewhat slow, but no help needed.
2 = Needs help to shower or bathe; or very slow in hygienic care.
3 = Requires assistance for washing, brushing teeth, combing hair,

going to bathroom.
4 = Foley catheter or other mechanical aids.

12. Turning in bed and adjusting bed clothes

0 = Normal.
1 = Somewhat slow and clumsy, but no help needed.
2 = Can turn alone or adjust sheets, but with great difficulty.
3 = Can initiate, but not turn or adjust sheets alone.
4 = Helpless.

13. Falling (unrelated to freezing)

0 = None.
1 = Rare falling.
2 = Occasionally falls, less than once per day.
3 = Falls an average of once daily.
4 = Falls more than once daily.

14. Freezing when walking

0 = None.
1 = Rare freezing when walking; may have start hesitation.
2 = Occasional freezing when walking.
3 = Frequent freezing. Occasionally falls from freezing.
4 = Frequent falls from freezing.

15. Walking

0 = Normal.
1 = Mild difficulty. May not swing arms or may tend to drag leg.
2 = Moderate difficulty, but requires little or no assistance.
3 = Severe disturbance of walking, requiring assistance.
4 = Cannot walk at all, even with assistance.

16. Tremor (Symptomatic complaint of tremor in any part of body)

0 = Absent.

1 = Slight and infrequently present.
2 = Moderate; bothersome to patient.
3 = Severe; interferes with many activities.
4 = Marked; interferes with most activities.

17. Sensory complaints related to parkinsonism

0 = None.
1 = Occasionally has numbness, tingling, or mild aching.
2 = Frequently has numbness, tingling, or aching; not distressing.
3 = Frequent painful sensations.
4 = Excruciating pain.

III Motor examination

18. Speech

0 = Normal.
1 = Slight loss of expression, diction and/or volume.
2 = Monotone, slurred but understandable; moderately impaired.
3 = Marked impairment, difficult to understand.
4 = Unintelligible.

19. Facial Expression (head, upper and lower extremities)

0 = Normal.
1 = Minimal hypomimia, could be normal "Poker Face".
2 = Slight but definitely abnormal diminution of facial expression.
3 = Moderate hypomimia; lips parted some of the time.
4 = Masked or fixed facies with severe or complete loss of facial expression; lips parted 1/4 inch or more.

20. Tremor at rest

0 = Absent.
1 = Slight and infrequently present.
2 = Mild in amplitude and persistent. Or moderate in amplitude, but only intermittently present.

3 = Moderate in amplitude and present most of the time.
4 = Marked in amplitude and present most of the time.

21. Action or Postural Tremor of hands (Judged on passive movement of major joints with patient relaxed in sitting position. Cogwheeling to be ignored.)

0 = Absent.
1 = Slight; present with action.
2 = Moderate in amplitude, present with action.
3 = Moderate in amplitude with posture holding as well as action.
4 = Marked in amplitude; interferes with feeding.

22. Rigidity (Patient taps thumb with index finger in rapid succession.)

0 = Absent.
1 = Slight or detectable only when activated by mirror or other movements.
2 = Mild to moderate.
3 = Marked, but full range of motion easily achieved.
4 = Severe, range of motion achieved with difficulty.

23. Finger Taps (Patient opens and closes hands in rapid succesion.)

0 = Normal.
1 = Mild slowing and/or reduction in amplitude.
2 = Moderately impaired. Definite and early fatiguing. May have occasional arrests in movement.
3 = Severely impaired. Frequent hesitation in initiating movements or arrests in ongoing movement.
4 = Can barely perform the task.

24. Hand Movements (Pronation-supination movements of hands, vertically and horizontally, with as large an amplitude as possible, both hands simultaneously.)

0 = Normal.
1 = Mild slowing and/or reduction in amplitude.

2 = Moderately impaired. Definite and early fatiguing. May have occasional arrests in movement.
3 = Severely impaired. Frequent hesitation in initiating movements or arrests in ongoing movement.
4 = Can barely perform the task.

25. Rapid Alternating Movements of Hands (Patient taps heel on the ground in rapid succession picking up entire leg. Amplitude should be at least 3 inches.)

0 = Normal.
1 = Mild slowing and/or reduction in amplitude.
2 = Moderately impaired. Definite and early fatiguing. May have occasional arrests in movement.
3 = Severely impaired. Frequent hesitation in initiating movements or arrests in ongoing movement.
4 = Can barely perform the task.

26. Leg Agility (Patient attempts to rise from a straightbacked chair, with arms folded across chest.)

0 = Normal.
1 = Mild slowing and/or reduction in amplitude.
2 = Moderately impaired. Definite and early fatiguing. May have occasional arrests in movement.
3 = Severely impaired. Frequent hesitation in initiating movements or arrests in ongoing movement.
4 = Can barely perform the task.

27. Arising from Chair

0 = Normal.
1 = Slow; or may need more than one attempt.
2 = Pushes self up from arms of seat.
3 = Tends to fall back and may have to try more than one time, but can get up without help.
4 = Unable to arise without help.

28. Posture

0 = Normal erect.
1 = Not quite erect, slightly stooped posture; could be normal for older person.
2 = Moderately stooped posture, definitely abnormal; can be slightly leaning to one side.
3 = Severely stooped posture with kyphosis; can be moderately leaning to one side.
4 = Marked flexion with extreme abnormality of posture.

29. Gait (Response to sudden, strong posterior displacement produced by pull on shoulders while patient erect with eyes open and feet slightly apart. Patient is prepared.)

0 = Normal.
1 = Walks slowly, may shuffle with short steps, but no festination (hastening steps) or propulsion.
2 = Walks with difficulty, but requires little or no assistance; may have some festination, short steps, or propulsion.
3 = Severe disturbance of gait, requiring assistance.
4 = Cannot walk at all, even with assistance.

30. Postural Stability (Combining slowness, hesitancy, decreased armswing, small amplitude, and poverty of movement in general.)

0 = Normal.
1 = Retropulsion, but recovers unaided.
2 = Absence of postural response; would fall if not caught by examiner.
3 = Very unstable, tends to lose balance spontaneously.
4 = Unable to stand without assistance.

31. Body Bradykinesia and Hypokinesia

0 = None.
1 = Minimal slowness, giving movement a deliberate character; could be normal for some persons. Possibly reduced amplitude.

2 = Mild degree of slowness and poverty of movement which is definitely abnormal. Alternatively, some reduced amplitude.
3 = Moderate slowness, poverty or small amplitude of movement.
4 = Marked slowness, poverty or small amplitude of movement.

IV. Complications of therapy (In the past week)

A. Dyskinesias

32. Duration: What proportion of the waking day are dyskinesias present ? (Historical information.)

0 = None
1 = 1-25% of day.
2 = 26-50% of day.
3 = 51-75% of day.
4 = 76-100% of day.

33. Disability: How disabling are the dyskinesias ? (Historical information; may be modified by office examination.)

0 = Not disabling.
1 = Mildly disabling.
2 = Moderately disabling.
3 = Severely disabling.
4 = Completely disabled.

34. Painful Dyskinesias: How painful are the dyskinesias ? (Historical information.)

0 = No painful dyskinesias.
1 = Slight.
2 = Moderate.
3 = Severe.
4 = Marked.

35. Presence of Early Morning Dystonia

0 = No
1 = Yes

B. Clinical fluctuations

36. Are "off" periods predictable?

0 = No
1 = Yes

37. Are "off" periods unpredictable?

0 = No
1 = Yes

38. Do "off" periods come on suddenly, within a few seconds?

0 = No
1 = Yes

39. What proportion of the waking day is the patient "off" on average?

0 = None
1 = 1-25% of day.
2 = 26-50% of day.
3 = 51-75% of day.
4 = 76-100% of day.

C. Other complications

40. Does the patient have anorexia, nausea, or vomiting ?

0 = No
1 = Yes

41. Any sleep disturbances, such as insomnia or hypersomnolence ? (Record the patient's blood pressure, height and weight on the scoring form)

0 = No
1 = Yes

42. Does the patient have symptomatic orthostasis?

0 = No
1 = Yes

[1] Recent Developments in Parkinson' Disease (Volume 2) [1987] (S.Fahn, C.D.Marsden, D.B.Calne, M.Goldstein) 153-163, 293- 304 - Unified Parkinson' Disease Rating Scale

Hoehn and Yahr

The Hoen and Yahr characterises patients according to five stages of severity, from Stage 1 (mild) to Stage 5 (incapacitated) [1, 2].

Stage One

1 Signs and symptoms on one side only
2 Symptoms mild
3 Symptoms inconvenient but not disabling
4 Usually presents with tremor of one limb
5 Friends have noticed changes in posture, locomotion and facial expression

Stage Two

1 Symptoms are bilateral
2 Minimal disability
3 Posture and gait affected

Stage Three

1 Significant slowing of body movements
2 Early impairment of equilibrium on walking or standing
3 Generalized dysfunction that is moderately severe

Stage Four

1 Severe symptoms
2 Can still walk to a limited extent
3 Rigidity and bradykinesia
4 No longer able to live alone
5 Tremor may be less than earlier stages

Stage Five

1 Cachectic stage
2 Invalidism complete
3 Cannot stand or walk
4 Requires constant nursing care

[1] Neurology [1967] 17 (5) : 427–442 (M.Hoehn, M.Yahr)

[2] Movement Disorders [2004] 19 (9) : 1020–1028 (C.G.Goetz, W. Poewe, O.Rascol, C.Sampaio, G.T.Stebbins, C.Counsell, N.Giladi, R. G.Holloway, C.G.Moore, G.K.Wenning, M.D.Yahr, L.Seidl)

MDS-UPDRS

The MDS-UPDRS is the Movement Disorder Society revision of the Unified Parkinson's Disease Rating Scale [1].

Permission is required to use the Scales (with the exception of personal or individual use). The MDS-UPDRS has four parts : Part I (non-motor experiences of daily living), Part II (motor experiences of daily living), Part III (motor examination) and Part IV (motor complications).

Part I has two components : IA concerns a number of behaviours that are assessed by the investigator with all pertinent information from patients and caregivers, and IB is completed by the patient with or without the aid of the caregiver, but independently of the investigator. These sections can be reviewed by the rater to ensure that all questions are answered clearly, and to help explain any perceived ambiguities.

Part II is designed to be a self-administered questionnaire like Part IB, but can be reviewed by the investigator to ensure completeness and clarity. Of note, the official versions of Part IA, Part IB and Part II of the MDS-UPDRS do not have separate on or off ratings. For individual programs the same questions can be used separately for on and off.

Part III has instructions for the rater to give or demonstrate to the patient; it is completed by the rater.

Part IV has instructions for the rater and also instructions to be read to the patient. This part integrates patient-derived information with the raters clinical observations and assessments and is completed by the rater [2].

[1] Movement Disorders [2010] 25 (9) : 1190–1194 (C.G.Goetz, G.T. Stebbins, T.A.Chmura, S.Fahn, W.Poewe, C.M.Tanner)

[2] The Movement Disorder Society, MDS-UPDRS Home [2011] : http://www.movementdisorders.org/updrs/

Modified Rankin Scale

The modified Rankin Scale (mRS) assesses the level of disability caused by neurological disorders, including Parkinson's Disease [1]. The modified Rankin Scale is scored 0-6 with lower scores reflecting less disability :

0 No symptoms

1 No significant disability : Able to carry out all usual activities, despite some symptoms.

2 Slight disability : Able to look after own affairs without assistance, but unable to carry out all previous activities.

3 Moderate disability : Requires some help, but able to walk unassisted.

4 Moderately severe disability : Unable to attend to own bodily needs without assistance. Unable to walk unassisted.

5 Severe disability : Requires constant nursing care and attention, bedridden, incontinent.

6 Dead

[1] Journal of Clinical Neuroscience [2013] 20 (9) : 1200-1203 (T. Simuni, S.T.Luo, K.L.Chou, H.Fernandez, B.He, S.Parashos)

PDQ39

The PDQ-39 assesses the quality of life. The PDQ-39 is the most widely used Parkinson's Disease specific measure of health status. It contains thirty nine questions, covering eight aspects of quality of life instead of being aimed specifically at the symptoms of Parkinson's Disease.

Scores on the PDQ range from 0 to 100, with higher scores reflecting greater problems [1]. Each question has five options with increasing levels of seriousness : Never, Occasionally, Sometimes, Often, Always or cannot do at all. Only one option can be chosen. Each question is begun "Due to having Parkinson' disease, how often during the last month have you...." [1].

1 Had difficulty doing the leisure activities which you would like to do ?

2 Had difficulty looking after your home, e.g. DIY, housework, cooking ?

3 Had difficulty carrying bags of shopping ?

4 Had problems walking half a mile ?

5 Had problems walking 100 yards ?

6 Had problems getting around the house as easily as you would like?

7 Had difficulty getting around in public ?

8 Needed someone else to accompany you when you went out ?

9 Felt frightened or worried about falling over in public ?

10 Been confined to the house more than you would like ?

11 Had difficulty washing yourself ?

12 Had difficulty dressing yourself ?

13 Had problems doing up your shoe lace ?

14 Had problems writing clearly ?

15 Had difficulty cutting up your food ?

16 Had difficulty holding a drink without spilling it ?

17 Felt depressed ?

18 Felt isolated and lonely ?

19 Felt weepy or tearful ?

20 Felt angry or bitter ?

21 Felt anxious ?

22 Felt worried about your future ?

23 Felt you had to conceal your Parkinson's from people ?

24 Avoided situations which involve eating or drinking in public ?

25 Felt embarrassed in public due to having Parkinson's Disease ?

26 Felt worried by other people's reaction to you ?

27 Had problems with your close personal relationships ?

28 Lacked support in the ways you need from your spouse or partner ? If you do not have a spouse or partner tick here

29 Lacked support in the ways you need from your family or close friends ?

30 Unexpectedly fallen asleep during the day ?

31 Had problems with your concentration, e.g. when reading or watching TV ?

32 Felt your memory was bad ?

33 Had distressing dreams or hallucinations ?

34 Had difficulty with your speech ?

35 Felt unable to communicate with people properly ?

36 Felt ignored by people ?

37 Had painful muscle cramps or spasms ?

38 Had aches and pains in your joints or body ?

39 Felt unpleasantly hot or cold ?

[1] The Parkinson's Disease Questionnaire : PDQ-39 User Manual (including PDQ-8 and the PDQ Summary Index) [2008] (C.Jenkinson, R. Fitzpatrick, V.Peto, R.Harris, P.Saunders)

PDQL

The PDQL is the Parkinson's Disease Quality of Life questionnaire. It is self administered and contains thirty seven questions concerning symptoms and quality of life for people with Parkinson's Disease. It includes sub-scales : Parkinsonian symptoms (P), systemic symptoms (Sys), emotional functioning (E), social functioning (Soc). An overall scale can be derived, with a higher score indicating better perceived quality of life [1]. Response options are : (1) All of the time, (2) Most of the time, (3) Some of the time, (4) A little of the time, (5) Never. How often during the last three months did you have trouble with :

1 stiffness (P)

2 feeling generally unwell (Sys)

3 that you are no longer able to do your hobbies (Soc)

4 being tense (P)

5 feeling insecure of yourself due to your physical limitations (E)

6 shaking of the hand(s) (P)

7 feeling worn out or having no energy (Sys)

8 difficulties in doing sport or leisure activities (Soc)

9 clumsiness (P)

10 feeling embarrassed because of your illness (E)

11 shuffling (P)

12 having to postpone or cancel social activities because of your illness (Soc)

13 a feeling of extreme exhaustion (Sys)

14 difficulties turning around while walking (P)

15 being afraid of possible progressing of the illness (E)

16 difficulties writing (P)

17 being less able to go on holiday than before your illness (Soc)

18 feeling insecure of yourself around others (E)

19 difficulties getting a good night's rest (Sys)

20 "on/off' periods (P)

21 difficulty with accepting your illness (E)

22 difficulties talking (P)

23 difficulties signing your name in public (Soc)

24 difficulties walking (Sys)

25 drooling (P)

26 feeling depressed or discouraged (E)

27 difficulty with sitting still (for long periods) (P)

28 often needing to urinate and/or wetting yourself (Sys)

29 difficulties with transport (Soc)

30 sudden extreme movements (P)

31 difficulties concentrating (E)

32 difficulties getting up from a chair (P)

33 constipation (Sys)

34 difficulties with your memory (E)

35 difficulties turning around in bed (P)

36 that your illness inhibits your sex life (Soc)

37 feeling worried about (the possible consequences of) an operation in connection with your illness (E)

[1] Age and Ageing [1999] 28 : 341-346 (P.Hobson, A.Holden, J. Meara)

SCHWAB AND ENGLAND

The Schwab and England Activities of Daily Living assesses patients in terms of their degree of independence concerning their functions - with a range a percentages from 100% to 0%. Rating can be assigned by the rater or the patient [1].

100%
Completely independent. Able to do all chores w/o slowness, difficulty, or impairment.

90%
Completely independent. Able to do all chores with some slowness, difficulty, or impairment. May take twice as long.

80%
Independent in most chores. Takes twice as long. Conscious of difficulty and slowing.

70%
Not completely independent. More difficulty with chores. 3 to 4 times as long on chores for some. May take large part of day for chores.

60%
Some dependency. Can do most chores, but very slowly and with much effort. Errors, some impossible.

50%
More dependant. Help with half of chores. Difficulty with everything.

40%
Very dependant. Can assist with all chores but few alone.

30%
With effort, now and then does a few chores alone or begins alone. Much help needed.

20%
Nothing alone. Can do some slight help with some chores. Severe invalid.

10%
Totally dependant, helpless.

0%
Vegetative functions such as swallowing, bladder and bowel function are not functioning. Bedridden.

[1] Third Symposium on Parkinson's Disease, Royal College of Surgeons in Edinburgh, May 20-22, [1968] : Schwab RS, England AC Jr. Projection techniques for evaluating surgery in Parkinson's Disease. pages 152-157; E. & S.Livingstone Ltd. [1969]

Webster scale

The Webster disability rating scale is a four point scale used to assess ten designated key criteria that have been identified as being indicative of the various stages and severity of Parkinson's Disease.

Bradykinesia of hands

0 - no involvement
1 - detectable slowing of the supination-pronation rate; beginning difficulty in handling tools buttoning clothes and with handwriting
2 - moderate slowing of the supination-pronation rate in one or both sides; moderate impairment of hand function; handwriting is greatly impaired micrographia present
3 - severe slowing of the supination-pronation rate; unable to write or button clothes; marked difficulty in handling utensils

Rigidity

0 - no involvement
1 - detectable rigidity in neck and shoulders; activation phenomenon is present; one or both arms show mild negative resting rigidity
2 - moderate rigidity in neck and shoulders; resting rigidity is present if patient is not on medications
3 - severe rigidity in neck and shoulders; resting rigidity cannot be reversed by medication

Posture

0 - normal posture; head flexed forward less than 4 inches
1 - beginning poker spine; head flexed forward more than 5 inches
2 - beginning arm flexion; head flexed forward up to 6 inches; one or both arms raised but still below waist
3 - onset of simian posture; head flexed forward more than 6 inches; one or both hands elevated above the waist; sharp flexion of hands beginning interphalangeal extension; beginning flexion of knees

Upper extremity swing

0 - swings both arms well
1 - one arm definitely decreased in amount of swing
2 - one arm fails to swing
3 - both arms fail to swing

Gait

0 - steps out well with 18-30 inch stride; turns about effortlessly
1 - gait shortened to 12-18 inch stride; beginning to strike one heel; turn around time slowing; requires several steps
2 - stride moderately shortened to 6-12 inches; both heels beginning to strike floor forcefully
3 - onset of shuffling gait; steps less than 3 inches; occasional stuttering-type or blocking gait; walks on toes; turns around very slowly

Tremor

0 - no detectable tremor found
1 - less than 1 inch of peak-to-peak tremor movement observed in limbs or head at rest or in either hand while walking or during the finger-to-nose testing
2 - maximum tremor envelope fails to exceed 4 inches; tremor is severe but not constant and patient retains some control of hands
3 - tremor envelope exceeds 4 inches; tremor is constant and severe; patient cannot get free of tremor while awake unless it is a pure cerebellar type; writing and feeding self are impossible

Facies

0 - normal; full animation; no stare
1 - detectable immobility; mouth remains closed; beginning features of anxiety or depression
2 - moderate immobility; emotion breaks through at markedly increased threshold; lips parted some of the time; moderate appearance of anxiety or depression; drooling may be present
3 - frozen facies; mouth opens >= 0.25 inches; drooling may be severe

Seborrhea

0 - none
1 - increased perspiration secretions remain thin

2 - obvious oiliness present and secretion much thicker
3 - marked seborrhea; entire face and head covered by thick secretion

Speech

0 - clear loud resonant easily understood
1 - beginning of hoarseness with loss of inflection and resonance; good volume and still easily understood
2 - moderate hoarseness and weakness; constant monotone unvaried pitch; beginning of dysarthria hesitance stuttering difficult to understand.
3 - marked harshness and weakness; very difficult to hear and to understand

Self-care

0 - no impairment
1 - still provides full self-care but rate of dressing definitely impeded; able to live alone and may be employable
2 - requires help in certain critical areas; very slow in performing most activities but manages by taking much time
3 - continuously disabled; unable to dress feed self or walk alone

Scale Disability

1-10 early illness

11-20 moderate

21-30 severe or advanced

[1] Modern Treatment [1968] 5 : 257-282 (D.D.Webster)

Systematic Screening of Handwriting Difficulties (SOS-test)

Method : The Systematic Screening of Handwriting Difficulties (SOS-test) is a method of assessing hand writing. Participants are asked to copy as much as possible of a text within five minutes. They are instructed to write as neatly and quickly as in daily life. Writing speed, size of handwriting and quality of handwriting are compared [1].

Efficacy : People with Parkinson's Disease had smaller and slower handwriting and showed worse writing quality. The outcomes of the SOS-test significantly correlated with fine motor skill performance and disease duration and severity [2]. People with Parkinson's Disease who had freezing of gait showed decreased writing amplitudes, increased variability and had a higher total score on the SOS test than those people with Parkinson's Disease who did not have freezing of gait [3].

[1] The Systematic Screening of Handwriting Difficulties (SOS-test) : validation for patients with Parkinson’s disease [2016] (S.Broeder, Sanne, A.Nieuwboer, E.Heremans, M.Pereira, B.Engelsman, E. Nackaerts)

[2] PLoS One [2017] 12 (3) : e0173157 (E.Nackaerts, E.Heremans, B.C.Smits-Engelsman, S.Broeder, W.Vandenberghe, B.Bergmans, A.Nieuwboer)

[3] Neurorehabilitation and Neural Repair [2016] 30 (10) : 911-919 (E. Heremans, E.Nackaerts, S.Broeder, G.Vervoort, S.P.Swinnen, A. Nieuwboer)

CHAPTER 33

DIAGNOSIS OF PARKINSON'S DISEASE

TECHNOLOGICAL METHODS

Diagnosis

Diagnosis is usually based on physical observation and questioning of the patients. The most commonly used symptom questionnaire is the Unified Parkinson Disease Rating Scale (UPDRS). Assessments can also involve the SPECT or PET scans, which are the most accurate methods of diagnosing Parkinson's Disease.

Misdiagnosis

SWEDD (scans without evidence for dopaminergic deficit) refers to somebody assumed to have Parkinson's Disease but whose scan shows the absence of dopamine deficiency. Most SWEDD cases are due to a misdiagnosis of Parkinson's Disease but a small proportion may still have Parkinson's Disease because of : a positive L-dopa response, clinical progression, imaging and genetic evidence [1].

[1] Journal of Neurology, Neurosurgery and Psychiatry [2016] 87 (3) : 319-323 (R.Erro, S.A.Schneider, M.Stamelou, N.P.Quinn, K.P.Bhatia)

Technological methods of diagnosis

Besides the SPECT scan [PAGE 404] and the PET scan [PAGE 406], less common technological methods that are available or in development include : dysphonia measures [PAGE 408], eye brain tracker [PAGE 409], Gaitrite [PAGE 409], laryngeal electromyography [PAGE 410], magnetic resonance imaging [PAGE 411], P3a wave [PAGE 412], Parkinson's Kineti Graph [PAGE 412], sensory pen [PAGE 413], smartphones [PAGE 414], smartwatch [PAGE 414], transcranial doppler sonography [PAGE 415], transcranial sonography [PAGE 416], ultrasound elastography [PAGE 419], vestibulography [PAGE 420], and wearable sensors [PAGE 420].

SPECT SCAN

Technology : A single-photon emission computerised tomography (SPECT) procedure allows the analysis of the function of the internal organs. A SPECT scan is a type of nuclear imaging test, which means it uses a radioactive substance and a special camera to create three dimensional images that show how the organs work. Most SPECT scans involve two steps : receiving a radioactive dye and then using a SPECT machine to scan a specific area of the body. Before undergoing the SPECT scan, patients receive a radioactive substance through an injection or through an intravenous (IV) infusion into a vein in the arm. The patient is positioned on a table in the room where they undergo the SPECT scan. Most SPECT scans take 30 to 90 minutes [1, 2, 3].

Efficacy : SPECT is often used as an aid in diagnosing Parkinson's Disease as it can show decreased dopamine activity. Although it is often claimed to show the extent of the loss of the dopaminergic neurons (the cells involved in Parkinson's Disease), it instead shows the level of activity in the existing cells. SPECT can distinguish Parkinson's Disease from healthy controls with excellent sensitivity and specificity [4]. A second SPECT scan after two years can reduce any remaining diagnostic uncertainty [5]. There is substantial agreement in diagnosis between the SPECT scan and the PET scan [6]. A single SPECT scan performed in the early stage of Parkinson's Disease can help to predict disease severity [7]. However, SPECT does not predict the progression of motor symptoms [8]. SPECT is relatively accurate in being able to distinguish between Parkinson's Disease and Vascular Parkinsonism, and also between Parkinson's Disease and Essential Tremor [9]. However, although a SPECT scan can be used to assist the diagnosis of Parkinsonism in order to differentiate Essential Tremor it is not conclusive [10]. Using the SPECT scan there was an 87% accuracy in the differential diagnosis between Parkinson's Disease, progressive supranuclear palsy, and corticobasal degeneration [11].

DaTSCAN

Technology : DaTSCAN is the name of a clear colourless solution used for injection in SPECT scans. Its active constituent is Ioflupane.

Ioflupane is cleared rapidly from the blood after intravenous injection. Only 5% of the administered activity remains in whole blood at 5 minutes post-injection. Uptake in the brain is rapid, reaching about 7% of injected activity at 10 minutes post-injection and decreasing to 3% after 5 hours. About 30% of the whole brain activity is attributed to striatal uptake. At 48 hours post-injection, approximately 60% of the injected radioactivity is excreted in the urine, with faecal excretion calculated at approximately 14% [12].

Efficacy : DaTSCAN is used in people with clinically uncertain Parkinsonian Syndromes in order to help differentiate Essential Tremor from Parkinsonian Syndromes related to idiopathic Parkinson's Disease, Multiple System Atrophy and Progressive Supranuclear Palsy. However, DaTSCAN is unable to discriminate between Parkinson's Disease, Multiple System Atrophy and Progressive Supranuclear Palsy. Ioflupane binds to the dopamine transporter. Medicines that bind to the dopamine transporter with high affinity may therefore interfere with DaTSCAN diagnosis. These include amphetamine, benzatropine, buproprion, cocaine, mazindol, methylphenidate, phentermine and sertraline. Common side effects of DaTSCAN include : increased appetite, headache, vertigo, and formication (paraesthesia). Uncommon side effects are injection site pain and intense pain following administration into small veins [11]. When a DaTscan was carried out on people with definite Parkinson's Disease, the DaTscan was markedly abnormal in 92% of people with Parkinson's Disease and normal in the remaining 8% [13].

[1] Grainger & Allison's Diagnostic Radiology [2014] (Andrew S.McQueen, Lee A.Grant, Jennifer F.Findlay, Sheetal Sharma, Vivek S.Shrivastava, Scott M.McDonald)

[2] Bradley's Neurology in Clinical Practice [2015] (Robert B.Daroff, Joseph Jankovic, John C.Mazziotta, Scott L.Pomeroy)

[3] Imaging in Parkinson's Disease [2011] (David Eidelberg)

[4] European Journal of Nuclear Medicine and Molecular Imaging [2009] 36 (3) : 454-462 (S.A.Eshuis, P.L.Jager, R.P.Maguire, S. Jonkman, R.A.Dierckx, K.L.Leenders)

[5] Movement Disorders [2007] 22 (16) : 2346-2351 (E.Tolosa, T.V. Borght, E.Moreno)

[6] Nuklearmedizin [2010] 49 (4) : 139-147 (R.Buchert)

[7] Neurological Science [2009] 30 (4) : 301-3055 (R.Djaldetti, T.A. Treves, I.Ziv, E.Melamed, Y.Lampl, M.Lorberboym)

[8] European Neurology [2011] 65 (4) : 187-192 (M.Hubbuch, G. Farmakis, A.Schaefer, S.Behnke, S.Schneider, D.Hellwig, K. Fassbender, C.M.Kirsch, U.Dillmann, J.Spiegel)

[9] BMC Neurology [2007] 7 : 27 (A.M.Vlaar, M.J.van Kroonenburgh, A.G.Kessels, W.E.Weber)

[10] Journal of Neuroimaging [2012] 22 (3) : 225-230 (R.A.Hauser, D. G.Grosset)

[11] Revue Neurologique [2009] 165 (5) : 440-448 (A.Kreisler, L. Defebvre, A.Duhamel, P.Lecouffe, K.Dujardin, MSteinling, F.Pasquier, A.Destée)

[12] GE Healthcare http://www.datscan.com

[13] Clinical Nuclear Medicine [2015] 40 (5) : 390-393 (I.Gayed, U. Joseph, M. Fanous, D.Wan, M.Schiess, W.Ondo, K.S.Won)

PET SCAN

Technology : Positron emission tomography (PET) is a nuclear medicine imaging technique that produces a three-dimensional image or map of functional processes in the body. The system detects pairs of gamma rays emitted indirectly by a positron-emitting radionuclide (tracer) that is introduced into the body on a biologically active molecule. It takes approximately 30 to 60 minutes for the radiotracer to travel through the body and to be absorbed by the organ or tissue being studied. The patient is then asked to rest quietly, avoiding movement and talking. The patient will then be moved into the PET scanner and then the imaging will begin. The patient will need to remain still during imaging. Actual scanning time is approximately 45 minutes. Images of tracer concentration in 3-dimensional space within the body are then reconstructed by computer analysis. The F-dopa PET scan is used as an aid in diagnosing Parkinson's Disease as it can show decreased dopamine activity in the basal ganglia. Although it is often claimed to show the extent of the loss of the dopaminergic neurons it instead shows the level of activity in the existing dopaminergic neurons [1, 2].

Efficacy : Positron emission tomography (PET) can detect Parkinson's Disease with excellent sensitivity and specificity [3] and can measure the rate of progression of Parkinson's Disease [4]. It can detect the presence of striatal, pallidal, midbrain, and cortical dopamine terminal dysfunction [5], and presynaptic dopamine insufficiency [6]. Putamen 18F-dopa uptake of patients with Parkinson's Disease is reduced by at least 35% at onset of symptoms [7]. There is substantial agreement in diagnosis using PET and SPECT scans [8]. PET can also assist in the differential diagnosis of types of Parkinsonism [9, 10] but the evidence is inconclusive [11]. Differential diagnosis between Parkinson's Disease and multiple system atrophy, progressive supranuclear palsy and corticobasal degeneration is not clearly determined using the PET scan [12].

[1] Nuclear Medicine and PET/CT : Technology and Techniques [2016] (Kristen M.Waterstram-Rich, David Gilmore)

[2] Imaging in Parkinson's Disease [2011] (David Eidelberg)

[3] European Journal of Nuclear Medicine and Molecular Imaging [2009] 36 (3) : 454-462 (S.A.Eshuis, P.L.Jager, R.P.Maguire, S. Jonkman, R.A.Dierckx, K.L.Leenders)

[4] Movement Disorders [2001] 16 (4) : 608-615 (E.Nurmi, H.M. Ruottinen, J.Bergman, M.Haaparanta, O.Solin, P.Sonninen, J.O.Rinne)

[5] Annals of the New York Academy of Sciences [2003] 991 : 22-35 (D.J.Brooks)

[6] Acta Neurologica Scandinavica (Supplement) [1991] 136 : 37-39 (S.M.Aquilonius)

[7] Neurology [1991] 41 (5 Supplement 2) : 24-27 (D.J.Brooks)

[8] Nuklearmedizin [2010] 49 (4) : 139-147 (R.Buchert)

[9] Brain and Cognition [1995] 28 (3) : 297-310 (H.Shinotoh, D.B. Calne)

[10] European Journal of Nuclear Medicine [1999] 26 (2) : 171-182 (J. Booij, G.Tissingh, A.Winogrodzka, E.A.van Royen)

[11] Revista Espanola Medicine Nuclear [2009] 28 (3) : 106-113 (J. Puñal-Riobóo, A.Serena-Puig, L.Varela-Lema, A.M.Alvarez-Páez, A. Ruano-Ravina)

[12] Neurophysiologie Clinique [2001] 31 (5) : 321-340 (S.Thobois, S. Guillouet, E.Broussolle)

Dysphonia measures

Technology : Dysphonia is an impairment in the ability to produce vocal sounds. A wide range of speech signal processing algorithms (dysphonia measures) aim at predicting Parkinson's Disease severity using speech signals. Researchers assessed how accurately such measures can be in indicating Parkinson's Disease. In total they found 132 measures of dysphonia from sustained vowels. They then used a large database of vocal samples from different people [1].

Efficacy : The researchers demonstrated that these measures of dysphonia can outperform standard methods of diagnosing Parkinson's Disease by reaching almost 99% overall classification accuracy. They achieved this by using only ten features of dysphonia [1]. This approach can be used by phone. Telephone monitoring using the cellular mobile telephone networks showed that the Parkinson's Disease (UPDRS) symptom score could be estimated to within about 3.5 points difference from the clinicians' assessment, which is useful because even different clinicians vary by as much as 4 to 5 points [2].

[1] IEEE Transactions on Biomedical Engineering [2012] 59 (5) : 1264-1271 (A.Tsanas, M.A.Little, P.E.McSharry, J. Spielman, L.O. Ramig)

[2] IEEE Transactions on Biomedical Engineering (submitted) [2013] (A.Tsanas, M.A.Little, P.E.McSharry, L.O.Ramig)

Eye Brain Tracker

Technology : Mobile Eye Brain Tracker (EBT) is available for the detection of Parkinson-plus diseases. Different areas of the brain are involved in producing eye movements, and so abnormalities that occur can be linked to dysfunction in certain areas of the brain. The equipment consists of : a recording device for high-frequency, accurate eye movement measurement, two screens, an introductory computer application for behavioural testing, and an automatic test analysis application. The Mobile EBT is non-invasive and costs less than regularly used imaging techniques. When an eye movement exam is conducted the tests are displayed on a screen. The subject's eye movements are recorded whilst he takes the test. Once the tests are completed the examiner may conduct a thoroughly automatic analysis with the option of manually adjusting the results to enhance quality. Based on this analysis, an eye movement report is automatically printed to aid the examiner in diagnosing patients' possible illnesses [1].

Efficacy : Results have shown that eye movements provide a more accurate early diagnosis than traditional clinical examinations [1].

[1] E(ye) Brain - http://eye-brain.com

GAITRite gait analysis

Technology : The GAITRite system is an electronic pathway that contains pressure sensitive sensors arranged in a grid-like pattern. The carpet used is portable and can be rolled up for transportation. There are several versions of the GAITRite device available with different lengths. It is used for laboratory evaluation and provides information regarding several gait parameters, such as walking speed, cadence and step length. Some safety precautions have been highlighted as needed, such as a wall fixed side rail or supervised gait [1].

Efficacy : The GAITRite gait analysis system was a moderately effective tool in evaluating parkinsonian bradykinesia. There were significant correlations between off-on improvement in gait parameters and in UPDRS III score [2]. The GaitRite system can be useful in detecting footfall patterns and selected time and distance measurements of persons with early stage Parkinson's Disease [3]. The quick timed test provided quantitative data for gait evaluation and was valid for clinical use [4].

[1] Journal of Neuroengineering and Rehabilitation [2016] 13 (1) : 24 (C.Godinho, J.Domingos, G.Cunha, A.T.Santos, R.M.Fernandes, D. Abreu, N.Gonçalves, H.Matthews, T.Isaacs, J.Duffen, et al)

[2] Parkinsonism & Related Disorders [2006] 12 (7) : 438-442 (S.L. Chien, S.Z.Lin, C.C.Liang, Y.S.Soong, S.H.Lin, Y.L.Hsin, C.W.Lee, S.Y.Chen)

[3] NeuroRehabilitation [2002] 17 (3) : 255-262 (A.J.Nelson, D.Zwick, S.Brody, C.Doran, L.Pulver, G.Rooz, M.Sadownick, R.Nelson, J. Rothman)

[4] International Journal of Rehabilitation Research [2015] 38 (1) : 88-91 (M.S.Bryant, C.D.Workman, G.R.Jackson)

Laryngeal electromyography

Technology : Laryngeal electromyography (LEMG) evaluates the integrity of the neuromuscular system in the larynx by recording action potentials generated in the laryngeal muscles during voluntary and involuntary contraction. LEMG is particularly useful for helping to differentiate between disorders involving upper motor neurons, lower motor neurons, peripheral nerves, the neuromuscular junction, muscle fibers, and the laryngeal cartilages and joints. LEMG is an extension of the physical examination, not an isolated laboratory procedure [1, 2].

Efficacy : Tremors were not detected on LEMG of the cricothyroid and thyroarytenoid muscles even in patients with clinical tremor. LEMG hypercontractility during voice rest was the typical result observed in over 90% of patients regardless of disease severity. Gender and age of subjects did not correlate with laryngeal electromyography results.

Patients with Parkinson's Disease presented spontaneous intrinsic laryngeal muscle activity during voice rest, regardless of disease severity [3]. LEMG hypertonicity during voice rest was the feature observed in 73% of the patients with Parkinson's Disease. The severity of the disease, diagnosis, and the time of treatment did not correlate with LEMG findings [4, 5]. Laryngeal tremor was not detected by LEMG although vocal tremor was detected by Voxmetria in 69% of the individuals tested and in 61% of them by perceptive-auditive analysis [5].

[1] Laryngeal Electromyography [2006] (R.T.Sataloff, S.Mandel, R. Manon-Espaillat, Y.Heman-Ackah, M.Abaza)

[2] Otolaryngolic Clinics of North America [2007] 40 (5) : 1003-1023 (Y.D.Heman-Ackah, S.Mandel, R.Manon-Espaillat, M.M.Abaza, R.T. Sataloff)

[3] Laryngoscope [2014] 124 (3) : 725-729 (A.P.Zarzur, A.de Campos Duprat, B.O.Cataldo, D.Ciampi, E.Fonoff)

[4] Laryngoscope [2007] 117 (5) : 831-834 (A.P.Zarzur, A.C.Duprat, G.Shinzato, C.A.Eckley)

[5] Brazilian Journal of Otorhinolaryngology [2010] 76 (1) : 40-43 (A. P.Zarzur, I.S.Duarte, N.Holanda Gdo, M.A.Martins)

Magnetic resonance imaging

Technology : Magnetic resonance imaging (MRI) is a type of scan that uses strong magnetic fields and radio waves to produce detailed images of the inside of the body. An MRI scanner is a large tube that contains powerful magnets. The patient lays inside the tube during the scan and is moved into the scanner either head or feet first. The MRI scanner is operated by a radiographer who controls the scanner using a computer [1, 2].

Efficacy : An evaluation was carried out of the substantia nigra (SN) of people who did and who did not have Parkinson's Disease. The substantia nigra (SN) is the area of the brain most affected by

Parkinson's Disease. Deviations from the normal appearance of the substantia nigra were described and indicated as abnormal. The abnormal architecture of the substantia nigra allowed a discrimination between people who did and who did not have Parkinson's Disease with a sensitivity and specificity of 100% and 96% respectively [3].

[1] Magnetic Resonance Imaging (MRI) for Technologist : Practical MRI Procedures and Techniques [2013] (Azmi Bani Baker)

[2] Magnetic Resonance Imaging in Movement Disorders : A Guide for Clinicians and Scientists [2013] (Paul Tuite, Alain Dagher)

[3] Radiology [2014] 271 (3) : 831-838 (M.Cosottini, D.Frosini, I. Pesaresi, M.Costagli, L.Biagi, R.Ceravolo, U.Bonuccelli, M.Tosetti)

P3a wave

Technology : The P3a wave, which is a scalp-recorded brain potential, is presently being assessed as a neurophysiological measure of Parkinson's Disease duration and severity. The P3a wave is an event-related potential associated with involuntary attention and dopaminergic function. P3a is reduced at initial stages of Parkinson's Disease [1].

Efficacy : The P3a amplitude was significantly lower in all stages of Parkinson's Disease. A regression analysis showed that the disease duration predicted inversely the P3a [1].

[1] Clinical Neurophysiology [2015] 126 (11) : 2142-2149 (R.Solís-Vivanco, M.Rodríguez-Violante, Y.Rodríguez-Agudelo, A.Schilmann, U.Rodríguez-Ortiz, J.Ricardo-Garcell)

Parkinson's KinetiGraph

Technology : The Parkinson's KinetiGraph system was commercialised by Global Kinetics Corporation. It consists of a sensor that is worn around the wrist of the patient to record data about their symptoms, and a computer unit which receives that data and analyses it. The device remotely records data about a person's movement and via algorithms, provides a report for their neurologist showing an objective measure of the presence and severity of bradykinesia and dyskinesia, the two key disabling symptoms of Parkinson's Disease. The device also reminds the person when to take their Parkinson's Disease drugs as prescribed by their medical practitioner [1].

Efficacy : No assessments concerning the efficacy have been published.

[1] http://www.greyinnovation.com/portfolio/medtech

Sensory pen

Technology : A means of diagnosing Parkinson's Disease is being developed by MANUS Neurodynamica using sensory pen technology. The system, combining sensor and computing technology, requires the patient to perform a set of writing tasks, drawing activities or a combination of both. The system records all movements of the pen as well as other parameters such as drawing pressure, plus acceleration and deceleration of movement, to identify patterns that are indicative of specific kinds of neuromotor disorder. The sensory pen can be used by non-specialists with minimal training so that large numbers of people would be able to be screened. The system's software records key features regarding the movement of the pen, relating it to the motion of the limb, particularly the role of the hand and fingers in co-ordinating overall pen motion. The recordings enable the operator to assess akinesia, bradykinesia, tremor, rigidity and other signs of motor deterioration that cannot be easily detected by other means. The software takes inputs from a variety of sensors in the pen and converts them, using proprietary algorithms, into outcome percentages that represent the likelihood of the presence of Parkinson's Disease or other neuromotor disorders [1].

Efficacy : No assessments concerning the efficacy have been published.

[1] MANUS Neurodynamica - http://www.manusneuro.com

SMARTPHONES

Technology : A smartphone is a mobile phone with an advanced mobile operating system. Participants are provided with smartphones with an Android operating system containing a smartphone application that assesses voice, posture, gait, finger tapping, and response time [1]. Another system uses applications to assess tremor. The system is based on measuring the acceleration from the hand of the person with Parkinson's Disease using a mobile cell phone accelerometer [2].

Efficacy : Patients underwent in-clinic assessments, including the Unified Parkinson's Disease Rating Scale (UPDRS). Participants then took the smart phones home to perform the five tasks four times a day for a month. Once a week they had a remote visit with a Parkinson's Disease specialist in which a modified UPDRS was performed. The analyses of the five tasks differed between those people with Parkinson's Disease and those who did not. There was a high degree of accuracy. In discriminating participants with Parkinson's Disease the mean sensitivity was 96% and the mean specificity was 96% [1]. In a separate study features were extracted forming a feature vector of 12 different elements. The features extracted from the subjects were classified using a neural networks classifier. The results obtained regarding tremor showed an accuracy of 95%. These results indicate that a cell phone accelerometer can accurately detect and record rest tremor in people with Parkinson's Disease [2].

[1] Parkinsonism & Related Disorders [2015] 21 (6) : 650-653 (S.Arora, V.Venkataraman, A.Hang, S.Donohue, K.M.Biglan, E.R. Dorsey, M.A. Little)

[2] Journal of Medical Engineering Technology [2016] 40 (3) : 127-134 (L.Fraiwan, R.Khnouf, A.R.Mashagbeh)

SMARTWATCH

Technology : A smartwatch is effectively a wearable computer with functions beyond those of a normal watch. Smart watches can be used for accelerometry assessments in order aid the diagnosis of Parkinson's Disease. Recordings are made with a smart watch device on the predominantly affected hand of people with Parkinson's Disease, and simultaneously with an analog accelerometer with hands at rest and outstretched [1].

Efficacy : Tremor peak frequency, peak power, and power of the first four harmonics was calculated and compared between the two devices. Mean power at the first four harmonics was calculated and used to classify tremor as parkinsonian or essential. Mean harmonic peak power was both highly sensitive and specific for the distinction of Parkinson's Disease postural tremor from essential tremor with an optimal threshold for the sample, with a sensitivity of 91% [1].

[1] Journal of Neuroscience Methods [2014] 230 : 1-4 (D.J.Wile, R. Ranawaya, Z.H.Kiss)

Transcranial doppler sonography

Technology : Transcranial Doppler sonography is a technique that uses a handheld, microprocessor-controlled, low-frequency, pulsed Doppler transducer to measure the velocity and pulsatility of blood flow within certain areas of the brain [1]. The value is determined of the enhanced substantia nigra echo in the diagnosis of Parkinson's Disease by analyzing the intensity and area of substantia nigra echo [2].

Efficacy : People without Parkinson's Disease were compared to people with early stage Parkinson's Disease using results of substantia nigra echo, which are graded I (the least) to V (the greatest). The sensitivity of substantia nigra echo in diagnosing Parkinson's Disease was 89% and the specificity was 93%. The levels were much higher in Parkinson's Disease. The figures for those people with Parkinson's Disease compared to those who did not have it were Grade V (19% v none), Grade IV (33% v none), Grade III (36% v 6%), Grade II (11% v 40%), Grade I (none v 53%). High grades were only present in people with Parkinson's Disease. Low grades were only present when there was no Parkinson's Disease. Analysis of substantia nigra echo is therefore of practical use for the diagnosis of early stage Parkinson's Disease [2].

[1] Transcranial Doppler Sonography [2013] (Rune Aaslid)

[2] European Review of Medical and Pharmacologial Sciences [2015] 19 (23) : 4621-4626 (J.J.Zhuang, Y.H.Zheng, X.W.Xu, L.Zhou)

Transcranial sonography

Technology : Transcranial sonography is a non-invasive, easy-to-repeat diagnostic technique that makes use of sound waves to create a digital image. The sound waves are typically produced by a transducer. Strong, short, electrical pulses from the ultrasound machine make the transducer ring at the desired frequency. Materials on the face of the transducer enable the sound to be transmitted efficiently into the body. The sound wave is partially reflected from layers between different tissues. Sound is reflected anywhere that there are density changes in the body. Some of the reflections return to the transducer. The return of the sound wave to the transducer results in the same process that it took to send the sound waves except that the process is in reverse. The return sound wave vibrates the transducer, which turns the vibrations into electrical pulses that travel to the ultrasonic scanner. In the ultrasonic scanner the electrical pulses are processed and transformed into a digital image [1, 2].

Efficacy : SPECT scanning is clearly more reliable than Transcranial Sonography in detecting Parkinson's Disease [3, 4], but due to its greater ease, Transcranial Sonography might be used as a screening tool before ordering a SPECT scan [3]. An abnormal hyperechogenicity of the substantia nigra is thought to be the most characteristic sonographic feature in Parkinson's Disease [5]. Hyperechogenecity of the substantia nigra was found in around 90% of people with Parkinson's Disease, and in patients and in around 10% of people who did not have Parkinson's Disease [5-21]. Some initially healthy subjects with substantia nigra hyperechogenicity eventually developed Parkinson's Disease [6]. Larger echogenic size of the substantia nigra correlated with younger age at onset of Parkinson's Disease, moderately or not at all with duration, but not with age, Parkinson's Disease duration or severity, or type of Parkinson's Disease [18, 22, 23, 24]. Diagnostic accuracy is 83% to 93% sensitivity and 85% to 87% specificity [29, 30]. It has been shown to quite a degree that Transcranial sonography can discriminate Parkinson's Disease from a number of similar disorders such as essential tremor, and atypical Parkinsonian syndromes [5, 7, 10, 23, 25, 26, 27]. However, the diagnostic accuracy of early stage Parkinson's Disease is not sufficient for routine clinical use [28].

[1] Transcranial Sonography and the Detection of Neurodegenerative Disease [2010] (Daniela Berg, Uwe Walter)

[2] Imaging in Parkinson's Disease [2011] (David Eidelberg)

[3] BMC Neurology [2008] 8 : 42 (A.M.Vlaar, T.de Nijs, M.J.van Kroonenburgh, W.H.Mess, A.Winogrodzka, S.C.Tromp, W.E.Weber)

[4] Movement Disorders [2008] 23 (3) : 405-410 (F.Doepp, M. Plotkin, L.Siegel, A.Kivi, D.Gruber, E.Lobsien, A.Kupsch, S.J. Schreiber)

[5] Zhurnal Nevrologii i Psikhiatrii imeni S.S.Korsakova [2011] 111 (1) : 49-55 (E.Fedotova, A.O.Chechetkin, M.I.Shadrina, P.A. Slominskii, I.A.Ivanova-Smolenskaia, S.N.Illarioshkin)

[6] Journal of Neural Transmission [2011] 118 (4) : 613-619 (D.Berg)

[7] Der Nervenarzt [2010] 81 (10) : 1189-1195 (JHagenah, G.Seidel)

[8] International Review of Neurobiology [2010] 90 : 81-92 (A. Gaenslen, D.Berg)

[9] BMC Neurology [2010] 10 : 9 (S.Mehnert, I.Reuter, K.Schepp, P. Maaser, E.Stolz, M.Kaps)

[10] Journal of Neurology [2009] 256 (4) : 530-538 (A.M.Vlaar, A. Bouwmans, W.H.Mess, S.C.Tromp, W.E.Weber)

[11] Medicina Clinica (Barcelona) [2008] 131 (8) : 285-289 (J. Herandez Vara, M.Rubiera del Fueyo, C.Lorenzo Bosquet, J.Castell Conesa, C.A.Molina Cateriano, F.M.Rodrguez)

[12] Vojnosanit Pregled [2008] 65 (8) : 601-605 (M.Mijajlovic, I. Petrovic, T.Stojkovic, M.Svetel, E.Stefanova, V.S.Kostic)

[13] Acta Neurologica Scandinavica [2009] 119 (1) : 17-21 (M. Budisic, Z.Trkanjec, J.Bosnjak, A.Lovrencic-Huzjan, V.Vukovic, D. Demarin)

[14] Lancet Neurology [2008] 7 (5) : 417-424 (A.Gaenslen, B. Unmuth, J.Godau, I.Liepelt, A.Di Santo, K.J.Schweitzer, T.Gasser, H.J. Machulla, M.Reimold, K.Marek, D.Berg)

[15] Internal Medicine [2007] 46 (18) : 1527-1531 (M.Okawa, H. Miwa, Y.Kajimoto, K.Hama, S.Morita, I.Nakanishi, T.Kondo)

[16] Journal of Neuroimaging [2007] 17 (2) : 164-167 (P.Ressner, D.Skoloudk, P.Hlustk, P.Kanovsk)

[17] Nature Clinical Practice Neurology [2008] 4 (10) : 536-537 (W.W. Martin)

[18] Movement Disorders [2007] 22 (1) : 48-54 (U.Walter, D. Dressler, A.Wolters, M.Wittstock, R.Benecke)

[19] Journal of Neural Transmission (Supplement) [2006] (70) : 249-254 (D.Berg)

[20] Movement Disorders [2006] 21 (10) : 1763-1765 (J.Prestel, K.J. Schweitzer, A.Hofer, T.Gasser, D.Berg)

[21] Journal of Ultrasound Medicine [2014] 33 (9) : 1635-1640 (E. Sanzaro, F.Iemolo, G.Duro, G.Malferrari)

[22] Movement Disorders [2007] 22 (13) : 1922-1926 (J.Y.Kim, S.T. Kim, S.H.Jeon, W.Y.Lee)

[23] Journal of Ultrasound Medicine [2014] 33 (12) : 2069-2074 (A. Alonso-Cánovas, J.L.López-Sendón, J.Buisán, A.de Felipe-Mimbrera, M.Guillán, N.García-Barragán, I.Corral, M.C.Matute-Lozano, et al)

[24] Journal of Neurological Science [2016] 364 : 9-11 (J.Jesus-Ribeiro, J.Sargento-Freitas, M.Sousa, F.Silva, A.Freire, C.Januário)

[25] Journal of Neurology [2007] 254 (4) : 501-507 (C.F.Tsai, R.M. Wu, Y.W.Huang, L.L.Chen, P.K.Yip, J.S.Jeng)

[26] Movement Disorders [2007] 22 (3) : 414-417 (H.Stockner, M. Sojer, K.S.K, J.Mueller, G.K.Wenning, C.Schmidauer, W.Poewe)

[27] Journal of Neural Transmission [2002] 109 (2) : 191-196 (U. Walter, M.Wittstock, R.Benecke, D.Dressler)

[28] BMJ Open [2013] 3 (4) (A.E.Bouwmans, A.M.Vlaar, W.H.Mess, A.Kessels, W.E.Weber)

[29] Journal of Ultrasound Medicine [2016] 35 (1) : 17-23 (T. Toomsoo, I.Liepelt-Scarfone, R.Kerner, L.Kadastik-Eerme, T.Asser, I. Rubanovits, D.Berg, P.Taba)

[30] Scientific Reports [2016] 6 : 20863 (D.H.Li, Y.C.He, J.Liu, S.D. Chen)

Ultrasound elastography

Technology : Ultrasound elastography is a means of assessing the mechanical properties of tissue, by applying stress and detecting tissue displacement using ultrasound. It provides information on tissue stiffness [1, 2, 3].

Efficacy : Ultrasound shear wave elastography has been used to assess muscle stiffness in people with Parkinson's Disease. The mean Young's modulus was 59 kPa in remarkably symptomatic arms, 47 kPa in mildly symptomatic arms, and 24 kPa in healthy controls. A significant difference was found between healthy controls and all people with Parkinson's Disease, thereby enabling it to be used as a quantitative assessment of muscle stiffness in people with Parkinson's Disease [4].

[1] Handbook of Ultrasound Elastography : Biomedical Applications and Medicine [2017] (James F.Greenleaf, Ivan Z.Nenadic, Mikael Tanter)

[2] British Journal of Radiology [2012] 85 (1019) : 1435-1445 (E.E. Drakonaki, G.M.Allen, D.J.Wilson)

[3] Diagnostic and Interventional Imaging [2013] 94 (5) 487-495 (J.-L. Gennisson, T.Deffieux, M.Fink, M.Tanter)

[4] Clinical Imaging [2016] 40 (6) : 1075-1080 (L.J.Du, W.He, L.G. Cheng, S.Li, Y.S.Pan, J.Gao)

Vestibulography

Technology : Electrovestibulography is a method of diagnosing Parkinson's Disease based on the analysis of electrovestibulography (EVestG) signals. Electrovestibulography signals are the vestibular response modulated by cortical brain signals. The brain signals are recorded from the ear canal in to which a receptor connected by a wire has easily been placed. This enables the signals to be recorded on a computer. So electrovestibulography can provide a quick and non-invasive method of diagnosis [1].

Efficacy : The results showed more than 95% accuracy for the diagnosis of Parkinson's Disease [1].

[1] Medical & Biological Engineering & Computing [2012] 50 (5) : 483-491 (Z.A.Dastgheib, B.Lithgow, Z.Moussavi)

Wearable sensors

Wearable sensors being used or assessed for the diagnosis of Parkinson's Disease include APDM Mobility Lab, Dynaport, Mercury, the Pedestrian Dead Reckoning (PDR) System, Perform, Rempark, the SENSE-PARK system, Stepwatch, and Trictrac RT3 Accelerometer.

APDM MOBILITY LAB

Technology : The APDM Mobility Lab uses wearable sensors and sophisticated signal processing to track subtle changes in gait, stride, balance, rotation, and efficiency and the range of movement in the limbs and torso. Sensors are simply strapped on to the subject on various parts of the body, including the chest, waist, wrists and the ankles. Subjects perform a standardised test and then a report is generated [1].

Efficacy : During an assessment each person performed iTUG (instrumented Timed-Up-and-Go) and iSway (instrumented Sway) using the APDM Mobility Lab. They were assessed according to a range of Parkinson's Disease scores. iTUG and iSway variables differentiated people with Parkinson's Disease. They correlated with all Parkinson's Disease severity measures. Objective scores correlated more strongly with iTUG than they did with iSway [1].

[1] Journal of Neurological Science [2014] 345 (1-2) : 131-138 (D.C. Dewey, S.Miocinovic, I.Bernstein, P.Khemani, R.B.Dewey, R.Querry, S.Chitnis, R.B.Dewey Jr)

DYNAPORT

Technology : The Dynaport enables the easy assessment of the physical activity status of people with Parkinson's Disease. With one small device, worn in an elastic strap on the lower back, the person's physical activity can be assessed for up to 14 days. It consists of a hardware unit, managing software, and one or more chosen analysis modules, accessible through a web service [1].

Efficacy : The DynaPort method overestimated gait duration by 10% and underestimated the number of steps by 7%. Accuracy decreased significantly as walking distance decreased. The accelerometry-based method is less speed dependent and is more appropriate in people with Parkinson's Disease for walking trajectories of 5 metres or more [1, 2].

[1] Age and Ageing [2008] 37 (4) : 436-441 (B.Dijkstra, W.Zijlstra, E.Scherder, Y.Kamsma)

[2] Journal of Neuroengineering and Rehabilitation [2016] 13 (1) : 24 (C.Godinho, J.Domingos, G.Cunha, A.T.Santos, R.M.Fernandes, D. Abreu, N.Gonçalves, H.Matthews, T.Isaacs, J.Duffen, et al)

MERCURY

Technology : Mercury is a wearable wireless sensor used as a means of enabling home monitoring of the motion of people with Parkinson's

Disease. Patients wear wireless nodes equipped with sensors for monitoring their movement and physiological conditions. Mercury consequently has the capability of analyzing sensor data in order to reliably estimate clinical scores capturing the severity of the patient's tremor, bradykinesia, and dyskinesia. The basic approach is to capture data from each limb segment (upper and lower arms and legs) using wearable sensors. The patient wears up to eight sensors each day and recharges the sensors at night. A laptop in the patient's home serves as a base station to collect and store sensor data. The data is then delivered via the Internet to the clinic where it is visualised and further processed by physicians. Signals are subjected to extensive processing in order to tie the sensor data to clinical measures that evaluate the patient's motor function and progression of the disease [1, 2, 3].

Efficacy : The method quantified tremor severity with 87 % accuracy, discriminated resting from postural tremor, and discriminated tremor from other Parkinsonian motor symptoms during daily activities [4].

[1] Mercury : A Wearable Sensor Network Platform for High-Fidelity Motion Analysis [2009] (Konrad Lorincz, Bor-rong Chen, Geoffrey Werner Challen, Atanu Roy Chowdhury, Shyamal Patel, Paolo Bonato, Matt Welsh)

[2] IEEE transactions on bio-medical engineering [2010] : 4411-4414 (S.Patel, T.Buckley, R.Rednic, D. McClure, L.Shih, D.Tarsy, M.Welsh, P.Bonato)

[3] IEEE transactions on bio-medical engineering [2011] 58 (3) : 831-836 (B.R.Chen, S.Patel, T.Buckley, R.Rednic, D.J.McClure, L. Shih, D.Tarsy, M.Welsh, P.Bonato)

[4] IEEE transactions on bio-medical engineering [2012] 16 (3) : 478-487 (G.Rigas, A.T.Tzallas, M.G.Tsipouras, P.Bougia, E.E.Tripoliti, D. Baga, D.I.Fotiadis, S.G.Tsouli, S.Konitsiotis)

PEDESTRIAN DEAD RECKONING SYSTEM

Technology : The pedestrian dead reckoning (PDR) system is a method that continuously monitors and records the patient's gait characteristics using a smartphone. It uses sensors in a smartphone to help to identify patients in early stages of neurological disease [1].

Efficacy : On average, the accuracy of the step length estimation was about 98%. Using a binary classification method, called support vector machine, they carried out a case study and showed that it was feasible to identify changes in the walking patterns of people with Parkinson's Disease patient with an accuracy of 94%. It provides a first step to experimentally show the possibility of applying smartphone sensor data to provide early warnings to people who might have Parkinson's Disease in order to encourage them to obtain a diagnosis earlier [1].

[1] Telemedicine Journal and e-health [2016] 22 (1) : 75-81 (P.Raknim, K.C.Lan)

PERFORM

Technology : PERFORM is a system aimed at the usage of low-cost wearable sensors that can continuously collect and process accelerometry signals in order to automatically detect and quantify the symptoms of the patient. The information is sent to a hospital to generate a daily report that will alert the doctor in case of any observation that is well outside of the expected range of values. This information is used to develop a support system for medical experts in order to help them manage the generated information, to build a disease profile for each patient, and to achieve a personalised treatment [1].

Efficacy : The performance of the system has been evaluated in real life conditions. The accuracy and acceptability of the system by people with Parkinson's Disease has been tested. A comparison with a routine clinical evaluation done by their physician has been carried out [2].

[1] Sensors [2014] 14 (9) : 17235-17255 (J.Cancela, M.Pastorino, A.T. Tzallas, M.G.Tsipouras, G.Rigas, M.T.Arredondo, D.I.Fotiadis)

[2] Sensors [2014] 14 (11) : 21329-21357 (A.T.Tzallas, M.G. Tsipouras, G.Rigas, D.G.Tsalikakis, E.C.Karvounis, M.Chondrogiorgi, F.Psomadellis, J.Cancela, M.Pastorino, M.T.Waldmeyer, et al)

REMPARK

Technology : REMPARK is a wearable system based on a belt-worn movement sensor, which detects alterations in the movements of the people wearing it. These activate an auditory cueing system controlled by a smartphone in order to improve a patient's gait. The belt-worn sensor analyzes patient's movement based on a database collected from people with Parkinson's Disease. Data collected during long periods of time enables the tailoring of medication to the patients needs.

Efficacy : The REMPARK system is presently being assessed for its accuracy in diagnosing Parkinson's Disease [1].

[1] Studies in Health Technology and Informatics [2014] 207 : 115-124 (A.Samà, C.Pérez-López, D.Rodríguez-Martín, J.M.Moreno-Aróstegui, J.Rovira, C.Ahlrichs, R.Castro, J.Cevada, R.Graça, V.Guimarães, et al)

SENSE-PARK SYSTEM

Technology : The SENSE-PARK System consists of wearable sensors, three of which are worn during the day and one of them worn at night, a smartphone-based App, and a balance board and computer software. The SENSE-PARK System enables an objective, continuous and relatively unobtrusive system that can be used to monitor Parkinson's Disease [1].

Efficacy : The SENSE-PARK System was tested 24/7 over 12 weeks in a study involving people with Parkinson's Disease. Patients obtained feedback about their performance but during the last eight weeks. The study included seven clinical visits with standardised interviews and regular phone contact. The participants rated the usability of the SENSE- PARK System favourably. The interviews revealed that most participants liked using the system and appreciated that it signalled changes in their health condition [1].

[1] BMC Neurology [2015] 15 : 89 (J.J.Ferreira, C.Godinho, A.T. Santos, J.Domingos, D.Abreu, R.Lobo, N.Gonçalves, M.Barra, F. Larsen, Ø.Fagerbakke, I.Akeren, H.Wangen, J.A.Serrano, et al)

STEPWATCH 3

Technology : The StepWatch step activity monitor is a highly accurate, unobtrusive instrument that is worn on the ankle. Consisting of a sensor, electronics and battery molded into a urethane case, the StepWatch is a durable, sealed, waterproof device. It neither requires nor allows any adjustment or maintenance by the subject. The StepWatch records step counts in short, adjustable time intervals over extended monitoring periods. It is normally used to collect in one minute time intervals for two to four weeks. This allows patterns of activity and rest to be measured, as well as overall activity [1, 2].

Efficacy : The StepWatch Step Activity Monitor (SAM) assessed the stride count of people with Parkinson's Disease. The participants took 3 passes over the GaitMat II while wearing the StepWatch Step Activity Monitor (SAM). Strides counted by GaitMat II were compared with strides counted by the StepWatch Step Activity Monitor (SAM). There was a 1.0 correlation coefficient between them, showing that the Stepwatch is a valid tool for assessing stride count in Parkinson's Disease [1].

[1] Journal of Geriatric Physical Therapy [2011] 34 (1) : 41-45 (A.L. Schmidt, M.L.Pennypacker, A.H.Thrush, C.I.Leiper, R.L.Craik)

[2] Journal of Neuroengineering and Rehabilitation [2016] 13 (1) : 24 (C.Godinho, J.Domingos, G.Cunha, A.T.Santos, R.M.Fernandes, D. Abreu, N.Gonçalves, H.Matthews, T.Isaacs, J.Duffen, et al)

TRITRAC RT3 ACCELEROMETER

Technology : The TriTrac RT3 accelerometer is a pager sized tri-axial accelerometer capable of measuring acceleration in three planes of movement. The TriTrac RT3 accelerometer can be hooked on to a belt easily and securely [1].

Efficacy : The accelerometer reliably measured free-living physical activity in people with Parkinson's Disease. It was found to distinguish between people who had varying levels of mobility better than a recall questionnaire [1, 2].

[1] Archives of Physical Medicine and Rehabilitation [2008] 89 (9) : 1765-1771 (L.A.Hale, J.Pal, I.Becker)

[2] Journal of Neuroengineering and Rehabilitation [2016] 13 (1) : 24 (C.Godinho, J.Domingos, G.Cunha, A.T.Santos, R.M.Fernandes, D. Abreu, N.Gonçalves, H.Matthews, T.Isaacs, J.Duffen, et al)

CHAPTER 34

DIAGNOSIS OF PARKINSON'S DISEASE

CHEMICAL METHODS

Diagnosis

Diagnosis is usually based on physical observation and questioning of the patients. The most commonly used symptom questionnaire is the Unified Parkinson Disease Rating Scale (UPDRS). Assessments can also involve the SPECT or PET scans, which are the most accurate methods of diagnosing Parkinson's Disease.

Chemical methods of diagnosis

Chemical methods of diagnosing Parkinson's Disease that are either available or are in development include : biomarkers [PAGE 427], a breath test [PAGE 428], PD2 peptoid [PAGE 429], saliva gland test [PAGE 429], and several types of smell test [PAGE 430].

Biomarkers

Technology : A biomarker is a substance used as an indicator of a biological state or illness [1]. These have included a selection of blood-borne autoantibody biomarkers with a higher prevalence in early Parkinson's Disease used to facilitate the diagnosis of early Parkinson's Disease. Antibodies are proteins produced by a person's immune system that allows their body to distinguish between "self" and "non-self" proteins [2].

Efficacy : A systematic review was undertaken to determine which biomarkers for disease progression in Parkinson's Disease exist. The sensitivity of the tests was an average of 71%, which is insufficient for Parkinson's Disease diagnosis. The range in sensitivity was between 51% and 86% showing that some of the methods were nearer to having a practical use [1]. More recently, selected, blood-borne autoantibody biomarkers with a higher prevalence in early Parkinson's Disease could distinguish early Parkinson's Disease with an overall accuracy of 88%, a sensitivity of 94% and a specificity of 85%. These biomarkers were also capable of differentiating people with early Parkinson's Disease from those with mild to moderate Parkinson's Disease with an overall accuracy of 97%. Biomarkers could also distinguish people with early Parkinson's Disease from those with other neurological disorders [2].

[1] BMC Neurology [2013] 13 : 35 (D.J.McGhee, P.L.Royle, P.A. Thompson, D.E.Wright, J.P.Zajicek, C.E. Counsell)

[2] Immunology Letters [2015] 168 (1) : 80-88 (C.A.DeMarshall, M. Han, E.P.Nagele, A.Sarkar, N.K.Acharya, G.Godsey, E.L.Goldwaser, M.Kosciuk, U.Thayasivam, B.Belinka, R.G.Nagele)

Breath test

Technology : A method of diagnosing Parkinson's Disease is being developed that uses breath testing. Alveolar breath is collected from people with Parkinson's Disease. Their breath is analyzed using sensors (organically functionalised carbon nanotubes and gold nanoparticles). Statistical differences were compared between the different groups, which was supported by chemical analysis of the breath samples using gas chromatography combined with mass spectrometry [1, 2].

Efficacy : Gas chromatography combined with mass spectrometry analysis was able to show statistically significant differences in the average level of volatile organic compounds in the breath of people with Parkinson's Disease. Parkinson's Disease could be distinguished from healthy states with an accuracy of 78% to 81% [1, 2].

[1] Nanomedicine [2013] 8 (1) : 43-56 (U.Tisch, I.Schlesinger, R. Ionescu, M.Nassar, N.Axelrod, D.Robertman, Y. Tessler, F.Azar, A. Marmur, J.Aharon-Peretz, H.Haick)

[2] Parkinsonism & Related Disorders [2015] 21 (2) : 150-153 (M.K. Nakhleh, S.Badarny, R.Winer, R.Jeries, J.Finberg, H.Haick)

PD2 Peptoid

Technology : Researchers have identified a peptoid called PD2, which significantly binds higher levels of IgG3 antibody in those people with Parkinson's Disease [1].

Efficacy : PD2 peptoid was found to be 68% accurate in identifying Parkinson's Disease, which is less accurate than existing methods. However, PD2 was 84% accurate in identifying new cases of Parkinson's Disease. It is new cases of Parkinson's Disease that existing methods are not so accurate with. PD2 levels are also positively correlated with the United Parkinson's Disease Rating Scale score, which is the primary symptom questionnaire for Parkinson's Disease [1].

[1] NPJ Parkinsons Disease [2016] 16012 Epub Jun 23 (U.Yazdani, S. Zaman, L.S.Hynan, L.S.Brown, R.B.Dewey, D.Karp, D.C.German)

Saliva gland test

Technology : Testing a portion of a person's saliva gland may be a means of diagnosing Parkinson's Disease. It was previously shown in autopsies of people with Parkinson's Disease that the abnormal proteins associated with Parkinson's are consistently found in the submandibular saliva glands, which are found under the lower jaw [1].

Efficacy : A study involved 15 people with an average age of 68 who had Parkinson's Disease for an average of 12 years who responded to Parkinson's Disease medication and who did not have known saliva gland disorders. Biopsies were taken of two different saliva glands. The abnormal Parkinson's Disease protein was detected in nine of the 11 patients who had enough tissue to study [1]. Oasis Diagnostics Corporation are attempting to validate the development of a non-invasive, saliva-based, rapid test for Parkinson's Disease detection and diagnosis. Research has shown that as few as three salivary biomarkers can lead to an accurate diagnosis of Parkinson's Disease using their technology [2].

[1] Mayo Clinic - http://newsnetwork.mayoclinic.org/discussion/saliva-gland-test-for-parkinsons-shows-promise-study-finds

[2] Oasis Diagnostics Corporation - http://4saliva.com

SMELL TESTS

Loss of olfactory function (sense of smell) is common in Parkinson's Disease [1] and is consequently used as a means of diagnosis. Smell tests being used are the University of Pennsylvania Smell Identification Test (UPSIT), Sniffin sticks and The Brief Smell Identification Tests (B-SIT).

UPSIT

Technology : The SIT, also known as the University of Pennsylvania Smell Identification Test (UPSIT), consists of four self-administered test booklets each containing ten stimuli for smell. Respondents pick from one of four multiple choices. The SIT provides a rapid and easy means of quantifying smell functioning. The SIT focuses on the comparative abilities of individuals to identify a number of odorants at the suprathreshold level. Test stimuli include a number of odorous components mimicking the types of stimuli usually experienced by individuals in the general population. An individual's test scores are compared to scores from people of equivalent age and gender using tables provided in the manual. The resulting percentile score provides a measure of the individual's performance that is easy to interpret [2].

Efficacy : The sensitivity of the University of Pennsylvania Smell Identification Test (UPSIT) was as much as 86%, which is not much different from the DaTSCAN at 92%. Although DaTSCAN is superior, UPSIT is considerably cheaper [3]. The University of Pennsylvania Smell Identification Test is moderately sensitive and specific for the differentiation of Parkinson's Disease from non-idiopathic Parkinson's Disease. The sensitivity was 77% to 86%, and the specificity was 83% to 85% [3-6]. However, at 62% it is less specific for distinguishing Parkinson's Disease from multiple system atrophy [6].

SNIFFIN STICKS

Technology : 'Sniffin' Sticks' is a test of nasal chemosensory performance based on pen-like odour dispensing devices. It comprises three tests of olfactory function, namely tests for odour threshold (n-butanol), odour discrimination (16 pairs of odorants, triple forced choice) and odour identification (16 common odorants, multiple forced choice from four verbal items per test odorant) [7].

Efficacy : The specificity of the 16-item identification test from Sniffin' Sticks (SS-16) when used in Parkinson's Disease was 87% to 90% with a sensitivity of 76% to 85% [4, 5, 8, 15]. Olfactory function was assessed using an extended version of the "Sniffin' Sticks", comprising 32-item odour identification and discrimination tasks. There was no significant difference in diagnostic accuracy between the 16-item and the 32-item versions of the odour identification or discrimination test [9]. The Sniffin' Sticks (SS-12) gave a sensitivity of 76% and specificity of 86% for the diagnosis of Parkinson's Disease [10]. The Colombo SS-12, which is an adaptation of the 16-item identification test from Sniffin' Sticks (SS-16), were correctly identified by at least 50% of the control subjects. The Colombo SS-12 specificity was 93% with a sensitivity of 91% [11].

B-SIT

Technology : The Brief Smell Identification Tests are a rapid and effective five minute screening test. It is a 12-item version of the UPSIT [12].

Efficacy : The B-SIT (brief smell identification test) differentiated Parkinson's Disease from controls with 71% sensitivity and 85% specificity [13]. The B-SIT improved the accuracy of Parkinson's Disease diagnosis using the DatSCAN [14].

[1] Parkinsons Disease [2011] : 450939 (A.Haehner, T.Hummel, H. Reichmann)

[2] SIT Administration Manual

[3] QJM [2010] 103 (12) : 941-952 (J.Deeb, M.Shah, N.Muhammed, R.Gunasekera, K.Gannon, L.J.Findley, C.H.Hawkes)

[4] Movement Disorders [2009] 24 (8) : 1144-1153 (L.Silveira-Moriyama, A.Petrie, D.R.Williams, A.Evans, R.Katzenschlager, E.R. Barbosa, A.J.Lees)

[5] Movement Disorders [2008] 23 (16) : 2328-2334 (L.Silveira-Moriyama, J.M. de Carvalho, R.Katzenschlager, A.Petrie, R.Ranvaud, E.R.Barbosa, A.J.Lees)

[6] Neurologist [2007] 13 (6) : 382-385 (J.H.McKinnon, B.M. Demaerschalk, J.N.Caviness, K.E.Wellik, C.H.Adler, D.M. Wingerchuk)

[7] Chemical Senses [1997] 22 (1) : 39-52 (T.Hummel, B.Sekinger, S. R.Wolf, E.Pauli, G.Kobal)

[8] Movement Disorders [2016] May 9 [Epub ahead of print] (P.Mahlknecht, R.Pechlaner, S.Boesveldt, D.Volc, B.Pinter B, E.Reiter, C.Müller, F.Krismer, H.W.Berendse, J.J.van Hilten, A.Wuschitz, et al)

[9] Movement Disorders [2009] 24 (1) : 85-90 (S.Boesveldt, R.J.de Muinck Keizer, D.L.Knol, E.Ch.Wolters, H.W.Berendse)

[10] Parkinsonism & Related Disorders [2014] 20 (8) : 830-833 (E. Antsov, L.Silveira-Moriyama, S.Kilk, L.Kadastik-Eerme, T.Toomsoo, A.Lees, P.Taba)

[11] Movement Disorders [2009] 24 (8) : 1229-1233 L.Silveira-Moriyama, D.Sirisena, P.Gamage, R.Gamage, R.de Silva, A.J.Lees)

[12] B-SIT Administration Manual

[13] Movement Disorders [2011] 26 (1) : 173-176 (M.Rodríguez-Violante, A.J.Lees, A.Cervantes-Arriaga, T.Corona, L.Silveira-Moriyama)

[14] Journal of Neurology [2015] 262 (9) : 2154-2163 (C. Georgiopoulos, A.Davidsson, M.Engström, E.M.Larsson, H. Zachrisson, N.Dizdar)

[15] Parkinsonism & Related Disorders [2016] Nov 21 [Epub ahead of print] (F.Krismer, B.Pinter, C.Mueller, P.Mahlknecht, M.Nocker, E.Reiter, A.Djamshidian-Tehrani, S.M.Boesch, G.K.Wenning, et al)

CHAPTER 35

CAUSES OF PARKINSON'S DISEASE

BIOCHEMICAL CAUSES

BIOCHEMICAL REACTIONS

Almost all biochemical reactions require the presence, in optimal quantities, of specific enzymes, substrates, coenzymes and cofactors. Consequently, the concentrations of those enzymes, substrates, coenzymes and cofactors determine the rate at which the biochemical reactions take place.

DOPAMINE BIOSYNTHESIS

Parkinson's Disease is primarily due to the insufficient biosynthesis of dopamine. The primary methods of treating Parkinson's Disease are based on this fact. So when the enzymes, substrates, coenzymes and cofactors required for dopamine biosynthesis are deficient the biosynthesis of dopamine is greatly reduced. The insufficient biosynthesis of dopamine causes Parkinson's Disease.

ENZYMES

Enzymes enable biochemical reactions to take place. Almost all biochemical reactions require an enzyme for the biochemical reaction to be completed. The level of activity of the enzyme determines the rate at which the biochemical reaction occurs. However, unless the enzymes have genetic errors, which is a rare occurrence, the enzymes will be present.

In people with Parkinson's Disease, the activity of the enzymes required for dopamine biosynthesis are substantially reduced, to very low levels in some people [1-6]. However, the activity of the enzymes can be greatly increased with the use of the substrate, coenzymes, and cofactors for those enzymes [7-15].

SUBSTRATES

The substrate is the substance on which an enzyme acts. The substrate bonds with the enzyme active site, and an enzyme-substrate complex is formed. The substrate is transformed into one or more products, which are then released from the active site.

The biosynthesis of dopamine requires only one substrate for its formation, which is L-tyrosine. L-tyrosine is essential for the biosynthesis of L-dopa via the enzyme tyrosine 3-monooxygenase [7-10]. The quantity of L-dopa formed increases or decreases according to the concentration of L-tyrosine [7-10].

COENZYMES

A coenzyme is a chemical compound that is essential for the biochemical activity of many but not all enzymes. The activity of the enzyme increases or decreases according to the concentration of the coenzyme. Most coenzymes are ultimately derived from vitamins.

The biosynthesis of dopamine requires four coenzymes : pyridoxal phosphate, tetrahydrofolic acid, NADPH, and NADP. Pyridoxal phosphate is essential for the formation of dopamine from L-dopa. Tetrahydrofolic acid is essential for the biosynthesis of L-dopa from L-tyrosine. Dopamine biosynthesis requires tetrahydrofolic acid, which requires NADPH, and pyridoxal phosphate, which requires NADP.

Pyridoxine is essential for the biosynthesis of pyridoxal phosphate [16, 17]. Folic acid is essential for the biosynthesis of tetrahydrofolic acid [18-21]. Nicotinamide is essential for the biosynthesis of the nicotinamide coenzymes NADPH and NADP [22-34].

COFACTORS

A cofactor is a chemical compound that is essential for the biochemical activity of many but not all enzymes. The activity of the enzyme increases or decreases according to the concentration of the cofactor. Most cofactors are mineral elements such as manganese and zinc.

The biosynthesis of dopamine requires three cofactors : ferrous iron, zinc, and manganese. Ferrous iron is an essential cofactor for the biosynthesis of L-dopa from L-tyrosine [7-10]. Zinc is an essential cofactor for the biosynthesis of pyridoxal phosphate, which is essential for the formation of dopamine [16, 17]. Manganese is an essential cofactor for the biosynthesis of NADP and NADPH, which are essential for dopamine biosynthesis [27-34].

Malnutrition

Even partial deficiencies of the substances that are necessary for dopamine formation will cause a reduction in dopamine biosynthesis [7-10]. The deficiency of more than one substance required for dopamine biosynthesis multiplies the detrimental effect on dopamine biosynthesis [7-10].

Up to 60% of people with Parkinson's Disease are at risk of malnutrition, and therefore the risk of not just partical deficiencies but serious deficiencies of the nutrients required for the biosynthesis of dopamine [35-41, 57].

The prevalence of serious malnutrition in people with Parkinson's Disease is as much as 25% [35-39, 42, 57]. Severe malnutrition occurs in about 2% of people with Parkinson's Disease [35, 36]. The prevalence of malnutrition in people with Parkinson's Disease worsened over time and was in relation to the severity of Parkinson's Disease [39].

Deficiencies

L-tyrosine is essential for the formation of dopamine. It is normally obtained in the diet in the form of protein. However, most people with Parkinson's Disease have a significantly lower protein intake [43, 44], and therefore a lower intake of L-tyrosine. Parkinson's Disease is also associated with the deficiency of all of the other substances that are essential for dopamine biosynthesis including zinc [45-50], iron [51, 52], manganese [53], folic acid [44, 54, 55], nicotinamide [54, 56], and pyridoxine [54, 56].

[1] Movement Disorders [1995] 10 (1) : 10-17 (X.H.Zhong, J.W. Haycock, K.Shannak, Y.Robitaille, J.Fratkin, A.H.Koeppen, O. Hornykiewicz, S.J.Kish)

[2] Klinische Wochenschrift [1960] 38 : 1236-1239 (H.Ehringer, O. Hornykiewicz)

[3] Journal of Neural Transmission (Supplement) [1978] (14) : 121-131 (P.Riederer, W.D.Rausch, W.Birkmayer, K.Jellinger, D.Seemann)

[4] Journal of Pharmacology and Experimental Therapeutics [1975] 195 (3) : 453-464 (K.G.Lloyd, L.Davidson, O.Hornykiewicz)

[5] Movement Disorders [1995] 10 (1) : 10-17 (X.H.Zhong, J.W. Haycock, K.Shannak, Y.Robitaille, J.Fratkin, A.H.Koeppen, O. Hornykiewicz, S.J.Kish)

[6] Journal of Neural Transmission [1988] 72 (1) : 77-82 (M.Mogi, M.Harada, K.Kiuchi, K.Kojima, T.Kondo, H.Narabayashi, D.Rausch, P.Riederer, K.Jellinger, T.Nagatsu)

[7] Nature [1983] 302 : 830-832 (S.El Mestikawy, J.Glowinski, M. Hamon)

[8] Archives of Biochemistry and Biophysics [1967] 120 : 420-427 (M.Ikeda, M.Levitt, S.Udenfriend)

[9] Journal of Biological Chemistry [1964] 239 : 2910-2917 (T. Nagatsu, M.Levitt, S.Udenfriend)

[10] Comptes Rendue des Academie Sciences Series 3 [1986] 302 : 435-438 (D. Pigeon, R.Drissi-Daoudi, F.Gros, J.Thibault)

[11] Proceedings of the National Academy of Sciences, USA [1972] 69 : 343-347 (J.G.Christenson, W.Dairman, S.Udenfriend)

[12] Journal of Biological Chemistry [1962] 237 : 89-93 (W. Lovenberg, H.Weissbach, S.Udenfriend)

[13] Journal of Biological Chemistry [1957] 227 : 617-624 (H. Weissbach, D.F.Bogdanski, B.G.Redfield, S.Udenfriend)

[14] Journal of Biological Chemistry [1948] 174 : 813-816 (R.W. McGilvery, P.P. Cohen)

[15] Hoppe-Seyler's Zeitschrift fur Physiologie Chemie [1963] 332 : 70-78 (C.E.Sekeris)

[16] Journal of Biological Chemistry [1961] 236 : 2076-2084 (D.B. McCormick, M.E.Gregory, E.E.Snell)

[17] Biulleten Eksperimental noi Biologii i Meditsiny [1946] 22 (6) : 40-43 (A.F.Trufanov, J.A.Krisanova)

[18] Journal of Biological Chemistry [1961] 236 : 1163 (R.L.Blakley, B.M.McDougall)

[19] Journal of Biological Chemistry [1982] 257 : 13650-13662 (J.T. Bolin, D.J.Filman, D.A.Matthews, J.Kraut)

[20] Journal of Biological Chemistry [1966] 241 : 1319-1328 (B.T. Kaufman, R.C.Gardiner)

[21] Biochimica et Biophysica Acta [1969] 177 : 401-411 (I.G.Young, F.Gibson)

[22] Journal of Biological Chemistry [1957] 225 : 759-770 (J.Preiss, P.Handler)

[23] Biochemical Journal [1961] 80 : 318-323 (M.R.Atkinson, J.F. Jackson, R.K.Morton)

[24] Archives of Biochemistry and Biophysics [1967] 120 : 440-450 (W.Dahmen, B.Webb, J.Preiss)

[25] Journal of Biological Chemistry [1951] 191 : 535-541 (A. Kornberg, W.E.Pricer)

[26] Biochemistry [1990] 29 (10) : 2501 (S.Ruggieri, L.Gregori, P.Natalini, A.Vita, M.Emanuelli, N.Raffaelli, G.Magni)

[27] International Journal of Biochemistry [1982] 14 : 839-844 (J.R. Butler, E.T.McGuinness)

[28] Journal of Biological Chemistry [1967] 242 : 1182-1186 (A.E. Chung)

[29] Journal of Biological Chemistry [1950] 182 : 805-813 (A. Kornberg)

[30] Journal of Biological Chemistry [1954] 206 : 311-325 (T.P.Wang, N.O.Kaplan)

[31] The Pyridine Nucleotide Coenzymes (J.Everse, B.M.Anderson, K.You) [1982] : 279 (R.R.Fisher, S.R.Earle)

[32] CRC Critical Reviews in Biochemistry [1985] 17 : 313 (K.S.You)

[33] Analytical Biochemistry [1986] 154 (1) : 64 (S.J.Berger, N.A. Berger)

[34] Enzyme and Microbial Technology [1994] 16 (3) : 236 (L.M. Simon, M.Kotorman, B.Szajani)

[35] Journal of Nutrition, Health and Aging [2014] 18 (6) : 601-607 (J.vanSteijn, B.van Harten, E.Flapper, E.Droogsma, P.van Walderveen, M.Blaauw, D.van Asselt)

[36] Parkinsonism & Related Disorders [2010] 16 (2) : 119-123 (G. Wang, Y.Wan, Q.Cheng, Q.Xiao, Y.Wang, J.Zhang, J.F.Ma, X.J. Wang, H.Y.Zhou, S.D.Chen)

[37] International Journal of Nursing Practice [2016] 22 (2) : 129-137 (S.R.Kim, S.J.Chung, S.H.Yoo)

[38] Nutrition Reviews [2011] 69 (9) : 520-532 (J.M.Sheard, S.Ash, P.A.Silburn, G.K.Kerr)

[39] Nutritional Neuroscience [2008] 11 (3) : 128-134 (M.Barichella, M.C.Villa, A.Massarotto, S.E.Cordara, A.Marczewska, A.Vairo, C. Baldo, A.Mauri, C.Savardi, G.Pezzoli)

[40] Journal of Parkinsons Disease [2014] 4 (3) : 473-481 (S.M. Fereshtehnejad, L.Ghazi, M.Sadeghi, D.Khaefpanah, G.A.Shahidi, A. Delbari, J.Lökk)

[41] Journal of Nutrition, Health and Aging [2013] 17 (2) : 148-151 (J.M.Sheard, S.Ash, P.A.Silburn, G.K.Kerr)

[42] Movement Disorders [2014] 29 (12) : 1543-1547 (A.Laudisio, D.L.Vetrano, E.Meloni, D.Ricciardi, F.Franceschi, A.R.Bentivoglio, R.Bernabei, G.Zuccalà)

[43] Topics in Spinal Cord Injury Rehabilitation [2103] 19 (3) : 229-235 (A.J.Pellicane, S.R.Millis, S.E.Zimmerman, E.J.Roth)

[44] Nutricion Hospitalaria [2015] 31 (6) : 2764-2770 (M.Zilli Canedo Silva, N.Carol Fritzen, M.de Oliveira, M.Paes da Silva, R.Rasmussen Petterle, H.A.Teive, C.de Mesquita Barros Almeida Leite, et al)

[45] Annals of Pharmacotherapy [2014] 48 (11) : 1515-1520 (M.J. Quiroga, D.W.Carroll, T.M.Brown)

[46] Neuroepidemiology [2011] 36 (4) : 240-244 (T.Fukushima, X.Tan, Y.Luo, H.Kanda)

[47] American Journal of Alzheimers Disease and other dementias [2010] 25 (7) : 572-575 (G.J.Brewer, S.H.Kanzer, E.A.Zimmerman, E.S.Molho, D.F.Celmins, S.M.Heckman, R.Dick)

[48] Journal of Neural Transmission (Supplement) [2006] (71) : 229-236 (G.A.Qureshi, A.A.Qureshi, S.A.Memon, S.H.Parvez)

[49] Medical Hypotheses [2001] 56 (5) : 641-645 (S.Johnson)

[50] Journal of Alternative and Complementary Medicine [1999] 5 (1) : 57-64 (L.Forsleff, A.G.Schauss, I.D.Bier, S.Stuart)

[51] Journal of Parkinsons Disease [2013] 3 (4) : 523-537 (N.P. Visanji, J.F.Collingwood, M.E.Finnegan, A.Tandon, E.House, L.N. Hazrati)

[52] Neurochemical Research [2012] 37 (7) : 1436-1441 (G.Madenci, S.Bilen, B.Arli, M.Saka, F.Ak)

[53] BioMed Research International [2015] 672838 (Z.S.Agim, J.R. Cannon)

[54] Nutrition Reviews [2016] 74 (5) : 281-300 (G.Sechi, E.Sechi, C. Fois, N.Kumar)

[55] Metabolic Brain Disease [2009] 24 (2) : 257-269 (E.F.dos Santos, E.N.Busanello, A.Miglioranza, A.Zanatta, A.G.Barchak, C.R.Vargas, J. Saute, C.Rosa, M.J.Carrion, D.Camargo, A.Dalbem, J.C.da Costa, et al)

[56] Clinical Science [1979] 56 (1) : 89-93 (D.A.Bender, C.J.Earl, A.J. Lees)

[57] Journal of Neurological Science [2017] 375 : 235-238 (S.Tomic, V.Pekic, Z. Popijac, T.Pucic, M.Petek, T.G.Kuric, S.Misevic, R.P. Kramaric)

CHAPTER 36

CAUSES OF PARKINSON'S DISEASE

TOXIC CAUSES

Toxic causes

A small proportion of cases have a toxic cause as the sole or a partial cause of Parkinson's Disease. The toxic exposure usually has to be acute or chronic. Symptoms normally develop when the toxic exposure occurs or soon after, or gradually increase over time when the exposure persists. Symptoms do not develop years later as is sometimes claimed. Avoidance of the source of toxicity can lead, in most cases, to a reduction in the symptoms but with some toxins this can take years.

Toxic causes of Parkinson's Disease include : Annonaceae [PAGE 440], Carbon disulfide [PAGE 442], Carbon monoxide [PAGE 443], Copper [PAGE 445], Cyanide [PAGE 446], Cycad seeds [PAGE 447], Dieldrin [PAGE 452], Hydrocarbons [PAGE 453], Lead [PAGE 454], Maneb [PAGE 456], Manganese [PAGE 457], Mercury [PAGE 459], MPTP [PAGE 461], N-hexane [PAGE 461], Nitrogen dioxide [PAGE 462], Octenol [PAGE 463], Organophosphorus pesticides [PAGE 464], Paraquat [PAGE 465], Rotenone [PAGE 468], Toluene [PAGE 469] and Trichloroethylene [PAGE 470]. No studies have proven Agent Orange to be a cause of Parkinson's Disease.

Annonaceae

Chemistry : Annonaceae is a family of flowering plants that is also called the custard apple family. Some annonaceae species produce edible fruits. Annonaceae contain acetogenins.

Common sources : In Guadeloupe, Annonaceae are consumed as herbal teas and fruits, especially soursop [1-8].

Means of toxicity : Annonacin, which is the most abundant acetogenin, is toxic to dopaminergic neurons in nanomolar concentrations [1-3]. Acetogenins are potent mitochondrial toxins, like other Parkinsonism inducing compounds [1, 2, 3, 5, 6, 9]. The concentrations of annonacin, the major acetogenin in Annona Muricata, are so high that one fruit or can of nectar per day is more in a year than induced brain lesions in rats receiving purified annonacin by intravenous infusion [3].

Symptoms : Parkinsonism is associated with the consumption of Annonaceae in Guadeloupe [1-9], and New Caledonia [10, 11]. Parkinsonism is unusually prevalent in Guadeloupe [9]. The symptoms are of an atypical akinetic-rigid syndrome with some similarity to Progressive Supranuclear Palsy that is unresponsive to L-dopa [1]. There is also symmetry of Parkinsonian features, early dysarthria, and frontolimbic cognitive impairment [2]. Within this group, early postural instability, dysarthria, frontal behaviour disorder, cortical or subcortical atrophy, pyramidal signs, axial rigidity, and family history of neurodegenerative disorders were associated with poorer prognosis [2].

[1] Journal of Neural Transmission (Supplement) [2006] (70) : 153-157 (A.Lannuzel, G.U.Hoglinger, P.Champy, P.P.Michel, E.C. Hirsch, M.Ruberg)

[2] Movement Disorders [2005] 20 (Supplement 12) : S114-S118 (D. Caparros-Lefebvre, A.J.Lees)

[3] Movement Disorders [2005] 20 (12) : 1629-1633 (P.Champy, A. Melot, V.Guerineau Eng, C.Gleye, D.Fall, G.U.Hoglinger, M.Ruberg, A.Lannuzel, O.Laprevote, A.Laurens, R.Hocquemiller)

[4] Journal of Chromatography, B. Analytical Technologies in the biomedical and life sciences [2004] 806 (1) : 75-78 (Y.Kotake, K. Okuda, M.Kamizono, N.Matsumoto, T.Tanahashi, H.Hara, et al)

[5] Journal of Neurochemistry [2004] 88 (1) : 63-69 (P.Champy, G.U. Hoglinger, J.Feger, C.Gleye, R.Hocquemiller, A.Laurens, V.Guerineau, O.Laprevote, F.Medja, A.Lombes, P.P.Michel, A.Lannuzel, et al)

[6] Neurosience [2003] 121 (2) : 287-296 (A.Lannuzel, P.P.Michel, G. U.Hoglinger, P.Champy, A.Jousset, F.Medja, A.Lombes, F.Darios, C. Gleye, A.Laurens, R.Hocquemiller, E.C.Hirsch, M.Ruberg)

[7] Lancet [1999] 354 (9175) : 281-286 (D.Caparros-Lefebvre, A. Elbaz)

[8] Movement Disorders [2002] 17 (1) : 84-90 (A.Lannuzel, P.P. Michel, D.Caparros-Lefebvre, J.Abaul, R.Hocquemiller, M.Ruberg)

[9] Brain [2002] 125 (Part 4) : 801-811 (D.Caparros-Lefebvre, N. Sergeant, A.Lees, A.Camuzat, S.Daniel, A.Lannuzel, A.Brice, E. Tolosa, A.Delacourte, C.Duyckaerts)

[10] Movement Disorders [2004] 19 (5) : 604 (D.Caparros-Lefebvre)

[11] Movement Disorders [2004] 19 (5) : 603-604 (G.Angibaud, C.Gaultier, O.Rascol)

CARBON DISULFIDE

Chemistry : Carbon disulfide is a colourless, flammable, and poisonous liquid with the chemical formula CS_2.

Common sources : Carbon disulfide is in pesticides used as fumigants [1], disulfiram, which is a drug used in the treatment of chronic alcoholism [2], industrial solvents [3], and solvents used in the production of viscose rayon and cellophane film [4, 5].

Means of toxicity : Carbon disulfide interferes with the enzyme pyridoxal 5-phosphate, which is essential for the formation of dopamine from L-dopa. So carbon disulfide might cause Parkinson's Disease symptoms by reducing the formation of L-dopa.

Symptoms : Atypical Parkinsonism with cerebellar signs, hearing loss, sensory changes, cogwheel rigidity, decreased associated movements, distal sensory shading, tremulousness, nerve conduction abnormalities [1]. Parkinsonism and frontal lobe-like syndrome associated with bilateral lesions of the lentiform nuclei [2]. Parkinsonism, pyramidal signs, mild cognitive decline, and unresponsiveness to L-dopa. Two patients had a predominantly axonal and sensory polyneuropathy of the lower legs with fasciculations in one of them. Parkinsonian features were progressive even after the patients had stopped work [3]. Balance problems, impotence, and irritability, without tremor, cogwheel rigidity, bradykinesia, changes in facial expression [6]. Encephalopathy with Parkinsonism, pyramidal signs, cerebellar ataxia, and cognitive impairment, as well as axonal polyneuropathy [7]. Parkinsonian features without polyneuropathy or cerebellar signs, polyneuropathy, tremor and encephalopathy [8]. Toxic effects of carbon disulfide can persist for several years after the exposure to carbon disulfide has ceased [9].

[1] Archives of Neurology [1988] 45 (5) : 537-540 (H.A.Peters, R.L. Levine, C.G.Matthews, L.J.Chapman)

[2] Journal of Neurology, Neurosurgery, and Psychiatry [1992] 55 (10) : 925-929 (D.Laplane, N.Attal N, B.Sauron, A.de Billy, B.Dubois)

[3] Journal of Neurology [1999] 246 (3) : 198-206 (G.Hageman, J.Van Der Hoek, M. Van Hout, G. Van Der Laan, E.J.Steur, W.De Bruin, K. Herholz)

[4] Journal of Neuropathology and Experimental Neurology [1945] 4 : 324 (R.Richter)

[5] British Journal of Industrial Medicine [1954] 11 : 235 (E.C. Vigliani)

[6] Environmental Health Perspectives [1998] 106 (9) : 611-613 (M. Frumkin)

[7] European Neurology [2003] (4) : 220-224 (M.C.Ku, C.C.Huang, H. C.Kuo, T.C.Yen, C.J.Chen, T.S.Shih, H.Y.Chang)

[8] Neurotoxicology [2004] 25 (3) : 341-347 (C.C.Huang, T.C.Yen, T. S.Shih, H.Y.Chang, N.S.Chu)

[9] Acta Neurologica Taiwanica [2004] (1) : 3-9 (C.C.Huang)

Carbon monoxide

Chemistry : Carbon monoxide is a colourless, odourless, and tasteless gas that is slightly less dense than air with the chemical formula CO. Carbon monoxide is produced from the partial oxidation of carbon containing compounds when there is not enough oxygen to produce carbon dioxide.

Common sources : Motor vehicle exhaust fumes, cigarette smoke. It also forms when fuels such as coal, paraffin, oil or wood, and especially natural gas, do not burn completely in appliances such as heaters, furnaces, stoves, water heaters, and ovens. Carbon monoxide toxicity is frequent due to the formation of carbon monoxide by very common means such as gas cookers and exhaust fumes. However, carbon monoxide rarely causes Parkinson's Disease. It normally requires the person having gone in to a coma as a result of the carbon monoxide poisoning before symptoms of Parkinson's Disease develop.

Means of toxicity : Carbon monoxide causes hemoglobin, which transports oxygen, to turn in to carboxyhemoglobin, which does not transport oxygen. Oxygen is required for the formation of L-dopa. So carbon monoxide may cause Parkinson's Disease symptoms by interfering with the availability of oxygen to the brain. The precise means by which it causes Parkinson's Disease has still not been proven.

Symptoms : A Parkinsonian state in which there is behavioural and cognitive impairment but in which the person could walk or in which they progressed further to an akinetic-mute state, and were bed-bound [1]. Delayed onset of Parkinsonism in some people from which they recovered [2]. Parkinson's Disease symptoms such as tremor and rigidity were experienced in only a small number of people [3]. In a small proportion of people, Parkinsonian symptoms occurred, such as gait disturbance, impaired mentality, urinary incontinence, and mutism. The most frequent signs were short-step gait, hypokinesia, masked face, increased muscle tone (rigidity), glabella sign, grasp reflex, and retropulsion. There was occasional intentional tremor, but no resting tremor [4]. Those people that had carbon monoxide intoxication had nine times the normal risk of developing Parkinson's Disease [5].

[1] Movement Disorders [1994] 9 (5) : 550-558 (M.S.Lee, C.D. Marsden)

[2] European Neurology [1999] 42 (3) : 141-144 (I.S.Choi, H.Y.Cheon)

[3] Seishin Shinkeigaku Zasshi [1999] 101 (7) : 592-618 (K.Mimura, M.Harada, S.Sumiyoshi, G.Tohya, M.Takagi, E.Fujita, A.Takata, S. Tatetsu)

[4] European Neurology [2002] 48 (1) : 30-33 (I.S.Choi)

[5] Journal of Pediatric Gastroenterology and Nutrition [2015] 94 (19) : 1-6 (C.Y.Lai, M.C.Chou, C.L.Lin, C.H.Kao)

Copper

Chemistry : Copper, whose chemical symbol is Cu, is a chemical element that is required as a nutrient, but which can be toxic in large quantities.

Common sources : Due to Wilson's Disease in which there is a genetic accumulation of copper, copper mines, copper cooking pots, copper plumbing, extreme consumption of nutritional supplements that contain copper.

Means of toxicity : Excessive copper can cause the formation of a copper-dopamine complex, which leads to the oxidation of dopamine to aminochrome [1].

Symptoms : Parkinsonism and depression when it is due to Wilson's Disease [2]. Parkinson's Disease is associated with Wilson's Disease, a genetic disorder in which copper accumulates. Exposure to large quantities of copper is also associated with symptoms of Parkinson's Disease [3].

[1] Journal of Neurochemistry [2001] 77 (2) : 519-529 (I.Paris, A. Dagnino-Subiabre, K.Marcelain, L.B.Bennett, P.Caviedes, R.Caviedes, C.O.Azar, J.Segura-Aguilar)

[2] Journal of Clinical Neuroscience [2005] 12 (3) : 303-305 (K.H. Chan, R.T.Cheung, K.M.Au-Yeung, W.Mak, T.S.Cheng, S.L.Ho)

[3] Neurology [1997] 48 (3) : 650-658 (J.M.Gorell, C.C.Johnson, B.A. Rybicki, E.L.Peterson, G.X.Kortsha, G.G.Brown, R.J.Richardson)

CYANIDE

Chemistry : Cyanide is any chemical compound that contains a cyano group, which consists of a carbon atom triple-bonded to a nitrogen atom. It has the chemical formula CN.

Common sources : Cyanide is contained in drugs such as potassium cyanide and sodium cyanide. Cyanides can also be produced by certain bacteria, fungi, and algae, and are found in a number of foods and plants. Cyanide occurs naturally in cassava roots (also known as manioc), which are potato-like tubers of cassava plants grown in tropical countries. They must be processed, usually by extended boiling, prior to consumption. Fruits that have a pit, such as cherries or apricots, often contain either cyanides or cyanogenic glycosides in the pit. Bitter almonds, from which almond oil and flavouring is made, also contain cyanide. Hydrogen cyanide is contained in vehicle exhaust and in tobacco smoke. The smoke of burning plastics contains hydrogen cyanide, and so house fires often result in cyanide poisonings. A deep blue pigment called Prussian blue, used in the making of blueprints, is iron (III) ferrocyanide. Cyanides are one of the very few soluble compounds of gold and thus are used in electroplating, gold mining, metallurgy and jewellery for chemical gilding, buffing, and extraction of gold. Cyanides and hydrogen cyanide are used in the production of chemicals, photographic development, making plastics, fumigating ships, and some mining processes. Potassium ferrocyanide is used to achieve a blue colour on cast bronze sculptures.

Means of toxicity : Cyanide interrupts the electron transport chain in the inner membrane of the mitochondrion because it binds more strongly than oxygen to the $Fe3^{+}$ in cytochrome a3, preventing this cytochrome from combining electrons with oxygen. Cyanide also occupies the place of oxygen in hemoglobin, which transports oxygen. Oxygen is required for the formation of L-dopa. So cyanide might cause Parkinson's Disease symptoms by interfering with the availability of oxygen to the brain.

Symptoms : Symptoms can include : Severe Parkinsonian syndrome [1-4] characterised primarily by akinesia and rigidity [1], or combined with progressive dystonia [2], profound micrographia and with hypersalivation [3], progressive Parkinsonism, dystonia and apraxia of eye opening [5], Parkinsonism that develops slowly after the poisoning apart from dysarthria, bradykinesia of the upper limbs and very brisk monosynaptic reflexes [6, 7].

[1] Neurology [1985] 35 (6) : 921-925 (R.J.Uitti, A.H.Rajput, E.M. Ashenhurst, B.Rozdilsky)

[2] Movement Disorders [1989] 4 (2) : 188-193 (F.Grandas, J.Artieda, J.A.Obeso)

[3] International Journal of Psychiatry in Medicine [1990] 20 (2) : 173-179 (J.M.Feldman, M.D.Feldman)

[4] Neurology [1989] 39 (1) : 142-144 (N.L.Rosenberg, J.A.Myers, W. R.Martin)

[5] Journal of Neurology, Neurosurgery, and Psychiatry [1988] 51 (10) : 1345-1348 (F.Carella, M.P.Grassi, M.Savoiardo, P.Contri, B.Rapuzzi, A.Mangoni)

[6] European Archives of Psychiatry and Neurological Sciences [1988] 237 (3) : 139-143 (B.Messing, B.Storch)

[7] Journal of Neural Transmission (Supplementum) [1991] 33 : 141-147 (B.Messing)

Cycad seeds

Chemistry : Cycad seeds of the Cycas micronesica contain ss-methylamino-L-alanine (BMAA), which have been implicated due to the involvement of a product of BMAA and a beta-carbamate [1].

Cycad seeds, by different means, can cause Amyotrophic lateral sclerosis (ALS) and Parkinsonism-dementia complex (PDC). This occurs in Guam which is in the Mariana islands, in the Pacific Ocean [2, 3], the Kii peninsula of Japan [4], and New Guinea [5, 6, 7], which is divided between Indonesia and Papua New Guinea.

[1] Rinsho Shinkeigaku [2002] 42 (11) : 1073-1076 (S.Kuzuhara)

[2] Neurology [2008] 70 (21) : 1984-1990 (J.C.Steele, P.L. McGeer)

[3] The Island of the Colorblind [1997] (Oliver Sacks)

[4] Archives of Neurology [2003] 60 (9) : 1257-1261 (Y.Kokubo, S. Kuzuhara)

[5] Movement Disorders [2005] 20 (Supplement 12) : S119-S126 (P.S. Spencer, V.S.Palmer, A.C.Ludolph)

[6] Geriatrics] [1991] 46 (Supplement 1) : 37-42 (P.S.Spencer, G.E. Kisby, A.C.Ludolph)

[7] Journal of Neurological Science [1998] 157 (1) : 37-41 (M.Yasui, K.Ota)

GUAM

In Guam and the Mariana islands there is a high, but declining, incidence of Amyotrophic lateral sclerosis (ALS) and Parkinsonism-dementia complex (PDC). It mostly occurs within the Chamorro people in Guam [1, 2]. It was referred to as Lytico-Bodig disease [2]. It was found to be one hundred times more common in Guam than it is in the U.S.A. [3].

Common means : Eating a species of Flying Fox called the Mariana Fruit Bat, which is a centuries old culinary delicacy in Guam amongst the Chamorro people [4]. Mariana Fruit Bats consume large quantities of the potentially toxic cycad seeds [2], which are implicated as a cause [5]. Served at weddings, festivals and birthdays, the etiquette of bat eating and preparation involves rinsing off the outside of the animal and then putting it in boiling water. The animals are served whole in coconut milk and are consumed in their entirety. Meat, internal organs, fur, eyes, and wing membranes are all eaten. As the number of Mariana Fruit Bats has declined in number so has the illness [6]. The people of Guam also used to depend heavily on flour that is made from the starch extracted from cycad seeds, and use that flour to make poultices for wounds.

Means of toxicity : A recurring hypothesis as to causation is exposure to Cycas micronesica, which is the false Sago palm known locally as fadang. However, this has been doubted [1]. BMAA occurs not only as a free amino acid but also can be released from a bound form. Within brain tissues the endogenous neurotoxic reservoir of bound BMAA can slowly release free BMAA thereby causing recurrent neurological damage over years or even decades, which may explain the long latency period for neurological disease onset among the Chamorro people [7]. BMAA occurs in much higher levels in the Flying Foxes in Guam than in the cycad seeds the flying foxes feed on [8, 9].

Symptoms : ALS-PDC is a complex of amyotrophic lateral sclerosis and parkinsonism dementia complex with additional symptoms of Alzheimer's Disease [10]. It manifests clinically with parkinsonism as well as dementia and is characterised neuropathologically by prominent cortical neuron loss in association with extensive telencephalic neurofibrillary tau pathology [11]. Tau pathology was observed in both grey and white matter with frontal and temporal lobes being the most severely affected [11]. Alpha-synuclein pathology affects the amygdala, and also the cerebellum, where it appears to involve both Purkinje cells and specialised astrocytes [12]. There is also a reduced sense of smell [13, 14].

[1] Neurology [2008] 70 (21) : 1984-1990 (J.C.Steele, P.L. McGeer)

[2] The Island of the Colorblind [1997] (Oliver Sacks)

[3] Annals of Neurology[1980] 8 (6) : 612-619 (R.M.Garruto, C. Gajdusek, K.M.Chen)

[4] Neurology [2002] 58 (6) : 956-959 (O.W.Sacks, P.A.Cox)

[5] Canadian Journal of Neurological Science [1987] 14 (3 Supplement) : 347-357 (P.S.Spencer)

[6] Conservation Biology [2003] June edition (Clark Monson, Sandra Banack, Paul Cox)

[7] Proceedings, National Academy of Sciences U.S.A. [2004] 101 (33) : 12228-12231 (S.K.Murch, P.A.Cox, S.A.Banack)

[8] Neurology [2003] 61 (3) : 387-389 (S.A.Banack, P.A.Cox)

[9] Proceedings, National Academy of Sciences U.S.A [2003] 100 (23) : 13380-13383 (P.A.Cox, S.A.Banack, S.J.Murch)

[10] Journal of Ethnopharmacology [2002] 82 (2-3) : 159-167 (D.M. Brownson, T.J.Mabry, S.W.Leslie)

[11] Acta Neuropathologica [2006] 111 (5) : 401-412 (M.J.Winton, S.Joyce, V.Zhukareva, D.Practico, D.P.Perl, D. Galasko, U.Craig, J.Q. Trojanowski, V.M.Lee)

[12] Acta Neuropathology [2004] 107 (6) : 497-503 (J.Sebeo, P.R.Hof, D.P.Perl)

[13] Geriatrics [1991] 46 (Supplement 1) : 47-51 (R.L.Doty, D.P.Perl, J.C.Steele, K.M.Chen, J.D.Pierce Jr, P.Reyes, L.T.Kurland)

[14] Neurology [1991] 41 (5) (Supplement 2) : 77-81 (R.L.Doty, D.P. Perl, J.C.Steele, K.M.Chen, J.D.Pierce Jr, P.Reyes, L.T.Kurland)

KII PENINSULA

The Kii Peninsula of Japan, together with Guam and West New Guinea, has one of the highest incidences of amyotrophic lateral sclerosis (ALS) and parkinsonism-dementia complex (PDC) in the world [1]. Kii paralysis was first described in Japan in the 1680s in Japanese folk literature [2].

Common means : A recurring hypothesis as to causation is exposure to Cycas Micronesica, which is the false Sago palm known locally as fadang. However, this has been doubted [3].

Means of toxicity : Seeds of the Cycas Micronesica contain ss-methylamino-L-alanine (BMAA), which has been implicated as the means of toxicity due to the involvement of a product of BMAA and a beta-carbamate [4]. The finding of an obvious decrease in cerebral blood flow of the frontal and temporal lobes in people with PDC and ALS with or without cerebral atrophy supports the concept that the two medical conditions are different manifestations of one single frontotemporal tauopathy [1].

Symptoms : The main features of Kii ALS/PDC consist of dementia and Parkinsonism [5, 6]. Family history was positive in more than 70% of patients [7]. The initial symptoms can be parkinsonian gait or hypobulia / amnesia, followed by akinesia, rigidity, occasional tremor, bradyphrenia, abulia and amnesia, and finally by akinetic mutism [8]. Parkinsonism can be followed by psychiatric symptoms [9]. Within several years most of the patients developed ALS symptoms such as muscle atrophy, bulbar palsy, and upper motor neuron signs [5, 8]. There was mild to severe atrophy of the frontal and temporal lobes and a marked decrease in cerebral blood flow [1, 8]. Marked loss of nerve cells was associated with abundant neurofibrillar tangles in the entire central nervous system, predominantly in the brainstem and temporal lobe. Concomitant ALS involving the upper and lower motor neurons was common. Senile plaques were absent in most cases [5-8,10].

[1] Archives of Neurology [2003] 60 (9) : 1257-1261 (Y.Kokubo, S. Kuzuhara)

[2] Brain Nerve [2011] 63 (2) : 119-129 (S.Kuzuhara)

[3] Neurology [2008] 70 (21) : 1984-1990 (J.C.Steele, P.L.McGeer)

[4] Journal of Ethnopharmacology [2002] 82 (2-3) : 159-167 (D.M. Brownson, T.J.Mabry, S.W.Leslie)

[5] Rinsho Shinkeigaku [2001] 41 (11) : 769-774 (Y.Kokubo, S. Kuzuhara)

[6] Annals of Neurology [2001] 49 (4) : 501-511 (S.Kuzuhara, Y. Kokubo, R.Sasaki, Y.Narita, T.Yabana, M.Hasegawa, T. Iwatsubo)

[7] Rinsho Shinkeigaku [2002] 42 (11) : 1073-1076 (S.Kuzuhara)

[8] Movement Disorders [2005] (Supplement 12) : S108-113 (S. Kuzuhara, Y.Kokubo)

[9] Journal of Neurology [2003] 250 (2) : 164-170 (M.Konagaya, T. Kato, M.Sakai, S.Kuru, Y.Matsuoka, Y.Konagaya, Y.Hashizume, T. Tabira)

[10] Folia Neuropathologica [2003] 41 (2) : 59-64 (A.Kowalska, M. Konagaya, M.Sakai, Y.Hashizume, T.Tabira)

New Guinea

ALS and Parkinsonism-dementia complex (PDC) is common in New Guinea (in Irian Jaya, Indonesia) [1, 2, 3], especially among the primitive Auyu and Jakai people [4, 5].

Common means : Parkinsonism in New Guinea is associated with the medical use of Cycad seeds [1, 2]. Topical use of cycad seed (termed kurru) gametophyte to treat large skin lesions is advanced as a plausible but unproven etiologic factor [1].

Means of toxicity : Two neurotoxins in the cycad seeds are recognised, one of which is cycasin [2]. Epidemiological surveys in the Western Pacific (Guam, and Kii Peninsula and West New Guinea) suggest that low calcium, low magnesium, high aluminium and high manganese in rivers, soil and drinking water may be implicated [3].

Symptoms : Parkinsonism is common in New Guinea [1-3], in association with Amyotrophic lateral sclerosis and dementia [1-5].

[1] Movement Disorders [2005] 20 (Supplement 12) : S119-S126 (P.S. Spencer, V.S.Palmer, A.C.Ludolph)

[2] Geriatrics] [1991] 46 (Supplement 1) : 37-42 (P.S.Spencer, G.E. Kisby, A.C.Ludolph)

[3] Journal of Neurological Science [1998] 157 (1) : 37-41 (M.Yasui, K.Ota)

[4] Neurology [1983] 33 (6) : 812 (H.Feit)

[5] Neurology [1982] 32 (2) : 107-126 (D.C.Gajdusek, A.M.Salazar)

Dieldrin

Chemistry : Dieldrin is an Organochlorine pesticide. It has the chemical formula $C_{12} H_8 Cl_6 O$.

Common sources : Dieldrin is used as a pesticide [1].

Means of toxicity : Dieldrin adversely affects cellular processes associated with Parkinson's Disease including mitochondrial function and reactive oxygen species production [2]. Dieldrin showed inhibitory effects on proteasome activities at low concentrations [3]. Dieldrin induces apoptosis in dopaminergic neurons via caspase-3-dependent proteolytic activation of protein kinase C delta (PKCdelta) [4, 5].

Symptoms : Dieldrin levels were above normal in brains of people with Parkinson's Disease [6, 7, 8]. Dieldrin was the most frequently detected Organochlorine pesticide in people with Parkinson's Disease thereby suggesting that dieldrin may be associated with Parkinson's Disease [1].

[1] ISRN Neurology [2013] : 371034 (N.Chhillar, N.K.Singh, B.D. Banerjee, K.Bala, M.Mustafa, D.Sharma, M.Chhillar)

[2] Chemical Research in Toxicology [2013] 26 (7) : 1043-1054 (E.M. Allen, V.R.Florang, L.L.Davenport, Y.Jinsmaa, J.A.Doorn)

[3] Neurobiology of Disease [2006] 23 (1) : 198-205 (X.F.Wang, S.Li, A.P.Chou, J.M.Bronstein)

[4] Molecular Brain [2008] Oct 22 (A.G.Kanthasamy, M.Kitazawa, Y. Yang, V.Anantharam, A.Kanthasamy)

[5] Neuroscience [2003] 119 (4) : 945-964 (M.Kitazawa, V. Anantharam, A.G.Kanthasamy)

[6] Journal of Toxicology and Environmental Health (Part A) [2000] 59 (4) : 229-234 (F.M.Corrigan, C.L.Wienburg, R.F.Shore, S.E.Daniel, D. Mann)

[7] Experimental Neurology [1998] 150 (2) : 339-342 (F.M.Corrigan, L.Murray, C.L.Wyatt, R.F.Shore)

[8] Annals of Neurol [1994] 36 (1) : 100-103 (L.Fleming, J.B.Mann, J. Bean, T.Briggle, J.R.Sanchez-Ramos)

Hydrocarbons

Chemistry : Hydrocarbons are organic compounds consisting entirely of hydrogen and carbon. The chemical formulae differ.

Common sources : Hydrocarbon poisoning such as that of benzene and petroleum usually occurs accidentally by their inhalation or ingestion. Sources of hydrocarbons include : natural gas, cooking gas, petrol, gasoline.

Means of toxicity : The means of toxicity is unknown.

Symptoms : People that have been subjected to exposure to petroleum products, especially when working with petroleum products increases the likelihood of developing Parkinson's Disease [1-4]. Hydrocarbon exposure increased the likelihood of Parkinson's Disease by 1.32 times normal [1]. Exposure to petroleum products increased the risk of Parkinson's Disease [2, 3] by 2.3 times [3]. Occupational exposure to hydrocarbons increased the likelihood of developing Parkinson's Disease to 1.61 times normal [1]. Working in a gas station (petrol station) increased the risk of Parkinson's Disease by 2.6 times [4].

[1] Parkinsonism & Related Disorders [2014] 21 (3) : 243-248 (O. Palin, C.Herd, K.E.Morrison, A.C.Jagielski, K.Wheatley, G.N.Thomas, C.E.Clarke)

[2] Canadian Journal of Neurological Science [1995] 22 (3) : 232-234 (S.Chaturvedi, T.Ostbye, A.J.Stoessl, H.Merskey, V.Hachinski)

[3] Neurology [1994] 44 (6) : 1051-1054 (J.W.Tetrud, J.W.Langston, I. Irwin, B.Snow)

[4] American Journal of Industrial Medicine [2014] 57 (2) : 163-171 (K.Teschke, S.A.Marion, J.K.Tsui, H.Shen, K.Rugbjerg, M.A.Harris)

Lead

Chemistry : Lead, whose chemical symbol is Pb, is a chemical element that is toxic in humans.

Common sources : Lead contaminated soil, ingestion of lead dust or chips from deteriorating lead-based paints. Air pollution from the processing of lead, food grown in contaminated soil, drinking water from plumbing and fixtures that are either made of lead or have trace amounts of lead in them. Lead can also be found in cosmetics in some countries, in some herbal remedies, and in toys such as many from China.

Means of toxicity : Due to the similarity of their structures lead can inadvertently replace iron in enzymatic reactions but it does not properly function as a cofactor. This might cause a reduction in L-dopa because iron is an essential cofactor for L-dopa formation. Most lead poisoning symptoms are thought to occur by interfering with the enzyme Delta-aminolevulinic acid dehydratase (ALAD), which is required for hemoglobin biosynthesis, as is ferrochelatase, which is also inhibited by lead. Hemoglobin transports oxygen, which is required for the formation of L-dopa. So carbon monoxide may also cause Parkinson's Disease symptoms by interfering with the availability of oxygen to the brain. However, the precise means by which it causes Parkinson's Disease has still not been proven.

Symptoms : Serious and chronic exposure to lead can more than double the likelihood of developing Parkinson's Disease. Milder exposure to lead did not increase the likelihood of Parkinson's Disease [1]. Prolonged exposure to lead can double the likelihood of developing Parkinson’s Disease [1]. Bone lead concentrations tend to be higher in people with Parkinson's Disease [2]. A higher risk of Parkinson's Disease (1.65 times greater) was associated with higher exposure to larger particles (PM10) of pollution. A higher risk of Parkinson's Disease (1.29 times) was also associated with exposure to smaller particles (PM2.5) of pollution. Women were more affected than men in this way [3].

Consequently, pollution, especially larger particles, is the cause of a moderate increase in the risk of Parkinson's Disease. The could be higher when the exposures to pollution are more intense or more prolonged.

[1] Environmental Health Perspective [2006] 114 (12) : 1872-1876 (S. Coon, A.Stark, E.Peterson, A.Gloi, G.Kortsha, J.Pounds, D.Chettle, J. Gorell)

[2] Environmental Health Perspectives [2010] 118 (11) : 1609-1613 (M.G.Weisskopf, J.Weuve, H.Nie, M.H.Saint-Hilaire, L.Sudarsky, D. K.Simon, B.Hersh, J.Schwartz, R.O.Wright, H.Hu)

[3] Environmental Health Perspectives [2016] 124 (11) : 1759-1765 (R.Liu, M.T. Young, J.C.Chen, J.D.Kaufman, H.Chen)

Maneb

Chemistry : The main active element of Maneb is manganese ethylene-bis-dithiocarbamate. It has the chemical formula ($C_4 H_6 Mn N_2 S_4$)n.
Common sources : Maneb is used as a fungicide. There is a greatly increased likelihood of developing symptoms by people involved in horticulture and agriculture [1].

Means of toxicity : As Maneb contains manganese it is possible that it causes Parkinson's Disease symptoms via the same means as manganese, which is by inhibiting tyrosine hydroxylation. Tyrosine hydroxylation is essential for the formation of dopamine. Maneb would, by this means, lower dopamine levels. The effects of Maneb are potentiated when there is simultaneous exposure to the pesticide Paraquat [2-6].

Symptoms : Combined exposure to maneb, paraquat and ziram was associated with 3 times the risk of Parkinson's Disease [7]. Risk from ambient workplace exposure is greater than residential exposure, and was especially high for people with younger onset Parkinson's Disease and when exposed in both locations [7]. Pesticides are associated with an increased rate of Parkinson's Disease [8]. Toxicity can cause plastic rigidity with cogwheel phenomenon, headache, fatigue, nervousness, memory complaints, and sleepiness, other neurologic signs, such as postural tremor, cerebellar signs, and bradykinesia [9]. It can cause damaging effects on the dopaminergic system [2-6], and can even have effect prior to birth [2-6]. This suggests that somebody could be affected by the fungicide because of their mother's exposure to it during pregnancy.

[1] Scandinavian Journal of Work, Environment & Health. [2000] 26 (4) : 359-362 (F.Tuchsen, A.A.Jensen)

[2] Birth Defects Research. Part A, Clinical and molecular teratology [2005] 73 (3) : 136-139 (D.A.Cory-Slechta, M.Thiruchelvam, E.K. Richfield, B.K.Barlow, A.I.Brooks)

[3] Developmental Neuroscience [2004] 26 (1) : 11-23 (B.K.Barlow, E. K.Richfield, D.A.Cory-Slechta, M.Thiruchelvam)

[4] European Journal of Neuroscience [2003] 18 (3) : 589-600 (M. Thiruchelvam, A.McCormack, E.K.Richfield, R.B.Baggs, A.W.Tank, D.A.Di Monte, D.A.Cory-Slechta)

[5] Neurotoxicology [2002] 23 (4-5) : 621-633 (M.Thiruchelvam, E.K. Richfield, B.M.Goodman, R.B.Baggs, D.A.Cory-Slechta)

[6] Journal of Neuroscience [2000] 20 (24) : 9207-9214 (M. Thiruchelvam, E.K.Richfield, R.B.Baggs, A.W.Tank, D.A.Cory-Slechta)

[7] European Journal of Epidemiology [2011] 26 (7) : 547-555 (A. Wang, S.Costello, M.Cockburn, X.Zhang, J.Bronstein, B. Ritz)

[8] Neurology [1998] 50 (5) : 1346-1350 (J.M.Gorell, C.C.Johnson, B. A.Rybicki, E.L.Peterson, R.J.Richardson)

[9] Neurology [1988] 38 (4) : 550-553 (H.B.Ferraz, P.H.Bertolucci, J.S. Pereira, J.G.Lima, L.A.Andrade)

Manganese

Chemistry : Manganese, whose chemical symbol is Mn, is a chemical element that is required as a nutrient but can be toxic in large quantities.

Common sources : Occupational exposures occur mainly in : welding, when highly exposed [1-4], which is dose dependent [12]. Mining as miners are surrounded by manganese dust and airborne manganese particles, alloy production, processing, ferro-manganese operations especially in which manganese ore or manganese compounds are turned into steel, and work with agrochemicals [2, 5]. Manganese exposures in welders are less than those associated with the reports of manganism in miners and smelter workers [2]. The towns and communities surrounding the areas of manganese heavy industry could also become affected by exposure to manganese. It could occur with very excessive use of manganese supplements. It is hypothesized but has not been proven that long-term exposure to naturally occurring manganese in shower water also puts people at risk. It has occurred in drug addicts who use intravenous methcathinone (ephedrone) contaminated with potassium permanganate [6].

Means of toxicity : Manganese inhibits tyrosine hydroxylation, which is essential for the formation of dopamine [7, 8]. So high levels of manganese causes Parkinson's Disease by lowering dopamine levels. It does not involve degeneration of dopaminergic neurons [8]. L-dopa is not an effective therapy [8].

Symptoms : A syndrome called Manganism, which is a fairly irreversible neurological disorder. Manganism is a medical disorder that is virtually no different in its symptoms from Parkinson's Disease [1, 3, 4, 9, 10, 11].

[1] Neurology 2001 (1) : 8-13 (B.A.Racette, L.McGee-Minnich, S.M. Moerlein, J.W.Mink, T.O.Videen, J.S.Perlmutter)

[2] Journal of Toxicological and Environmental Health (Part B - Critical Reviews) [2007] 10 (6) : 417-465 (A.B.Santamaria, C.A. Cushing, J.M.Antonini, B.L.Finley, F.S.Mowat)

[3] International Journal of Hygiene and Environmental Health [2009] 212 (5) : 459-469 (M.R.Flynn, P.Susi)

[4] Bratislavské Lekárske Listy [2009] 110 (6) : 358-360 (J.Y.Fang, F.T. Phibbs, T.L.Davis)

[5] International Journal of Occupational and Environmental Health [2003] 9 (2) : 153-163 (B.S.Levy, W.J.Nassetta)

[6] Addiction [2012] 108 (4) : 771-779 (A.Djamshidian, Y.Sanotsky, Y.Matviyenko, S.S.O'Sullivan, S.Sharman, M.Selikhova, L. Fedoryshyn, Y.Filts, J.Bearn, A.J.Lees, B.B.Averbeck)

[7] FASEB Journal [2010] 24 (12) : 4989-5002 (K.Sriram, G.X.Lin, A. M.Jefferson, J.R.Roberts, O.Wirth, Y.Hayashi, K.M. Krajnak, J.M. Soukup, A.J.Ghio, S.H.Reynolds, V.Castranova, A.E. Munson, et al)

[8] Environmental Health Perspectives [2010] 118 (8) : 1071-1080 (T. R.Guilarte)

[9] Safety and Health at Work [2013] 4 (3) : 123-135 (R.M.Park)

[10] Parkinsonism & Related Disorders [2014] S1353-S8020 (14) 00456-00458 (J.H.Yoon, Y.S.Ahn)

[11] International Journal of Environmental Research and Public Health [2015] 12 (7) : 7519-7540 (G.F.Kwakye, M.M.Paoliello, S. Mukhopadhyay, A.B.Bowman, M.Aschner)

[12] Neurology [2016] Dec 28 [Epub ahead of print] (B.A.Racette, S.Searles Nielsen, S.R.Criswell, L.Sheppard, N.Seixas, M.N.Warden, H.Checkoway)

Mercury

Chemistry : Mercury, whose chemical symbol is Hg, is a chemical element that is toxic in humans.

Common sources : Dietary fish intake, ethnic over-the-counter medications, occupational exposures to mercury vapour, dental amalgam fillings, gold production, skin ointment, and some soaps.

Means of toxicity : One of the chief means is via the enzyme pyruvate dehydrogenase (PDH), which is irreversibly inhibited by several mercury compounds. The lipoic acid component of the multienzyme complex binds mercury compounds tightly and thus inhibits PDH. However, the cause of the symptoms of Parkinson's Disease is likely to be due to the fact that mercury potently causes the release of dopamine, thereby lowering dopamine levels.

Symptoms : Parkinson’s Disease [1], tremor [2, 3], hand tremor, balance and gait disturbance with bradykinesia, paresthesias of the upper extremities, neurobehavioral abnormalities, slight memory loss, and spatial disorientation [4]. Psychoneurological examination revealed dementia, Parkinson's syndrome and ataxia of the lower limbs [4]. Tremor, paralysis, excessive salivation, tooth loss, skin problems, and pulmonary complaints [5]. Fine hand tremor, depression, hypochondria symptoms, introvert behaviour, concentration difficulty, psychomotor, perceptual and motor co-ordination disturbances [6]. Tremor, loss of memory, sleeplessness, and metallic taste [7]. Emotional changes (depression and anxiety) and neurological changes (amnesia, insomnia and tremor of the tongue) [8]. Impaired short term verbal and spatial memory, impaired sustained and divided attention, impaired motor speed, psychiatric symptoms, including anxiety, depression and phobic avoidance, and tremor, weakness in the limbs, and excessive sweating [9]. Intention tremor, dysdiadochokinesis and mild rigidity [10]. Tremor and reduced coordination ability [11].

[1] Neuroepidemiology [1989] (3) : 128-141 (C.H.Ngim, G. Devathasan)

[2] Neurotoxicology [1999] 20 (6) : 945-952 (H.Biernat, S.A.Ellias, L. Wermuth, D.Cleary, E.C.De Oliveira Santos, P.J.Jorgensen, R.G. Feldman, P.Grandjean)

[3] Neurotoxicology [2005] 26 (2) : 149-157 (N.Auger, O.Kofman, T. Kosatsky, B.Armstrong)

[4] Neurologia i Neurochirurgia Polska [2003] 37 (Supplement 5) : 31-38 (K.Miller, S.Ochudlo, G.Opala, W.Smolicha, J.Siuda)

[5] Neurology [2004] 62 (6) : 963-966 (M.J.Doherty)

[6] La Medicina del Lavoro [2003] 94 (6) : 531-541 (N.Pranjic, O. Sinanovic, R.Jakubovic)

[7] The Science of the Total Environment [2003] 307 (1-3) : 71-82 (S. Bose-O'Reilly, G.Drasch, C.Beinhoff, S.Maydl, M.R.Vosko, G.Roider, D.Dzaja)

[8] Revista de Neurologia [2000] 31 (8) : 712-716 (V.Tirado, M.A. Garcia, J.Moreno, L.M.Galeano, F.Lopera, A.Franco)

[9] Brain Injury [2000] 14 (9) : 797-814 (T.J.Powell)

[10] Occupational Medicine [1998] 48 (6) : 413-415 (A.M.Donoghue)

[11] Neurotoxicology and Teratology [1996] 18 (4) : 505-509 (B. Netterstrom, B.Guldager, J.Heeboll)

MPTP

Chemistry : MPTP (1-methyl 4-phenyl 1,2,3,6-tetrahydropyridine) is a chemical that may be produced accidentally during illicit manufacture of the recreational drug MPPP, which is a synthetic heroin substitute. It has the chemical formula $C_{12} H_{15} N$.

Common sources : The recreational drug MPPP (Desmethylprodine). It was also developed but unused as a herbicide. It is also an industrial toxin.

Means of toxicity : MPTP inhibits tyrosine hydroxylation, which is essential for the formation of dopamine. So MPTP causes Parkinson's Disease by lowering dopamine levels.

Symptoms : Parkinson's Disease [1, 2].

[1] Neurology [1989] 39 (11) : 1483-1487 (J.W.Tetrud, J.W.Langston, P.L.Garbe, A.J.Ruttenber)

[2] Neurology [1993] 43 (2) : 456-457 (J.W.Tetrud, J.W.Langston)

N-Hexane

Chemistry : N-Hexane is an alkane. It may refer to any of five structural isomers or to a mixture of them but is the unbranched isomer. It has the chemical formula $C_6 H_{14}$.

Common sources : Most of the n-hexane used in industry is mixed with solvents. The major use for solvents containing n-hexane is to extract vegetable oils from crops such as soybeans. These solvents are also used as cleaning agents in the printing, textile, furniture, and shoemaking industries. Use by chemists. Certain glues used in the roofing and shoe and leather industries also contain n-hexane. Several consumer products contain n-hexane, such as gasoline, spot removers, quick-drying glues used in various hobbies, and rubber cement.

Means of toxicity : The precise means is not known.

Symptoms : Parkinsonism [1, 2, 3].

[1] Neurological Science [2000] 21 (1) : 49-52 (N.Vanacore, M. Gasparini, I.Brusa, G.Meco)

[2] Annals of Neurology [1996] 40 (6) : 922-925 (G.Pezzoli, O. Strada, V.Silani, A.Zecchinelli, L.Perbellini, F.Javoy-Agid, P.Ghidoni, E.D. Motti, T.Masini, G.Scarlato, Y.Agid, E.C.Hirsch)

[3] Lancet [1989] 2 (8667) : 874 (G.Pezzoli, S.Barbieri, C.Ferrante, A. Zecchinelli, V.Foa)

NITROGEN DIOXIDE

Chemistry : Nitrogen dioxide is a chemical compound with the formula NO_2. It is one of several nitrogen oxides.

Common sources : Nitrogen dioxide is an intermediate in the industrial synthesis of nitric acid, millions of tons of which are produced each year. At higher temperatures nitrogen dioxide is a reddish-brown gas that has a characteristic sharp, biting odour and is a prominent air pollutant.

Means of toxicity : Exposure of nitrogen dioxide to tyrosine hydroxylase results in the nitration of its tyrosine residues [1].

Symptoms : High exposure to nitrogen dioxide, largely because of pollution, trebled the risk of Parkinson's Disease [2]. Lower exposures did not significantly increase the risk [2, 3, 4, 5].

[1] Journal of Biological Chemistry [2003] 278 (31) : 28736-28742 (S.Park, T.J.Geddes, J.A.Javitch, D.M.Kuhn)

[2] Environmental Research [2016] 151 : 713-720 (P.C.Lee, O. Raaschou-Nielsen, C.M.Lill, L.Bertram, J.S.Sinsheimer, J.Hansen, B. Ritz)

[3] Environmental Health Perspectives [2016] Jun 10 [Epub ahead of print] (R.Liu, M.T.Young, J.C.Chen, J.D.Kaufman, C.H.Chen)

[4] Environmental Health Perspectives [2016] 124 (3) : 351-356 (B.Ritz, P.C.Lee, J.Hansen, C.F.Lassen, M.Ketzel, M.Sørensen, O. Raaschou-Nielsen)

[5] Environmental Research [2007] 104 (3) : 420-432 (M.M. Finkelstein, M.Jerrett)

Octenol

Chemistry : Octenol (1-octen-3-ol), which is commonly known as mushroom alcohol, is produced by several plants and fungi [1]. It has the chemical formula $C_8 H_{16} O$.

Common sources : Octenol can often be inhaled by humans after being produced in damp, mouldy or water damaged buildings [1].

Means of toxicity : Octenol interferes with two genes involved in the creation of dopamine : the human plasma membrane dopamine transporter (DAT) and the human VMAT ortholog (VMAT2). This demonstrates that 1-octen-3-ol exerts toxicity via disruption of dopamine homeostasis [1].

Symptoms : It may represent a naturally occurring cause of Parkinsonism.

[1] Proceedings of the National Academy of Sciences USA [2013] 110 (48) : 19561-19566 (A.A.Inamdar, M.M.Hossain, A.I.Bernstein, G.W. Miller, J.R.Richardson, J.W.Bennett)

Organophosphorus Pesticides

Chemistry : Organophosphorus compounds are degradable organic compounds containing carbon-phosphorus bonds.

Common sources : Organophosphorous pesticides are used primarily in pest control as alternatives to chlorinated hydrocarbons, which can persist in the environment. Organophosphorous pesticides are often used in agriculture [1]. Organophosphorus chemicals have also been used as active ingredients in household pesticides for several decades [2].

Means of toxicity : The means by which toxicity is caused is unknown. Human paraoxonase 1 (PON1) is a high-density lipoprotein (HDL)-associated enzyme that protects against exposure to organophosphorus pesticides by hydrolyzing their toxic oxon metabolites [3, 4].

Symptoms : Organophosphorus pesticides were significantly associated with Parkinson's Disease [1, 5, 6]. For every 1.0 μg per litre of pesticide in groundwater, the risk of Parkinson's Disease increases by 3% [7]. The frequent use of household pesticides that contain organophosphorus chemicals increased the chances of developing Parkinson's Disease by 71% [2]. Exposure can lead to Parkinsonism [8-10].

[1] Roczniki Panstwowego Zakladu Higieny [2015] 66 (1) : 21-26 (S. Norkaew, S.Lertmaharit, W.Wilaiwan, W.Siriwong, H.M.Pérez, M.G. Robson)

[2] International Journal of Epidemiology [2013] 42 (5) : 1476-1485 (S. Narayan, Z.Liew, K.Paul, P.C.Lee, J.S.Sinsheimer, J.M.Bronstein, B. Ritz)

[3] Chemico-biological Interactions [2010] 187 (1-3) : 355-361 (C.E. Furlong, S.M.Suzuki, R.C.Stevens, J.Marsillach, R.J.Richter, G.P. Jarvik, H.Checkoway, A.Samii, L.G.Costa, A.Griffith, et al)

[4] Toxicology and Applied Pharmacology [2011] 256 (3) : 418-424 (V.P.Androutsopoulos, K.Kanavouras, A.M.Tsatsakis)

[5] BMC Neurology [2008] 8 : 6 (D.B.Hancock, E.R.Martin, G.M. Mayhew, J.M.Stajich, R.Jewett, M.A.Stacy, B.L.Scott, J.M.Vance, W. K.Scott)

[6] Occupational and Environmental Medicine [2014] 71 (4) : 275-281 (A.Wang, M.Cockburn, T.T.Ly, J.M.Bronstein, B.Ritz)

[7] International Journal of Toxicology [2015] 34 (3) : 266-273 (K.A. James, D.A.Hall)

[8] Neurology [1999] 52 (7) : 1467-1471 (M.H.Bhatt, M.A.Elias, A.K. Mankodi)

[9] Journal of Neurology, Neurosurgery and Psychiatry [1999] 66 (2) : 253-254 (K.R.Müller-Vahl, H.Kolbe, R.Dengler)

[10] Journal of Nervous and Mental Disease [1978] 166 (3) : 222-225 (K.L.Davis, J.A.Yesavage, P.A.Berger)

PARAQUAT

Chemistry : Paraquat is the trade name for N,N'-Dimethyl-4, 4'-bipyridinium dichloride, which is a quaternary ammonium herbicide. It has the chemical formula $[(C_5 H_4 N)_2] Cl_2$. Other members of this class of herbicides include diquat, cyperquat, diethamquat, difenzoquat and morfamquat.

Common sources : Paraquat is used as a herbicide. There is a greatly increased likelihood of developing symptoms by people involved in horticulture and agriculture [1]. People with Parkinson’s Disease are more than twice as likely to report heavy exposure to pesticides over their lifetime as family members without Parkinson's Disease. Those people affected were usually those who used a lot of pesticides in their homes and in their hobbies rather than those who routinely used pesticides for their occupation [2]. Pesticides are known to affect well water [3].

Means of toxicity : Paraquat structurally resembles MPTP and its metabolite MPP+. MPTP and MPP+ are neurotoxic chemicals, that can induce Parkinson's Disease in people exposed to it. Paraquat therefore might, as MPTP and MPP+ do, inhibit tyrosine hydroxylation, which is the enzyme reaction essential for the formation of dopamine. Some evidence suggests that paraquat may cause toxicity through oxidative stress [4].

Symptoms : Combined exposure to paraquat and ziram was associated with a 80% increased risk of Parkinson's Disease [5]. Risk estimates for workplace exposure were greater than for residential exposure and were especially high for people with younger onset Parkinson's Disease and when exposed in both locations [5]. There is a positive association between Parkinson's Disease and pesticide use related to dose and the duration of use [6]. Insecticide exposure increased the likelihood of Parkinson's Disease in men, particularly with late onset Parkinson's Disease, and when the doses are higher [6]. Pesticides are known to be associated with an increased rate of Parkinson's Disease [7], sometimes only marginally [8]. However, the levels of most pesticides are not significantly increased in people with Parkinson's Disease [9, 10]. No connection was found between high-dose paraquat exposure and the development of Parkinsonism [11]. Paraquat can kill dopaminergic neurons in mice [12, 13], and is associated with the symptoms of Parkinson's Disease in humans [14]. However, it is claimed that paraquat only potentiates the effect of Maneb [15, 16], and that it has no effect on humans on its own [11, 17]. Paraquat caused hypokinesia in rodents, but did not have the effects that would be expected if it caused Parkinson's Disease [18].

[1] Scandinavian Journal of Work, Environment & Health. [2000] 26 (4) : 359-362 (F.Tuchsen, A.A.Jensen)

[2] BMC Neurology [2008] 8 : 6 (D.B.Hancock, E.R. Martin, G.M. Mayhew, J.M.Stajich, R.Jewett, M.A.Stacy, B.L.Scott, J. M.Vance, W.K.Scott)

[3] Environmental Health Perspectives [2009] 117 (6) : 964-969 (N.M. Gatto, M.Cockburn, J.Bronstein, A.D.Manthripragada, B.Ritz)

[4] Journal of Toxicology and Environmental Health, Part A [2005] 68 (22) : 1939-1961 (W.Yang, E.Tiffany-Castiglioni)

[5] European Journal of Epidemiology [2011] 26 (7) : 547-555 (A. Wang, S.Costello, M.Cockburn, X.Zhang, J.Bronstein, B.Ritz)

[6] Annals of Neurology [2009] 66 (4) : 494-504 (A.Elbaz, J.Clavel, P. J.Rathouz, F.Moisan, J.P.Galanaud, B.Delemotte, A.Alpérovitch, C. Tzourio)

[7] Neurology [1998] 50 (5) : 1346-1350 (J.M.Gorell, C.C.Johnson, B. A.Rybicki, E.L.Peterson, R.J.Richardson)

[8] Neurology [2012] 79 (20) : 2061-2066 (P.C.Lee, Y.Bordelon, J. Bronstein, B.Ritz)

[9] Archives of Neurology [2009] 66 (7) : 870-875 (J.R.Richardson, S. L.Shalat, B.Buckley, B.Winnik, P.O'Suilleabhain, R.Diaz-Arrastia, J. Reisch, D.C.German)

[10] Neurology [2010] 74 (13) : 1055-1061 (M.G.Weisskopf, P.Knekt, E.J.O'Reilly, J.Lyytinen, A.Reunanen, F.Laden, L.Altshul, A.Ascherio)

[11] Journal of Occupational and Environmental Medicine [2011] 53 (11) : 1332-1336 (J.Brent, T.H.Schaeffer)

[12] Antioxidants & Redox Signaling [2005] 7 (5-6) : 649-653 (D. Bonneh-Barkay, W.J.Langston, D.A.Di Monte)

[13] Brain Research [1999] 823 (1-2) : 1-10 (A.I.Brooks, C.A. Chadwick, H.A.Gelbard, D.A.Cory-Slechta, H.J.Federoff)

[14] Neurology [1997] 48 (6) : 1583-1588 (H.H.Liou, M.C.Tsai, C.J. Chen, J.S.Jeng, Y.C.Chang, S.Y.Chen, R.C.Chen)

[15] Journal of Neuroscience [2000] 20 (24) : 9207-9214 (M. Thiruchelvam, E.K.Richfield, R.B.Baggs, A.W.Tank, D.A.Cory -Slechta)

[16] Brain Research [2000] 873 (2) : 225-234 (M.Thiruchelvam, B.J. Brockel, E.K.Richfield, R.B.Baggs, D.A.Cory-Slechta)

[17] Klinische Wochenschrift [1988] 66 (22) : 1138-1141 (T. Zilker, F. Fogt, M.Von Clarmann)

[18] Experimental Neurology [2007] 208 (1) : 120-126 (A.I.Rojo, C. Cavada, M.R. de Sagarra, A.Cuadrado)

ROTENONE

Chemistry : Rotenone occurs naturally in the seeds and stems of several plants. It has the chemical formula $C_{23} H_{22} O_6$.

Common sources : Rotenone is used as an insecticide. There is a greatly increased likelihood of developing symptoms by people involved in horticulture and agriculture [1]. People with Parkinson's Disease are more than twice as likely to report heavy exposure to pesticides over their lifetime as family members without Parkinson's Disease. Those affected were usually those who used a lot of pesticides in their homes and in their hobbies, rather than those who routinely used pesticides for their occupation [2]. Insecticides are also known to affect well water [3]. Rotenone is commonly used in powdered form to treat parasitic mites on chickens and other fowl, and so can be found in poultry. Rotenone is used to eradicate exotic fish from their non-native habitats. Rotenone is produced by extraction from the roots, seeds, and leaves of certain tropical legumes. People have been known to catch fish by extracting rotenone from plants and then release the rotenone into water.

Means of toxicity : Rotenone inhibits tyrosine hydroxylation, which is essential for the formation of dopamine. So Rotenone causes Parkinson's Disease by lowering dopamine levels. [4].

Symptoms : The neurochemical, neuropathological and behavioural features of Parkinson's Disease [5], including hypokinesia and rigidity [6]. However, some rotenone treated mice and rats remained without any symptoms [7]. Pesticides are known to be associated with an increased rate of Parkinson's Disease [8], as are some pesticides that are found in well water (such as methomyl, chlorpyrifos, propargite) [9]. The levels of most pesticides are not increased in people with Parkinson's Disease [10]. However, there is a positive association between Parkinson's Disease and professional pesticide use that is related to the dose and duration of use [11]. Insecticide exposure increased the likelihood of Parkinson's Disease in men, particularly when the onset of Parkinson's Disease was at an older age, and when the doses are higher [11].

[1] Scandinavian Journal of Work, Environment & Health. [2000] 26 (4) : 359-362 (F.Tuchsen, A.A.Jensen)

[2] BMC Neurology [2008] 8 : 6 (D.B.Hancock, E.R.Martin, G.M. Mayhew, J.M.Stajich, R.Jewett, M.A.Stacy, B.L.Scott, J.M.Vance, W. K.Scott)

[3] International Journal of Toxicology [2015] 34 (3) 266-273 (K.A. James, D.A.Hall)

[4] Toxicology [2005] 216 (1) : 9-14 (Y.Hirata, T.Nagatsu)

[5] Behavioural Brain Research [2002] 136 (1) : 317-324 (M.Alam, W. J.Schmidt)

[6] Nature Neuroscience [2000] 3 (12) : 1301-1306 (R.Betarbet, T.B. Sherer, G.MacKenzie, M.Garcia-Osuna, A.V.Panov, J.T. Greenamyre)

[7] Experimental Neurology [2007] 208 (1) : 120-126 (A.I.Rojo, C. Cavada, M.R.de Sagarra, A.Cuadrado)

[8] Neurology [1998] 50 (5) : 1346-1350 (J.M.Gorell, C.C.Johnson, B. A.Rybicki, E.L.Peterson, R.J.Richardson)

[9] Environmental Health Perspectives [2009] 117 (12) : 1912-1918 (N. M.Gatto, M.Cockburn, J.Bronstein, A.D.Manthripragada, B.Ritz)

[10] Neurology [2010] 74 (13) : 1055-1061 (M.G.Weisskopf, P.Knekt, E.J.O'Reilly, J.Lyytinen, A.Reunanen, F.Laden, L.Altshul, A.Ascherio)

[11] Annals of Neurology [2009] 66 (4) : 494-504 (A.Elbaz, J.Clavel, P.J.Rathouz, F.Moisan, J.P.Galanaud, B.Delemotte, A.Alpérovitch, C. Tzourio)

Toluene

Chemistry : Toluene is an aromatic hydrocarbon consisting of a methyl group bonded to a benzene ring. It has the chemical formula C_7H_8.

Common sources : Toluene is used as an octane booster in fuel, as a solvent in paints, paint thinners, chemical reactions, rubber, printing, adhesives, lacquers, leather tanning, disinfectants, producing phenol and TNT. Toluene is also used as a raw material for toluene diisocyanate, which is used in the manufacture of polyurethane foams. Toluene is also used in the manufacture of dyes. Dyes are highly associated with the symptoms of Parkinson's Disease [1].

Means of toxicity : The means of toxicity is unknown.

Symptoms : Parkinsonism, pyramidal signs, mild cognitive decline, and no response to L-dopa, a predominantly axonal and sensory polyneuropathy of the lower legs with fasciculations in one of them. Parkinsonian features were progressive, even after the patients had stopped work [2]. Toluene has been shown to cause Parkinson's Disease or has been associated with Parkinson's Disease [2, 3].

[1] International Journal of Neuroscience [2010] 120 (5) : 361-367 (V. D.Hristina, S.B.Sipetic, J.M.Maksimovic, J.M.Marinkovic, E.D. Dzoljic, I.S.Ratkov, V.S.Kostic)

[2] Journal of Neurology [1999] 246 (3) : 198-206 (G.Hageman, J.Van Der Hoek, M.Van Hout, G.Van Der Laan, E.J.Steur, W.De Bruin, K. Herholz)

[3] European Journal of Epidemiology [2003] 18 (12) : 1133-1142 (P. Pals, B.Van Everbroeck, B.Grubben, M.K.Viaene, R.Dom, C.Van Der Linden, P.Santens, J.J.Martin, P.Cras)

TRICHLOROETHYLENE

Chemistry : Trichloroethylene is a solvent with a sweet smell that is a clear non-flammable liquid. Trichloroethylene has the chemical formula $C_2 HCl_3$.

Common sources : Trichloroethylene is a solvent that is used in industry and the military and is a common environmental contaminant. It has been used to extract vegetable oils, in coffee decaffeination, and the preparation of flavouring extracts from hops and spices.

Means of toxicity : The means of toxicity is unknown.

Symptoms : Workers with workstations adjacent to the source of trichloroethylene and who were subjected to chronic inhalation and dermal exposure from handling trichloroethylene-soaked metal parts all had Parkinson's Disease. Lesser chronic respiratory exposure to trichloroethylene led to many features of Parkinsonism, including significant motor slowing [1]. Trichloroethylene multiplied the risk of Parkinson's Disease by six times [2].

[1] Annals of Neurology [2008] 63 (2) : 184-192 (D.M.Gash, K. Rutland, N.L.Hudson, P.G.Sullivan, G.Bing, W.A.Cass, J.D.Pandya, M.Liu, D.Y.Choi, R.L.Hunter, G.A.Gerhardt, C.D.Smith, et al)

[2] Annals of Neurology [2012] 71 (6) : 776-784 (S.M.Goldman, P.J. Quinlan, G.W.Ross, C.Marras, C.Meng, G.S.Bhudhikanok, K.Comyns, M.Korell, A.R.Chade, M.Kasten, B.Priestley, K.L.Chou, et al)

CHAPTER 37

CAUSES OF PARKINSON'S DISEASE

GENETIC CAUSES

GENETIC CAUSES

A small proportion of cases of Parkinson's Disease have a genetic cause. Most genetic causes make Parkinson's Disease more likely rather than make it inevitable. Genetic disorders normally occur due to inheritance, either autosomal recessive (from both parents) or autosomal dominant (from one parent), but can arise spontaneously. Having relatives with Parkinson's Disease does not mean that it has been inherited. Relatives can have similar environmental factors as each other that causes their Parkinson's Disease. Most but not all genetic causes are identified by a PARK number.

Genetic causes of Parkinson's Disease with a PARK number include : PARK 1 (Alpha-Synuclein) [PAGE 473], PARK 2 (Parkin) [PAGE 477], PARK 3 (Lewy body) [PAGE 484], PARK 5 (UCHL1) [PAGE 484], PARK 6 (Pink 1) [PAGE 485], PARK 7 (DJ-1) [PAGE 487], PARK 8 (LRRK2) [PAGE 488], PARK 9 (ATP13A2) [PAGE 491], PARK 10 (USP24) [PAGE 493], PARK 11 (GIGYF2) [PAGE 495], PARK 12 [PAGE 497], PARK 13 (HtrA2) [PAGE 498], PARK 14 (PLA2G6) [PAGE 499], PARK 15 (FBXO7) [PAGE 501], PARK 16 [PAGE 502], PARK 17 (VPS35) [PAGE 503], PARK 18 (EIF4G1) [PAGE 505], PARK 19 (DNAJC6) [PAGE 506], PARK 20 (SYNJ1) [PAGE 506], PARK 21 (DNAJC13) [PAGE 508], PARK 22 (CHCHD2) [PAGE 509], PARK 23 (VPS13C) [PAGE 510].

Genetic causes of Parkinson's Disease without a PARK number include : Tyrosine Hydroxylase [PAGE 511], Dopa decarboxylase [PAGE 514], ADORA1 [PAGE 515], CYP2D6 [PAGE 515], DRD2 [PAGE 516], DRD3 [PAGE 517], GLIS1 [PAGE 518], HLA [PAGE 519], LINGO1 [PAGE 521], MAPT [PAGE 522], MCCC1 [PAGE 524], NR4A2 [PAGE 525], PDE8B [PAGE 525], PITX3 [PAGE 526], PTRHD1 [PAGE 527], RAB39B [PAGE 528], RIT2 [PAGE 530], STH [PAGE 531], TMEM230 [PAGE 532].

PARK 1

Gene : Alpha-Synuclein (SNCA) [1]

Chromosome : 4 (q21-q23) [1-5]

Biochemical function : Alpha-Synuclein appears to be involved in dopamine biosynthesis, storage, release, and uptake [6].

Type of inheritance : Autosomal dominant [1, 7-14]

Symptoms : Increased risk of developing Parkinson's Disease [15-30], at an early age of onset [31]. Over half of the cases had early-onset parkinsonism and non-motor features, such as dysautonomia, rapid eye movement sleep behaviour disorder (RBD), hallucinations (usually visual) and cognitive deficits leading to dementia [32].

Prevalence : China [15, 18, 19, 21, 23, 26, 31, 33, 34, 35, 42, 43], Taiwan [16], Iran [17], India [20], Italy [22, 36], Australia [31], Poland [37], Tunisian Berbers [38], Japan [39], Korea [40], Mexican Mestizos [41], Brazil [44]

Genetic tests : PARK1 Parkinsonism (by Centogene AG), SNCA Complete sequencing (by Instituto de Medicina Genomica Paterna), SNCA MLPA testing (by Instituto de Medicina Genomica Paterna), Parkinson disease type 1 (by Bioarray), Parkinson disease 1/4 (by CGC Genetics), CSingle gene testing SNCA (by CeGaT GmbH) [45]

[1] Annals of Neurology [1998] 44 (3 Supplement 1) : S63-S64 (M.H. Polymeropoulos)

[2] Movement Disorders [2000] 15 (6) : 1075-1083 (M.Farrer, T. Destée, E.Becquet, F.Wavrant-DeVrièze, V.Mouroux, F.Richard, L. Defebvre, S.Lincoln, J.Hardy, P.Amouyel, M.C.Chartier-Harlin)

[3] Annals of Neurology [1999] 46 (3) : 374-381 (K.Markopoulou, Z.K.Wszolek, R.F.Pfeiffer, B.A.Chase)

[4] Neurology [1998] 50 (1) : 270-273 (J.J.Higgins, I.Litvan, L.T.Pho, W.Li, L.E.Nee)

[5] Human Molecular Genetics [1997] 6 (10) : 1687-1691 (R.L. Nussbaum, M.H.Polymeropoulos)

[6] Molecular Neurobiology [2005] 31 (1-3) : 243-254 (S.Yu, K.Ueda, P.Chan)

[7] Parkinsons Disease [2015] : 546462 (R.Ferese, N.Modugno, R. Campopiano, M.Santilli, S.Zampatti, E.Giardina, A.Nardone, D. Postorivo, F.Fornai, G.Novelli, E.Romoli, S.Ruggieri, S.Gambardella)

[8] JAMA Neurology [2014] 71 (12) : 1535-1539 (J.Trinh, I.Guella, M.J.Farrer)

[9] Parkinsonism & Related Disorders [2012] 18 (Supplement 1) : S7-S10 (C.Sundal, S.Fujioka, R.J.Uitti, Z.K.Wszolek)

[10] Neurogenetics [2008] 9 (4) : 263-269 (J.M.Choi, M.S.Woo, H.I. Ma, S.Y.Kang, Y.H.Sung, S.W.Yong, S.J.Chung, J.S.Kim, H.W.Shin, C.H.Lyoo, P.H.Lee, J.S.Baik, S.J.Kim, M.Y.Park, Y.H.Sohn, et al)

[11] European Journal of Neurology [2007] 14 (1) : 7-11 (G. Xiromerisiou, G.M.Hadjigeorgiou, V.Gourbali, J.Johnson, I. Papakonstantinou, A.Papadimitriou, A.B.Singleton)

[12] Brain [2003] 126 (Part 1) : 32-42 (H.Kobayashi, R.Krüger, K. Markopoulou, Z.Wszolek, B.Chase, H.Taka, R.Mineki, K.Murayama, O.Riess, Y.Mizuno, N.Hattori)

[13] Cellular and Molecular Life Sciences [2000] 57 (13-14) : 1894-1908 (C.B.Lücking, A.Brice)

[14] Annals of Neurology [1998] 43 (3) : 394-397 (M.Farrer, F. Wavrant-DeVrieze, R.Crook, L.Boles, J.Perez-Tur, J.Hardy, W.G. Johnson, J.Steele, D.Maraganore, K.Gwinn, T.Lynch)

[15] American Journal of Medical Genetics B [2013] 162B (5) : 452-456 (N.N.Li, X.Y.Mao, X.L.Chang, D.M.Zhao, J.H.Zhang, Q. Liao, W.J.Yu, E.K.Tan, R.Peng)

[16] Parkinsonism & Related Disorders [2013] 19 (2) : 251-255 (Y.H. Wu-Chou, Y.T.Chen, T.H.Yeh, H.C.Chang, Y.H.Weng, S.C.Lai, C.L. Huang, R.S.Chen, Y.Z.Huang, C.C.Chen, J.Hung, W.L.Chuang, et al)

[17] Neurological Sciences [2016] 37 (5) : 731-736 (S.Rahimi-Aliabadi, N.Shahmohammadibeni, J.Jamshidi, B.Emamalizadeh, H.A. Shahmohammadibeni, A.Zare Bidoki, H.Akhavan-Niaki, et al)

[18] Genetic Testing and Molecular Biomarkers [2015] 19 (9) : 481-487 (X.B.Li, R.Y.Huang, S.L.Shi, Y.Wu, C.Qin, J.Chen, Y.M. Zhang, S.Wang, Y.L.Feng, S.N.Zhou)

[19] Neurobiology of Aging [2015] 36 (4) : 1765 (J.F.Guo, K.Li, R.L.Yu, Q.Y.Sun, L.Wang, L.Y.Yao, Y.C.Hu, Z.Y.Lv, L.Z.Luo, L.Shen, H.Jiang, X.X.Yan, Q.Pan, K.Xia, B.S.Tang)

[20] Parkinsonism & Related Disorders [2012] 18 (6) : 801-802 (M. Vishwanathan Padmaja, M.Jayaraman, A.V.Srinivasan, C.R.Srikumari Srisailapathy, A.Ramesh)

[21] Parkinsonism & Related Disorders [2012] 18 (5) : 632-634 (F.Pan, H.Dong, H.Ding, M.Ye, W.Liu, Y.Wu, X.Zhang, Z.Chen, Y.Luo, X. Ding)

[22] Parkinsonism & Related Disorders [2012] 18 (3) : 257-262 (L.Trotta, I.Guella, G.Soldà, F.Sironi, S.Tesei, M.Canesi, G.Pezzoli, S .Goldwurm, S.Duga, R.Asselta)

[23] Movement Disorders [2011] 26 (12) : 2283-2286 (H.Ding, A.K. Sarokhan, S.S.Roderick, R.Bakshi, N.E.Maher, P.Ashourian, C.G. Kan, S.Chang, A.Santarlasci, K.E.Swords, B.M.Ravina, et al)

[24] European Journal of Neurology [2011] 18 (6) : 876-881 (C.Wider, C.Vilariño-Güell, M.G.Heckman, B.Jasinska-Myga, A.I.Ortolaza-Soto, N.N.Diehl, J.E.Crook, S.A.Cobb, J.A.Bacon, J.O.Aasly, et al)

[25] Archives of Neurology [2010] 67 (11) : 1350-1356 (I.F.Mata, M. Shi, P.Agarwal, K.A.Chung, K.L.Edwards, S.A.Factor, D.R. Galasko, C.Ginghina, A.Griffith, D.S.Higgins, D.M.Kay, H.Kim, et al)

[26] Brain Research [2010] 1346 : 262-265 (L.Yu, P.Xu, X.He, F.Hu, Z.Lin, M.Zhu, Z.Liu, L.He, Y.Xu)

[27] Annals of Human Genetics [2010] 74 (2) : 97-109 (T.L.Edwards, W.K.Scott, C.Almonte, A.Burt, E.H.Powell, G.W.Beecham, L.Wang, S.Züchner, I.Konidari, G.Wang, C.Singer, F.Nahab, B.Scott, et al)

[28] Neurology [2007] 69 (18) : 1745-1750 (S.Winkler, J.Hagenah, S. Lincoln, M.Heckman, K.Haugarvoll, K.Lohmann-Hedrich, V.Kostic, M.Farrer, C.Klein)

[29] Neurology [2004] 62 (1) : 128-131 (E.K.Tan, A.Chai, Y.Y.Teo, Y.Zhao, C.Tan, H.Shen, V.R.Chandran, M.L.Teoh, Y.Yih, R.Pavanni, M.C.Wong, K.Puvan, Y.L.Lo, E.Yapp)

[30] American Journal of Medical Genetics [2008] 147B (7) : 1222-1230 (D.M.Kay, S.A.Factor, A.Samii, D.S.Higgins, A.Griffith, J.W.Roberts, B.C.Leis, J.G.Nutt, J.S.Montimurro, R.G.Keefe, et al)

[31] Biomed Research International [2015] : 135674 (Y.Huang, G. Wang, D.Rowe, Y.Wang, J.B.Kwok, Q.Xiao, F.Mastaglia, J.Liu, S.D. Chen, G.Halliday)

[32] Parkinsonism & Related Disorders [2016] 22 (Supplement 1) : S1-S6 (T.Konno, O.A.Ross, A.Puschmann, D.W.Dickson, Z.K. Wszolek)

[33] Parkinsonism & Related Disorders [2016] 24 : 89-94 (G.Wang, Y. Huang, Wei Chen, S.Chen, Y.Wang, Q.Xiao, J.Liu, V.S.Fung, G. Halliday, S.Chen)

[34] Neurology India [2013] 61 (4) : 360-364 (F.Pan, H.Ding, H.Dong, M.Ye, W.Liu, G.Cui, J.Chen, Y.Wu, H.Wang, X.Dai, H.Shi, X.Ding)

[35] American Journal of Medical Genetics [2013] 162B (5) : 452-456 (N.N.Li, X.Y.Mao, X.L.Chang, D.M.Zhao, J.H.Zhang, Q.Liao, W.J.Yu, E.K.Tan, R.Peng)

[36] Parkinsons Disease [2015] : 546462 (R.Ferese, N.Modugno, R. Campopiano, M.Santilli, S.Zampatti, E.Giardina, A.Nardone, D. Postorivo, F.Fornai, G.Novelli, E.Romoli, S.Ruggieri, S.Gambardella)

[37] Neurologia i Neurochirurgia Polska [2013] 47 (4) : 319-324 (D.Koziorowski, D.Hoffman-Zacharska, J.Slawek, Z.Jamrozik, P.Janik, A.Potulska-Chromik, A.Roszmann, R.Tataj, J.Bal, A.Friedman)

[38] European Journal of Neurology [2014] 21 (11) : e91-e92 (J.Trinh, E.K.Gustavsson, I.Guella, C.Vilariño-Güell, D.Evans, M.Encarnacion, H.Sherman, F.Hentati, M.J.Farrer)

[39] Movement Disorders [2010] 25 (16) : 2871-2875 (T.Sekine, H.Kagaya, M.Funayama, Y.Li, H.Yoshino, H.Tomiyama, N.Hattori)

[40] Neurogenetics [2008] 9 (4) : 263-269 (J.M.Choi, M.S.Woo, H.I. Ma, S.Y.Kang, Y.H.Sung, S.W.Yong, S.J.Chung, J.S.Kim, H.W.Shin, C.H.Lyoo, P.H.Lee, J.S.Baik, S.J.Kim, M.Y.Park, Y.H.Sohn, et al)

[41] Arquivos de Neuro-Psiquiatria [2016] 74 (6) : 445-449 (S.García, G.Chavira-Hernández, M.P.Gallegos-Arreola, L.Dávila-Maldonado, F.García Martínez, L.A.Montes Almanza, C.Palma-Flores, et al)

[42] Parkinsons Disease [2016] : 3474751 (J.Fang, K.Yi, M.Guo, X.An, H.Qu, Q.Lin, M.Bi, Q.Ma)

[43] Human Molecular Genetics [2016] Dec 22 [Epub ahead of print] (J.N.Foo, L.C.Tan, I.D.Irwan, W.L.Au, H.Q.Low, K.M.Prakash, A.Ahmad-Annuar, J.Bei, A.Y.Chan, C.M.Chen, Y.C.Chen, et al)

[44] Frontiers in Aging Neuroscience [2017] 9 : 198 (C.L.CCampêlo, F.C.Cagni, D.de Siqueira Figueredo, L.G.Oliveira, A.B.Silva-Neto, P.T.Macêdo, J.R.Santos, G.S.Izídio, A.M.Ribeiro, et al)

[45] Genetic Testing Registry

PARK 2

Gene : Parkin RBR E3 ubiquitin protein ligase (Parkin)

Chromosome : 6 (q25.2-q27) [1-4]

Biochemical function : PARK2 is an E3 ubiquitin ligase [5-9], that can selectively translocate to dysfunctional mitochondria to promote their removal by autophagy [6]. PARK2 has an important role as a tumor suppressor in melanoma predisposition and progression. This could explain the link between Parkinson's Disease and melanoma [10].

Type of inheritance : Autosomal recessive [8, 9, 11-14]

Symptoms : Juvenile Parkinsonism [15, 16], early onset Parkinson's Disease [8, 13-15, 17-23]. Late onset Parkinson's Disease has been associated with PARK2 mutations [18], but not in another study [24].

Prevalence : U.S.A. (rare) [25], Czech [26-27], Denmark [28], France [29], Norway [30], Germany [30, 31], Italy [32, 33], Portugal [34], Russia [35], Serbia [36], Turkey [37], 8% of early onset in the U.K. [38], 4.7% of early onset in Poland [39-40], as many as 4% of people with Parkinson's Disease in Poland [41], Han Chinese [42-48], Taiwan [49, 50], Uyghur [51, 52], Korea [53, 54], Tunisia [55], Jordan [56], Iran [57], South India [58], 7.2% of people with Parkinson's Disease in East India [59], 2.9% of early onset Parkinson's Disease in Brazil [60-62], Mexican-mestizo [63], South Africa [64]

Genetic test : PARK2 Parkinsonism (by Centogene AG) [65]

[1] Nature [1998] 392 (6676) : 605-608 (T.Kitada, S.Asakawa, N. Hattori, H.Matsumine, Y.Yamamura, S.Minoshima, M.Yokochi, Y. Mizuno, N.Shimizu)

[2] American Journal of Human Genetics [1998] 63 (1) : 80-87 (A.C. Jones, Y.Yamamura, L.Almasy, S.Bohlega, B.Elibol, J.Hubble, S. Kuzuhara, M.Uchida, T.Yanagi, D.E.Weeks, T.G.Nygaard)

[3] Annals of Neurology [1998] 44 (6) : 935-941 (N.Hattori, T.Kitada, H.Matsumine, S.Asakawa, Y.Yamamura, H.Yoshino, T.Kobayashi, M. Yokochi, M.Wang, A.Yoritaka, T.Kondo, S.Kuzuhara, et al)

[4] National Genetics [2010] 42 (1) : 77-82 (S.Veeriah, B.S.Taylor, S. Meng, F.Fang, E.Yilmaz, I.Vivanco, M.Janakiraman, N.Schultz, A.J. Hanrahan, W.Pao, M.Ladanyi, C.Sander, A.Heguy, E.C.Holland, et al)

[5] Neuron [2015] 87 (2) : 371-381 (A.M.Pickrell, C.H.Huang, S.R. Kennedy, A.Ordureau, D.P.Sideris, J.G.Hoekstra, J.W.Harper, R.J. Youle)

[6] Cancer Research [2015] 75 (9) : 1815-1827 (D.C.Lin, L.Xu, Y. Chen, H.Yan, M.Hazawa, N.Doan, J.W.Said, L.W.Ding, L.Z.Liu, H. Yang, S.Yu, M.Kahn, D.Yin, H.P.Koeffler)

[7] Biochemical Journal [2014] 460 (1) : 127-139 (A.Kazlauskaite, C.Kondapalli, R.Gourlay, D.G.Campbell, M.S.Ritorto, K.Hofmann, D.R.Alessi, A.Knebel, M.Trost, M.M.Muqit)

[8] Journal of Biological Chemistry [2007] 282 (17) : 12842-12850 (E.Avraham, R.Rott, E.Liani, R.Szargel, S.Engelender)

[9] Human Molecular Genetics [2003] 12 (20) : 2587-2597 (D.P. Huynh, D.R.Scoles, D.Nguyen, S.M.Pulst)

[10] Journal of the National Cancer Institute [2015] 108 (3) pii : djv340 (H.H.Hu, C.Kannengiesser, S.Lesage, J.André, S.Mourah, L.Michel, V. Descamps, N.Basset-Seguin, M.Bagot, A.Bensussan, C.Lebbé, et al)

[11] Science [2013] 340 (6139) : 1451-1455 (J.F.Trempe, V.Sauvé, K. Grenier, M.Seirafi, M.Y.Tang, M.Ménade, S.Al-Abdul-Wahid, J.Krett, K.Wong, G.Kozlov, B.Nagar, E.A.Fon, K.Gehring)

[12] American Journal of Medical Genetics Part B : Neuropsychiatric Genetics [2014] 165B (3) : 235-244 (N.Monroy-Jaramillo, J.L. Guerrero-Camacho, M.Rodríguez-Violante, M.C.Boll-Woehrlen, et al)

[13] Movement Disorders [2003] 18 (7) : 758-763 (L.C.Tan, C.M. Tanner, R.Chen, P.Chan, M.Farrer, J.Hardy, J.W.Langston)

[14] Neurological Sciences [2002] 23 (Supplement 2) : S59-S60 (V. Bonifati, M.C.Dekker, N.Vanacore, G.Fabbrini, F.Squitieri, R.Marconi, A.Antonini, P.Brustenghi, A.Dalla Libera, M.De Mari, F.Stocchi, et al)

[15] American Journal of Medical Genetics [2002] 114 (5) : 584-591 (A.West, M.Periquet, S.Lincoln, C.B.Lücking, D.Nicholl, V.Bonifati, N.Rawal, T.Gasser, E.Lohmann, J.F.Deleuze, D.Maraganore, et al)

[16] Annals of Neurology [2006] Dec 22 [Epub ahead of print] (D. M.Kay, D.Moran, L.Moses, P.Poorkaj, C.P.Zabetian, J.Nutt, S.A. Factor, C.E.Yu, J.S.Montimurro, R.G.Keefe, G.D.Schellenberg, et al)

[17] JAMA Neurology [2014] 71 (1) : 62-67 (R.N.Alcalay, E. Caccappolo, H.Mejia-Santana, M.X.Tang, L.Rosado, M.Orbe Reilly, D.Ruiz, E.D.Louis, C.L.Comella, M.A.Nance, S.B.Bressman, et al)

[18] Neuroscience Letters [2010] 468 (3) : 264-266 (H.R.Martínez, H.González-González, L.Cantú-Martínez, R.Rangel-Guerra, C.D. Hernández-Castillo, J.J.Vergara-Saavedra, M.R.Ramos-Gonzalez, et al)

[19] Neurology [2009] 73 (4) : 279-286 (N.Pankratz, D.K.Kissell, M.W.Pauciulo, C.A.Halter, A.Rudolph, R.F.Pfeiffer, K.S.Marder, T.Foroud, W.C.Nichols)

[20] Archives of Neurology [2006] 63 (4) : 548-552 (L.N.Clark, S.Afridi, E.Karlins, Y.Wang, H.Mejia-Santana, J.Harris, E.D.Louis, L. J.Cote, H.Andrews, S.Fahn, C.Waters, B.Ford, S.Frucht, et al)

[21] Brain [2003] 126 (Part 6) : 1271-1278 (M.Periquet, M.Latouche, E.Lohmann, N.Rawal, G.De Michele, S.Ricard, H.Teive, V.Fraix, M. Vidailhet, D.Nicholl, P.Barone, N.W.Wood, S.Raskin, et al)

[22] Nature [2013] 496 (7445) : 372-376 (S.A.Sarraf, M.Raman, V. Guarani-Pereira, M.E.Sowa, E.L.Huttlin, S.P.Gygi, J.W.Harper)

[23] Movement Disorders [2005] 20 (4) : 424-431 (A.M.Bertoli-Avella, J.L.Giroud-Benitez, A.Akyol, E.Barbosa, O.Schaap, H.C.van der Linde, E.Martignoni, L.Lopiano, P.Lamberti, E.Fincati, et al)

[24] Neurology [2001] 57 (2) : 359-362 (R.L.Oliveri, M.Zappia, G. Annesi, D.Bosco, F.Annesi, P.Spadafora, A.A.Pasqua, C.Tomaino, G. Nicoletti, D.Pirritano, A.Labate, A.Gambardella, G.Logroscino, et al)

[25] Parkinsonism & Related Disorders [2003] 9 (5) : 309-312 (R. Chen, N.S.Gosavi, J.W.Langston, P.Chan)

[26] PLoS One [2014] 9 (9) : e107585 (O.Fiala, D.Zahorakova, L. Pospisilova, J.Kucerova, M.Matejckova, P.Martasek, J.Roth, E. Ruzicka)

[27] Neuro Endocrinology Letters [2010] 31 (2) : 187-192 (O.Fiala, L. Pospisilova, J.Prochazkova, M.Matejckova, P.Martasek, L.Novakova, J.Roth, E.Ruzicka)

[28] European Journal of Neurology [2006] 13 (4) : 385-390 (J.M. Hertz, K.Ostergaard, I.Juncker, S.Pedersen, A.Romstad, L.B.Møller, F. Güttler, E.Dupont)

[29] Journal of Medical Genetics [2008] 45 (1) : 43-46 (S.Lesage, E. Lohmann, F.Tison, F.Durif, A.Dürr, A.Brice)

[30] Acta Neurologica Scandinavica [2006] 113 (1) : 9-13 (A.M. Schlitter, M.Kurz, J.P.Larsen, D.Woitalla, T.Müller, J.T.Epplen, G. Dekomien)

[31] Annals of Neurology [2002] 51 (5) : 621-625 (M.Kann, H.Jacobs, K.Mohrmann, K.Schumacher, K.Hedrich, J.Garrels, K.Wiegers, E. Schwinger, P.P.Pramstaller, X.O.Breakefield, L.J.Ozelius, et al)

[32] Neurotoxicology [2007] 28 (3) : 698-701 (I.Ghione, A.Di Fonzo, F.Saladino, R.Del Bo, N.Bresolin, G.P.Comi, M.Rango)

[33] European Journal of Human Genetics [2005] 13 (9) : 1086-1093 (C.Klein, A.Djarmati, K.Hedrich, N.Schäfer, C.Scaglione, R.Marchese, N.Kock, B.Schüle, A.Hiller, T.Lohnau, S.Winkler, K.Wiegers, et al)

[34] BMC Neurology [2008] 8 : 1 (J.Bras, R.Guerreiro, M.Ribeiro, A. Morgadinho, C.Januario, M.Dias, A.Calado, C.Semedo, C.Oliveira, J. Hardy, A.Singleton)

[35] Movement Disorders [2012] 27 (1) : 139-142 (E.V.Semenova, M.I.Shadrina, P.A.Slominsky, I.A.Ivanova-Smolenskaya, G.Bagyeva, S.N.Illarioshkin, S.A.Limborska)

[36] Human Mutation [2004] 23 (5) : 525 (A.Djarmati, K.Hedrich, M. Svetel, N.Schäfer, V.Juric, S.Vukosavic, R.Hering, O.Riess, S.Romac, C.Klein, V.Kostic)

[37] European Journal of Neurology [2012] 19 (5) : 769-775 (E. Lohmann, B.Dursun, S.Lesage, H.A.Hanagasi, G.Sevinc, A.Honore, B. Bilgic, H.Gürvit, O.Dogu, H.Kaleagasi, G.Babacan, J.Yazici, et al)

[38] Movement Disorders [2012] 27 (12) : 1522-1529 (L.L.Kilarski, J.P.Pearson, V.Newsway, E.Majounie, M.D.Knipe, A.Misbahuddin, P. F.Chinnery, D.J.Burn, C.E.Clarke, M.H.Marion, A.J.Lewthwaite, et al)

[39] Neurologia i Neurochirurgia Polska [2013] 47 (4) : 319-324 (D. Koziorowski, D.Hoffman-Zacharska, J.Slawek, Z.Jamrozik, P.Janik, A.Potulska-Chromik, A.Roszmann, R.Tataj, J.Bal, A.Friedman)

[40] Parkinsonism & Related Disorders [2010] 16 (2) : 136-138 (D. Koziorowski, D.Hoffman-Zacharska, J.Slawek, W.Szirkowiec, P.Janik, J.Bal, A.Friedman)

[41] Current Genomics [2015] 16 (4) : 215-223 (A.Oczkowska, J. Florczak-Wyspianska, A.Permoda-Osip, M.Owecki, M.Lianeri, W. Kozubski, J.Dorszewska)

[42] Neuroscience Letters [2010] 477 (1) : 19-22 (B.R.Zhang, Z.X.Hu, X.Z.Yin, M.Cai, G.H.Zhao, Z.R.Liu, W.Luo)

[43] Journal of Neurology [2010] 257 (7) : 1170-1175 (J.F.Guo, X.W. Zhang, L.L.Nie, H.N.Zhang, B.Liao, J.Li, L.Wang, X.X.Yan, B.S. Tang)

[44] Journal of Neural Transmission [2008] 115 (5) : 715-719 (D.K. Chan, V.Mok, P.W.Ng, J.Yeung, J.B.Kwok, Z.M.Fang, R.Clarke, L. Wong, P.R.Schofield, N.Hattori)

[45] Zhonghua Yi Xue Yi Chuan Xue Za Zhi [2007] 24 (1) : 38-41 (R.Peng, W.J.Chen, Y.Wu, M.Liu, X.H.Lai, J.H.Zhang, G.G.Yuan, Y. R.Gou, T.Li, Y.C.Wang)

[46] Parkinsonism & Related Disorders [2005] 11 (3) : 173-180 (W.C. Shyu, S.Z.Lin, M.F.Chiang, C.Y.Pang, S.Y.Chen, Y.L.Hsin, P.Thajeb, Y.J.Lee, H.Li)

[47] Zhonghua Yi Xue Yi Chuan Xue Za Zhi [2004] 21 (3) : 219-223 (H.Q.Zou, B.Chen, Q.L.Ma, X.Li, J.F.Yang, X.L.Feng, X.M.Dong, Y.J. Li)

[48] European Neurology [2003] 49 (2) : 85-89 (R.Peng, Y.Gou, Q. Yuan, T.Li, H.Latsoudis, G.Yuan, D.Luo, X.Liu, D.A.Collier)

[49] Movement Disorders [2009] 24 (1) : 104-108 (M.J.Lee, I.F.Mata, C.H.Lin, K.Y.Tzen, S.J.Lincoln, R.Bounds, P.J.Lockhart, M.M. Hulihan, M.J.Farrer, R.M.Wu)

[50] Archives of Neurology [2005] 62 (1) : 82-87 (R.M.Wu, R.Bounds, S.Lincoln, M.Hulihan, C.H.Lin, W.L.Hwu, J.Chen, K.Gwinn-Hardy, M.Farrer)

[51] Journal of Neurological Science [2014] Mar 31 [Epub ahead of print] (H.Li, A.Yusufujiang, S.Naser, Y.Zhu, M.Maimaiti, X.He, J.Bu, X.Meng, M.Wang, J.Li, B.Dina, L.Yang, Z.Nayi, H.Dang, et al)

[52] Journal of the Neurological Sciences [2014] 342 (1-2) : 21-24 (H.Li, A.Yusufujiang, S.Naser, Y.Zhu, M.Maimaiti, X.He, J.Bu, X. Meng, M.Wang, J.Li, B.Dina, L.Yang, Z.Nayi, H.Dang, C.Wang, et al)

[53] Journal of Neurology [2011] 258 (12) : 2260-2267 (H.J.Kim, J.Y. Lee, J.Y.Yun, S.Y.Kim, S.S.Park, B.S.Jeon)

[54] Neurogenetics [2008] 9 (4) : 263-269 (J.M.Choi, M.S.Woo, H.I. Ma, S.Y.Kang, YH.Sung, S.W.Yong, S.J.Chung, J.S.Kim, H.W.Shin, C.H.Lyoo, P.H.Lee, J.S.Baik, S.J.Kim, M.Y.Park, Y.H.Sohn, et al)

[55] Journal of Neurology, Neurosurgery, and Psychiatry [2010] 81 (4) : 391-395 (K.Nishioka, M.Kefi, B.Jasinska-Myga, C.Wider, C. Vilariño-Güell, O.A.Ross, M.G.Heckman, L.T.Middleton, et al)

[56] BMC Neurology [2008] 8 : 47 (R.Myhre, S.Steinkjer, A.Stormyr, G.L.Nilsen, H.Abu Zayyad, K.Horany, M.K.Nusier, H.Klungland)

[57] Movement Disorders [2011] 26 (1) : 80-89 (F.Ghazavi, Z.Fazlali, S.S.Banihosseini, S.R.Hosseini, M.H.Kazemi, S.Shojaee, K.Parsa, H. Sadeghi, F.Sina, M.Rohani, G.A.Shahidi, N.Ghaemi, M.Ronaghi, et al)

[58] Neuroscience Letters [2012] 523 (2) : 145-147 (M.V.Padmaja, M. Jayaraman, A.V.Srinivasan, C.R.Srisailapathy, A.Ramesh)

[59] Parkinsonism & Related Disorders [2006] 12 (7) : 420-426 (A. Biswas, A.Gupta, T.Naiya, G.Das, R.Neogi, S.Datta, S.Mukherjee, S.K.Das, K.Ray, J.Ray)

[60] Disease Markers [2013] 35 (3) : 181-185 (K.C.Moura, M.Campos Junior, A.I.de Rosso, D.H.Nicaretta, J.S.Pereira, D.J.Silva, F.L.dos Santos, C.Rodrigues Fda, C.B.Santos-Rebouças, M.M.Pimentel)

[61] Arquivos de Neuro-Psiquiatria [2009] 67 (1) : 7-11 (O.G. Barsottini, A.C.Felício, C.Aguiar Pde, C.Godeiro-Junior, M.C.Shih, M.Q.Hoexter, R.A.Bressan, H.B.Ferraz, L.A.Andrade)

[62] Movement Disorders [2008] 23 (9) : 1228-1233 (C.Aguiar Pde, P.S.Lessa, C.Jr.Godeiro, O.Barsottini, A.C.Felício, V.Borges, S.M. Silva, R.A.Saba, H.B.Ferraz, C.A.Moreira-Filho, L.A.Andrade)

[63] Movement Disorders [2012] 27 (8) : 1047-1051 (J.L.Guerrero Camacho, N.Monroy Jaramillo, P.Yescas Gómez, M.Rodríguez Violante, C.Boll Woehrlen, M.E.Alonso Vilatela, M.López López)

[64] Parkinsonism & Related Disorders [2012] 18 (1) : 89-92 (W.L. Haylett, R.J.Keyser, M.C.du Plessis, C.van der Merwe, J.Blanckenberg, D.Lombard, J.Carr, S.Bardien)

[65] Genetic Testing Registry

PARK 3

Gene : Parkinson disease 3 (autosomal dominant, Lewy body) [1]

Chromosome : 2 (p13) [2]

Biochemical function : Unknown

Type of inheritance : Autosomal dominant [2]

Symptoms : Parkinson's Disease susceptibility [3]

Prevalence : European origin [3], Germany [4]

Genetic tests : None [5]

[1] The HUGO Gene Nomenclature Committee (HGNC)

[2] American Journal of Human Genetics [2002] 70 (5) : 1089-1095 (A.L.DeStefano, M.F.Lew, L.I.Golbe, M.H.Mark, A.M.Lazzarini, M. Guttman, E.Montgomery, C.H.Waters, C.Singer, R.L.Watts, et al)

[3] Nature Genetics [1998] 18 (3) : 262-265 (B.Müller-Myhsok, Z.K. Wszolek, R.Oehlmann, D.B.Calne, V.Bonifati, B.Bereznai, E.Fabrizio, P.Vieregge, R.D.Horstmann)

[4] Journal of Medical Genetics [2006] 43 (7) : 557-562 (M.Sharma, J.C.Mueller, A.Zimprich, P.Lichtner, A.Hofer, P.Leitner, S.Maass, D.Berg, A.Dürr, V.Bonifati, G.De Michele, B.Oostra, A.Brice, et al)

[5] Genetic Testing Registry

PARK 5

Gene : UCHL1 (ubiquitin carboxyl-terminal esterase L1) [1]

Chromosome : 4 (p14-p15.1) [2]

Biochemical function : UCH-L1 inhibits alpha-synuclein expression and distribution [3]

Type of inheritance : Autosomal dominant [4]

Symptoms : Increased likerlihood of Parkinson's Disease [5, 6]

Prevalence : Germany [7], China [8, 9]

Genetic tests : PARK5 Parkinsonism (by Centogene AG) [10]

[1] The HUGO Gene Nomenclature Committee (HGNC)

[2] Journal of Clinical Neuroscience [2004] 11 (2) : 119-123 (D.J.Cordato, D.K.Chan)

[3] PLoS One [2012] 7 (4) : e34713 (A.E.Cartier, K.Ubhi, B.Spencer, R.A.Vazquez-Roque, K.A.Kosberg, L.Fourgeaud, P.Kanayson, C. Patrick, E.Rockenstein, G.N.Patrick, E.Masliah)

[4] Medical Science [2003] 19 (5) : 613-619 (O.Corti, A.Brice)

[5] Biomolecular NMR Assignments [2011] 5 (2) : 165-168 (H.S.Tse, H.Y.Hu, K.H.Sze)

[6] Cell [2002] 111 (2) : 209-218 (Y.Liu, L.Fallon, H.A.Lashuel, Z.Liu, P.T.Lansbury Jr.)

[7] Neuroscience Letters [1999] 270 (1) : 1-4 (B.S.Harhangi, M.J. Farrer, S.Lincoln, V.Bonifati, G.Meco, G.De Michele, A.Brice, A. Dürr, M.Martinez, T.Gasser, B.Bereznai, J.R.Vaughan, et al)

[8] Journal of Clinical Neuroscience [2011] 18 (4) : 541-544 (L. Wang, J.F.Guo, L.L.Nie, L.Luo, X.Zuo, L.Shen, H.Jiang, X.X.Yan, K. Xia, Q.Pan, B.S.Tang)

[9] Movement Disorders [2002] 17 (4) : 767-771 (J.Wang, C.Y.Zhao, Y.M.Si, Z.L.Liu, B.Chen, L.Yu)

[10] Genetic Testing Registry

PARK 6

Gene : Pink 1 (PTEN induced putative kinase 1) [1, 2, 3]

Chromosome : 1 (p35-p36) [1]

Biochemical function : Pink 1 can protect the cells from damage mediated mitochondrial dysfunction, oxidative stress, and cell apoptosis [4].

Type of inheritance : Autosomal recessive [1]

Symptoms : Sporadic early-onset of parkinsonism with a slow progression of symptoms and an excelleent response to L-dopa [5].

Prevalence : Italians [5], not in Sub Saharan Africa [6]

Genetic tests : PARK6 Parkinsonism (by Centogene AG), Parkinson's Disease, Early Onset via the PINK1 Gene (by PreventionGenetics), PINK1 Complete sequencing (by Instituto de Medicina Genomica), Parkinson disease type 6 (by Bioarray), Parkinson disease type 6 (by CGC Genetics), Single gene testing PINK1 (by CeGaT GmbH), PINK1 (by Fulgent Clinical Diagnostics Lab), PINK1 DNA Sequencing Test (by Athena Diagnostics Inc), PINK1 Deletion Test (by Athena Diagnostics Inc) [7]

[1] Archives of Neurology [2004] 61 (12) : 1898-1904 (E.Rogaeva, J. Johnson, A.E.Lang, C.Gulick, K.Gwinn-Hardy, T.Kawarai, C.Sato, A. Morgan, J.Werner, R.Nussbaum, A.Petit, M.S.Okun, et al)

[2] Journal of Biological Chemistry [2009] 284 (24) : 16482- 16491 (J. Sämann, J.Hegermann, E.von Gromoff, S.Eimer, R.Baumeister, E. Schmidt)

[3] Biochemical and Biophysical Research Communications [2008] 377 (3) : 975-980 (Y.Kim, J.Park, S.Kim, S.Song, S.K.Kwon, S.H.Lee, T.Kitada, J.M.Kim, J.Chung)

[4] Oxidative Medicine and Cellular Longevity [2013] : 601587 (S. Matsuda, Y.Kitagishi, M.Kobayashi)

[5] Annals of Neurology [2004] 56 (3) : 336-341 (E.M.Valente, S. Salvi, T.Ialongo, R.Marongiu, A.E.Elia, V.Caputo, L.Romito, A. Albanese, B.Dallapiccola, A.R.Bentivoglio)

[6] Journal of Neurological Science [2013] 335 (1-2) : 22-25 (J. Blanckenberg, S.Bardien, B.Glanzmann, N.U.Okubadejo, J.A.Carr)

[7] Genetic Testing Registry

PARK 7

Gene : DJ1 [1]

Chromosome : 1 (p36) [2]

Biochemical function : DJ-1 is a protein deglycase that repairs methylglyoxal-glycated and glyoxal-glycated amino acids and proteins by acting on early glycation intermediates, and releases repaired proteins and lactate or glycolate, respectively [1].

Type of inheritance : Autosomal recessive [2]

Symptoms : Early-onset of parkinsonism with a low risk for cognitive decline and a pathological process usually restricted to the brainstem [3]. Early-onset of Parkinson's Disease [4]. Early onset L-dopa responsive parkinsonism with some signs of amyotrophic lateral sclerosis [5].

Prevalence : Turkey [5], none in Turkey in another study [6], very rare in Italy [7]

Genetic tests : Single gene testing PARK7 (by CeGaT GmbH) [8]

[1] Journal of Biological Chemistry [2015] 290 (3) : 1885-1897 (G. Richarme, M.Mihoub, J.Dairou, L.C.Bui, T.Leger, A. Lamouri)

[2] American Journal of Human Genetics [2001] 69 (3) : 629-634 (C. M.van Duijn, M.C.Dekker, V.Bonifati, R.J.Galjaard, J.J.Houwing-Duistermaat, P.J.Snijders, L.Testers, G.J.Breedveld, M.Horstink, et al)

[3] Parkinsonism & Related Disorders [2013] 19 (4) : 407-415 (A. Puschmann)

[4] Parkinsonism & Related Disorders [2007] 13 (Supplement 3) : S229- S232 (C.Wider, Z.K.Wszolek)

[5] Parkinsonism & Related Disorders [2016] [Epub ahead of print] (A.Hanagasi, A.Giri, G.Guven, B.Bilgiç, A.K.Hauser, M.Emre, P. Heutink, N.Basak, T.Gasser, J.Simón-Sánchez, E.Lohmann)

[6] European Journal of Neurology [2012] 19 (5) : 769-775 (E. Lohmann, B.Dursun, S.Lesage, H.A.Hanagasi, G.Sevinc, A.Honore, B. Bilgic, H.Gürvit, O.Dogu, H.Kaleagasi, G.Babacan, J.Yazici, et al)

[7] Neuroscience Letters [2013] 557 (Part B) : 165-170 (F.Sironi, P. Primignani, S.Ricca, S.Tunesi, M.Zini, S.Tesei, R.Cilia, G.Pezzoli, M. Seia, S.Goldwurm)

[8] Genetic Testing Registry

PARK 8

Gene : LRRK2

Chromosome : 1 (2p11.23-12q13.11) [1, 2]

Biochemical function : The biochemical function of the LRRK2 gene is to encode a protein with an ankryin repeat region, a leucine-rich repeat (LRR) domain, a kinase domain, a DFG-like motif, a RAS domain, a GTPase domain, an MLK-like domain, and a WD40 domain. The protein is present largely in the cytoplasm but it also associates with the mitochondrial outer membrane [3].

Type of inheritance : Autosomal dominant [1, 2, 4-8]

Symptoms : Susceptibility to Parkinson's Disease [1, 9]. Early and late onset Parkinson's Disease [10]. Late onset Parkinson's Disease [6].

Prevalence : Japan [1, 5], Malaysia [11], Canadian [12], American [12], U.S.A. [13], Brazil [14, 15], Norway [16], Thailand [9], China [17, 18, 22], Maltese [19], Colombia [20]. The G2019S LRRK2 mutation, is up to 20 times more common in Arabs than in Europeans and North

Americans, suggesting that it originated amongst Arabs. It is by far the most common form of genetic Parkinson's Disease in Arabs, causing about 40% of genetic Parkinson's Disease, in comparison to only 2%-3% in Europeans and North Americans [21].

Genetic tests : PARK8 Parkinsonism (by Centogene AG) [23]

[1] Annals of Neurology [2002] 51 (3) : 296-301 (M.Funayama, K. Hasegawa, H.Kowa, M.Saito, S.Tsuji, F.Obata)

[2] Neuron [2004] 44 (4) : 601-607 (A.Zimprich, S.Biskup, P.Leitner, P.Lichtner, M.Farrer, S.Lincoln, J.Kachergus, M.Hulihan, R.J.Uitti, D. B.Calne, A.J.Stoessl, R.F.Pfeiffer, N.Patenge, I.C.Carbajal, et al)

[3] Biochemical Journal [2015] 470 (3) : e21-e24 (H.L.Melrose)

[4] Annals of Neurology [2005] 57 (3) : 453-456 (D.G.Hernandez, C. Paisán-Ruíz, A.McInerney-Leo, S.Jain, A.Meyer-Lindenberg, E.W. Evans, K.F.Berman, J.Johnson, G.Auburger, A.A.Schäffer, et al)

[5] Annals of Neurology [2005] 57 (6) : 918-921 (M.Funayama, K. Hasegawa, E.Ohta, N.Kawashima, M.Komiyama, H.Kowa, S.Tsuji, F. Obata)

[6] Neuroscience Letters [2005] 382 (3) : 309-311 (I.F.Mata, J.P. Taylor, J.Kachergus, M.Hulihan, C.Huerta, C.Lahoz, M.Blazquez, L. M.Guisasola, C.Salvador, R.Ribacoba, C.Martinez, M.Farrer, et al)

[7] Journal of Neurological Science [2015] 353 (1-2) : 59-62. (M.Z. Jankovic, N.D.Kresojevic, V.S.Dobricic, V.V.Markovic, I.N.Petrovic, I.V.Novakovic, V.S.Kostic)

[8] Lancet [2005] 365 (9457) : 415-416 (W.P.Gilks, P.M.Abou-Sleiman, S.Gandhi, S.Jain, A.Singleton, A.J.Lees, K.Shaw, K.P.Bhatia, V.Bonifati, N.P.Quinn, J.Lynch, D.G.Healy, J.L.Holton, et al)

[9] Parkinsonism & Related Disorders [2014] 20 (9) : 1018-1021 (T. Pulkes, C.Papsing, A.Thakkinstian, S.Pongpakdee, K.Kulkantrakorn, S. Hanchaiphiboolkul, S.Tiamkao, P.Boonkongchuen)

[10] Lancet [2005] 365 (9457) : 412-415 (A.Di Fonzo, C.F.Rohé, J. Ferreira, H.F.Chien, L.Vacca, F.Stocchi, L.Guedes, E.Fabrizio, M. Manfredi, N.Vanacore, S.Goldwurm, G.Breedveld, C.Sampaio, et al)

[11] Biomed Research International [2014] : 867321 (A.A.Gopalai, S. Y.Lim, J.Y.Chua, S.Tey, T.T.Lim, N.Mohamed Ibrahim, A.H.Tan, G. B.Eow, Z.Abdul Aziz, S.D.Puvanarajah, S.Viswanathan, I.Looi, et al)

[12] American Journal of Human Genetics [2004] 74 (1) : 11-19 (A. Zimprich, B.Müller-Myhsok, M.Farrer, P.Leitner, M.Sharma, M. Hulihan, P.Lockhart, A.Strongosky, J.Kachergus, D.B.Calne, et al)

[13] Lancet [2005] 365 (9457) : 410-412 (W.C.Nichols, N.Pankratz, D. Hernandez, C.Paisán-Ruíz, S.Jain, C.A.Halter, V.E.Michaels, T.Reed, A.Rudolph, C.W.Shults, A.Singleton, T.Foroud)

[14] Neuroscience Letters [2008] 433 (1) : 17-21 (M.M.Pimentel, K.C. Moura, C.B.Abdalla, J.S.Pereira, A.L.de Rosso, D.H.Nicaretta, M. Campos Jr, R.M. de Almeida, J.M.dos Santos, I.C.Bastos, et al)

[15] Neuroscience Lettes [2016] Oct 21 [Epub ahead of print] (G.M. Abreu, D.C.Valença, M.J.Campos, C.P.da Silva, J.S.Pereira, M.A. Araujo Leite, A.L.Rosso, D.H.Nicaretta, L.F.Vasconcellos, et al)

[16] Annals of Neurology [2005] 57 (5) : 762-765 (J.O.Aasly, M.Toft, I.Fernandez-Mata, J.Kachergus, M.Hulihan, L.R.White, M.Farrer)

[17] Human Mutation [2010] 31 (5) : 561-568 (E.K.Tan, R.Peng, Y.Y. Teo, L.C.Tan, D.Angeles, P.Ho, M.L.Chen, C.H.Lin, X.Y.Mao, X.L. Chang, K.M.Prakash, J.J.Liu, W.L.Au, W.D.Le, J.Jankovic, et al)

[18] Neurobiology of Aging [2015] 36 (10) : 2908 (K.Li, B.S.Tang, Z.H.Liu, J.F.Kang, Y.Zhang, L.Shen, N.Li, X.X.Yan, K.Xia, J.F.Guo)

[19] BMC Med Genetics [2016] 17 (1) : 65 (C.Zahra, C.Tabone, G.Camilleri, A.E.Felice, R.Farrugia, S.Bezzina Wettinger)

[20] Colombia Medica [2015] 46 (3) : 117-121 (A.F.Duque, J.C.Lopez, B.Benitez, H.Hernandez, J.J.Yunis, W.Fernandez, H.Arboleda, G. Arboleda)

[21] Movement Disorders [2008] 23 (9) : 1205-1210 (H.T. Benamer, R.de Silva, K.A.Siddiqui, D.G.Grosset)

[22] Human Molecular Genetics [2016] Dec 22 [Epub ahead of print] (J.N.Foo, L.C.Tan, I.D.Irwan, W.L.Au, H.Q.Low, K.M.Prakash, A.Ahmad-Annuar, J.Bei, A.Y.Chan, C.M.Chen, Y.C.Chen, et al)

[23] Genetic Testing Registry

PARK 9

Gene : ATP13A2 [1]

Chromosome : 1 (p36) [2]

Biochemical function : ATP13A2 encodes a member of the P5 subfamily of ATPases which transports inorganic cations and other substrates [3, 4].

Type of inheritance : Autosomal recessive [1, 5]

Symptoms : Mutations in this gene are associated with Kufor-Rakeb syndrome (KRS), which is a rare form of early-onset, L-dopa responsive parkinsonism [1, 6]. Kufor-Rakeb syndrome has additional signs that distinguishes it from Parkinson's Disease, including supranuclear vertical gaze palsy, myoclonic jerks, pyramidal signs, and cognitive impairment [7]. Early onset L-dopa-responsive dystonia-parkinsonism with pyramidal signs and eye movement abnormalities. There was also generalised atrophy and putaminal and caudate iron accumulation bilaterally [5].

Prevalence : Han Chinese - none [8, 9], Chile [6], Italy [10], Brazil - none [11], Japan - none [12], Chinese [13, 14, 15], Chinese - rare [15], Chinese - none [16, 17], Germany, mostly European ethnic origin - none [18], Germany - none [19], Tunisia - none [20], Eastern Asia [21]. One sporadic case from Brazil with juvenile parkinsonism at the age of twelve with L-dopa-responsive severe akinetic-rigid parkinsonism, L-dopa-induced motor fluctuations and dyskinesias, severe visual hallucinations, and supranuclear vertical gaze paresis, but no pyramidal deficit nor dementia [22]. There are two Italian cases with young onset Parkinson's Disease that do not have any additional atypical features [22].

Genetic tests : PARK9 Parkinsonism (by Centogene AG), ATP13A2 Complete sequencing (by Instituto de Medicina Genomica), ATP13A2 Gene Sequencing (by DDC Molecular Diagnostics Laboratory DDC Clinic), Single gene testing ATP13A2 (CeGaT GmbH) [23]

[1] Human Mutation [2011] 32 (8) : 956-964 (J.S.Park, P.Mehta, A.A. Cooper, D.Veivers, A.Heimbach, B.Stiller, C.Kubisch, V.S.Fung, D. Krainc, A.Mackay-Sim, C.M.Sue)

[2] Neuroscience Letters [2009] 455 (3) : 159-161 (H.Tomiyama, Y.Li, H.Yoshino, Y.Mizuno, S.Kubo, T.Toda, N.Hattori)

[3] Human Molecular Genetics [2012] 21 (8) : 1725-1743 (D.Ramonet, A.Podhajska, K.Stafa, S.Sonnay, A.Trancikova, E.Tsika, O.Pletnikova, J.C.Troncoso, LGlauser, D.J.Moore)

[4] Journal of Neuroscience [2012] 32 (12) : 4240-4246 (M.Usenovic, E.Tresse, J.R.Mazzulli, J.P.Taylor, D.Krainc)

[5] Movement Disorders [2010] 25 (8) : 979-984 (S.A.Schneider, C.Paisan-Ruiz, N.P.Quinn, A.J.Lees, H.Houlden, J.Hardy, K.P.Bhatia)

[6] Archives of Neurology [2010] 67 (11) : 1357-1363 (N.Brüggemann, J.Hagenah, K.Reetz, A.Schmidt, M.Kasten, I.Buchmann, S.Eckerle, M.Bähre, A.Münchau, A.Djarmati, J.van der Vegt, H.Siebner, et al)

[7] Movement Disorders [2010] 25 (12) : 1791-1800 (C.Paisán-Ruiz, R.Guevara, M.Federoff, H.Hanagasi, F.Sina, E.Elahi, S.A.Schneider, P.Schwingenschuh, N.Bajaj, M.Emre, A.B.Singleton, J.Hardy, et al)

[8] Chinese Medical Journal [2012] 125 (4) : 588-592 (L.H.Zhu, X.G. Luo, Y.S.Zhou, F.R.Li, Y.C.Yang, Y.Ren, H.Pang)

[9] Neuroscience Letters [2010] 475 (2) : 61-63 (Q.Z.Fei, L.Cao, Q. Xiao, T.Zhang, L.Zheng, X.J.Wang, G.Wang, H.Y.Zhou, Y.Wang, S.D. Chen)

[10] Neurogenetics [2011] 12 (1) : 33-39 (L.Santoro, G.J.Breedveld, F. Manganelli, R.Iodice, C.Pisciotta, M.Nolano, F.Punzo, M.Quarantelli, S.Pappatà, A.Di Fonzo, B.A.Oostra, V.Bonifati)

[11] Neuroscience Letters [2010] 485 (2) : 121-124 (A.V.Dos Santos, C.P.Pestana, K.R.Diniz, M.Campos, C.B.Abdalla-Carvalho, A.L.de Rosso, J.S.Pereira, D.H.Nicaretta, W.L.de Carvalho, et al)

[12] Movement Disorders [2010] 25 (14) : 2434-2437 (M.Funayama, H.Tomiyama, R.M.Wu, K.Ogaki, H.Yoshino, Y.Mizuno, N.Hattori)

[13] Chinese Medical Journal [2009] 122 (24) : 3082-3085 (H.N. Zhang, L.Shen, H.Jiang, Q.Pan, K.Xia, B.S.Tang, X.X.Yan)

[14] Neurology [2008] 71 (21) : 1727-1732 (C.H.Lin, E.K.Tan, M.L. Chen, L.C.Tan, H.Q.Lim, G.S.Chen, R.M.Wu)

[15] Parkinsonism & Related Disorders [2010] 16 (3) : 235-236 (X.Y. Mao, J.M.Burgunder, Z.J.Zhang, X.L.Chang, R.Peng, J.M.Burgunder, Y.Yang, Y.C.Wang, T.Li, Z.J.Zhang)

[16] Zhonghua Yi Xue Yi Chuan Xue Za Zhi [2009] 26 (5) : 567-570 (D.He, J.F.Guo, L.Wang, Z.Q.Xiao, L.L.Nie, X.W.Zhang, B.S.Tang)

[17] Movement Disorders [2008] 23 (14) : 2074-2079 (J.F.Guo, B. Xiao, B.Liao, X.W.Zhang, L.L.Nie, Y.H.Zhang, L.Shen, H.Jiang, K. Xia, Q.Pan, X.X.Yan, B.S.Tang)

[18] Movement Disorders [2009] 24 (14) : 2104-2111 (A.Djarmati, J. Hagenah, K.Reetz, S.Winkler, M.I.Behrens, H.Pawlack, K.Lohmann, A.Ramirez, V.Tadic, N.Brüggemann, D.Berg, H.R.Siebner, et al)

[19] Movement Disorders [2009] 24 (3) : 429-433 (A.Rakovic, B.Stiller, A.Djarmati, A.Flaquer, J.Freudenberg, M.R.Toliat, M. Linnebank, V.Kostic, K.Lohmann, S.Paus, P.Nürnberg, et al)

[20] Human Mutation [2009] 30 (3) : 406-410 (C.Vilariño-Güell, A.I. Soto, S.J.Lincoln, S.Ben Yahmed, M.Kefi, M.G.Heckman, M.M. Hulihan, H.Chai, N.N.Diehl, R.Amouri, A.Rajput, D.C.Mash, et al)

[21] Neurology [2008] 70 (16 Part 2) : 1491-1493 (Y.P.Ning, K.Kanai, H.Tomiyama, Y.Li, M.Funayama, H.Yoshino, S.Sato, M.Asahina, S. Kuwabara, A.Takeda, T.Hattori, Y.Mizuno, N.Hattori)

[22] Neurology [2007] 68 (19) : 1557-1562 (A.Di Fonzo, H.F.Chien, M.Socal, S.Giraudo, C.Tassorelli, G.Iliceto, G.Fabbrini, R.Marconi, E. Fincati, G.Abbruzzese, P.Marini, F.Squitieri, M.W.Horstink, et al)

[23] Genetic Testing Registry

PARK 10

Gene : Human immunodeficiency virus type I enhancer binding protein 3 (HIVEP3) [1] or Ubiquitin specific peptidase 24 (USP24) [2].

Chromosome : 1 (p32) [3]

Biochemical function : USP24 belongs to a family of cysteine proteases that are deubiquitinating enzymes. Modification of cellular proteins by ubiquitin is controlled by ubiquitin-conjugating and deubiquitinating enzymes [4]. HIVEP3 is a transcription factor and can regulate nuclear factor kappaB mediated transcription by binding the kappaB motif in target genes. HIVEP3 binds the recombination signal sequence that flanks the V, D, and J regions of immunoglobulin and T-cell receptors [5].

Type of inheritance : Unknown

Symptoms : Parkinson's Disease susceptibility [3, 6, 7]

Prevalence : Iceland [2], Norway [2], Ireland [2, 8], U.S.A. [2], U.S.A. (not proven) [8], Norway (not proven) [8]

Genetic tests : None [9]

[1] Annals of Human Genetics [2007] 71 (5) : 639-647 (Y.J.Li, J.Deng, G.M.Mayhew, J.W.Grimsley, X.Huo, J.M.Vance)

[2] European Journal of Human Genetics [2009] 17 (3) : 336-343 (K. Haugarvoll, M.Toft, L.Skipper, M.G.Heckman, J.E.Crook, A.Soto, O. A.Ross, M.M.Hulihan, J.M.Kachergus, S,B.Sando, L.R.White, et al)

[3] Annals of Neurology [2002] 52 (5) : 549-555 (A.A.Hicks, H. Pétursson, T.Jónsson, H.Stefánsson, H.S.Jóhannsdóttir, J.Sainz, M.L. Frigge, A.Kong, J.R.Gulcher, K.Stefánsson, S.Sveinbjörnsdóttir)

[4] Biochemical and Biophysical Research Communications [2004] 314 (1) : 54-62 (V.Quesada, A.Díaz-Perales, A.Gutiérrez-Fernández, C. Garabaya, S.Cal, C.López-Otín)

[5] Genomics [2001] 71 (1) : 89-100 (M.D.Hicar, Y.Liu, C.E.Allen, L. C.Wu), Proceedings, National Academy Sciences U.S.A. [1990] 87 (22) : 8707-8710 (A.K.Rustgi, L.J.Van 't Veer, R.Bernards)

[6] American Journal of Human Genetics [2005] 77 (5) : 685-693 (D. M.Maraganore, M.de Andrade, T.G.Lesnick, K.J.Strain, M.J.Farrer, W. A.Rocca, P.V.Pant, K.A.Frazer, D.R.Cox, D.G.Ballinger)

[7] Neurology [2015] 84 (10) : 972-980 (G.W.Beecham, D.W. Dickson, W.K.Scott, E.R.Martin, G.Schellenberg, K.Nuytemans, E. B.Larson, J.D.Buxbaum, J.Q.Trojanowski, V.M.Van Deerlin, et al)

[8] Movement Disorders [2007] 22 (4) : 585-587 (K.Haugarvoll, M. Toft, O.A.Ross, J.T.Stone, M.G.Heckman, L.R.White, T.Lynch, J.M. Gibson, Z.K.Wszolek, R.J.Uitti, J.O.Aasly, M.J.Farrer)

[9] Genetic Testing Registry

PARK 11

Gene : GRB10 interacting GYF protein 2 (GIGYF2) [1-6]

Chromosome : 2 (q36-q37) [7]

Biochemical function : The Grb10 gene binds to the intracellular domains of the activated tyrosine kinase receptors. Grb10 and GIGYFs might act cooperatively in order to regulate the signalling of receptors [8].

Type of inheritance : Autosomal recessive [9, 10, 11]

Symptoms : Parkinson's Disease susceptibility [11]

Prevalence : North America [2, 6], Japan - unproven [12], Caucasian [13], China [14], China - unproven [15, 16], Belgium - unproven [3, 9], Portugal - unproven [6], Spain - unproven [17], France - unproven [18], Italy - unproven [1, 5, 10, 18], U.S.A. - unproven [4], rare in two Asian countries [19], Australia - unproven [20], Brazil - unproven [21]

Genetic tests : None [22]

[1] Movement Disorders [2009] 24 (12) : 1867-1868 (M.Bonetti, A. Ferraris, M.Petracca, A.R.Bentivoglio, B.Dallapiccola, E.M.Valente)

[2] Neuroscience Letters [2009] 454 (3) : 209-211 (Y.Guo, J.Jankovic, S.Zhu, W.Le, Z.Song, W.Xie, D.Liao, H.Yang, H.Deng)

[3] Neurobiologial Aging [2011] 32 (2) : 308-312 (B.Meeus, K. Nuytemans, D.Crosiers, S.Engelborghs, P.Pals, B.Pickut, K.Peeters, M. Mattheijssens, E.Corsmit, P.Cras, P.P.De Deyn, J.Theuns, et al)

[4] Neurology [2009] 72 (22) : 1886-1892 (W.C.Nichols, D.K.Kissell, N.Pankratz, M.W.Pauciulo, V.E.Elsaesser, K.A.Clark, C.A.Halter, A. Rudolph, J.Wojcieszek, R.F.Pfeiffer, T.Foroud)

[5] Movement Disorders [2009] 24 (4) : 619-620 (C.Vilariño-Güell, O.A.Ross, A.I.Soto, M.J.Farrer, K.Haugarvoll, J.O.Aasly, R.J.Uitti, Z.K.Wszolek)

[6] Human Molecular Genetics [2009] 18 (2) : 341-346 (J.Bras, J. Simón-Sánchez, M.Federoff, A.Morgadinho, C.Januario, M.Ribeiro, L. Cunha, C.Oliveira, A.B.Singleton)

[7] American Journal of Human Genetics [2003] 72 (4) : 1053-1057 (N.Pankratz, W.C.Nichols, S.K.Uniacke, C.Halter, A.Rudolph, C. Shults, P.M.Conneally, T.Foroud)

[8] Journal of Biological Chemistry [2003] 278 (34) : 31564-31573 (B.Giovannone, E.Lee, L.Laviola, F.Giorgino, K.A.Cleveland, R.J. Smith)

[9] Neurobiological Aging [2010] 31 (6) : 1069-1071 (S.Lesage, C. Condroyer, E.Lohman, A.Troiano, F.Tison, F.Viallet, P.Damier, C. Tranchant, M.Vidhaillet, A.M.Ouvrard-Hernandez, A.Dürr, A.Brice)

[10] Parkinsonism & Related Disorders [2009] 15 (9) : 703-705 (A.Di Fonzo, E.Fabrizio, A.Thomas, E.Fincati, R.Marconi, M.Tinazzi, G.J. Breedveld, E.J.Simons, H.F.Chien, J.J.Ferreira, M.W.Horstink, et al)

[11] HUGO Gene Nomenclature Committee (GIGYF2)

[12] Neuroscience Letters [2010] 479 (3) : 245-248 (L.Li, M. Funayama, H.Tomiyama, Y.Li, H.Yoshino, R.Sasaki, Y.Kokubo, S. Kuzuhara, Y. Mizuno, N.Hattori)

[13] Neurological Science [2015] 36 (11) : 2073-2079 (Y.Zhang, Q.Y. Sun, R.H.Yu, J.F.Guo, B.S.Tang, X.X.Yan)

[14] Neuroscience Letters [2010] 473 (2) : 131-135 (L.Wang, J.F.Guo, W.W.Zhang, Q.Xu, X.Zuo, C.H.Shi, L.Z.Luo, J.Liu, L.Hu, Y.C.Hu, L. She, H.Jiang, X.X.Yan, K.Xia, Q.Pan, B.S.Tang)

[15] Parkinsonism & Related Disorders [2010] 16 (4) : 294-297 (L. Cao, T.Zhang, L.Zheng, Y.Wang, G.Wang, J.Zhang, Q.Z.Fei, P.J.Cui, X.J.Wang, J.F.Ma, Q.Xiao, S.D.Chen)

[16] Neuroscience Letters [2009] 463 (3) : 172-175 (Y.Zhang, L. Zheng, T.Zhang, Y.Wang, Q.Xiao, Q.Z.Fei, P.J.Cui, L.Cao, S.D. Chen)

[17] European Journal of Neurology [2010] 17 (2) : 321-325 (L. Samaranch, E.Lorenzo, M.A.Pastor, M.Riverol, M.R.Luquin, M.C. Rodríguez-Oroz, J.A.Obeso, P.Pastor)

[18] American Journal of Human Genetics [2008] 82 (4) : 822-833 (C. Lautier, S.Goldwurm, A.Dürr, B.Giovannone, W.G.Tsiaras, G.Pezzoli, A.Brice, R.J.Smith)

[19] Human Genetics [2009] 126 (3) : 425-430 (E.K.Tan, C.H.Lin, C. H.Tai, L.C.Tan, M.L.Chen, R.Li, H.Q.Lim, R.Pavanni, Y.Yuen, K.M. Prakash, Y.Zhao, R.M.Wu)

[20] Movement Disorders [2009] 24 (3) : 449-452 (G.T.Sutherland, G. A.Siebert, J.R.Newman, P.A.Silburn, R.S.Boyle, J.D.O'Sullivan, G.D. Mellick)

[21] Neuroscience Letters [2010] 485 (2) : 121-124 (A.V.Dos Santos, C.P.Pestana, K.R.Diniz, M.Campos, C.B.Abdalla-Carvalho, A.L.de Rosso, J.S.Pereira, D.H.Nicaretta, W.L.de Carvalho, et al)

[22] Genetic Testing Registry

PARK 12

Gene : Unknown [1]

Chromosome : X (q21-q25) [1]

Biochemical function : Unknown [1]

Type of inheritance : Unknown [1]

Symptoms : Parkinson's Disease susceptibility [1]

Prevalence : U.S.A. [1]

Genetic tests : None [2]

[1] Human Molecular Genetics [2003] 12 (20) : 2599-2608 (N. Pankratz, W.C.Nichols, S.K.Uniacke, C.Halter, J.Murrell, A. Rudolph, C.W.Shults, P.M.Conneally, T.Foroud)

[2] Genetic Testing Registry

PARK 13

Gene : HtrA2 (HtrA serine peptidase 2) [1]

Chromosome : 2 p12 [2]

Biochemical function : HtrA serine peptidase 2 cleaves UCH-L1 and inhibits tyrosine hydroxylase [3].

Type of inheritance : Unknown

Symptoms : Parkinson's Disease [1, 4, 5, 6]

Prevalence : Taiwan [1], Han Chinese [4], Belgium [5], Germany [6], U.S.A. - unproven [7], North America - unproven [8], Italy [9, 10].

Genetic tests : Parkinson disease 13 (by CGC Genetics), PARK13 Parkinsonism (by Centogene AG) [11]

[1] Cell Death and Differentiation [2012] 19 (2) : 257-266 (J.C. Fitzgerald, M.D.Camprubi, L.Dunn, H.C.Wu, N.Y.Ip, R.Kruger, L.M. Martins, N.W.Wood, H.Plun-Favreau)

[2] Journal of Biological Chemistry [2000] 275 (4) : 2581-2588 (L. Faccio, C.Fusco, A.Chen, S.Martinotti, J.V.Bonventre, A.S.Zervos)

[3] Biochemical and Biophysical Research Communications [2011] 415 (1) : 24-29 (D.W.Park, M.K.Nam, H.Rhim)

[4] Journal of Pineal Research [2011] 50 (3) : 281-291 (F.Han, R.R. Tao, G.S.Zhang, Y.M.Lu, L.L.Liu, Y.X.Chen, Y.J.Lou, K.Fukunaga, Z.H.Hong)

[5] Human Mutation [2008] 29 (6) : 832-840 (V.Bogaerts, K. Nuytemans, J.Reumers, P.Pals, S.Engelborghs, B.Pickut, E.Corsmit, K. Peeters, J.Schymkowitz, P.P.De Deyn, P.Cras, F.Rousseau, et al)

[6] Human Molecular Genetics [2005] 14 (15) : 2099-2111 (K.M. Strauss, L.M.Martins, H.Plun-Favreau, F.P.Marx, S.Kautzmann, D. Berg, T.Gasser, Z.Wszolek, T.Müller, A.Bornemann, H.Wolburg, et al)

[7] Parkinsonism & Related Disorders [2008] 14 (7) : 539-543 (O.A. Ross, A.I.Soto, C.Vilariño-Güell, M.G.Heckman, N.N.Diehl, M.M. Hulihan, J.O.Aasly, S.Sando, J.M.Gibson, T.Lynch, et al)

[8] Human Molecular Genetics [2008] 17 (13) : 1988-1993 (J. Simón-Sánchez, A.B.Singleton)

[9] Journal of Alzheimers Disease [2014] 38 (2) : 351-357 (M.Anfossi, R.Colao, M.Gallo, L.Bernardi, M.E.Conidi, F. Frangipane, F.Vasso, G.Puccio, A.Clodomiro, M.Mirabelli, S.A. Curcio, et al)

[10] Parkinsonism & Related Disorders [2014] 20 (8) : 911-914 (R. Cilia, C.Siri, D.Rusconi, R.Allegra, A.Ghiglietti, G.Sacilotto, M.Zini, A.L.Zecchinelli, R.Asselta, S.Duga, A.M.Paganoni, G.Pezzoli, et al)

[11] Genetic Testing Registry

PARK 14

Gene : PLA2G6 (phospholipase A2, group VI, cytosolic, calcium-independent) [1-7]

Chromosome : 22 (q12-q13) [8]

Biochemical function : Calcium-independent group VI phospholipase A(2) [1, 8]

Type of inheritance : Autosomal recessive [2]

Symptoms : L-dopa-responsive early onset Parkinson's Disease [1], early onset parkinsonism [2], adult-onset L-dopa responsive dystonia-parkinsonism [7, 9], presenting with rapidly progressive parkinsonism that is L-dopa responsive but which later on caused cognitive decline and loss of L-dopa responsiveness [6], L-dopa-responsive parkinsonism with dementia, in which there was a rapid rate of progression [4].

Prevalence : In a small proportion of people with early onset Parkinson's Disease [1, 4], Han Chinese [10], mainland China [2], Japan (in a small number) [3], Saudi Arabia [9]

Genetic tests : Parkinson disease 14 (by Praxis fuer Humangenetik Wien), Parkinson disease 14 (sequence analysis of PLA2G6 gene) (by CGC Genetics), PARK14 Parkinsonism (by Centogene AG) [11]

[1] Movement Disorders [2011] 26 (13) : 2415-2417 (K.M.Kauther, C. Höft, I.Rissling, W.H.Oertel, J.C.Möller)

[2] Neurology [2011] 77 (1) : 75-81 (C.H.Shi, B.S.Tang, L.Wang, Z.Y. Lv, J.Wang, L.Z.Luo, L.Shen, H.Jiang, X.X.Yan, Q.Pan, K.Xia, J.F. Guo)

[3] Journal of Human Genetics [2011] 56 (5) : 401-403 (H.Tomiyama, H.Yoshino, K.Ogaki, L.Li, C.Yamashita, Y.Li, M. Funayama, R. Sasaki, Y.Kokubo, S.Kuzuhara, N.Hattori)

[4] Neurology [2010] 75 (15) : 1356-1361 (H.Yoshino, H.Tomiyama, N.Tachibana, K.Ogaki, Y.Li, M.Funayama, T.Hashimoto, S. Takashima, N.Hattori)

[5] PLoS One [2010] 5 (9) : e12897 (L.A.Engel, Z.Jing, D.E.O'Brien, M.Sun, P.T.Kotzbauer)

[6] Movement Disorders [2010] 25 (12) : 1791-1800 (C.Paisán-Ruiz, R.Guevara, M.Federoff, H.Hanagasi, F.Sina, E.Elahi, S.A.Schneider, P. Schwingenschuh, N.Bajaj, M.Emre, A.B.Singleton, J.Hardy, et al)

[7] Annals of Neurology [2009] 65 (1) : 19-23 (C.Paisan-Ruiz, K.P. Bhatia, A.Li, D.Hernandez, M.Davis, N.W.Wood, J.Hardy, H. Houlden, A.Singleton, S.A.Schneider)

[8] Nature Genetics [2006] 38 (7) : 752-754 (N.V.Morgan, S.K. Westaway, J.E.Morton, A.Gregory, P.Gissen, S.Sonek, H.Cangul, J. Coryell, N.Canham, N.Nardocci, G.Zorzi, S.Pasha, D.Rodriguez, et al)

[9] BMC Research Notes [2016] 9 (1) : 295 (S.A.Bohlega, B.R. Al-Mubarak, E.A.Alyemni, M.Abouelhoda, D.Monies, A.E.Mustafa, D.S.Khalil, S.Al Haibi, H.Abou Al-Shaar, T.Faquih, et al)

[10] Parkinsonism & Related Disorders [2013] 19 (1) : 21-26 (Y.X.Gui, Z.P.Xu, Wen-Lv, H.M.Liu, J.J.Zhao, X.Y.Hu)

[11] Genetic Testing Registry

PARK 15

Gene : F-box protein 7 (FBXO7) [1]

Chromosome : 22 (q12-q13) [2]

Biochemical function : SCF-type E3 ubiquitin ligases are crucial regulators of cell cycle progression. F-box protein is the substrate specifying subunit of this family of ligases. So their availability dictates the timing and the location of the ubiquitination of substrates [3].

Type of inheritance : Autosomal recessive [1]

Symptoms : Presents with severe L-dopa-responsive parkinsonism and pyramidal disturbances [1]. Early-onset and progressive parkinsonism and pyramidal tract signs [4]. Progressive speech problems, severe apathy, chorea, and tics at presentation. Very mild parkinsonism after developed after three years. Young onset asymmetric tremor-dominant parkinsonism with features, such as postural instability, tics, and also tachyphemic speech [5]. Typical Parkinson's Disease that presents with features such as rapid eye movement sleep disorders, depression, and anxiety [6].

Prevalence : In a Dutch family [1] and an Italian family [1]. Rare in Spain [7]. In a Kurdish family [6], and a Turkish family [6].

Genetic tests : PARK15 Parkinsonism (by Centogene AG), Parkinson disease 15 (PARK15, sequence analysis of FBXO7 gene) (by CGC Genetics) [8]

[1] PLoS One [2011] 6 (2) : e16983 (T.Zhao, E.De Graaff, G.J. Breedveld, A.Loda, L.A.Severijnen, C.H.Wouters, F.W.Verheijen, M. C.Dekker, P.Montagna, R.Willemsen, B.A.Oostra, V.Bonifati)

[2] Cold Spring Harbor Perspectives in Medicine [2012] 2 (1) : a008888 (C.Klein, A.Westenberger)

[3] Journal of Biological Chemistry [2011] 286 (22) : 19804-19815 (D. E.Nelson, H.Laman)

[4] Neurology [2009] 72 (3) : 240-245 (A.Di Fonzo, M.C.Dekker, P. Montagna, A.Baruzzi, E.H.Yonova, L.Correia Guedes, A.Szczerbinska, T.Zhao, L.O.Dubbel-Hulsman, C.H.Wouters, et al)

[5] Parkinsonism & Related Disorders [2014] 20 (11) : 1253-1256 (A.Gündüz, A.G.Eken, B.Bilgiç, H.A.Hanagasi, K.Bilgüvar, M. Günel, A.N.Basak, S.Ertan)

[6] Movement Disorders [2015] 30 (8) : 1130-1133 (E.Lohmann, A.S. Coquel, A.Honoré, H.Gurvit, H.Hanagasi, M.Emre, A.L.Leutenegger, V.Drouet, M.Sahbatou, G.Guven, et al)

[7] Neurobiology of Aging [2014] 35 (3) : 727 (P.Gómez-Garre, S.Jesús, F.Carrillo, M.T.Cáceres-Redondo, I.Huertas-Fernández, I. Bernal-Bernal, M.Bonilla-Toribio, L.Vargas-González, et al)

[8] Genetic Testing Registry

PARK 16

Gene : Unknown [1]

Chromosome : 1 (q32) [1]

Biochemical function : Unknown

Type of inheritance : Unknown [2]

Symptoms : PARK 16 is more likely in Parkinson's Disease [1, 2].

Prevalence : Han population of Suzhou, China [2], Japan [3], China [3], Chile [4], Malaysia [5] Han Chinese [6, 7]

Genetic tests : None

[1] PLoS Genetics [2011] 7 (6) : e1002142 (V.Plagnol, M.A.Nalls, J.M.Bras, D.G.Hernandez, M.Sharma, U.M.Sheerin, M.Saad, J.Simón-Sánchez, C.Schulte, S.Lesage, S.Sveinbjörnsdóttir, P.Amouyel, et al)

[2] Zhonghua Yi Xue Za Zhi [2011] 91 (5) : 296-300 (D.H.Li, J.Wang, C.J.Mao, W.D.Hu, L.Xiao, Y.P.Yang, Z.H.Qin, C.F.Liu)

[3] Neurology [2010] 75 (6) : 508-512 (E.K.Tan, H.H.Kwok, L.C.Tan, W.T.Zhao, K.M.Prakash, W.L.Au, R.Pavanni, Y.Y.Ng, W. Satake, Y.Zhao, T.Toda, J.J.Liu)

[4] Parkinsonism & Related Disorders [2011] 17 (1) : 70-71 (A. Ramirez, A.Ziegler, S.Winkler, J.Kottwitz, R.Giesen, F.Daz-Grez, M. Miranda, P.Venegas, O.T.Godoy, R.Avello, M.I.Behrens, et al)

[5] American Journal of Medical Genetics - B Neuropsychiatric Genetics [2016] May 13 [Epub ahead of print] (A.A.Gopalai, A.Ahmad-Annuar, H.H.Li, Y.Zhao, S.Y.Lim, A.H.Tan, T.T.Lim, et al)

[6] Neurobiology of Aging [2013] 34 (10) : 2442 (K.H.Chang, C.M. Chen, Y.C.Chen, R.K.Lyu, H.S.Chang, L.S.Ro, G.J.Lee-Chen, Y.R. Wu)

[7] Genetics and Molecular Research [2015] 14 (2) : 2978-2985 (H. Xia, Q.Luo, X.X.Li, X.L.Yang)

[8] Genetic Testing Registry

PARK 17

Gene : VPS35 [1]

Chromosome : 16 (q13-q21) [2]

Biochemical function : VPS35 mediates vesicle transport between the mitochondria and peroxisomes [3].

Type of inheritance : Autosomal dominant [3], and Autosomal recessive [4]

Symptoms : The mean age of onset of Parkinson's Disease in the affected individuals was 53 years old [4]. Tremor predominant dopa-responsive parkinsonism with a mean onset of 50 years old could also occur [1].

Causes of symptoms : VPS35 is a component of the retromer complex and mediates retrograde transport between endosomes and the trans-Golgi network [4].

Prevalence : In a Dutch family [4]. In a Swiss family [3]. In Japanese [5], Indians (rare) [6]. It must be rare because it occurred in only one man out of one assessment of 1774 people with Parkinson's Disease [7].

Genetic tests : Park17 Parkinson (by Centogene AG), Single gene testing VPS35 (by CeGaT GmbH), Parkinson disease 17 (by CGC Genetics Porto), VPS35 (by Fulgent Clinical Diagnostics Lab), VPS35 (by Institute for Human Genetics) [8]

[1] American Journal of Human Genetics [2011] 89 (1) : 162-167 (C.Vilariño-Gell, C.Wider, O.A.Ross, J.C.Dachsel, J.M.Kachergus, S.J. Lincoln, A.I.Soto-Ortolaza, S.A.Cobb, G.J.Wilhoite, et al)

[2] Genomics [2000] 70 (2) : 253-257 (P.Zhang, L.Yu, L.Gao, Q.Fu, F.Dai, Y.Zhao, L.Zheng, S.Zhao)

[3] Current Biology [2010] 20 (14) : 1310-1315 (E.Braschi, V.Goyon, R.Zunino, A.Mohanty, L.Xu, H.M.McBride)

[4] American Journal of Human Genetics [2011] 89 (1) : 168-175 (A. Zimprich, A.Benet-Pagès, W.Struhal, E.Graf, S.H.Eck, M.N. Offman, D.Haubenberger, S.Spielberger, E.C.Schulte, P.Lichtner, et al)

[5] Movement Disorders [2012] 27 (11) : 1413-1417 (M.Ando, M. Funayama, Y.Li, K.Kashihara, Y.Murakami, N.Ishizu, C.Toyoda, K.Noguchi, T.Hashimoto, N.Nakano, R.Sasaki, Y.Kokubo, et al)

[6] Neurobiology of Aging [2013] pii: S0197-S4580 (13) 00193-0 (S.Sudhaman, M.Behari, S.T.Govindappa, U.B.Muthane, R.C.Juyal, B.K.Thelma)

[7] Archives of Neurology [2012] : 1-5 (K.R.Kumar, A.Weissbach, M.Heldmann, M.Kasten, S.Tunc, C.M.Sue, M.Svetel, V.S.Kostic, J. Segura-Aguilar, A.Ramirez, D.K.Simon, P.Vieregge, T.F.Münte, et al)

[8] Genetic Testing Registry

PARK 18

Gene : EIF4G1 (Eukaryotic translation initiation factor 4-gamma) [1]

Chromosome : 3 (q26-q28) [1]

Biochemical function : mRNA translation initiation [1]

Type of inheritance : Autosomal dominant [1]

Symptoms : Parkinson's Disease susceptibility [1]. One study suggests that it is not a cause of Parkinson's Disease because the mutation was more common in people that did not have Parkinson's Disease [2].

Prevalence : Different countries [1]

Genetic tests : EIF4G1 (by Fulgent Clinical Diagnostics Lab), Parkinson Syndrome autosomal dominant Panel (by CeGaT GmbH) [3]

[1] American Journal of Human Genetics [2011] 89 (3) : 398-406 (M. C.Chartier-Harlin, J.C.Dachsel, C.Vilario-Gell, S.J.Lincoln, F.Leprtre, M.M.Hulihan, J.Kachergus, A.J.Milnerwood, L.Tapia, et al)

[2] Neurobiology of Aging [2015] 36 (8) : 2444 (N.Nichols, J.M.Bras, D.G.Hernandez, I.E.Jansen, S.Lesage, S.Lubbe, A.B.Singleton)

[3] Genetic Testing Registry

PARK 19

Gene : DNAJC6 [1]

Chromosome : 1 (p31.3) [1]

Biochemical function : DNAJC6 encodes the HSP40 Auxilin, which is a protein that is specifically expressed in neurons and which confers specificity to the ATPase activity of its partner Hcs70 in clathrin uncoating [2].

Type of inheritance : unknown

Symptoms : Juvenile Parkinsonism that presented with mental retardation, pyramidal signs and epilepsy, as well as varying degrees of a progressive neurological disease [1]. Juvenile Parkinsonism [2].

Prevalence : Turkey [1], Israel [2].

Genetic tests : Park19 Parkinson (by Centogene AG), DNAJC6 Gene Sequencing (by DDC Molecular Diagnostics Laboratory), Parkinson disease 19 (by CGC Genetics) [3]

[1] Parkinsonism & Related Disorders [2013] 19 (3) : 320-324 (C. Köroglu, L.Baysal, M.Cetinkaya, H.Karasoy, A.Tolun)

[2] PLoS One [2012] 7 (5) : e36458 (S.Edvardson, Y.Cinnamon, A.Ta-Shma, A.Shaag, Y.I.Yim, S.Zenvirt, C.Jalas, S.Lesage, A.Brice, A. Taraboulos, K.H.Kaestner, L.E.Greene, O.Elpeleg)

[3] Genetic Testing Registry

PARK 20

Gene : SYNJ1 (synaptojanin 1) [1]

Chromosome : 21 (q22) [2]

Biochemical function : Encodes a phosphoinositide phosphatase that regulates phosphatidylinositol-4, 5-bisphosphate. So the enzyme may affect synaptic transmission and membrane trafficking [3, 4].

Type of inheritance : Autosomal recessive [5, 6]

Symptoms : Early onset Parkinsonism [6, 7, 8], dystonia, and cognitive deterioration, poor response to L-dopa, brain atrophy, nigrostriatal dopaminergic defects, cerebral hypometabolism [6].

Prevalence : Italian [6, 8], Iranian [7].

Genetic tests : Park20 Parkinson (by Centogene AG), SYNJ1 Gene Sequencing (by DDC Molecular Diagnostics Laboratory), Parkinson disease 20 (by CGC Genetics) [9]

[1] Journal of Alzheimers Disease [2014] 42 (3) : 767-775 (S.B. Martin, A.L.Dowling, J.Lianekhammy, I.T.Lott, E.Doran, M.P. Murphy, T.L.Beckett, F.A.Schmitt, E.Head)

[2] Psychiatry Research [2004] 127 (1-2) : 157-161 (P.Stopkova, J. Vevera, I.Paclt, I.Zukov, H.M.Lachman)

[3] Biomed Research International [2014] : 289728 (V.Drouet, S. Lesage)

[4] Journal of Biomolecular Screening [2014] 19 (4) : 585-594 (L.B. McIntire, K.I.Lee, B.Chang-Ileto, G.Di Paolo, T.W.Kim)

[5] Neurogenetics [2014] 15 (3) : 183-188 (S.Olgiati, A.De Rosa, M. Quadri, C.Criscuolo, G.J.Breedveld, M.Picillo, S.Pappatà, M. Quarantelli, P.Barone, G.De Michele, V.Bonifati)

[6] Human Mutation [2013] 34 (9) : 1208-1215 (M.Quadri, M.Fang, M.Picillo, S.Olgiati, G.J.Breedveld, J.Graafland, B.Wu, F.Xu, R.Erro, M.Amboni, S.Pappatà, M.Quarantelli, G.Annesi, A.Quattrone, et al)

[7] Human Mutation [2013] 34 (9) : 1200-1207 (C.E.Krebs, S. Karkheiran, J.C.Powell, M.Cao, V.Makarov, H.Darvish, G.Di Paolo, R. H.Walker, G.A.Shahidi, J.D.Buxbaum, P.De Camilli, Z.Yue, et al)

[8] Parkinsonism & Related Disorders [2016] 23 : 102-105 (A.De Rosa, T.Pellegrino, S.Pappatà, M.Lieto, V.Bonifati, V.Palma, A.Topa, L.Santoro, L.Bilo, A.Cuocolo, G.De Michele)

[9] Genetic Testing Registry

PARK 21

Gene : DNAJC13 (DnaJ heat shock protein family (Hsp40) member C13) [1].

Chromosome : 3 (q22.1) [1]

Biochemical function : Encodes one of the Dnaj protein family. They are co-chaperones of a partner heat-shock protein by binding to the latter and stimulating ATP hydrolysis. The encoded protein associates with the heat-shock protein Hsc70 and plays a role in clathrin-mediated endocytosis. It may be involved in post-endocytic transport mechanisms with proteins including the sorting nexin SNX1 [2].

Type of inheritance : autosomal dominant [3, 4]

Symptoms : Parkinson's Disease susceptibility [5, 6]

Prevalence : French [5], French Canadian [5], Mennonites (Dutch, German, Russian) [6], Caucasian (uncommon) [7], Chinese (rare) [8]

Genetic tests : Park21 Parkinson (by Centogene AG) [9]

[1] Journal of Biological Chemistry [2005] 280 : 40135-40143 (M. Girard, V.Poupon, F.Blondeau, P.S.McPherson)

[2] Journal of Biological Chemistry [2015] 290 (35) : 21676-21689 (B.Xhabija, P.O.Vacratsis)

[3] European Journal of Neurology [2015] 22 (9) : 1323-1325 (O. Lorenzo-Betancor, K.Ogaki, A.I.Soto-Ortolaza, C.Labbe, R.L.Walton, A.J.Strongosky, J.A.van Gerpen, R.J.Uitti, P.J.McLean, et al)

[4] Human Molecular Genetics [2014] 23 (7) : 1794-1801 (C. Vilariño-Güell, A.Rajput, A.J.Milnerwood, B.Shah, C.Szu-Tu, J.Trinh, I.Yu, M.Encarnacion, L.N.Munsie, L.Tapia, E.K.Gustavsson EK, et al)

[5] Neurobiology of Aging [2016] May 3 [Epub ahead of print] (J.P. Ross, N.Dupre, Y.Dauvilliers, S.Strong, A.Ambalavanan, D. Spiegelman, A.Dionne-Laporte, E.Pourcher, M.Langlois, et al)

[6] Movement Disorders [2014] 29 (13) : 1684-1687 (S.Appel-Cresswell, A.H.Rajput, V.Sossi, C.Thompson, V.Silva, J. McKenzie, Dinelle, S.E.McCormick, C.Vilariño-Güell, A.J.Stoessl, et al)

[7] European Journal of Neurology [2015] 22 (9) : 1323-1325 (O. Lorenzo-Betancor, K.Ogaki, A.I.Soto-Ortolaza, C.Labbe, R.L. Walton, A.J.Strongosky, J.A.van Gerpen, R.J.Uitti, P.J.McLean, et al)

[8] Neurobiology of Aging [2014] 35 (4) : 935 (J.N.Foo, H.Liany, L.C.Tan, W.L.Au, K.M.Prakash, J.Liu, E.K.Tan)

[9] Genetic Testing Registry

PARK 22

Gene : CHCHD2 (Coiled-coil-helix-coiled-coil-helixdomain containing 2) [1]

Chromosome : 7 (p11.2) [2]

Biochemical function : Mediates oxygen-dependent expression of cytochrome c oxidase subunit 4-2 gene expression [3]

Type of inheritance : Autosomal dominant [1, 4]

Symptoms : Associated with Parkinson's Disease [1, 4]

Prevalence : Japanese [1], Han Chinese (none) [5], Han Chinese (rare) [6], Taiwanese (none) [7], Italy (none) [8]

Genetic tests : none [9]

[1] The Lancet Neurology [2015] 14 (3) : 274-282 (M.Funayama, K. Ohe, T.Amo, N.Furuya, J.Yamaguchi, S.Saiki, Y.Li, K.Ogaki, M.Ando, H.Yoshino, H.Tomiyama, K.Nishioka, K.Hasegawa, H.Saiki, et al)

[2] Meta Gene [2014] 2 : 274-282 (K.Varvagiannis, I.Papoulidis, T. Koromila, K.Kefalas, M.Ziegler, T.Lieher, M.B.Petersen, Y. Gyftodimou, E.Manolakos)

[3] Nucleic Acids Research [2013] 41 (4) : 2255-2266 (S.Aras, O.Pak, N.Sommer, R.Finley Jr, M.Hüttemann, N.Weissmann, L.Grossman)

[4] Neurobiology of Aging [2015] Nov 6 [Epub ahead of print] (C.H.Shi, C.Y.Mao, S.Y.Zhang, J.Yang, B.Song, P.Wu, C.T.Zuo, Y.T. Liu, Y.Ji, Z.H.Yang, J.Wu, Z.P.Zhuang, Y.M.Xu)

[5] Neurobiology of Aging [2015] Aug 15 [Epub ahead of print] (Z. Liu, J.Guo, K.Li, L.Qin, J.Kang, L.Shu, Y.Zhang, Y.Wei, N.Yang, Y. Luo, Q.Sun, Q.Xu, X.Yan, B.Tang)

[6] Parkinsonism & Related Disorders [2016] May 30 [Epub ahead of print] (X.Yang, Q.Zhao, R.An, J.Zheng, S.Tian, Y.Chen, Y.Xu)

[7] Neurobiology of Aging [2015] Dec 8 [Epub ahead of print] (T.S. Fan, H.I.Lin, C.H.Lin, R.M.Wu)

[8] Neurobiology of Aging [2017] Jan 5 [Epub ahead of print] (E. Rubino, L.Brusa, M.Zhang, S.Boschi, F.Govone, A.Vacca, A.Gai, L.Pinessi, L.Lopiano, E.Rogaeva, I.Rainero)

[9] Genetic Testing Registry

PARK 23

Gene : VPS13C (vacuolar protein sorting 13 homolog C) [1]

Chromosome : 15 (q) [2]

Biochemical function : Silencing of VPS13C is associated with lower mitochondrial membrane potential, mitochondrial fragmentation, increased respiration rates, exacerbated PINK1/Parkin-dependent mitophagy, and transcriptional upregulation of PARK2 in response to mitochondrial damage [3].

Type of inheritance : Autosomal recessive [3]

Symptoms : VPS13C mutations are associated with a distinct form of early-onset parkinsonism that is characterised by rapid and severe Parkinson's Disease progression and early cognitive decline. The pathological features are striking and reminiscent of diffuse Lewy body disease [3].

Prevalence : Uncommon [3], Han Chinese (none known) [4], Taiwan (none known) [5]

Genetic tests : None [6]

[1] The HUGO Gene Nomenclature Committee (HGNC)

[2] American Journal of Physiology - Endocrinology and Metabolism [2016] Jun 21 [Epub ahead of print] (Z.B.Mehta, N.Fine, T.J.Pullen, M.C.Cane, M.Hu, P.Chabosseau, G.Meur, A.Velayos-Baeza, et al)

[3] American Journal of Human Genetics [2016] 98 (3) : 500-513 (S. Lesage, V.Drouet, E.Majounie, V.Deramecourt, M.Jacoupy, A.Nicolas, F.Cormier-Dequaire, S.M.Hassoun, C.Pujol, S.Ciura, et al)

[4] American Journal of Medical Genetics [2016] 171B (3) : 342-347 (L.Wang, L.Cheng, N.N.Li, W.J.Yu, X.Y.Sun, R.Peng)

[5] Neurobiology of Aging [2016] 39 : 221.e1-e5 (C.M.Chen, Y.C. Chen, M.C.Chiang, H.C.Fung, K.H.Chang, G.J.Lee-Chen, Y.R.Wu)

[6] Genetic Testing Registry

Tyrosine Hydroxylase Deficiency

Gene : Tyrosine Hydroxylase (TH) [1]

Chromosome : 11 (p15.5) [1]

Biochemical function : L-dopa biosynthesis [2]

Type of inheritance : Autosomal recessive [1, 3]

Symptoms : There are two types : an infantile onset, progressive, hypokinetic-rigid syndrome with dystonia (type A), and a complex encephalopathy with neonatal onset (type B). Most of them can be successfully treated with L-dopa [2, 4-7], but some have a poor or no response [2]. There can be mild mental retardation [6]. Symptoms can also include dystonia [3] and L-dopa responsive myoclonus with dystonia [8], L-dopa responsive dystonia, and a sustained response to low-dose L-dopa therapy [9]. There can also be generalised tremor, brisk reflexes, hypokinesia, rigidity, distal chorea, and athetosis [10, 11]. Early-onset severe encephalopathy can be accompanied with : stagnation of psychomotor development, paroxysmal dystonic postures and movements of limbs, hypokinesia [12], and by poor treatment or infantile parkinsonism with motor delay or myopathy [13].

Prevalence : very rare [4], Czech Republic [5], Netherlands [6], Taiwan [9], Italy [12], China [13, 14], Greece [15]

Genetic tests : Segawa syndrome (sequence analysis of TH gene) (by CGC Genetics) [16]

[1] Molecular Genetics and Metabolism [2009] 97 (1) : 18-20 (D.I. Zafeiriou, M.A.Willemsen, M.M.Verbeek, E.Vargiami, A.Ververi, R. Wevers)

[2] Prenatal Diagnosis [2005] 25 (8) : 671-675 (L.B.Møller, A. Romstad, M.Paulsen, P.Hougaard, A.Ormazabal, M.Pineda, N.Blau, F. Güttler, R.Artuch)

[3] Journal of Neurosurgery Pediatrics [2011] (6) : 650-653 (M.J. Tormenti, N.D.Tomycz, K.A.Coffman, D.Kondziolka, D.J.Crammond, E.C.Tyler-Kabara)

[4] Brain [2010] 133 (Part 6) : 1810-1822 (M.A.Willemsen, M.M. Verbeek, E.J.Kamsteeg, J.F.de Rijk-van Andel, A.Aeby, N. Blau, A. Burlina, M.A.Donati, B.Geurtz, P.J.Grattan-Smith, M.Haeussler, et al)

[5] Prague Medical Report [2012] 113 (2) : 136-146 (K.Szentiványi, H.Hansíková, J.Krijt, K.Vinšová, M.Tesarová, E.Rozsypalová, P. Klement, J.Zeman, T.Honzík)

[6] Neurology [2000] 55 (12) : 1926-1928 (J.F.de Rijk-Van Andel, F.J. Gabreëls, B.Geurtz, G.C.Steenbergen-Spanjers, L.P.van Den Heuvel, J.A.Smeitink, R.A.Wevers)

[7] Annals of Neurology [2003] 54 (Supplement 6) : S56-S65 (G.F. Hoffmann, B.Assmann, C.Bräutigam, C.Dionisi-Vici, M.Häussler, J.B. de Klerk, M.Naumann, G.C.Steenbergen-Spanjers, et al)

[8] Neurology [2012] 79 (5) : 435-441 (M.Stamelou, N.E.Mencacci, C. Cordivari, A.Batla, N.W.Wood, H.Houlden, J.Hardy, K.P.Bhatia)

[9] Neurology [2004] 63 (8) : 1524-1526 (A.Schiller, R.A.Wevers, G. C.Steenbergen, N.Blau, H.H.Jung)

[10] Pediatric Neurology [2012] 46 (2) : 77-82 (C.S.Chi, H.F.Lee, C.R. Tsai)

[11] Movement Disorders [2002] 17 (2) : 354-359 (P.F.Grattan- Smith, R.A.Wevers, G.C.Steenbergen-Spanjers, V.S.Fung, J.Earl, B. Wilcken)

[12] Journal of Child Neurology [2012] 27 (4) : 523-525 (T. Giovanniello, D.Claps, C.Carducci, C.Carducci, N.Blau, F.Vigevano, I. Antonozzi, V.Leuzzi)

[13] Journal of Child Neurology [2011] 26 (2) : 179-187 (W.L.Yeung, V.C.Wong, K.Y.Chan, J.Hui, C.W.Fung, E.Yau, C.H.Ko, C.W.Lam, C. M.Mak, S.Siu)

[14] Molecular Genetics and Metabolism [2010] 99 (4) : 431-433 (C.M.Mak, C.W.Lam, T.S.Siu, K.Y.Chan, W.K.Siu, W.L.Yeung, J.Hui, V.C.Wong, L.C.Low, C.H.Ko, C.W.Fung, S.P.Chen, Y.P.Yuen, et al)

[15] Movement Disorders [2010] 25 (8) : 1086-1090 (R.Pons, M. Serrano, A.Ormazabal, C.Toma, A.Garcia-Cazorla, E.Area, M.Ribasés, E.Kanavakis, K.Drakaki, A.Giannakopoulos, I.Orfanou, et al)

[16] Genetic Testing Registry

Aromatic L-amino acid Decarboxylase Deficiency

Gene : Dopa decarboxylase (aromatic L-amino acid decarboxylase) (DDC) [1]

Chromosome : 7 (p12.2) [2]

Biochemical function : Dopamine biosynthesis [1]

Type of inheritance : unknown

Symptoms : Aromatic L-amino acid decarboxylase (AADC) deficiency is a disorder of amine metabolism resulting in generalised combined deficiency of serotonin, dopamine and catecholamines. The main clinical features are developmental delay, muscular hypotonia, dystonia, oculogyric crises and additional extraneurological symptoms Response to therapy is variable and unsatisfactory. Later, main neurological features were truncal muscular hypotonia, hypokinesia, oculogyric crises, and rigor. Patients presented with distinct extra-neurological symptoms, such as hypersalivation, hyperhidrosis, nasal congestion, sleep disturbances and hypoglycaemia. All patients have decreased concentrations of homovanillic and 5-hydroxyindoleacetic acid and an elevated concentration of 3-ortho-methyldopa in the CSF. Diagnosis is confirmed by measurement of plasma AADC activity. No patients completely recover from neurological symptoms, but partial improvement of mobility and mood can be achieved in some [1].

Prevalence : unknown

Genetic tests : none [3]

[1] Journal of Inherited Metabolic Disease [2009] 32 (3) : 371-380 (C.Manegold, G.F.Hoffmann, I.Degen, H.Ikonomidou, A.Knust, M.W. Laaß, M.Pritsch, E.Wilichowski, F.Hörster)

[2] Schizophrenia Research [2014] 159 (2-3) : 333-339 (J.Li, H.Y. Meltzer)

[3] Genetic Testing Registry

ADORA1

Gene : ADORA1 (adenosine A1 receptor) [1]

Chromosome : 1 (q32.1) [2]

Biochemical function : The type A1 receptors inhibit adenylyl cyclase. Functions of ADORA1 include its interaction with dopamine receptor D1 and its inhibitory effect on dopamine receptor D1 [1]. ADORA1 is located in the Parkinson's Disease locus PARK16. So ADORA1 may be the gene for susceptibility to Parkinson's Disease within this locus [1].

Type of inheritance : unknown

Symptoms : Parkinsonism and cognitive dysfunction can occur [1].

Prevalence : Iran [1]

Genetic tests : none [3]

[1] Movement Disorders [2016] 31 (7) : 1004-1011 (E.Jaberi, M. Rohani, G.A.Shahidi, S.Nafissi, E.Arefian, M.Soleimani, A. Moghadam, M.K.Arzenani, F.Keramatian, B.Klotzle, J.B.Fan, et al)

[2] Genomics [1995] 26 (2) : 423-425 (A.Townsend-Nicholson, E. Baker, P.R.Schofield, G.R.Sutherland)

[3] Genetic Testing Registry

CYP2D6

Gene : CYP2D6 [1]

Chromosome : 22 (q13) [2]

Biochemical function : cytochrome P450, family 2, subfamily D, polypeptide 6 [1]

Type of inheritance : unknown

Symptoms : Increased susceptibility to Parkinson's Disease [3, 4, 5]

Prevalence : Caucasians [3, 4], none in Asians [6], none in Chinese [7]

Genetic tests : none [8]

[1] Drug Metabolism and Pharmacokinetics [2014] 29 (1) : 29-43 (Z.Zahari, R.Ismail)

[2] Annals of Neurology [1997] 41 (6) : 813-817 (K.Wilhelmsen, D.Mirel, K.Marder, M.Bernstein, A.Naini, S.M.Leal, L.J.Cote, M.X. Tang, G.Freyer, J.Graziano, R.Mayeux)

[3] PLoS One [2013] 8 (12) : e84413 (Y.Lu, C.Mo, Z.Zeng, S.Chen, Y.Xie, Q.Peng, Y.He, Y.Deng, J.Wang, L.Xie, J.Zeng, S.Li, X.Qin)

[4] Journal of Neurological Science [2014] 336 (1-2) : 161-168 (Y.Lu, Q.Peng, Z.Zeng, J.Wang, Y.Deng, L.Xie, C.Mo, J.Zeng, X.Qin, S.Li)

[5] American Journal of Medical Genetics [1996] J67 (4) : 361-365 G.Lucotte, J.C.Turpin, N.Gérard, S.Panserat, R.Krishnamoorthy)

[6] Neuroepidemiology [2003] 22 (6) : 357-361 (A.S.Persad, T. Stedeford, S.Tanaka, L.Chen, M.Banasik)

[7] Journal of Neurology, Neurosurgery and Psychiatry [1998] 65 (5) : 781-784 (D.K.Chan, J.Woo, S.C.Ho, C.P.Pang, L.K.Law, P.W.Ng, W. T.Hung, T.Kwok, E.Hui, K.Orr, M.F.Leung, R.Kay)

[8] Genetic Testing Registry

DRD2

Gene : DRD2 (Dopamine receptor D2) [1]

Chromosome : 11 (q23) [2]

Biochemical function : Encodes the D2 subtype dopamine receptor [2].

Type of inheritance : unknown

Symptoms : Increased susceptibility to Parkinson's Disease [3, 4, 5].

Prevalence : Spain [1], Europeans [3], Italian [4].

Genetic tests : none [6]

[1] Neuroscience Letters [1999] 273 (3) : 151-154 (P.Pastor, E. Muñoz, V.Obach, M.J.Martí, R.Blesa, R.Oliva, E.Tolosa)

[2] Molecular Psychiatry [2009] 14 (9) : 885-893 (S.J.Glatt, S.V. Faraone, J.A.Lasky-Su, T.Kanazawa, H.G.Hwu, M.T.Tsuang)

[3] Biomedical Reports [2014] 2 (2) : 275-281 (D.Dai, Y.Wang, L.Wang, J.Li, Q.Ma, J.Tao, X.Zhou, H.Zhou, Y.Jiang, G.Pan, L.Xu, P.Ru, D. Lin, J.Pan, L.Xu, M.Ye, S.Duan)

[4] Movement Disorders [2000] 15 (1) : 127-131 (R.L.Oliveri, G. Annesi, M.Zappia, D.Civitelli, E.V.De Marco, A.A.Pasqua, F.Annesi, P.Spadafora, A.Gambardella, G.Nicoletti, D.Branca, et al)

[5] Neurology [1997] 48 (6) : 1589-1593 (V.Planté-Bordeneuve, D. Taussig, F.Thomas, G.Said, N.W.Wood, C.D.Marsden, A.E.Harding)

[6] Genetic Testing Registry

DRD3

Gene : DRD3 (Dopamine receptor D3) [1]

Chromosome : 3 (q13.3) [2]

Biochemical function : DRD3 encodes the D3 subtype dopamine receptor [1].

Type of inheritance : unknown

Symptoms : Increased susceptibility to Parkinson's Disease [1, 3], and impulse control and related behaviours (ICRB) [4].

Prevalence : China [1], India [3], Korea [4]

Genetic tests : none [5]

[1] Biomedical Reports [2014] 2 (2) : 275-281 (D.Dai, Y.Wang, L. Wang, J.Li, Q.Ma, J.Tao, X.Zhou, H.Zhou, Y.Jiang, G.Pan, L.Xu, P. Ru, D. Lin, J.Pan, L.Xu, M.Ye, S.Duan)

[2] European Journal of Human Genetics [2009] 17 (6) : 766-773 (D. Lorenz, S.Klebe, G.Stevanin, S.Thier, A.Nebel, J.Feingold, H. Frederiksen, E.Denis, K.Christensen, S.Schreiber, A.Brice, et al)

[3] Neurogenetics [2006] 7 (4) : 223-229 (R.C.Juyal, M.Das, S.Punia, M.Behari, G.Nainwal, S.Singh, P.V.Swaminath, S.T.Govindappa, S. Jayaram, U.B.Muthane, B.K.Thelma)

[4] Movement Disorders [2009] 24 (12) : 1803-1810 (J.Y.Lee, E.K. Lee, S.S..Park, J.Y.Lim, H.J.Kim, J.S.Kim, B.S.Jeon)

[5] Genetic Testing Registry

GLIS1

Gene : GLIS1 (GLIS family zinc finger 1) [1]

Chromosome : 1 (p32.3) [2]

Biochemical function : GLIS1 is an activator and repressor of transcription [1]

Type of inheritance : unknown

Symptoms : Increased risk of developing late onset Parkinson's Disease [3]

Prevalence : Han Chinese [3]

Genetic tests : none [4]

[1] Journal of Biological Chemistry [2002] 277 (34) : 30901-30913 (Y. S.Kim, M.Lewandoski, A.O.Perantoni, S.Kurebayashi, G.Nakanishi, A.M.Jetten)

[2] Circulation Cardiovascular Genetics [2013] 6 (1) : 97-105 (J. Divers, N.D.Palmer, L.Lu, T.C.Register, J.J.Carr, P.J.Hicks, R.C. Hightower, S.C.Smith, J.Xu, A.J.Cox, K.A.Hruska, et al)

[3] European Neurology [2012] 68 (2) : 89-92 (W.Song, Y.P.Chen, R. Huang, K.Chen, P.L.Pan, J.Li, Y.Yang, H.F.Shang)

[4] Genetic Testing Registry

HLA

Gene : Major histocompatibility complex [1]

Chromosome : 6 (p21.3) [2]

Biochemical function : HLA plays a central role in the function of the immune system

Type of inheritance : unknown

Symptoms : Increased risk of Parkinson's Disease [1, 3-7], but not in all studies [8, 9]

Prevalence : Iran [3], French [10], Chinese [4, 5, 11] but not in all studies [12], not in Taiwanese [13, 14]

Genetic tests : none [15]

[1] American Journal of Human Genetics [2013] 93 (5) : 984-993 (W. T.Wissemann, E.M.Hill-Burns, C.P.Zabetian, S.A.Factor, N. Patsopoulos, B.Hoglund, C.Holcomb, R.J.Donahue, G.Thomson, et al)

[2] Brain Research [2012] 1466 : 152-157 (T.Botta-Orfila, A.Sànchez-Pla, M.Fernández, F.Carmona, M.Ezquerra, E.Tolosa)

[3] International Journal of Immunogenetics (2014) 41 (6) : 508-511 (J.Jamshidi, A.Movafagh, B.Emamalizadeh, A.Zare Bidoki, A.Manafi, S.Ghasemi Firouzabadi, G.A.Shahidi, S.Kazeminasab, et al)

[4] Parkinsonism & Related Disorders [2013] 19 (7) : 701-702 (C.Ran, T.Willows, O.Sydow, A.Johansson, P.Söderkvist, N.Dizdar, A.Ahmadi, L.Olson, A.C.Belin)

[5] PLoS One [2012] 7 (11) : e48594 (C.Sun, L.Wei, F.Luo, Y.Li, J.Li, F.Zhu, P.Kang, R.Xu, L.Xiao, Z.Liu, P.Xu)

[6] PLoS One [2011] 6 (11) : e27109 (E.M.Hill-Burns, S.A.Factor, C.P. Zabetian, G.Thomson, H.Payami)

[7] Journal of Neurology, Neurosurgery, and Psychiatry [2010] 81 (8) : 890-891 (M.Saiki, A.Baker, C.H.Williams-Gray, T.Foltynie, R.S. Goodman, C.J.Taylor, D.A.Compston, R.A.Barker, S.J.Sawcer, et al)

[8] European Review for Medical and Pharmacological Sciences [2015] 19 (3) : 423-432 (R.L.Zhu, X.C.Lu, L.J.Tang, B.S.Huang, W. Yu, S.Li, L.X.Li)

[9] Clinical Genetics [2013] 84 (5) : 501-504 (Y.Zhao, A.A.Gopalai, A. Ahmad-Annuar, E.W.Teng, K.M.Prakash, L.C.Tan, W.L.Au, H.H.Li, S.Y.Lim, S.K.Lim, Y.B.Chong, L.P.Tan, N.M.Ibrahim, E.K.Tan)

[10] Movement Disorders [2012] 27 (9) : 1104-1110 (I.Ahmed, R. Tamouza, M.Delord, R.Krishnamoorthy, C.Tzourio, C.Mulot, M. Nacfer, J.C.Lambert, P.Beaune, P.Laurent-Puig, M.A.Loriot, et al)

[11] Neuroscience Letters [2011] 501 (3) : 185-187 (Y.Guo, X.Deng, W.Zheng, H.Xu, Z.Song, H.Liang, J.Lei, X.Jiang, Z.Luo, H.Deng)

[12] The International Journal of Neuroscience [2015] 125 (4) : 241-246 (Z.G.Ma, T.W.Liu, Y.L.Bo)

[13] American Journal of Medical Genetics. Part B [2013] 162B (8) : 841-846 (C.H.Lin, M.L.Chen, Y.C.Tai, C.Y.Yu, R.M.Wu)

[14] Parkinsonism & Related Disorders [2012] 18 (4) : 391-393 (H.L. Chiang, G.J.Lee-Chen, C.M.Chen, Y.C.Chen, C.M.Lee, M.H.Liao, Y. R.Wu)

[15] Genetic Testing Registry

LINGO1

Gene : LINGO1 [1]

Chromosome : 15 [2]

Biochemical function : LINGO-1 is associated with the Nogo-66 receptor complex and endowed with a canonical EGF receptor (EGFR)-like tyrosine phosphorylation site [1].

Type of inheritance : unknown

Symptoms : Susceptibility to Parkinson's Disease [3-6]

Prevalence : Italy [3], Spain [4], U.S.A. [5, 6]

Genetic tests : none [7]

[1] Proceedings, National Academy Sciences U.S.A. [2007] 104 (36) : 14430-14435 (H.Inoue, L.Lin, X.Lee, Z.Shao, S.Mendes, P.Snodgrass -Belt, H.Sweigard, T.Engber, B.Pepinsky, L.Yang, M.F.Beal, et al)

[2] European Journal of Neuroscience [2003] 18 (12) : 3167-3182 (L. Carim-Todd, M.Escarceller, X.Estivill, L.Sumoy)

[3] Parkinsonism & Related Disorders [2011] 17 (8) : 638-641 (F. Annesi, E.V.De Marco, F.E.Rocca, A.Nicoletti, P.Pugliese, G.Nicoletti, G. Arabia, P.Tarantino, M.De Mari, P.Lamberti, S.Gallerini, et al)

[4] Movement Disorders [2011] 26 (4) : 722-727 (O.Lorenzo-Betancor, L.Samaranch, E.García-Martín, S.Cervantes, J.A.Agúndez, F.J.Jiménez-Jiménez, H.Alonso-Navarro, A.Luengo, F.Coria, et al)

[5] Neurogenetics [2010] 11 (4) : 401-408 (C.Vilariño-Güell, C.Wider, O.A.Ross, B.Jasinska-Myga, J.Kachergus, S.A.Cobb, A.I.Soto-Ortolaza, B.Behrouz, M.G.Heckman, N.N.Diehl, C.M.Testa, et al)

[6] Parkinsonism & Related Disorders [2010] 16 (2) : 109-111 (C. Vilariño-Güell, O.A.Ross, C.Wider, B.Jasinska-Myga, S.A.Cobb, A.I. Soto-Ortolaza, J.M.Kachergus, B.H.Keeling, J.C.Dachsel, et al)

[7] Genetic Testing Registry

MAPT

Gene : MAPT (microtubule-associated protein tau) [1]

Chromosome : 17 (q21) [2]

Biochemical function : The MAPT gene encodes the microtubule-associated protein tau (MAPT) whose transcript undergoes complex, regulated and alternative splicing, giving rise to several types of mRNA [1].

Type of inheritance : unknown

Symptoms : Associated with Parkinson's Disease [2-15]

Prevalence : China [1, 16], Caucasian [8, 10], India [11], Iran [17]
Genetic tests : MAPT (by Fulgent Clinical Diagnostics Lab) [18]

[1] BMC Neuroscience [2014] 15 : 54 (L.Yu , J.Huang, D.Zhai, L. Liu, K.Guo, X.Long, J.Xiong, Z.Zhang, Y.Wang, Y.Zhao, P.Wu, D. Wang, Z.Lin, J.Wu, N.Xiong, T.Wang)

[2] Journal of Applied Genetics [2010] 51 (4) : 509-514 (K.S.Wang, J. E.Mullersman, X.F.Liu)

[3] Frontiers in Genetics [2014] 5 : 382 (J.M.Taymans, V.Baekelandt)

[4] European Journal of Neurology [2014] 21 (11) : e91-e92 (J.Trinh, E. K.Gustavsson, I.Guella, C.Vilariño-Güell, D.Evans, M.Encarnacion, H. Sherman, F.Hentati, M.J.Farrer)

[5] JAMA Neurology [2014] 71 (4) : 429-435 (J.M.Shulman, L.Yu, A. S.Buchman, D.A.Evans, J.A.Schneider, D.A.Bennett, P.L.De Jager)

[6] Journal of Neural Transmission [2014] 121 (4) : 353-356 (M.E.Di Battista, E.Pascale, C.Purcaro, F.Passarelli, E.Passarelli, R.Guglielmi, N.Vanacore, G.Meco)

[7] Archives of Neurology [2011] 68 (3) : 359-364 (N.Setó-Salvia, J.Clarimón, J.Pagonabarraga, B.Pascual-Sedano, A.Campolongo, O. Combarros, J.I.Mateo, D.Regaña, M.Martínez-Corral, et al)

[8] European Journal of Neurology [2011] 18 (6) : 876-881 (C.Wider, C.Vilariño-Güell, M.G.Heckman, B.Jasinska-Myga, A.I.Ortolaza-Soto, N.N.Diehl, J.E.Crook, S.A.Cobb, J.A.Bacon, J.O.Aasly, et al)

[9] Nature Genetics [2009] 41 (12) : 1308-1312 (J.Simón-Sánchez, C.Schulte, J.M.Bras, M.Sharma, J.R.Gibbs, D.Berg, C.Paisan-Ruiz, P. Lichtner, S.W.Scholz, D.G.Hernandez, R.Krüger, M.Federoff, et al)

[10] European Journal of Neurology [2010] 17 (3) : 483-486 (C. Wider, C.Vilariño-Güell, B.Jasinska-Myga, M.G.Heckman, A.I.Soto-Ortolaza, S.A.Cobb, J.O.Aasly, J.M.Gibson, T.Lynch, R.J.Uitti, et al)

[11] Neuroscience Letters [2009] 460 (1) : 16-20 (G.Das, A.K.Misra, S. K.Das, K.Ray, J.Ray)

[12] Neurology [2008] 71 (1) : 28-34 (J.E.Tobin, J.C.Latourelle, M.F. Lew, C.Klein, O.Suchowersky, H.A.Shill, L.I.Golbe, M.H.Mark, J.H. Growdon, G.F.Wooten, B.A.Racette, J.S.Perlmutter, R.Watts, et al)

[13] Annals of Neurology [2004] 55 (3) : 329-334 (J.B.Kwok, E.T. Teber, C.Loy, M.Hallupp, G.Nicholson, G.D.Mellick, D.D. Buchanan, P.A.Silburn, P.R.Schofield)

[14] Annals of Neurology [2007] 62 (2) : 137-144 (C.P.Zabetian, C.M. Hutter, S.A.Factor, J.G.Nutt, D.S.Higgins, A.Griffith, J.W. Roberts, B.C.Leis, D.M.Kay, D.Yearout, J.S.Montimurro, et al)

[15] Annals of Neurology [2007] 62 (2) : 145-153 (A.Goris, C.H. Williams-Gray, G.R.Clark, T.Foltynie, S.J.Lewis, J.Brown, M.Ban, M. G.Spillantini, A.Compston, D.J.Burn, P.F.Chinnery, R.A.Barker, et al)

[16] Neurobiology of Aging [2014] 35 (7) : 1780.e7-1780.e10 (X.Dan, C.Wang, J.Ma, X.Feng, T.Wang, Z.Zheng, P.Chan)

[17] Neurobiology of Aging [2014] 35 (12) : e27-e28 (B. Emamalizadeh, A.Movafagh, M.Akbari, S.Kazeminasab, A.Fazeli, M. Motallebi, G.A. Shahidi, P.Petramfar, R.Mirfakhraie, H.Darvish)

[18] Genetic Testing Registry

MCCC1

Gene : MCCC1 (methylcrotonoyl-CoA carboxylase 1) [1]

Chromosome : 3 (q27.1) [2]

Biochemical function : The biochemical function of MCCC1 is to function as a heterodimer and catalyzes the carboxylation of 3-methylcrotonyl-CoA to form 3-methylglutaconyl-CoA. [3]

Type of inheritance : Autosomal recessive [1]

Symptoms : Sporadic Parkinson's Disease [4], motor progression [5]

Prevalence : Han Chinese [4, 5, 6]

Genetic tests : none [7]

[1] International Journal of Biochemistry and Cell Biology [2016] 78 : 116-129 (L.Zandberg, H.van Dyk, F.H.van der Westhuizen, A.A.van Dijk)

[2] Human Genetics [2010] 128 (1) : 39-49 (N.Phasukkijwatana, B. Kunhapan, J.Stankovich, W.L.Chuenkongkaew, R.Thomson, T. Thornton, M.Bahlo, T.Mushiroda, Y.Nakamura, et al)

[3] Biochemische Zeitschrift [1961] 335 : 101-122 (J.Knappe, H.G.Schlegel, F.Lynen)

[4] Journal of Neural Transmission [2016] 123 (4) : 425-430 (L. Wang, L.Cheng, Z.J.Lu, X.Y.Sun, J.Y.Li, R.Peng)

[5] Neurobiology of Aging [2016] 37 : 209 (A.A.Davis, K.M. Andruska, B.A.Benitez, B.A.Racette, J.S.Perlmutter, C.Cruchaga)

[6] Human Molecular Genetics [2016] Dec 22 [Epub ahead of print] (J.N.Foo, L.C.Tan, I.D.Irwan, W.L.Au, H.Q.Low, K.M.Prakash, A. Ahmad-Annuar, J.Bei, A.Y.Chan, C.M.Chen, Y.C.Chen, et al)

[7] Genetic Testing Registry

NR4A2 (NURR1)

Gene : NRA42 (NURR1) [1]

Chromosome : 2 (q22-q23) [1]

Biochemical function : Essential in the development of mesencephalic dopaminergic neurons [2, 3].

Type of inheritance : unknown

Symptoms : Increased risk of Parkinson's Disease in males [4]. An increased risk of Parkinson's Disease in women, in people who are 60 years old or older, and in people of Caucasian origin [5].

Prevalence : China [4]

Genetic tests : NR4A2 (by Fulgent Clinical Diagnostics Lab) [6]

[1] American Journal of Medical Genetics [2002] 114 (1) : 15-23 H.Ishiguro, Y.Okubo, T.Ohtsuki, K.Yamakawa-Kobayashi, T.Arinami)

[2] Progress in Neurobiology [2005] 77 (1-2) : 128-138 (J.Jankovic, S.Chen, W.D.Le)

[3] Neuroscience Letters [2003] 347 (3) : 139-142 (E.K.Tan, H. Chung, Y.Zhao, H.Shen, V.R.Chandran, C.Tan, M.L.Teoh, Y.Yih, R. Pavanni, M.C.Wong)

[4] European Journal of Neurology [2012] 19 (6) : 870-875 (H.Liu, L.Wei, Q.Tao, H.Deng, M.Ming, P.Xu, W.Le)

[5] Journal of Neurological Science [2008] 273 (1-2) : 29-33 (W.Le, T.Pan, M.Huang, P.Xu, W.Xie, W.Zhu, X.Zhang, H.Deng, J.Jankovic)

[6] Genetic Testing Registry

PDE8B

Gene : PDE8B (Nucleotide phosphodiesterase 8B) [1]

Chromosome : 5 (q13.3-q14.1) [2]

Biochemical function : PDE8B is necessary for phosphodiesterase, which degrades cyclic AMP [2].

Type of inheritance : Autosomal dominant [1, 2]

Symptoms : Slowly progressive parkinsonism [1]. The symptoms can include bradykinesia, dysarthria, muscle rigidity, but not tremor [2].

Prevalence : Japan [1], Germany [2]

Genetic tests : none [3]

[1] Movement Disorders [2015] 30 (14) : 1964-1967 (R.Azuma, K. Ishikawa, K.Hirata, Y.Hashimoto, M.Takahashi, K.Ishii, A.Inaba, T. Yokota, S.Orimo)

[2] American Journal of Human Genetics [2010] 86 (1) : 83-87 (S. Appenzeller, A.Schirmacher, H.Halfter, S.Bäumer, M.Pendziwiat, V. Timmerman, P.De Jonghe, K.Fekete, F.Stögbauer, P.Lüdemann, et al)

[3] Genetic Testing Registry

PITX3

Gene : PITX3 (Paired-like homeodomain 3) [1]

Chromosome : 10 (q24.32) [2]

Biochemical function : PITX3 is a transcription factor that is important for the differentiation and survival of midbrain dopaminergic neurons during their development [3].

Type of inheritance : unknown

Symptoms : Increased risk of Parkinson's Disease [4-8], particularly in older people [9], and younger onset Parkinson's Disease [3, 10].

Prevalence : Asians [4], China [5, 7, 9]

Genetic tests : none [11]

[1] Swiss Medical Weekly [2012] 142 : w13521 (Y.Gui, Y.Zhao, H. Liu, J.Fu, Z.Xu, X.Hu)

[2] American Journal of Medical Genetics B [2012] 159B (2) : 236-242 (K.Derwinska, H.Mierzewska, A.Goszczanska, E.Szczepanik, Z.Xia, K.Kusmierska, J.Tryfon, A.Kutkowska-Kazmierczak, E.Bocian, et al)

[3] Neurobiology of Aging [2011] 32 (4) : 750-753 (W.Le, D. Nguyen, X.W.Lin, P.Rawal, M.Huang, Y.Ding, W.Xie, H.Deng, J.Jankovic)

[4] Neuroscience Letters [2014] 561 : 128-133 (G.Qiu, C.Fu, G.H. Liang)

[5] Brain Research [2011] 1392 :116-120 (J.Liu, Q.Y.Sun, B.S.Tang, L.Hu, R.H.Yu, L.Wang, C.H.Shi, X.X.Yan, Q.Pan, K.Xia, J.F.Guo)

[6] Movement Disorders [2011] 26 (9) : 1729-1732 (Y.Guo, W.D.Le, J.Jankovic, H.R.Yang, H.B.Xu, W.J.Xie, Z.Song, H.Deng)

[7] European Journal of Neurology [2011] 18 (5) : 778-783 (L.H.Yu, Z.F.Lin, Y.Liu, F.Y.Hu, X.H.He, Z.L.Liu, Y.M.Xu)

[8] Neurobiology of Aging [2009] 30 (5) : 731-738 (J.Fuchs, J.C. Mueller, P.Lichtner, C.Schulte, M.Munz, D.Berg, U.Wüllner, T.Illig, M.Sharma, T.Gasser)

[9] European Journal of Neurology [2012] 19 (6) : 870-875 (H.Liu, L. Wei, Q.Tao, H.Deng, M.Ming, P.Xu, W.Le)

[10] Neurobiology of Aging [2010] 31 (1) : 114-117 (O.Bergman, A. Håkansson, L.Westberg, K.Nordenström, A.Carmine Belin, O.Sydow, L.Olson, B.Holmberg, E.Eriksson, H.Nissbrandt)

[11] Genetic Testing Registry

PTRHD1

Gene : PTRHD1[1]

Chromosome : 2 (p23.3) [1]

Biochemical function : PTRHD1 is a peptidyl-tRNA hydrolase domain containing 1 [2].

Type of inheritance : Autosomal recessive [1]

Symptoms : Parkinsonism and intellectual disability [1].

Prevalence : Iran (individual family) [1]

Genetic tests : none [3]

[1] Movement Disorders [2016] Oct 18 [Epub ahead of print] (H. Khodadadi, L.J.Azcona, V.Aghamollaii, M.D.Omrani, M.Garshasbi, S.Taghavi, A.Tafakhori, G.A.Shahidi, J.Jamshidi, et al)

[2] Protein Expression and Purification [2016] 126 : 49-54 (G.L.Burks, H.McFeeters, R.L.McFeeters)

[3] Genetic Testing Registry

RAB39B

Gene : RAB39B [1]

Chromosome : Xq28 [2]

Biochemical function : Rab proteins are involved in the regulation of vesicular trafficking [3]. They are able to promote the clearance of alpha-synuclein and rescue alpha-synuclein induced toxicity [4].

Type of inheritance : Autosomal dominant [5]

Symptoms : Loss of RAB39B resulted in pathologically confirmed Parkinson's Disease. There was widespread classic Lewy body pathology. Additional features included cortical Lewy bodies, brain iron accumulation, tau immunoreactivity, and axonal spheroids.

Mutations in RAB39B cause intellectual disability and pathologically confirmed early-onset Parkinson's Disease [3, 6]. Juvenile Parkinsonism [11].

Prevalence : Caucasians (rare) [1], rare [7], Han Chinese (none) [8, 9], Taiwanese (none) [10], Chinese [11]

Genetic tests : none [12]

[1] Neurobiology of Aging [2016] 45 : 107-108 (K.Hodges, S.S. Brewer, C.Labbé, A.I.Soto-Ortolaza, R.L.Walton, A.J.Strongosky, R.J. Uitti, J.A.van Gerpen, N.Ertekin-Taner, K.Kantarci, V.J.Lowe, et al)

[2] Cytogenetic and Genome Research [2002] 97 (1-2) : 72-75 (H.Cheng, Y.Ma, X.Ni, M.Jiang, L.Guo, K.Ying, Y.Xie, Y.Mao)

[3] Neurology Genetics [2015] 1 (1) : e9 (S.Lesage, J.Bras, F.Cormier-Dequaire, C.Condroyer, A.Nicolas, L.Darwent, R.Guerreiro, E. Majounie, M.Federoff, P.Heutink, N.W.Wood, T.Gasser, J.Hardy, et al)

[4] PLoS Genetics [2016] 12 (4) : e1005995 (S.A.Gonçalves, D. Macedo, H.Raquel, P.D.Simões, F.Giorgini, J.S.Ramalho, D.C.Barral, L.Ferreira Moita, T.F.Outeiro)

[5] Molecular Neurodegeneration [2015] 10 : 50 (I.F.Mata, Y.Jang, C.H.Kim, D.S.Hanna, M.O.Dorschner, A.Samii, P.Agarwal, J.W. Roberts, O.Klepitskaya, D.R.Shprecher, K.A.Chung, S.A.Factor, et al)

[6] American Journal of Human Genetics [2014] 95 (6) : 729-735 (G.R.Wilson, J.C.Sim, C.McLean, M.Giannandrea, C.A.Galea, J.R. Riseley, S.E.Stephenson, E.Fitzpatrick, S.A.Haas, K.Pope, et al)

[7] Parkinsonism & Related Disorders [2016] 23 : 116-117 (T.Löchte, N.Brüggemann, E.J.Vollstedt, P.Krause, A.Domingo, R.Rosales, L.V. Lee, F.Hopfner, A.Westenberger, A.Kühn, C.Klein, K.Lohmann, et al)

[8] Neurobiol of Aging [2015] 36 (10) : 2907 (L.Yuan, X.Deng, Z. Song, Z.Yang, B.Ni, Y.Chen, H.Deng)

[9] Scientific Reports [2016] 6 : 34502 (J.F.Kang, Y.Luo, B.S.Tang, C.M.Wan, Y.Yang, K.Li, Z.H.Liu, Q.Y.Sun, Q.Xu, X.X.Yan, J.F.Guo)

[10] Neurobiology of Aging [2016] Oct 21 [Epub ahead of print] (H.H. Lin, R.M.Wu, H.I.Lin, M.L.Chen, C.H.Tai, C.H.Lin)

[11] Movement Disorders [2016] 31 (12) : 1905-1909 (C.H.Shi, S.Y.Zhang, Z.H.Yang, J.Yang, D.D.Shang, C.Y.Mao, H.Liu, H.M.Hou, M.M.Shi, J.Wu, Y.M.Xu)

[12] Genetic Testing Registry

RIT2

Gene : RIT2 [1]

Chromosome : 18 [1]

Biochemical function : GTP-binding protein [2]

Type of inheritance : unknown [1]

Symptoms : A moderately increased risk of Parkinson's Disease [1, 3-6].

Prevalence : Chinese [3-6], none in Han Chinese [7]

Genetic tests : none [8]

[1] Annals of Neurology [2012] 71 (3) : 370-384 (N.Pankratz, G.W. Beecham, A.L.DeStefano, T.M.Dawson, K.F.Doheny, S.A.Factor, T.H. Hamza, A.Y.Hung, B.T.Hyman, A.J.Ivinson, D.Krainc, et al)

[2] Journal of Neuroscience [1996] 16 (21) : 6784-6794 (C.H.Lee, N.G.Della, C.E.Chew, D.J.Zack)

[3] Parkinsonism & Related Disorders [2014] S1353-S8020 (14) 00478-7 (J.Wang, M.Gong, Y.Ye, J.Ye , G.Lin, Q.Zhuang, X.Zhang, J.Zhu)

[4] Neuroscience Letters [2015] 602 : 167-171 (X.Zhang, M.Niu, H.Li, A.Xie)

[5] Neurobiology of Aging [2015] 36 (3) : 1600 (Z.H.Liu, J.F.Guo, Y.Q.Wang, K.Li, Q.Y.Sun, Q.Xu, X.X.Yan, C.S.Xu, B.S.Tang)

[6] Neurobiology of Aging [2015] 36 (3) : 1603 (K.Nie, S.J.Feng, H.M. Tang, G.X.Ma, R.Gan, X.Zhao, J.H.Zhao, L.M.Wang, Z.H.Huang, J. Huang, L.Gao, Y.W.Zhang, R.M.Zhu, Z.P.Duan, Y.H.Zhang, et al)

[7] Neurological Science [2016] Nov 26 [Epub ahead of print] (J.Y.Li, J.H.Zhang, N.N.Li, L.Wang, Z.J.Lu, L.Cheng, X.Y.Sun, R.Peng)

[8] Genetic Testing Registry

STH

Gene : STH (Saitohin) [1]

Chromosome : 17 (q21.31) [2]

Biochemical function : unknown [3]

Type of inheritance : unknown

Symptoms : An increased risk of Parkinson's Disease that was 1.8 times greater when the age of onset was less than 65 years old, and two times greater when the age of onset was older than 65 years old [1].

Prevalence : Turkey [1]

Genetic tests : none [4]

[1] Cellular and Molecular Neurobiology [2014] Aug 29 [Epub ahead of print] (E.Sonmez, M.D.Ozel, E.E.Islek, A.Sazci, H.A.Idrisoglu)

[2] Gene [2012] 492 (1) : 319-324 (S.Kitsiou-Tzeli, H.Frysira, K. Giannikou, A.Syrmou, K.Kosma, G.Kakourou, E.Leze, C.Sofocleous, E.Kanavakis, M.Tzetis)

[3] Journal of Cellular Biochemistry [2011] 112 (11) : 3482-3488 (Y. Wang, L.Gao, C.G.Conrad, A.Andreadis)

[4] Genetic Testing Registry

TMEM230

Gene : TMEM230 [1]

Chromosome : 20 (20pter-p12) [1]

Biochemical function : The biochemical function of TMEM230 is to produce vesicles involved in packaging the neurotransmitter dopamine in the dopaminergic neurons and then secreting it [1].

Type of inheritance : Autosomal dominant [1]

Symptoms : Typical of Parkinson's Disease [1].

Prevalence : North America and Asia, including China [1]

Genetic tests : none [2]

[1] Nature Genetics [2016] 48 (7) : 733-739 (H.X.Deng, Y.Shi, Y. Yang, K.B.Ahmeti, N.Miller, C.Huang, L.Cheng, H.Zhai, S.Deng, K. Nuytemans, N.J.Corbett, M.J.Kim, H.Deng, B.Tang, Z.Yang, et al)

[2] Genetic Testing Registry

CHAPTER 38

CAUSES OF PARKINSON'S DISEASE

PHARMACOLOGICAL CAUSES

PHARMACOLOGICAL CAUSES

A small proportion of cases of Parkinson's Disease have a pharmacological cause. To varying extents some drugs can also be a partial cause or the sole cause of Parkinson's Disease. The use of the drugs must usually be persistent in order to cause Parkinson's Disease. The withdrawal or gradual reduction of the dosage of these drugs can lead, in most cases but not with all drugs, to the reduction in the Parkinson's Disease symptoms they cause or contribute to.

The drugs that can cause or worsen Parkinson's Disease symptoms include : Amiodarone (an anti-arrhythmic agent) [PAGE 533], Amphetamines and methamphetamines [PAGE 534], Aripiprazole (an anti-psychotic) [PAGE 535], Benzamides [PAGE 536], Calcium channel blockers [PAGE 537], Dopamine antagonists [PAGE 541], Ephedrone (which is manganese containing) [PAGE 543], Estrogen (an oral contraceptive) [PAGE 545], Lithium [PAGE 546], Phenothiazines (drugs with anti-psychotic effects) [PAGE 548], Trimetazidine (an anti-ischaemic agent) [PAGE 550], Valproic acid (a drug used for the treatment of a variety of psychiatric and neurological disorders including epilepsy) [PAGE 551], and Zolpidem [PAGE 553].

AMIODARONE

Pharmacology : Amiodarone is the most widely used anti-arrhythmic agent [1]. Use of Amiodarone causes a marked increase in the duration of transmembrane action potential [2].

Adverse effects : Use of Amiodarone is associated with Parkinsonism [3-6], which can revert after withdrawal of Amiodarone [6].

Causes of symptoms : Amiodarone can cause Parkinson's Disease symptoms because amiodarone is able to inhibit the dopamine D1 and D2 receptors and can therefore reduce dopaminergic activity [7].

[1] Expert Opinion on Drug Safety [2012] 11 (2) : 191-214 (P. Santangeli, L.Di Biase, J.D.Burkhardt, R.Bai, P.Mohanty, A.Pump, A. Natale)

[2] Journal of Clinical Pharmacology [1989] 29 (5) : 405-412 (P. Somani)

[3] Clinical Neuropathology [2010] 29 (2) : 84-88 (S.Ishida, M.Sugino, T.Hosokawa, T.Sato, D.Furutama, A.Fukuda, F.Kimura, H.Kuwabara, Y.Shibayama, T.Hanafusa)

[4] Movement Disorders [1995] 10 (2) : 233-234 (M.T.Dotti, A. Federico)

[5] Fundamental and Clinical Pharmacology [1994] 8 (4) : 293-306 (J. L.Montastruc, M.E.Llau, O.Rascol, J.M.Senard)

[6] Annals of Neurology [1989] 25 (6) : 630-632 (E.G.Werner, C.W. Olanow)

[7] Journal of Pharmacology and Experimental Therapeutics [1998] 287 (2) : 725-732 (A.Matsui, H.Matsuo, H.Takanaga, S.Sasaki, M. Maeda, Y.Sawada)

Amphetamines and Methamphetamines

Pharmacology : Amphetamines and methamphetamines are central nervous stimulants. They are also often used as recreational drugs. In certain parts of the brain amphetamines and methamphetamines can have some of their effects by increasing the concentration of dopamine in the synaptic cleft [1].

Adverse effects : In methamphetamine and amphetamine users there was nearly a three fold increased risk of Parkinson's Disease, indicating them as a cause of Parkinson's Disease [2, 3]. Prolonged amphetamine exposure made Parkinson's Disease eight times more likely [4].

Causes of symptoms : Methamphetamine, but not amphetamine, prevented the dopamine induced increase in the spontaneous firing of dopaminergic neurons [5].

[1] Journal of Neurochemistry [2011] 116 (2) : 164-176 (G.M.Miller)

[2] Drug and Alcohol Dependence [2015] 146 : 30-38 (K.Curtin, A.E. Fleckenstein, R.J.Robison, M.J.Crookston, K.R.Smith, G.R. Hanson)

[3] Parkinsonism & Related Disorders [2016] 25 : 27-32 (G.Todd, V. Pearson-Dennett, R.A.Wilcox, M.T.Chau, K.Thoirs, D.Thewlis, A.P. Vogel, J.M.White)

[4] Neurotoxicology [2006] 27 (6) : 1003-1006 (E.R.Garwood, W. Bekele, C.E.McCulloch, C.W.Christine)

[5] Journal of Biological Chemistry [2014] 289 (32) : 22246-22257 (K. Saha, D.Sambo, B.D.Richardson, L.M.Lin, B.Butler, L.Villarroel, H. Khoshbouei)

Aripiprazole

Pharmacology : Aripiprazole is a novel atypical neuroleptic used in the treatment of psychosis [1].

Adverse effects : The use of Aripiprazole is associated with Parkinsonism [1-4, 7]. Neuroleptics generally tripled the risk of developing Parkinson's Disease [5].

Causes of symptoms : Aripiprazole can cause Parkinson's Disease symptoms because it acts as a D2 dopamine receptor antagonist and can therefore reduce dopaminergic activity [6].

[1] Journal of Medical Case Reports [2009] 3 : 6448 (L.L.Lua, L. Zhang)

[2] Journal of Clinical Psychopharmacology [2016] Aug 6 [Epub ahead of print] (K.D.Jakobsen, C.H.Bruhn, A.K.Pagsberg, A.Fink-Jensen, J. Nielsen)

[3] Movement Disorders [2006] 21 (9) : 1538-1539 (I.M.Ali, M. Wickremaratchi, H.R.Morris)

[4] Tijdschrift voor Psychiatrie [2011] 53 (5) : 299-303 (P.De Schutter, F.Bouckaert, J.Peuskens)

[5] Neurology [2012] 79 (15) : 1615-1616 (A.Foubert-Samier, C. Helmer, F.Perez, M.Le Goff, S.Auriacombe, A.Elbaz, J.F.Dartigues, F. Tison)

[6] International Journal of Neuropsychopharmacology [2014] 18 (4) (G.F.Ma, N.Raivio, J.Sabrià, J.Ortiz)

[7] Neurologist [2017] 22 (1) : 24-28 (K.Selfani, V.L.Soland, S. Chouinard, P.Huot)

BENZAMIDES

Pharmacology : Cisapride is a benzamide derivative that is used as a gastroprokinetic agent as it increases the motility in the upper gastrointestinal tract. Levosulpiride is a substituted benzamide that is widely used for the management of dyspepsia and emesis [1].

Adverse effects : Cisapride worsened Parkinson's Disease [2, 3]. Sulpiride is implicated as a cause of Parkinsonism [1, 4, 5], which ceases in most people after discontinuation of sulpiride [5]. Benzamide derivatives including cisapride, sulpiride, tiapride, and metoclopramide are the main causes of drug-induced parkinsonism in recent years in Japan [6].

Causes of symptoms : Benzamides can cause Parkinson's Disease symptoms because benzamides bind to D2 dopamine receptors, especially D2Sh and can therefore reduce dopaminergic activity [7].

[1] Movement Disorders [2009] 24 (15) : 2249-2253 (H.W.Shin, M.J. Kim, J.S.Kim, M.C.Lee, S.J.Chung)

[2] Nihon Ronen Igakkai Zasshi [1994] 31 (11) : 899-902 (Y.Naito, S. Kuzuhara)

[3] Clinical Neuropharmacology [1995] 18 (1) : 76-78 (A.P.Sempere, J. Duarte, C.Cabezas, L.E.Clavería, F.Coria)

[4] Parkinsonism & Related Disorders [1996] 2 (3) : 145-149 (F.J. Jiménez-Jiménez, M.Ortí-Pareja, L.Ayuso-Peralta, T.Gasalla, F. Cabrera-Valdivia, A.Vaquero, J.Tejeiro, E.García-Albea)

[5] Neurologia [1996] 11 (1) : 10-15 (J.F.Martí Massó, J.J.Poza)

[6] Nihon Rinsho [2000] 58 (10) : 2049-2053 (S.Kuzuhara)

[7] Psychiatry Research [2013] 214 (3) : 175-180 (P.Seeman)

CALCIUM CHANNEL BLOCKERS

Pharmacology : Calcium channel blockers are used as antihypertensive drugs. Calcium channel blockers disrupt the movement of calcium (Ca^{2+}) through calcium channels.

Adverse effects : Calcium channel blockers can cause Parkinsonism [1-4]. Parkinsonism can cease in most people after withdrawal of Calcium channel blockers but tremor [3], and sometimes most symptoms [4] persist. However, some dihydropyridine calcium channel blockers can instead lessen the likelihood of developing Parkinson's Disease [5-9]. Calcium channel blockers are one of the most common pharmacological causes of Parkinson's Disease [10]. Cinnarizine is a piperazine derivative with calcium channel blocker and anticonvulsant properties and is used widely in the treatment of vertigo and circulatory disorders [11]. Cinnarizine can cause Parkinsonism [12-32, 47] which improves after discontinuation of the Cinnarizine [28-32]. It also inhibits NADH oxidation in submitochondrial particles and causes an NADH dependent generation of superoxide [11]. Flunarizine is a piperazine derivative with both calcium antagonist and anticonvulsant properties. Flunarizine is used widely in the treatment of vertigo and circulatory disorders [12]. Flunarizine can cause Parkinsonism [33-45, 47], whose symptoms improve after ceasing Flunarazine [41-45].

Causes of symptoms : Cinnarizine could cause the symptoms of Parkinsonism because it interferes with dopamine D2 receptors [46].

Cinnarizine also inhibits NADH oxidation in submitochondrial particles and causes NADH dependent generation of superoxide [11]. Flunarizine could cause the symptoms of Parkinsonism because it interferes with dopamine D2 receptors [46].

[1] Parkinsonism & Related Disorders [1996] 2 (3) : 145-149 (F.J. Jiménez-Jiménez, M.Ortí-Pareja, L.Ayuso-Peralta, T.Gasalla, F. Cabrera-Valdivia, A.Vaquero, J.Tejeiro, E.García-Albea)

[2] Revista de Neurologia [1995] 23 (123) : 961-963 (J.F.Horga, M. Navarro, V.Peiró, M.Hernández)

[3] Parkinsonism & Related Disorders [1998] 4 (4) : 211-214 (P.J. Garci´a-Ruiz, F.Javier Jiménez-Jiménez, J.Garci´a de Yébenes)

[4] Clinical Neuropharmacology [1992] 15 (1) : 19-26 (P.J. García-Ruiz, J.García de Yébenes, F.J.Jiménez-Jiménez, A.Vázquez, D.García Urra, B.Morales)

[5] Annals of Neurology [2012] 71 (3) : 362-369 (C.Marras, A. Gruneir, P.Rochon, X.Wang, G.Anderson, J.Brotchie, C.M.Bell, S.Fox, P.C.Austin)

[6] American Journal of Epidemiology [2012] 175 (7) : 627-635 (B. Pasternak, H.Svanström, N.M.Nielsen, L.Fugger, M.Melbye, A.Hviid)

[7] Annals of Neurology [2010] 67 (5) : 600-606 (B.Ritz, S.L.Rhodes, L.Qian, E.Schernhammer, J.H.Olsen, S.Friis)

[8] Neurology [2008] 70 (16 Part 2) : 1438-1444 (C.Becker, S.S.Jick, C.R.Meier)

[9] Parkinsonism & Related Disorders [1996] 2 (3) : 145-149 (F.J. Jiménez-Jiménez, M.Ortí-Pareja, L.Ayuso-Peralta, T.Gasalla, F. Cabrera-Valdivia, A.Vaquero, J.Tejeiro, E.García-Albea)

[10] Pharmacoepidemiology and Drug Safety [2015] 24 (6) : 559-566 (Y.Lang, D.Gong, Y.Fan)

[11] Molecular Pharmacology [1994] 45 (1) : 158-163 (K.Veitch, L. Hue)

[12] Zhurnal Nevrol Psikhiatr Im S S Korsakova [2012] 112 (8) : 76-81 (O.S.Levin, N.N.Shindriaeva, M.A.Anikina)

[13] Arquivos de Neuro-Psiquiatria [2009] 67 (3B) : 957 (H.A.Teive, R.P.Munhoz, H.B.Ferraz)

[14] Parkinsonism & Related Disorders [2004] 10 (4) : 243-245 (H.A. Teive, A.R.Troiano, F.M.Germiniani, L.C.Werneck)

[15] Revue Neurologique [1999] 28 (9) : 876-878 (S.Stucchi-Portocarrero, J.M.Vega-Dienstmaier, J.E.Saavedra, A.Sagástegui)

[16] Movement Disorders [1999] 14 (3) : 534-535 (A.Negrotti, S. Calzetti)

[17] Revue Neurologique [1998] 27 (155) : 35-39 (J.M.Errea-Abad, J.R.Ara-Callizo, C.Aibar-Remón)

[18] Nihon Rinsho [1997] 55 (1) : 112-117 (S.Kuzuhara)

[19] Movement Disorders [1997] 12 (1) : 107-110 (A.Negrotti, S. Calzetti)

[20] Fundamental and Clinical Pharmacology [1994] 8 (4) : 293-306 (J. L.Montastruc, M.E.Llau, O.Rascol, J.M.Senard)

[21] Clinical Neuropharmacology [1991] 14 (2) : 156-164 (S. Giménez-Roldán, D.Mateo)

[22] British Medical Journal [1988] 297 (6650) : 722-723 (D.Capellà, J.R.Laporte, J.M.Castel, C.Tristán, A.Cos, F.J.Morales-Olivas)

[23] Journal of Neurology, Neurosurgery and Psychiatry [1988] 51 (1) : 158-159 (M.Fernandez Pardal, J.Fernandez Pardal, F.Micheli)

[24] Neurologia [1987] 2 (4) : 194-195 (F.Micheli, M.Fernández Pardal, G.Paradiso, R.Pikielny)

[25] Journal of Neurology, Neurosurgery and Psychiatry [1987] 50 (6) : 158-159 (J.F.Martí Massó, J.A.Obeso, N.Carrera, J.M.Martínez-Lage)

[26] Medicina Clinica [1985] 85 (15) : 614-616 (J.F.Martí Massó, N. Carrera, E.de la Puente)

[27] Neurologia [1996] 11 (1) : 10-15 (J.F.Martí Massó, J.J.Poza)

[28] Nederlands Tijdschrift voor Geneeskunde [2009] 153 : A336 (M. Louter, S.C.Tromp)

[29] Movement Disorders [1998] 13 (3) : 453-456 (J.F.Martí-Massó, J.J.Poza)

[30] Revue Neurologique [1994] 150 (11) : 757-762 (M.E.Llau, L. Nguyen, J.M.Senard, O.Rascol, J.L.Montastruc)

[31] Movement Disorders [1989] 4 (2) : 139-146 (F.E.Micheli, M.M. Pardal, R.Giannaula, M.Gatto, I.Parera, G.Paradiso, M.Torres, R. Pikielny, J.Pardal)

[32] Neurology [1987] 37 (5) : 881-884 (F.Micheli, M.F.Pardal, M. Gatto, M.Torres, G.Paradiso, I.C.Parera, R.Giannaula)

[33] Arquivos de Neuro-Psiquiatria [2009] 67 (3B) : 957 (H.A.Teive, R.P.Munhoz, H.B.Ferraz)

[34] Parkinsonism & Related Disorders [2004] 10 (4) : 243-245 (H.A. Teive, A.R.Troiano, F.M.Germiniani, L.C.Werneck)

[35] Nihon Rinsho [1997] 55 (1) : 112-117 (S.Kuzuhara)

[36] Movement Disorders [1997] 12 (1) : 107-110 (A.Negrotti, S. Calzetti)

[37] Arquivos de Neuro-Psiquiatria [1993] 51 (4) : 546-548 (I. Galhardo, M.O.Coutinho, E.S.De Albuquerque, O.Medeiros Lde)

[38] Neurotoxicology [1992] 13 (1) : 261-264 (A.Negrotti, S.Calzetti, E.Sasso)

[39] Rinsho Shinkeigaku [1989] 29 (6) : 681-686 (S.Kuzuhara, N. Kohara, Y.Ohkawa, S.Fuse, H.Yamanouchi)

[40] British Medical Journal [1988] 297 (6650) : 722-723 (D.Capellà, J.R.Laporte, J.M.Castel, C.Tristán, A.Cos, F.J.Morales-Olivas)

[41] Arquivos de Neuro-Psiquiatria [1989] 47 (4) : 471-473 (P.N.de Sá, L.M.Heinisch)

[42] Journal of Clinical Pharmacology [1988] 28 (7) : 600-608 (F. Benvenuti, A.Baroni, S.Bandinelli, L.Ferrucci, R.Corradetti, T. Pantaleo)

[43] Italian Journal of Neurological Sciences [1988] 9 (3) : 295-297 (A.Moretti, C.Lucantoni)

[44] Neurology [1987] 37 (5) : 881-884 (F.Micheli, M.F.Pardal, M. Gatto, M.Torres, G.Paradiso, I.C.Parera, R.Giannaula)

[45] Functional Neurology [1987] 2 (1) : 47-50 (A.E.Di Rosa, L. Morgante, M.Meduri, R.Musolino, N.Leggiadro, M.Coraci, A. Crisafulli, R.Di Perri)

[46] Rinsho Shinkeigaku [1990] 30 (11) : 1221-1226 (N.Ogawa, M.Asanuma, H.Takayama, H.Sato, I.Nukina)

[47] European Journal of Clinical Pharmacology [2016] Dec 16 [Epub ahead of print] (H.L.Lin, H.C.Lin, Y.F.Tseng, S.C.Chen, C.Y.Hsu)

Dopamine antagonists

Pharmacology : Dopamine D2 receptor antagonists include haloperidol [1], metoclopramide [2], clebopride [3], and lurasidone [4-7]. Dopamine antagonists inhibit the dopamine receptors.

Adverse effects : Haloperidol is one of the commonest drugs related to Drug Induced Parkinsonism [8]. Haloperidol can cause a significant increase in Parkinsonism [1, 8-14]. Use of 1mg per day or more of haloperidol made Parkinson's Disease 6 times more likely [14]. Clebopride can cause Parkinsonism but there is no suggestion that its withdrawal reverses Parkinsonism [15-19]. Metoclopramide can cause the symptoms of Parkinson's Disease [2, 20-24] but they can cease after withdrawal of Metoclopramide [2, 20, 21, 24]. Metoclopramide users were three times more likely to begin use of L-dopa compared with nonusers [25]. Increased risk of Parkinsonism is one of the most common adverse effects of lurasidone [4-7].

Causes of symptoms : Dopamine antagonists inhibit the dopamine receptors, and can therefore reduce dopaminergic activity.

[1] Neurology [1999] 52 (7 Supplement 3) : S10-S13 (E.C.Wolters)

[2] Nederlands Tijdschrift voor Geneeskunde [2013] 157 (26) : A6037 (M.W.Ade Ronde, H.J.Kingma, A.G.Munts)

[3] Bulletin of Experimental Biology and Medicine [2012] 153 (2) : 182-185 (K.K.Tanaeva, Y.V.Dobryakova, V.A.Dubynin, A.A. Kamensky)

[4] Pharmacological Reports [2016] 68 (4) : 748-755 (R.R.Jaeschke, M.Sowa-Kucma, P.Panczyszyn-Trzewik, P.Misztak, K.Styczen, W. Datka)

[5] Annals of Pharmacotherapy [2012] 46 (7-8) : 1033-1046 (V. Risbood, J.R.Lee, J.Roche-Desilets, M.A.Fuller)

[6] Clinical Schizophrenia and Related Psychoses [2012] 6 (2) : 76-85 (L.Citrome)

[7] International Journal of Clinical Practice [2011] 65 (2) : 189-210 (L.Citrome)

[8] Arquivos de Neuro-Psiquiatria [1998] 56 (2) : 171-175 (F.Cardoso, S.T.Camargos, G.A.Silva Júnior)

[9] European Neuropsychopharmacology [1991] 1 (4) : 541-548 (H. Lublin, J.Gerlach, U.Hagert, B.Meidahl, C.Mølbjerg, V.Pedersen, C. Rendtorff, E.Tolvanen)

[10] Journal of Gerontology [1985] 40 (3) : 303-308 (A.Aoba, Y. Kakita, N.Yamaguchi, M.Shido, T.Tsuneizumi, M.Shibata, K.Kitani, K.Hasegawa)

[11] Journal of Neurology, Neurosurgery and Psychiatry [1974] 37 (4) : 427-430 (H.L.Jr.Klawans, W.J.Weiner)

[12] The Quarterly Journal of Medicine [1986] 59 (230) : 549-556 (D.N.Bateman, M.D. Rawlins, J.M.Simpson)

[13] Southern Medical Journal [1990] 83 (5) : 525-532 (L.G.Miller, J. Jankovic)

[14] Archives of Internal Medicine [1994] 154 (10) : 1113-1117 (J. Avorn, M.Monane, D.E. Everitt, M.H.Beers, D.Fields)

[15] Movement Disorders [1994] 9 (1) : 114-115 (A.P.Sempere, J. Duarte, J.M.Palomares, F.Coria, L.E.Clavería)

[16] Movement Disorders [1992] 7 (1) : 89-90 (P.Montagna, A.S. Gabellini, L.Monari, E.Lugaresi)

[17] Revista Espanola de Enfermedades Digestivas [2011] 103 (3) : 161-162 (L.Berriozabal Diaz, L.Zubiaurre Lizarralde, A.Castiella Eguzkiza, E.Zapata Morcillo)

[18] Parkinsonism & Related Disorders [1996] 2 (3) : 145-149 (F.J. Jiménez-Jiménez, M.Ortí-Pareja, L.Ayuso-Peralta, T.Gasalla, F. Cabrera-Valdivia, A.Vaquero, J.Tejeiro, E.García-Albea)

[19] Movement Disorders [1993] 8 (2) : 246-247 (F.J.Jiménez-Jiménez, F.Cabrera-Valdivia, L.Ayuso-Peralta, J.Tejeiro, A.Vaquero, E.García- Albea)

[20] Archives of Internal Medicine [1986] 146 (10) : 2070-2071 (R.A. Sirota, P.L.Kimmel, M.D.Trichtinger, B.F.Diamond, H.D.Stein, M. Yudis)

[21] Archives of Neurology [1982] 39 (8) : 494-496 (T.Indo, K.Ando)

[22] Canadian Medical Association Journal [1982] 126 (1) : 23-25 (J. D.Grimes, M.N.Hassan, D.N.Preston)

[23] Nederlands Tijdschrift voor Geneeskunde [2002] 146 (4) : 175-177 (A.Hoogendam, J.Hofmeijer, C.J.Frijns, M.Heeringa, S.L.Schouten -Tjin a Tsoi, P.A.Jansen)

[24] South Medical Journal [1989] 82 (12) : 1581-1582 (K.D.Sethi, B. Patel, K.J.Meador)

[25] JAMA [1995] 274 (22) : 1780-1782 (J.Avorn, J.H.Gurwitz, R.L. Bohn, H.Mogun, M.Monane, A.Walker)

EPHEDRONE

Pharmacology : Ephedrone is intravenous methcathinone that is prepared using potassium permanganate.

Adverse effects : Ephedrone can cause the symptoms of Parkinsonism [1-10]. Ephedrone abusers also have widespread white matter damage with the greatest severity of damage underlying executive motor areas [11]. Ephedrone can cause a mixed hypokinetic-dystonic dysarthria after about eight months [12].

Causes of symptoms : Ephedrone, due to including manganese, can cause Manganism [1-10]. Manganese inhibits tyrosine hydroxylation, which is essential for the formation of dopamine [13, 14]. So manganese can cause Parkinson's Disease by lowering dopamine levels.

[1] Journal of Addiction Medicine [2013] 7 (4) : 302-303 (S.Fudalej, I. Kolodziejczyk, T.Gajda, B.Majkowska-Zwolinska, M.Wojnar)

[2] Journal of Medical Case Reports [2012] 6 (1) : 52 (M.Iqbal, T. Monaghan, J.Redmond)

[3] European Journal of Neurology [2009] 16 (6) : e114-e115 (C. Colosimo, M.Guidi)

[4] Acta Neurologica Scandinavica [2007] 115 (6) : 385-389 (K.Sikk, P.Taba, S.Haldre, J.Bergquist, D.Nyholm, G.Zjablov, T.Asser, S.M. Aquilonius)

[5] Addiction [2013] 108 (4) : 771-779 (A.Djamshidian, Y.Sanotsky, Y.Matviyenko, S.S.O'Sullivan, S.Sharman, M.Selikhova, Y.Filts, L. Fedoryshyn, J.Bearn, A.J.Lees, B.B.Averbeck)

[6] Parkinsons Disease [2011] : 865319 (K.Sikk, S.Haldre, S.M. Aquilonius, P.Taba)

[7] Movement Disorders [2008] 23 (15) : 2224-2231 (M.Selikhova, L. Fedoryshyn, Y.Matviyenko, I.Komnatska, M.Kyrylchuk, L.Krolicki, A. Friedman, A.Taylor, H.R.Jäger, A.Lees, Y.Sanotsky)

[8] New England Journal of Medicine [2008] 358 (10) : 1009-1017 (A. Stepens, I.Logina, V.Liguts, P.Aldins, I.Eksteina, A.Platkajis, I. Martinsone, E.Terauds, B.Rozentale, M.Donaghy)

[9] Archives of Neurology [2007] 64 (6) : 886-889 (R.M.de Bie, R.M. Gladstone, A.P.Strafella, J.H.Ko, A.E.Lang)

[10] Zhurnal Nevrologii i Psikhiatrii imeni S.S. Korsakova [2005] 105 (7) : 12-20 (O.S.Levin)

[11] Brain [2010] 133 (Part 12) : 3676-3684 (A.Stepens, C.J.Stagg, A. Platkajis, M.H.Boudrias, H.Johansen-Berg, M.Donaghy)

[12] Clinical Neurology and Neurosurgery [2016] 147 : 71-77 (M.Selikhova, E.Tripoliti, L.Fedoryshyn, Y.Matvienko, H.Stanetska, M.Boychuk, I.Komnatska, A.J.Lees, Y.Sanotsky)

[13] FASEB Journal [2010] 24 (12) : 4989-5002 (K.Sriram, G.X.Lin, A. M.Jefferson, J.R.Roberts, O.Wirth, Y.Hayashi, K.M. Krajnak, J.M. Soukup, A.J.Ghio, S.H.Reynolds, V.Castranova, A.E. Munson, et al)

[14] Environmental Health Perspectives [2010] 118 (8) : 1071-1080 (T. R.Guilarte)

Estrogen

Pharmacology : Oral contraceptives, which includes estrogen and progestin, are widely prescribed to women in order to prevent pregnancy.

Adverse effects : Oral contraceptives used by people with Parkinson's Disease were classified as conjugated estrogens, esterified estrogens, or progestin. Having used a hormone therapy demonstrated a suggested elevated risk with esterified estrogen use that was three times the normal. However, there was no increase in the risk of developing Parkinson's Disease in those people who had taken conjugated estrogen. Restricting this analysis to prescriptions that included progestin greatly increased the risk associated with esterified estrogen use, making Parkinson's Disease seven times more likely. Progestin also moderately increased the risk of developing Parkinson's Disease in those people who had taken conjugated estrogen [1]. Estrogen was associated with a moderate increase in Parkinson's Disease in some studies [2-5], but a mild improvement in other studies [5-8]. Current hormone users for less than 5 years showed a higher risk of developing Parkinson's Disease, which was anywhere between 11% more likely to more than twice as likely. However, this association disappeared for current hormone users after 5 years of use. Oral contraceptive use for ten years was associated with a lower risk of developing Parkinson's Disease, down to 59% of what would otherwise be expected [9].

Causes of symptoms : Estrogen decreases the levels of the dopamine

D2 receptors [10], which has an effect on Parkinson's Disease by decreasing dopaminergic activity.

[1] Movement Disorders [2014] 29 (13) : 1631-1636 (J.I.Lundin, T.G. Ton, A.Z.LaCroix, W.T.Longstreth, G.M.Franklin, P.D.Swanson, T. Smith-Weller, B.A.Racette, H.Checkoway)

[2] Parkinsonism & Related Disorders [2014] 20 (11) : 1149-1156 (N. M.Gatto, D.Deapen, S.Stoyanoff, R.Pinder, S.Narayan, Y.Bordelon, B. Ritz)

[3] Parkinsonism & Related Disorders [2013] 19 (4) : 457-460 (K. Rugbjerg, J.Christensen, A.Tjønneland, J.H.Olsen)

[4] Movement Disorders [2011] 26 (14) : 2563-2566 (A.Nicoletti, G. Nicoletti, G.Arabia, G.Annesi, M.De Mari, P.Lamberti, L.Grasso, R. Marconi, A.Epifanio, L.Morgante, A.Cozzolino, P.Barone, et al)

[5] Neuropsychiatric Disease and Treatment [2014] 11 : 59-66 (P. Wang, J.Li, S.Qiu, H.Wen, J.Du)

[6] Neurology [2000] 54 (12) : 2292-2298 (K.L.Tsang, S.L.Ho, S.K. Lo)

[7] Neurology [1999] 52 (7) : 1417-1421 (R.Saunders-Pullman, J. Gordon-Elliott, M.Parides, S.Fahn, H.R.Saunders, S.Bressman)

[8] European Journal of Neurology [2014] 21 (9) : 1168-1177 (N. Greene, C.F.Lassen, K.Rugbjerg, B.Ritz)

[9] Movement Disorders [2013] 29 (7) : 889-896 (R.Liu, D.Baird, Y. Park, N.D.Freedman, X.Huang, A.Hollenbeck, A.Blair, H. Chen)

[10] Brain Research [2010] 1321 : 51-59 (C.Chavez, M.Hollaus, E.Scarr, G.Pavey, A.Gogos, M.van den Buuse)

Lithium

Pharmacology : Lithium, usually as lithium carbonate, is used as a mood stabiliser for the treatment of bipolar disorder, which includes mania, depression and reducing the risk of suicide [1].

Adverse effects : Lithium can make Parkinson's Disease more likely [2] or can cause Parkinsonism [3-7]. The symptoms can improve after Lithium has been discontinued [8-10] but the symptoms do not always improve [11].

Causes of symptoms : Lithium appears to cause Parkinsonism by diminishing dopaminergic activity. This is probably due to a direct action on the G proteins, thereby reducing the capacity of the G proteins, once they are activated, in order to stimulate adenylyl cyclase [12].

[1] CNS Drugs [2013] 27 (2) : 135-153 (G.S.Malhi, M.Tanious, P.Das, C.M.Coulston, M.Berk)

[2] American Journal of Geriatric Psychiatry [2016] 24 (4) : 301-309 (C.Marras, N.Herrmann, H.D.Fischer, K.Fung, A.Gruneir, P.A.Rochon, S.Rej, S.Vigod, D.Seitz, K.I.Shulman)

[3] Movement Disorders [2011] 26 (12) : 2226-2231 (E.Bondon-Guitton, S.Perez-Lloret, H.Bagheri, C.Brefel, O.Rascol, J.L. Montastruc)

[4] Acta Neurologica Taiwanica [2007] 16 (4) : 231-233 (H.C.Shen, J. Y.Li, Y.K.Lo)

[5] Journal of Neurology, Neurosurgery and Psychiatry [2006] 77 (6) : 781-783 (M.Brandt-Christensen, K.Kvist, F.M.Nilsson, P.K.Andersen, L.V.Kessing)

[6] International Clinical Psychopharmacology [1994] 9 (2) : 127-129 (D.Lecamwasam, B.Synek, K.Moyles, K.Ghose)

[7] Der Nervenarzt [1997] 68 (7) : 586-590 (A.J.Fallgatter, W.K.Strik)

[8] Tijdschrift voor Psychiatrie [2009] 51 (2) : 123-127 (T.R. Walrave, C.Bulens)

[9] Journal of Geriatric Psychiatry and Neurology [1995] 8 (2) : 118-119 (S.Holroyd, D.Smith)

[10] Neurologia i Neurochirurgia Polska [1987] 21 (4-5) : 412-414 (K. Gajkowski, D.Werkowicz-Pelczyk, I.Masiak, A.Rysz)

[11] Journal of Clinical Neuroscience [2002] 9 (3) : 310-311 (C. Dallocchio, P.Mazzarello)

[12] Neurochemistry International [1994] 24 (1) : 13-22 (M.Carli, M.B. Anand-Srivastava, E.Molina-Holgado, K.M.Dewar, T.A.Reader)

PHENOTHIAZINES

Pharmacology : Phenothiazines used as antipsychotics are dopamine D2 receptor antagonists.

Adverse effects : Phenothiazines used as antipsychotics can cause Parkinson's Disease symptoms. These include chlorpromazine, which is a neuroleptic used in the treatment of psychosis. Chlorpromazine can block dopamine receptors and therefore reduce the effects of dopamine [1]. From around 30% to 61% of people can develop mild to moderate Parkinson's Disease symptoms as a result of taking chlorpromazine [2-5]. Parkinson's Disease symptoms can cease after discontinuation of chlorpromazine [6]. The other phenothiazines that can cause Parkinson's Disease symptoms are : fluphenazine [7-10], perphenazine [11, 12], prochlorperazine [13, 14], thioridazine [15, 16], and also trifluoperazine [17-20]. Although thiethylperazine is not normally used as an anti-psychotic, thiethylperazine can have anti-psychotic effects. Thiethylperazine can cause Parkinsonism [21, 22, 23], which can sometimes cease after thiethylperazine has been discontinued [23].

Causes of symptoms : Phenothiazines can cause Parkinson's Disease symptoms by decreasing the effect of dopamine on the dopamine receptors.

[1] British Journal of Nursing [1998] 7 (14) : 832-834, 836, 838-841 (J.Birtwistle, D.Baldwin)

[2] Journal of Clinical Psychopharmacology [1999] 19 (4) : 322-328 (M.P.Caligiuri, J.P.Lacro, D.V.Jeste)

[3] Archives of Internal Medicine [1994] 154 (10) : 1113-1117 (J. Avorn, M.Monane, D.E. Everitt, M.H.Beers, D.Fields)

[4] Southern Medical Journal [1990] 83 (5) : 525-532 (L.G.Miller, J. Jankovic)

[5] Journal of Mental Deficiency Research [1989] 33 (Part 1) : 81-86 (J. M.Rao, V.A.Cowie, B.Mathew)

[6] Canadian Journal of Psychiatry [1986] 31 (9) : 865-866 (J.H.Moss, D.E.Stewart)

[7] Journal of Clinical Psychiatry [1979] 40 (3) : 147-152 (G. Chouinard, L.Annable, A.Ross-Chouinard, M.L.Kropsky)

[8] British Journal of Psychiatry [1977] 130 : 581-585 (R.H.Mindham, P.Lamb, R.Bradley)

[9] Journal of International Medical Research [1976] 4 (6) : 435-440 (N.Capstick, H.Pudney)

[10] British Medical Journal [1973] 1 (5854) : 633-637 (S.R.Hirsch, R.Gaind, P.D.Rohde, B.C.Stevens, J.K.Wing)

[11] Southern Medical Journal [1990] 83 (5) : 525-532 (L.G.Miller, J. Jankovic)

[12] Psychopharmacology [1986] 90 (4) : 423-429 (No authors listed)

[13] Quaterly Journal of Medicine [1989] 71 (264) : 307-311 (D.N. Bateman, W.M.Darling, R.Boys, M.D.Rawlins)

[14] Quaterly Journal of Medicine [1986] 59 (230) : 549-556 (D.N. Bateman, M.D.Rawlins, J.M.Simpson)

[15] Southern Medical Journal [1990] 83 (5) : 525-532 (L.G.Miller, J. Jankovic)

[16] Archives of General Psychiatry [1981] 38 (6) : 668-675 (T.J. Crowley, M.Hydinger Macdonald)

[17] Journal of the Association of Physicians India [1986] 34 (6) : 455 (G.Srikant, L.Kantharaj, P.R.Rao)

[18] Journal of Geriatric Psychiatry and Neurology [1996] 9 (3) : 133-135 (G.Bashford, P.Bradd)

[19] American Journal of Psychiatry [1976] 133 (6) : 703-706 (T.J. Crowley, C.O.Rutledge, M.M.Hoehn, M.A.Stallings, S.Sundell)

[20] Archives of General Psychiatry [1978] 35 (1) : 97-104 (T.J. Crowley, M.M.Hoehn, C.O.Rutledge, M.A.Stallings, R.K.Heaton, S. Sundell, D.Stilson)

[21] Wiadomosci Lekarskie [1979] 32 (13) : 939-941 (A.Prusinski, H. Chmielewski)

[22] Parkinsonism & Related Disorders [1996] 2 (3) : 145-149 (F.J. Jiménez-Jiménez, M.Ortí-Pareja, L.Ayuso-Peralta, T.Gasalla, F. Cabrera-Valdivia, A.Vaquero, J.Tejeiro, E.García-Albea)

[23] European Journal of Neurology [2004] 11 (10) : 709-710 (C. Briani, A.Cagnin, F.Chierichetti, M.Tiberio, L.Battistin, G.Pizzolato)

TRIMETAZIDINE

Pharmacology : Trimetazidine is an anti-ischaemic agent, which provides symptom relief and functional improvement in patients with angina pectoris [1]. Trimetazidine inhibits beta-oxidation of fatty acids, which enhances glucose oxidation [2].

Adverse effects : The use of trimetazidine can cause Parkinsonism [3-7]. However, the symptoms of Parkinsonism can revert after the withdrawal of Trimetazidine [5, 6, 7].

Causes of symptoms : Trimetazidine can cause Parkinson's Disease symptoms because trimetazidine is able to blockade the dopamine D2 receptors and can therefore reduce dopaminergic activity [7].

[1] Drugs [1999] 58 (1) : 143-157 (K.J.McClellan, G.L.Plosker)

[2] Circulation Research [2000] 86 (5) : 580-588 (P.F.Kantor, A. Lucien, R.Kozak, G.D.Lopaschuk)

[3] Therapie [2005] 60 (6) : 603-605 (K.Masmoudi, V.Gras-Champel, Y.Douadi, H.Masson, M.Andréjak)

[4] Therapie [2005] 60 (4) : 419-422 (J.F.Martí Massó, I.Martí, N. Carrera, J.J.Poza, A.López de Munain)

[5] Neurologia [2004] 19 (7) : 392-395 (J.F.Martí Massó)

[6] Prescrire International [2006] 15 (84) : 136

[7] Fundamental and Clinical Pharmacology [2012] 26 (2) : 198-203 (K.Masmoudi, H.Masson, V.Gras, M.Andréjak)

VALPROIC ACID

Pharmacology : Valproic acid is a drug used for the treatment of a variety of psychiatric and neurological disorders including for the treatment of epilepsy [1].

Adverse effects : Valproic Acid can cause the symptoms of Parkinson's Disease [1-20]. The estimates as to what proportion of people taking valproic acid develop the symptoms of Parkinson's Disease differ enormously [20]. However, the symptoms of Parkinson's Disease can reduce after the withdrawal of the use of valproic acid [1, 2, 4, 7, 9, 11-18].

Causes of symptoms : Valproic acid increases the levels of GABA [21], which has an effect on Parkinson's Disease by decreasing dopaminergic neuron activity [22].

[1] Parkinsonism & Related Disorders [2013] 19 (8) : 758-760 (M. Silver, S.A.Factor)

[2] American Journal of Geriatric Pharmacotherapy [2011] 9 (6) : 405-412 (F.Mahmoud, R.R.Tampi)

[3] Movement Disorders [2011] 26 (12) : 2226-2231 (E.Bondon-Guitton, S.Perez-Lloret, H.Bagheri, C.Brefel, O.Rascol, J.L. Montastruc)

[4] Tijdschrift voor Gerontologie en Geriatrie [2009] 40 (1) : 29-33 (L. Schreur, C.W.Middeljans-Tijssen, G.J.Hengstman, M.G.Olde Rikkert)

[5] Progress in Neuropsychopharmacology and Biological Psychiatry [2008] 32 (5) : 1351-1352 (G.P.Sechi, M.Conti, G.F.Sau, G.A.Cocco)

[6] Movement Disorders [2007] 22 (8) : 1211 (G.J.Macphee, D.A. Stewart)

[7] Epilepsia [2006] 47 (12) : 2183-2185 (A.J.Ristic, N.Vojvodic, S. Jankovic, A.Sindelic, D.Sokic)

[8] Movement Disorders [2007] 22 (1) : 130-133 (D.Jamora, S.H. Lim, A.Pan, L.Tan, E.K.Tan)

[9] Pharmacopsychiatry [2006] 39 (1) : 9-12 (K.Masmoudi, V.Gras-Champel, H.Masson, M.Andréjak)

[10] Journal of Clinical Psychiatry [2002] 63 (1) : 75 (M.Iijima)

[11] Journal of Neurology [1998] 245 (12) : 794-796 (M.Onofrj, A. Thomas, C.Paci)

[12] No To Shinkei [1998] 50 (1) : 81-84 (Y.C.Park-Matsumoto, T. Tazawa)

[13] Neurologia [1995] 10 (9) : 381-383 (M.A.del Real Francia, J. Sanz Martínez, J.Vaamonde Gamo, M.Gudín Rodríguez-Magariños, R. Ibáñez Alonso, V.Riñón)

[14] Neurology [1996] 47 (3) : 626-635 (C.Armon, C.Shin, P.Miller, S.Carwile, E.Brown, J.D.Edinger, R.G.Paul)

[15] Epilepsia [1994] 35 (2) : 391-393 (E.Sasso, S.Delsoldato, A. Negrotti, D.Mancia)

[16] Australia and New Zealand Journal of Medicine [1994] 24 (4) : 413-414 (P.R.Froomes, M.R.Stewart)

[17] Clinical Neuropharmacology [1993] 16 (5) : 451-455 (M.J. Alvarez-Gomez, J.Vaamonde, J.Narbona, M.Barao, P.Barona, T. Brannan, M.Gudin, R.Ibañez)

[18] Nederlands Tijdschrift voor Geneeskunde [1989] 133 (24) : 1230-1232 (A.van der Zwan Jr.)

[19] Psychogeriatrics [2016] Jan 12 [Epub ahead of print] (H.Tada, T.Ogihara, D.Nakamura, D.Sasayama, N.Sugiyama, Y.Takahashi, S.Washizuka, N.Amano)

[20] CNS Drugs [2016] Jun 2 [Epub ahead of print] (F.Brugger, K.P.Bhatia, F.M.Besag)

[21] Psychopharmacology Bulletin [2003] 37 (Supplement 2) : 17-24 (M.J.Owens, C.B.Nemeroff)

[22] Neuron [2012] 73 (6) : 1184-1194 R.van Zessen, J.L.Phillips, E.A. Budygin, G.D.Stuber)

Zolpidem

Pharmacology : Zolpidem is a non-benzodiazepine hypnotic for the treatment of insomnia that potentiates GABA.

Adverse effects : Zolpidem marginally increases the risk of developing Parkinson's Disease, which increased to some extent according to the number of cumulative daily doses of zolpidem [1]. Parkinson's Disease is more prevalent amongst zolpidem users but not after 5 years. The risk of Parkinson's Disease was even higher in those people that had depression. The risk of Parkinson's Disease increased according to the dose of zolpidem [2].

Causes of symptoms : Zolpidem increases the activity of GABA [3], which has an effect on Parkinson's Disease by decreasing dopaminergic neuron activity [4].

[1] Journal of Psychiatric Research [2014] 58 : 84-88 (Y.W.Yang, T.F.Hsieh, C.H.Yu, Y.S.Huang, C.C.Lee, T.H.Tsai)

[2] Journal of Clinical Psychiatry [2015] 76 (1) : e104-e110 (H.C. Huang, C.H.Tsai, C.H.Muo, K.H.Lin, M.K.Lu, F.C.Sung, C.H.Kao)

[3] Scientific Reports [2016] 6 : 28674 (A.T.Che Has, N.Absalom, P.S. van Nieuwenhuijzen, A.N.Clarkson, P.K.Ahring, M.Chebib)

[4] Neuron [2012] 73 (6) : 1184-1194 R.van Zessen, J.L.Phillips, E.A. Budygin, G.D.Stuber)

CHAPTER 39

CAUSES OF PARKINSON'S DISEASE

MEDICAL CAUSES

MEDICAL CAUSES

There are other medical disorders that can cause symptoms, some of which coincide with those of Parkinson's Disease. In most cases the medical disorder is called a Parkinsonism. Somebody that has one of these medical disorders can be wrongly diagnosed with Parkinson's Disease due to some of the symptoms resembling those of Parkinson's Disease. Muscular injury and muscular strain can also cause symptoms similar to those of Parkinson's Disease but only in the affected muscles and whilst the muscular injury or muscular strain lasts.

These medical disorders can include : Acquired hepatolenticular degeneration [PAGE 554], Cerebellar Thoracic Outlet Syndrome [PAGE 556], Corticobasal Degeneration [PAGE 557], Creutzfeldt-Jakob Disease [PAGE 558], Encephalitis Lethargica [PAGE 559], Fahr's Syndrome [PAGE 560], FTDP-17 [PAGE 561], FXTAS [PAGE 562], Gaucher's Disease [PAGE 564], Hallervorden-Spatz Disease [PAGE 566], Head trauma [PAGE 567], HIV/AIDS [PAGE 570], Hydrocephalus [PAGE 570], Hypothermia [PAGE 572], Multiple System Atrophy [PAGE 572], Phenylketonuria [PAGE 574], Progressive Supranuclear Palsy [PAGE 575], Rett Syndrome [PAGE 576], Vascular Parkinsonism [PAGE 577], Wilson's Disease [PAGE 579], and X-Linked Dystonia-Parkinsonism [PAGE 580].

ACQUIRED HEPATOLENTICULAR DEGENERATION

Pathophysiology : Repeated episodes of liver failure or chronic liver cirrhosis may cause acquired hepatocerebral degeneration [1]. Acquired hepatolenticular degeneration is also known as "Parkinsonism in cirrhosis" [2 - 5]. Liver transplantation is usually effective. Reports of post-transplant residual symptoms suggest an element of irreversibility in some cases [2].

Symptoms : Acquired hepatolenticular degeneration is characterised by extrapyramidal symptoms including hypokinesia, dystonia and rigidity that are rapidly progressive and may be independent of the severity of cognitive dysfunction [2]. Typical features included rapid progression over several months, symmetric akinetic-rigid syndrome, postural but not resting tremor, and early postural impairment and gait impairment. Neuropsychiatric manifestations are minimal [3]. Some patients have minimal or absent tremors [5]. Another had a masked face, rigidity on bilateral arms and legs, and a lack of balance [6]. Parkinsonism is increased in cirrhosis [7], with estimates of the prevalence being as high as 21 % [2, 3], down to 4% [8]. Parkinsonism was 2.65 times more likely in cirrhosis [5]. In some patients L-dopa [2, 3, 8], bromocriptine [2], and other dopamine agonists [5] can be beneficial.

Causes of symptoms : The cause of Acquired hepatolenticular degeneration has been attributed to manganese deposition in basal ganglia structures, which leads to dopaminergic dysfunction [2]. Whole blood and cerebrospinal fluid manganese concentrations were several fold above the reference range [3]. The toxic effects of manganese are the major cause of basal ganglia dysfunction [3, 4]. There is evidence of damage to, or dysfunction of, presynaptic dopamine transporters together with a loss of post-synaptic dopamine receptors in basal ganglia of affected patients [2].

[1] Handbook of Clinical Neurology [2011] 100 : 193-197 (W. Meissner, F.Tison)

[2] Metabolic Brain Disease [2012] 28 (2) : 261-267 (R.F. Butterworth)

[3] Archives of Neurology [2003] 60 (4) : 521-528 (P.R.Burkhard, J. Delavelle, R.Du Pasquier, L.Spahr)

[4] Industrial Health [2007] 45 (3) : 497-500 (J.Kim, J.M.Kim, Y.K. Kim, J.W.Shin, S.H.Choi, S.E.Kim, Y.Kim)

[5] Annals of Indian Academy of Neurology [2008] 11 (3) : 179-181 (M.L.Noone, V.G.Kumar, K.Ummer, L.Achambat, K.A.Salam)

[6] Rinsho Shinkeigaku [2012] 52 (8) : 581-584 (T.Ishihara, M.Ito, H. Watanabe, M.Ishigami, T.Kiuchi, G.Sobue)

[7] Liver International [2011] 31 (5) : 592-594 (K.Weissenborn)

[8] Journal of Hepatology [2013] 58 (4) : 698-705 (A.B.Tryc, A. Goldbecker, G.Berding, S.Rümke, K.Afshar, G.H.Shahrezaei, H. Pflugrad, H.Barg-Hock, C.P.Strassburg, H.Hecker, K.Weissenborn)

Cerebellar Thoracic Outlet Syndrome

Pathophysiology : The Thoracic Outlet is a space between the rib cage (thorax) and the collar bone (clavicle) through which the main blood vessels and nerves pass from the neck and thorax into the arm. The nerves and blood vessels leave the neck between the two muscles (the scalene muscles) [1].

Symptoms : Thoracic outlet syndrome causes a combination of pain, numbness, tingling, weakness, or coldness in the upper extremity caused by pressure on the nerves and/or blood vessels in the thoracic outlet. Cerebellar Thoracic Outlet Syndrome (CTOS) patients had associated neurological lesions as a result of hypo-perfusion and hypo-metabolism in certain areas of the brain and cerebellum. The chronic hypoxia produces different results depending on the area of the brain and cerebellum affected [1]. Thoracic outlet syndrome can cause the symptoms of Parkinson's Disease [2, 3].

Causes of symptoms : When the chronic hypoxia affects the basal ganglia in the putamen, a decrease in the biosynthesis of dopamine takes place, which is what causes the symptoms of Parkinson's Disease [2, 3].

[1] The Official Patient's Sourcebook on Thoracic Outlet Syndrome [2002] (James N.Parker, Philip M.Parker)

[2] Journal of Cardiovascular Surgery [1996] 37 (6 Supplement 1) : 155-166 (E.I.Fernandez Noda, J.Nunez-Arguelles, J.Perez Fernandez, J.Castillo, M.Perez Izquierdo, H.Rivera Luna)

[3] Rinsho Kyobu Geka [1987] 7 (3) : 271-275 (E.I.Noda Fernandez, A.Lugo, E.Berrios, J.R.del Valle, F.Alvardo, M.S.Buch, J.P.Fernandez)

CORTICOBASAL DEGENERATION

Pathophysiology : Corticobasal degeneration (CBD) is quite a rare neurological disease in which parts of the brain deteriorate or degenerate. The cortex, or outer layer of the brain, is severely affected, especially the fronto-parietal regions, which are located near the centre-top of the head. Other deeper brain regions are also affected including parts of the basal ganglia, hence the name "corticobasal" degeneration. The combined loss of brain tissue in all of these areas causes the symptoms and findings seen in people with Corticobasal degeneration [1].

Symptoms : The initial symptoms of Corticobasal degeneration are often stiffness, shakiness, jerkiness, slowness, and clumsiness, in either the upper or lower extremities. Other initial symptoms may include dysphasia (difficulty with speech generation), dysarthria (difficulty with articulation), difficulty controlling the muscles of the face (hypomimia) and mouth, or walking and balance difficulties. The symptoms usually begin on one side of the body, and then spread gradually to the other side. Some of those people with Corticobasal degeneration, probably more than was commonly recognised in the past, may have memory or behavioural problems as the earliest or the presenting symptoms. Symptoms of Corticobasal degeneration usually begin after the age of sixty [1]. People with Corticobasal degeneration usually exhibit some or all of the symptoms of Parkinson's Disease [2, 3, 4].

Causes of symptoms : Parkinson's Disease symptoms can be caused by Corticobasal degeneration because of the deterioration or degeneration occurring in the part of the brain concerning Parkinson's Disease in the dopaminergic neurons.

[1] The Official Patient's Sourcebook on Corticobasal Degeneration [2002] (James N.Parker, Philip M.Parker)

[2] Archives Neurology [1998] 55 (7) : 957-961 (K.Kompoliti, C.G. Goetz, B.F.Boeve, D.M.Maraganore, J.E.Ahlskog, C.D.Marsden, K.P. Bhatia, P.E.Greene, S.Przedborski, E.C.Seal, R.S.Burns, et al)

[3] Brain [1994] 117 (Part 5) : 1183-1196 (J.O.Rinne, M.S.Lee, P.D. Thompson, C.D.Marsden)

[4] Ideggyógyászati Szemle [2005] 58 (1-2) : 45-51 (M.Farsang, A. Takts, I.Szirmai, T.Kovcs)

Creutzfeldt-Jakob Disease

Pathophysiology : Creutzfeldt-Jakob Disease is a rare, degenerative, invariably fatal brain disorder. It is one of a family of diseases known as transmissible spongiform encephalopathies. Spongiform refers to the appearance of infected brains, which become filled with holes until they resemble sponges under a microscope [1, 2].

Symptoms : Creutzfeldt-Jakob Disease is characterised by rapidly progressive dementia. Initially, patients experience problems with their muscular co-ordination; personality changes, including impaired memory, judgement, and thinking; and impaired vision. They may also experience insomnia, depression, or unusual sensations. The patients mental impairment eventually becomes severe. They often develop myoclonus, and may go blind. They eventually lose the ability to move and speak, and enter a coma. Pneumonia and other infections often occur and can lead to death [1, 2]. Parkinson's Disease symptoms can sometimes occur simultaneously with Creutzfeldt-Jakob Disease [3-7].

Causes of symptoms : Parkinson's Disease symptoms can occur as a result of the neuronal loss that Creutzfeldt-Jakob Disease can cause [7].

[1] Creutzfeldt-Jakob Disease : New Research [2007] (Mic J.Stones)

[2] The Official Patient's Sourcebook on Creutzfeldt-Jakob Disease [2003] (James N.Parker, Philip M.Parker)

[3] Parkinsonism & Related Disorders [2006] 12 (2) : 65-71 (D.Maltete, L.Guyant-Marechal, B. Mihout, D.Hannequin)

[4] Neuropathology [2001] 21 (4) : 294-297 (T.Ida, K.Doh-ura, T. Kawashima, H.Abe, T.Iwaki)

[5] Neurology [1998] 51 (2) : 617-619 (F.J.Vingerhoets, I.Hegyi, A. Aguzzi, P.Myers, G.Pizzolato, T.Landis)

[6] Canadian Journal of Neurological Science [1985] 12 (3) : 272-273 (C.Ezrin-Waters, LResch, A.E.Lang)

[7] Neuropsychiatry, Neuropsychology Behavioral Neurology [1997] 10 (2) : 120-124 (O.L.Lopez, M.L.Berthier, J.T.Backer, F. Boller)

Encephalitis Lethargica

Pathophysiology : People who have Encephalitis Lethargica have autoantibodies reactive against human basal ganglia antigens [1]. Between 1917 and 1928 Encephalitis Lethargica affected thousands of people of all ages. Although an epidemic of Encephalitis Lethargica has not recurred since then, occasional cases of Encephalitis Lethargica are still seen [2].

Symptoms : Encephalitis Lethargica could cause death in a short period or cause sleep that might last for days, weeks or months. Its symptoms were thought to encompass almost anything imaginable, which made its diagnosis very difficult [2]. Some of the symptoms of Parkinson's Disease often occur in Encephalitis Lethargica [1, 3-9]. It has been proposed that Encephalitis Lethargica was caused by influenza [10], and that influenza may be responsible for the formation of Lewy bodies and the subsequent death of neurons [11]. Severe influenza is associated with a doubling of the likelihood of Parkinson's Disease [12]. Recent influenza was associated with a trebling of the likelihood of Parkinson symptoms. The number of previous attacks increased the likelihood of Parkinson symptoms. However, influenza did not increase the likelihood of actual Parkinson's Disease [13].

Causes of symptoms : Encephalitis Lethargica may be able to cause Parkinson's Disease symptoms by affecting the function of the dopaminergic neurons in the basal ganglia.

[1] Brain [2004] 127 (Part 1) : 21-33 (R.C.Dale, A.J.Church, R.A. Surtees, A.J.Lees, J.E.Adcock, B.Harding, B.G.Neville, G.Giovannoni)

[2] Encephalitis Lethargic : During and After the Epidemic [2011] (Joel Vilensky)

[3] Movement Disorders [2006] 21 (1) : 1-8 (J.A.Vilensky, C.G. Goetz, S.Gilman)

[4] Clinical Neuropathology [2001] 20 (1) : 2-7 (M.Kiley, M.M.Esiri)

[5] Movement Disorders [1996] 11 (5) : 567-570 (F.Picard, A.de Saint-Martin, E.Salmon, E.Hirsch, C.Marescaux)

[6] Canadian Journal of Psychiatry [1992] 37 (2) : 140-142 (J.D. Dolan, R.Kamil)

[7] Developmental Medicine and Child Neurology [1991] 33 (2) : 158-161 (A.F.Mellon, R.E.Appleton, D.Gardner-Medwin, A.Aynsley-Green)

[8] Brain [1976] 99 (1) : 27-42 (A.M.Whiteley, M.Swash, H.Urich)

[9] Journal Neuropsychiatry Clinical Neuroscience [1995] 7 (2) : 125-134 (S.R.Cheyette, J.L.Cummings)

[10] Epidemiology and Infection [2009] 137 (4) : 449-455 (P.P. Mortimer)

[11] Japan Journal of Infectious Diseases [1999] 52 (3) : 89-98 (M. Takahashi, T.Yamada)

[12] Movement Disorders [2012] 27 (9) : 1111-1117 (M.A.Harris, J.K. Tsui, S.A.Marion, H.Shen, K.Teschke)

[13] Influenza and other Respiratory Viruses [2011] 5 (5) : 328-333 (S. Toovey, S.S.Jick, C.R.Meier)

FAHR'S SYNDROME

Pathophysiology : Fahr's Syndrome is a rare inherited neurological disorder. It is characterised by abnormal deposits of calcium in areas of the brain that control movement, including the basal ganglia and the cerebral cortex [1, 2]

Symptoms : Fahr's Syndrome can present with a wide spectrum of symptoms, including those of Parkinson's Disease. Symptoms that are similar to those of Parkinson's Disease include deterioration of motor function, dementia, dysarthria, tremors, muscle rigidity, a mask-like face, shuffling gait, and "pill-rolling" motion of the fingers. These symptoms usually occur later on. The more common symptoms include dystonia (disordered muscle tone) and chorea (involuntary, rapid, jerky movements). The age of onset is typically in the 40s or 50s but can occur during childhood or adolescence [1, 2].

Causes of symptoms : Fahr's Syndrome may be able to cause the symptoms of Parkinson's Disease by affecting the function of the dopaminergic neurons in the basal ganglia.

[1] The Official Patient's Sourcebook on Fahr's Syndrome [2002] (Icon Health Publications)

[2] Journal of the College of Physicians and Surgeons - Pakistan [2014] 24 (5) : S104-S106 (N.Dildar, H.Akram, I.M.Qasmi, M.N.Qureshi, S. Khan)

FTDP-17

Pathophysiology : Frontotemporal dementia is a clinical syndrome caused by degeneration of the frontal lobe of the brain and may extend back to the temporal lobe [1]. Frontotemporal dementia and parkinsonism linked to chromosome 17 (FTDP-17) is a genetic disorder. It is caused by mutations in the tau gene, which encodes a microtubule-binding protein.

Symptoms : FTDP-17 has three cardinal features : behavioural changes, cognitive impairment, and Parkinsonism. FTDP-17 can be further differentiated from Parkinson's Disease by there being a poor symptomatic response to L-dopa, progressive speech difficulties from the onset, and seizures that are poorly controlled with standard anticonvulsant therapy [2, 3].

Causes of symptoms : FTDP-17 may be able to cause Parkinson's Disease symptoms because of the degeneration of the frontal lobe of the brain, which would also affect the function of the dopaminergic neurons.

[1] Frontotemporal Dementia Syndromes [2011] (John R.Hodges)

[2] Orphanet Journal of Rare Disorders [2006] 1 : 30 (Z.K.Wszolek, Y. Tsuboi, B.Ghetti, S.Pickering-Brown, Y.Baba, W.P.Cheshire)

[3] Neurologia i Neurochirurgia Polska [2003] 37 (1) : 173-184 (Z.K. Wszolek, A.Krygowska-Wajs, M.Barcikowska)

Fragile X -Associated Tremor / Ataxia Syndrome

Pathophysiology : Fragile X-associated tremor / Ataxia Syndrome (FXTAS) is a genetic disorder caused by mutation of the FMR1 gene on the X chromosome. Carriers of premutation (CGG) expansions of the fragile X gene are generally thought to be spared most of the problems associated with the full mutation. However, a neurological disorder involving progressively severe tremor and difficulty with walking and balance appears to specifically affect some older premutation carriers [1].

Symptoms : The main features of FXTAS are cerebellar ataxia and/or intention tremor. Other documented symptoms are short-term memory loss, executive function deficits, parkinsonism, cognitive decline, peripheral neuropathy, lower limb proximal muscle weakness, and autonomic dysfunction. The clinical presentation of these patients, coupled with a specific lesion visible on magnetic resonance imaging and with neuropathological findings distinguishes it from other movement disorders [2]. Peripheral neuropathy is common among people with FXTAS, and can be the first or the only symptom [3]. The unique pathological feature - appearance of the intranuclear inclusions in the neurons and astrocytes, is discriminatory from those in other neurodegenerative disorders [4]. Males with FXTAS were more agitated, aggressive, depressed, apathetic, disinhibited, and irritable [5]. FXTAS also involves impairment of general intellectual functioning, with marked impairment of executive cognitive abilities [6, 7]. Cognitive deficits in FXTAS were found to occur in 50% of men, but none of the women. Cognitive deficits were on a similar scale to those found in Alzheimer's Disease but varied regarding the symptoms that were more prominent [8]. Tremor usually occurs first at approximately 60 years of age. From the onset of the initial motor sign, median delay of onset of ataxia was 2 years, onset of falls was 6 years, dependence on a walking aid was 15 years, and death was 21 years. Preliminary data on life expectancy is variable, with a range from 5 to 25 years [9]. The disorder affects at least one-third of carrier males over 50 years of age and, with an estimated carrier frequency of approximately 1 in 800 males [10]. Being a male carrier made somebody 13 times more likely of developing symptoms. Older men were much more likely to develop symptoms. Female carriers were only marginally likely to develop symptoms [11]. Among those female carriers with FXTAS there was an increased prevalence of thyroid disease, hypertension, seizures, peripheral neuropathy, fibromyalgia, and the typical symptoms of FXTAS-tremor and ataxia. In female carriers without the core features of FXTAS there were more complaints of chronic muscle pain, persistent paraesthesias in extremities, and of more tremor than is normal [12]. Medication can improve some symptoms of FXTAS [13].

Causes of symptoms : Parkinson's Disease symptoms could occur in FXTAS because the FMR1 gene is overexpressed and interferes with brain function.

[1] The Fragile X-Associated Tremor Ataxia Syndrome (FXTAS) [2010] (Flora Tassone, Elizabeth M.Berry-Kravis)

[2] American Journal of Medical Genetics [2003] 72 (4) : 869-878 (S. Jacquemont, R.J.Hagerman, M.Leehey, J.Grigsby, L.Zhang, J.A. Brunberg, C.Greco, V.Des Portes, T.Jardini, R.Levine, et al)

[3] American Journal of Medical Genetics Part A [2007] 143 (19) : 2256-2260 (R.J.Hagerman, S.M.Coffey, R.Maselli, K.Soontarapornchai J.A.Brunberg, M.A.Leehey, L.Zhang, L.W.Gane, et al)

[4] Current Opinion in Neurology [2005] 18 (4) : 393-398 (Y.Baba, R.J.Uitti)

[5] Journal of Clinical Psychiatry [2006] 67 (1) : 87-94 (S.Bacalman, F.Farzin, J.A.Bourgeois, J.Cogswell, B.L.Goodlin-Jones, L.W.Gane, J. Grigsby, M.A.Leehey, F.Tassone, R.J.Hagerman)

[6] Journal of Neurological Science [2006] 248 (1-2) : 227-233 (J. Grigsby, A.G.Brega, S.Jacquemont, D.Z.Loesch, M.A.Leehey, G.K. Goodrich, R.J.Hagerman, J.Epstein, R.Wilson, J.B.Cogswell, et al)

[7] Movement Disorders [2007] 22 (5) : 645-650 (J.Grigsby, A.G. Brega, M.A.Leehey, G.K.Goodrich, S.Jacquemont, D.Z.Loesch, J.B. Cogswell, J.Epstein, R.Wilson, T.Jardini, E.Gould, et al)

[8] American Journal of Medical Genetics Part B - Neuropsychiatric Genetics [2008] 147B (7) : 1138-1144 (A.L.Seritan, D.V.Nguyen, S.T. Farias, L.Hinton, J.Grigsby, J.A.Bourgeois, R.J. Hagerman)

[9] Movement Disorders [2007] 22 (2) : 203-206 (M.A.Leehey, E. Berry-Kravis, S.J.Min, D.A.Hall, C.D.Rice, L.Zhang, J.Grigsby, C.M. Greco, A.Reynolds, R.Lara, J.Cogswell, S.Jacquemont, et al)

[10] RNA Biology [2004] 1 (2) : 103-105 (F.Tassone, C.Iwahashi, P.J. Hagerman)

[11] JAMA [2004] 291 (24) : 2945-2946 (S.Jacquemont, R.J. Hagerman, M.A.Leehey, D.A.Hall, R.A.Levine, J.A.Brunberg, L. Zhang, T.Jardini, L.W.Gane, S.W.Harris, K.Herman, J.Grigsby, et al)

[12] American Journal of Medical Genetics Part A [2008] 146 (8) : 1009-1016 (S.M.Coffey, K.Cook, N.Tartaglia, F.Tassone, D.V.Nguyen, R.Pan, H.E.Bronsky, J.Yuhas, M.Borodyanskaya, J.Grigsby, et al)

[13] Movement Disorders [2006] 21 (10) : 1741-1744 (D.A.Hall, E. Berry-Kravis, R.J.Hagerman, P.J.Hagerman, C.D.Rice, M.A.Leehey)

Gaucher's disease

Pathophysiology : Gaucher's disease is a genetic disease in which lipid accumulates in some cells and organs. It is the most common of the lysosomal storage diseases. It is caused by a genetic deficiency of the enzyme glucocerebrosidase, which acts on glucocerebroside. When the enzyme is defective, glucocerebroside (GBA) accumulates, particularly in the mononuclear leukocytes [1].

Symptoms : Mutations in the Glucocerebrosidae gene are more frequent in Parkinson's Disease [2]. Gaucher's Disease has been found to make Parkinson's Disease four to five times more likely [3, 4]. Gaucher's Disease is an inherited metabolic disorder in which harmful quantities of a substance called glucocerebroside can accumulate in the spleen, liver, lungs, bone marrow, and the brain. Glucocerebroside accumulates because glucocerebrosidase (the chemical that breaks it down) is deficient in Gaucher's Disease. Around 1 in 100 people are a carrier for Gaucher's Disease, often without realising it. In Ashkenazi Jews as many as 1 in 15 are a carrier. People that had Gaucher's Disease and Parkinson's Disease developed Parkinson's Disease at an earlier age, were more likely to have affected relatives, and atypical clinical manifestations [4], and Parkinson's Disease generally [5], and had more rapid disease progression of motor impairment and cognitive decline [6] presenting symptoms of GBA related Parkinson's Disease are little different from those of Parkinson's Disease [7].

Causes of symptoms : Although it is known what causes Gaucher's Disease, it is not known how that can also cause the symptoms of Parkinson's Disease [3].

[1] Gaucher Disease [2006] (Anthony H.Futerman, Ari Zimran)

[2] Parkinsonism & Related Disorders [2014] 20 (11) : 1215-1220 (R. Asselta, V.Rimoldi, C.Siri, R.Cilia, I.Guella, S.Tesei, G. Soldà, G. Pezzoli, S.Duga, S.Goldwurm)

[3] European Journal of Neurology [2013] 20 (2) 402-405 (K.R.Kumar, A.Ramirez, A.Göbel, N.Kresojevic, M.Svetel, K.Lohmann, C.M.Sue, A.Rolfs, J.R.Mazzulli, R.N.Alcalay, D.Krainc, C.Klein, V.Kostic, et al)

[4] New England Journal of Medicine [2009] 361 (17) : 1651-1661 (E.Sidransky, M.A.Nalls, J.O.Aasly, J.Aharon-Peretz, G.Annesi, E.R. Barbosa, A.Bar-Shira, D.Berg, J.Bras, A.Brice, C.M.Chen, et al)

[5] Parkinsonism & Related Disorders [2014] 20 (9) : 986-991 (T. Pulkes, L.Choubtum, S.Chitphuk, A.Thakkinstian, S.Pongpakdee, K. Kulkantrakorn, S.Hanchaiphiboolkul, S.Tiamkao, et al)

[6] Movement Disorders [2015] 30 (3) : 407-411 (K.Brockmann, K. Srulijes, S.Pflederer, A.K.Hauser, C.Schulte, W.Maetzler, T.Gasser, D.Berg)

[7] Parkinsonism & Related Disorders [2015] 21 (7) : 804-807 (N. Kresojevic, M.Jankovic, I.Petrovic, K.R.Kumar, N.Dragaševic, V. Dobricic, I.Novakovic, M.Svetel, C.Klein, T.Pekmezovic, V.S.Kostic)

Hallervorden-Spatz Disease

Pathophysiology : Hallervorden-Spatz Disease is a rare, inherited, neurological disorder characterised by the progressive degeneration of the nervous system [1]. It is sometimes also called Pantothenate kinase associated neurodegeneration [1]. It is caused by mutations in the gene encoding pantothenate kinase 2 (PARK2), which causes pantothenate kinase associated neurodegeneration [2].

Symptoms : Hallervorden-Spatz syndrome is characterised by dystonia, parkinsonism, and iron accumulation in the brain [2]. There is progressive difficulty with movement, typically beginning in childhood, and can result in death in early adulthood. Movement abnormalities include involuntary muscle spasms, rigidity, and trouble with walking that worsens over time. Many people with Hallervorden-Spatz syndrome also develop problems with speech and some develop a loss of vision. Those people affected by Hallervorden-Spatz Disease may experience a loss of intellectual function, including dementia, and develop psychiatric symptoms such as behavioural problems, personality changes, and depression [1]. Hallervorden-Spatz Disease can also cause people to develop the symptoms of Parkinson's Disease [3-11].

Causes of symptoms : The symptoms of Parkinson's Disease could occur as a result of a degeneration of the part of the brain in which dopamine is produced.

[1] The Official Patient's Sourcebook on Hallervorden-Spatz Disease [2002] (James N.Parker, Philip M.Parker)

[2] Basic and Clinical Neuroscience [2016] 7 (2) : 165-166 (S. Gothwal, S.Nayan)

[3] Movement Disorders [2005] 20 (7) : 819-821 (Y.H.Zhang, B.S. Tang, A.L.Zhao, K.Xia, Z.G.Long, J.F.Guo, S.K.Westaway, S.J. Hayflick)

[4] Movement Disorders [2003] 18 (11) : 1351-1353 (J.L.Molinuevo, M.J.Marti, R.Blesa, E.Tolosa)

[5] Folia Neuropathologia [1999] 37 (4) : 235-238 (J.Dymecki, E. Bertrand, Z.Tomankiewicz, H.Szuniewicz)

[6] Journal of Neurological and Neurosurgical Psychiatry [1996] 61 (5) : 523-537 (P.J.Tuite, J.P.Provias, A.E.Lang)

[7] Archives Françaises de Pédiatrie [1993] 50 (1) : 35-37 (J.M. Pedespan, D.Fontan, J.F.Castell, P.Langlade, J.M.Guillard)

[8] Chinese Medical Journal [1990] 103 (8) : 686-688 (L.N.Wang, K. W.Huang, Z.Y.Liu)

[9] Journal of Neurological and Neurosurgical Psychiatry [1987] 50 (12) : 1665-1668 (R.Alberca, E.Rafel, I.Chinchon, J.Vadillo, A. Navarro)

[10] Neurology [1985] 35 (2) : 227-234 (J.Jankovic, J.B.Kirkpatrick, K. A.Blomquist, P.J.Langlais, E.D.Bird)

[11] Journal of Neurology [1984] 231 (3) : 112-116 (C.Kessler, K. Schwechheimer, R.Reuther, J.A.Born)

Head trauma

Pathophysiology : Head trauma refers to any damage to the scalp, skull or brain caused by injury. A closed injury refers to damage that does not break the skull or penetrate the brain tissue. Although the skull is not broken, this type of injury can still cause brain damage in the form of swelling or bruising. An open injury refers to damage that penetrates the skull causing problems such as bleeding in the brain, skull fracture or the pressing of bones against structures in the brain.

Symptoms : A prior head injury with amnesia or loss of consciousness was associated with an increased risk of developing Parkinson's Disease [1-14], but not in all studies [15]. The risk was increased further after subsequent head injuries and with head injuries requiring hospitalisation [8]. Mild head trauma with only amnesia did not increase the risk of developing Parkinson's Disease. People who experienced a mild head trauma with loss of consciousness or a more severe trauma greatly increased the risk of developing Parkinson's Disease [9, 16]. Mild traumatic brain injury on its own had little or no effect on the likelihood of developing Parkinson's Disease [17]. The linking of head injury and Parkinson's Disease greatly increased when the head injury occurred in the months before Parkinson's Disease symptoms first occurred. Head injuries years before symptoms began were of little significance. Severe head injuries make Parkinson's Disease even more likely, except when those injuries are caused by fractured skulls or intracranial haemorrhage [10]. Recall bias might have an effect on the outcome of these studies because many people with Parkinson's Disease reflect on the cause of their illness and so may remember head trauma more readily than those that do not have Parkinson's Disease [11].

Causes of symptoms : Head trauma can cause the symptoms of Parkinson's Disease by causing a loss of dopaminergic neurons [18].

[1] Archives in Neurology [1991] 48 (9) : 903-907 (M.Stern, E. Dulaney, S.B.Gruber, L.Golbe, M.Bergen, H.Hurtig, S.Gollomp, P. Stolley)

[2] Movement Disorders [2013] 28 (9) : 1222-1229 (S.Jafari, M. Etminan, F.Aminzadeh, A.Samii)

[3] Journal of Neurological and Neurosurgical Psychiatry [2010] 81 (11) : e58 (M.Perera, Y.Ben Shlomo, M.M.Wickremaratchi, R. Salmon, H.R.Morris)

[4] Neurology [2012] 79 (20) : 2061-2066 (P.C.Lee, Y.Bordelon, J. Bronstein, B.Ritz)

[5] Journal of Occupational and Environmental Medicine [2013] 70 (12) : 839-844 (M.A.Harris, H.Shen, S.A.Marion, J.K.Tsui, K.Teschke)

[6] Movement Disorders [2012] 27 (13) : 1632-1635 (F.Fang, H.Chen, A.L.Feldman, F.Kamel, W.Ye, K.Wirdefeldt)

[7] Neurology [2012] 79 (19) : 1970-1974 (E.J.Lehman, M.J.Hein, S.L. Baron, C.M.Gersic)

[8] Annals of Neurology [2006] 60 (1) : 65-72 (S.M.Goldman, C.M. Tanner, D.Oakes, G.S.Bhudhikanok, A.Gupta, J.W.Langston)

[9] Neurology [2003] 60 (10) : 1610-1615 (J.H.Bower, D.M. Maraganore, B.J.Peterson, S.K.McDonnell, J.E.Ahlskog, W.A.Rocca)

[10] BMJ [2008] 337 : a2494 (K.Rugbjerg, B.Ritz, L.Korbo, N. Martinussen, J.H.Olsen)

[11] Movement Disorders [1991] 6 (3) : 225-229 (S.A.Factor, W.J. Weiner)

[12] Parkinsonism & Related Disorders [2015] S1353-S8020 (15) 00003-00006 (J.Gao, R.Liu, E.Zhao, X.Huang, M.A.Nalls, A.B. Singleton, H. Chen)

[13] Parkinsonism & Related Disorders [2015] Dec 19 [Epub ahead of print] (K.M.Taylor, M.H.Saint-Hilaire, L.Sudarsky, D.K.Simon, B. Hersh, D.Sparrow, H.Hu, M.G.Weisskopf)

[14] JAMA Neurology [2016] Jul 11 [Epub ahead of print] (P.K.Crane, L.E.Gibbons, K.Dams-O'Connor, E.Trittschuh, J.B.Leverenz, C.D. Keene, J.Sonnen, T.J.Montine, D.A.Bennett, S.Leurgans, et al)

[15] Neurology [2015] 84 (11) : 1098-1103 (L.Kenborg, K.Rugbjerg, P.C.Lee, L.Ravnskjær, J.Christensen, B.Ritz, C.F.Lassen)

[16] Annals of Neurology [2015] 77 (6) : 987-995 (R.C.Gardner, J.F. Burke, J.Nettiksimmons, S.Goldman, C.M.Tanner, K.Yaffe)

[17] Archives of Physical Medicine and Rehabilitation [2014] 95 (3S) : S238-S244 (C.Marras, C.A.Hincapié, V.L.Kristman, C.Cancelliere, S. Soklaridis, A.Li, J.Borg, J.L.Geijerstam, J.D.Cassidy)

[18] Journal of Neurotrauma [2011] 28 (9) : 1783-1801 (C.B.Hutson, C.R.Lazo, F.Mortazavi, G.C.Giza, D.Hovda, M.F.Chesselet)

HIV/AIDS

Pathophysiology : Human immunodeficiency virus or HIV is a retrovirus that can cause Acquired Immunodeficiency Syndrome (AIDS), in which the immune system begins to fail [1].

Symptoms : HIV/AIDS can lead to potentially fatal infections [1]. Symptoms of Parkinson's Disease can sometimes occur as a result of HIV/AIDS [2-5].

Causes of symptoms : Subclinical nigral degeneration is common in AIDS and would explain the heightened susceptibility to Parkinsonism, because this would lead to dopaminergic dysfunction [6, 7].

[1] HIV/AIDS: A Very Short Introduction [2016] (Alan Whiteside)

[2] Arquivos de Neuro-Psiquiatria [2002] 60 (3-A) : 525-530 (J.P. Mattos, A.L.Rosso, R.B.Correa, S.A.Novis)

[3] Movement Disorders [2000] 15 (5) : 1032-1033 (M.Tanaka, K. Endo, T.Suzuki, A. Kakita, H.Takahashi, T.Sata)

[4] Arquivos de Neuro-Psiquiatria [1993] 51 (4) : 491-497 (J.P.De Mattos, A.L.Rosso, R.B.Correa, S.Novis)

[5] Neurology [1987] 37 (1) : 37-41 (A.Nath, J.Jankovic, L.C. Pettigrew)

[6] Acta Neuropathologica [1991] 82 (1) : 39-44 (M.G.Reyes, F. Faraldi, C.S.Senseng, C.Flowers, R.Fariello)

[7] Parkinsonism & Related Disorders [2004] 10 (6) : 323-334 (W.Tse, M.G.Cersosimo, J.M.Gracies, S.Morgello, C.W.Olanow, W.Koller)

Hydrocephalus

Pathophysiology : Hydrocephalus is a medical disorder in which there is an abnormal accumulation of cerebrospinal fluid within the ventricles or subarachnoid space of the brain [1]. Hydrocephalus can be caused by congenital or acquired factors [2].

Symptoms : In infancy, the most obvious indication of hydrocephalus is often the rapid increase in head circumstance or an unusually large head size. In older children and adults, symptoms may include headache followed by vomiting, nausea, papilledema (swelling of the optic disk, which is part of the optic nerve), downward deviation of the eyes (called "sunsetting"), problems with balance, poor coordination, gait disturbance, urinary incontinence, slowing or loss of development in children, lethargy, drowsiness, irritability, or other changes in personality or cognition, including memory loss [1]. Symptoms of Parkinson's Disease, most commonly gait disorders, can often occur simultaneously with hydrocephalus [3, 4, 5], and can be due to the effects of hydrocephalus [4, 6, 7, 8].

Causes of symptoms : Parkinson's Disease symptoms may be caused by hydrocephalus due to increased intracranial pressure reducing blood flow to the basal ganglia where dopamine is produced in the dopaminergic neurons [8].

[1] Hydrocephalus : A Guide for Patients, Families and Friends [1999] (Chuck Toporek, Kellie Robinson)

[2] Lancet [2016] 387 (10020) :788-799 (K.T.Kahle, A.V.Kulkarni, D.D.Limbrick, B.C.Warf)

[3] Journal of Neurology, Neurosurgery and Psychiatry [2001] 70 (3) : 289-297 (H.Stolze, J.P.Kuhtz-Buschbeck, H.Drucke, K.Johnk, M.Illert, G.Deuschl)

[4] Movement Disorders [1997] 12 (1) : 52-60 (J.K.Krauss, J.P.Regel, D.W.Droste, M.Orszagh, J.J.Borremans, W.Vach)

[5] Movement Disorders [1994] 9 (5) : 508-520 (T.Curran, A.E.Lang)

[6] Movement Disorders [1986] 1 (1) : 59-64 (J.Jankovic, M.Newmark, P.Peter)

[7] Canadian Journal of Neurological Science [1985] 12 (3) : 255-258 (L.Berger, S.Gauthier, R.Leblanc)

[8] Pediatric Neurology [1988] 4 (2) : 117-119 (E.Shahar, R.Lambert, P.A.Hwang, H.J.Hoffman)

Hypothermia

Pathophysiology : Hypothermia is due to reduced body temperature. It occurs when the body gets cold and loses heat faster than the body can produce it.

Symptoms : Hypothermia is usually a result of exposure to cold air, water, wind or rain. It can cause symptoms some of which coincide with those of Parkinson's Disease, including shaking, muscle stiffness, unsteadiness, and slurred speech. Other symptoms it often causes are : cold skin, poor judgement, numbness, and in severe hypothermia : slow pulse, shallow and slower breathing, weakness or sleepiness, confusion and loss of consciousness [1, 2]. The inclination towards symptoms some of which coincide with Parkinson's Disease is probably why people with Parkinson's Disease can tend towards increased symptoms during colder weather. The effect of the cold is adding to the symptoms that they already have.

Cause of symptoms : At low temperatures greater force can be attained by the contractile proteins but the contractile velocity is reduced thereby reducing muscular function [3].

[1] Minnesota Medicine [2001] 84 (11) : 30-36 (L.E.Wittmers)

[2] Hypothermia, Frostbite and Other Cold Injuries : Prevention, Survival, Rescue and Treatment [2006] (Gordon G.Giesbrecht, James A.Wilkerson, Andrea R.Gravatt)

[3] The Journal of Experimental Biology [1985] 115 : 333-344 (A.F. Bennett)

Multiple System Atrophy

Pathophysiology : Multiple System Atrophy is associated with the degeneration of nerve cells in specific areas of the brain that shrink (atrophy). When brain tissue of a person with Multiple System Atrophy is examined under a microscope, structures called glial inclusion bodies can be seen. Other terms were formally used to refer to Multiple

System Atrophy, based on the most prominent systems : Striatonigral degeneration - in which the substantia nigra is only mildly affected, while other areas of the brain show more severe damage, primarily causing the symptoms of Parkinsonism; Shy-Drager syndrome, which is characterised by Parkinsonism and more pronounced autonomic dysfunction; and Olivopontocerebellar atrophy, which is characterised by difficulty in articulating words [1].

Symptoms : This cell degeneration causes problems with movement such as stiffness, rigidity and tremor, and also loss of balance and coordination, impaired speech, breathing and swallowing difficulties, blurred vision, male impotence, constipation, urinary difficulties, orthostatic or postural hypotension (an excessive drop in blood pressure when the patient stands up that causes dizziness or momentary blackouts) [1]. Symptoms of Parkinson's Disease can occur in people with Multiple System Atrophy [2-8], with greater severity and disability compared with Parkinson's Disease [5]. Differences between Multiple System Atrophy and Parkinson's Disease include far more frequent falling [5], far less limb tremor [5], less facial expression [5], atypical rest, postural or action tremor [5], more symmetrical symptoms [5], greatly reduced response to L-dopa [5-7], early motor fluctuations [6], absence of dementia [6], autonomic features [6, 8], faster disease progression [8]. In Multiple System Atrophy up to 80% of people have tremor, half have postural tremor, a third have resting tremor, but only 10% have typical parkinsonian "pill-rolling" rest tremor [9].

Causes of symptoms : The degeneration of nerve cells in specific areas could cause Parkinson's Disease if they affect the dopaminergic neurons.

[1] Multiple System Atrophy [2011] (Gregor Wenning, Florian Krismer, Nadia Stefanova)

[2] Annals of the Academy of Medicine, Singapore [2005] 34 (9) : 553-557 (R.D.Jamora, A.Gupta, A.K.Tan, L.C.Tan)

[3] Journal of Neurology [2005] 252 (1) : 91-96 (K.Seppi, F.Yekhlef, A.Diem, E.Wolf Luginger, J.Mueller, F.Tison, N.P.Quinn, W.Poewe, G.K.Wenning)

[4] Parkinsonism & Related Disorders [2003] 9 (3) : 169-174 (T. Gurevich, N.Giladi)

[5] Movement Disorders [2002] 17 (4) : 701-709 (F.Tison, F.Yekhlef, V.Chrysostome, E.Balestre, N.P.Quinn, W.Poewe, G.K.Wenning)

[6] Journal of Neurological and Neurosurgical Psychiatry [2000] 68 (4) : 434-440 (G.K.Wenning, Y.Ben-Shlomo, A.Hughes, S.E.Daniel, A. Lees, N.P.Quinn)

[7] Clinical Neuropharmacology [1993] 16 (2) : 139-144 (E.A.Parati, V.Fetoni, G.C.Geminiani, P.Soliveri, P.Giovannini, D.Testa, S. Genitrini, T.Caraceni, F.Girotti)

[8] Brain [1994] 117 (4) : 835-845 (G.K.Wenning, Y.Ben Shlomo, M. Magalhaes, S.E.Daniel, N.P.Quinn)

[9] Tremor and other Hyperkinetic Movements [2013] Sep 3 (C. Kaindlstorfer, R.Granata, G.K.Wenning)

Phenylketonuria

Pathophysiology : Phenylketonuria (PKU) is an autosomal recessive metabolic disorder due to mutations in the phenylalanine hydroxylase gene, which converts L-phenylalanine to L-tyrosine. Although it is principally a childhood disorder, in rare cases, the first signs of Phenylketonuria may develop in late adulthood resembling common neurological diseases [1].

Symptoms : Phenylketonuria, if it is untreated, can lead to seizures, tremors, or trembling and shaking, stunted growth, hyperactivity, skin conditions, such as eczema, a musty odour of their breath, skin or urine. If treated it can lead to depression, anxiety and phobias [2]. Signs of Parkinsonism can sometimes occur in Phenylketonuria, particularly with age [1, 3, 4, 5].

Causes of symptoms : The reduced formation of L-tyrosine from L-phenylalanine can lead to a reduction in the levels of dopamine from what L-tyrosine is ultimately formed [3].

[1] Neurocase [2016] 22 (3) : 273-275 (Z.Tufekcioglu, A.Cakar, B. Bilgic, H.Hanagasi, H.Gurvit, M.Emre)

[2] Overcoming a bad gene : The story of the discovery and successful treatment of Phenylketonuria, a genetic disease that causes mental retardation [2004] (Seymour Kaufman)

[3] JIMD Reports [2015] 20 : 35-38 (M.Velema, E.Boot, M.Engelen, C.Hollak)

[4] Revue Neurologique [2014] 170 (4) : 280-287 (LDaelman, F.Sedel, A.Tourbah)

[5] Movement Disorders [2004] 19 (10) : 1232-1236 (A.H.Evans, D.C. Costa, S.Gacinovic, R.Katzenschlager, J.D.O'sullivan, S.Heales, P.Lee, A.J.Lees)

Progressive supranuclear palsy

Pathophysiology : Progressive supranuclear palsy (PSP) is a rare brain disorder that causes serious and permanent problems with the control of gait and balance [1].

Symptoms : The most frequent first symptom of Progressive Supranuclear Palsy is a loss of balance while walking. Patients may have unexplained falls or a stiffness and awkwardness in gait. The most obvious sign of the disease is an inability to aim the eyes properly, which occurs because of lesions in the area of the brain that coordinates eye movements. Patients often show alterations of mood and behaviour, including depression and apathy as well as progressive mild dementia [1]. The symptoms of Parkinson's Disease can occur in people with Progressive Supranuclear Palsy, and can initially even be the sole manifestation [2]. In addition to gaze palsy and early postural instability in Progressive Supranuclear Palsy, the absence of L-dopa induced dyskinesia, frontalis muscle overactivity, primitive reflexes, visuo-spatial impairment, and substantial frontal behavioural disturbances differentiated almost all those patients who had Progressive Supranuclear Palsy from those people who had Parkinson's Disease [3].

Causes of symptoms : There is a gradual deterioration of brain cells in a few small locations in the brainstem, including the substantia nigra, which is also affected in Parkinson's Disease. Damage to this region of the brain accounts for most of the motor symptoms that Progressive Supranuclear Palsy and Parkinson's Disease have in common [3].

[1] The Official Patient's Sourcebook on Progressive Supranuclear Palsy [2002] (James N.Parker, Philip M.Parker)

[2] Revue neurologique [1993] 149 (1) : 30-36 (G.Fenelon, A. Guillard, S.Romatet, A.Feve, F.Mahieux)

[3] Movement Disorders [2006] 21 (5) : 632-638 (N.J.Cordato, G.M. Halliday, D.Caine, J.G.Morris)

Rett Syndrome

Pathophysiology : Rett syndrome (RTT) is caused by mutations in the gene MECP2, which is located on the X chromosome. Rett Syndrome is a rare genetic disorder of the grey matter of the brain that almost exclusively affects females but has also been found in males [1].

Symptoms : The clinical features of Rett Syndrome include small hands and feet and a deceleration of the rate of head growth. Repetitive stereotyped hand movements, such as wringing or repeatedly putting hands into the mouth also occur. People with Rett syndrome are prone to gastrointestinal disorders. Up to 80% of them have seizures. They typically have no verbal skills, and about 50% of affected individuals do not walk [1]. In Rett Syndrome, Parkinsonian rigidity common occurs and frequently increases in its extent with age [2]. Several other Parkinsonian symptoms, including gait disturbance, can occur in Rett Syndrome [3, 4].

Causes of symptoms : Parkinsonian symptoms can occur because the gene MECP2 is essential for the normal function of nerve cells. MECP2 maintains dopamine content in a non-cell autonomous manner in the rostral striatum, which is critical for psychomotor control [5]. It also causes dysfunction in terminal dopamine release [6].

[1] Rett Syndrome : Therapeutic Interventions [2012] (Meir Lotan, Joav Merrick)

[2] Canadian Journal of Neurological Science [2016] 43 (4) : 567-573 (P.Humphreys, N.Barrowman)

[3] Neurology [1990] 40 (2) : 293-295 (P.M.FitzGerald, J.Jankovic, D.G.Glaze, R.Schultz, A.K.Percy)

[4] Movement Disorders [1990] 5 (3) : 195-202 (P.M.FitzGerald, J.Jankovic, A.K.Percy)

[5] Journal of Neuroscience [2015] 35 (15) : 6209-6220 (S.H.Su, F.C. Kao, Y.B.Huang, W.Liao)

[6] Journal of Neuroscience [2011] 31 (35) : 12629-12637 (S.C.Gantz, C.P.Ford, K.A.Neve, J.T.Williams)

Vascular Parkinsonism

Pathophysiology : Vascular Parkinsonism is produced by strokes that affect the basal ganglia. A stroke is the loss of activity of a discreet brain area (lesion) because of blockage of the blood supply to that brain region [1].

Symptoms : Vascular diseases are associated with a higher prevalence of Parkinson's Disease [2]. There are three different pathologic states that produce Vascular Parkinsonism (VP), including multiple lacunar infarctions in the basal ganglia area [3,4], subcortical arteriosclerotic changes (Binswanger's disease) [3,4] and a single vascular lesion that present a clinical picture indistinguishable from Parkinson's Disease [3, 4, 5]. Parkinson's Disease symptoms can occur in Vascular Parkinsonism [6-15]. However, the resting tremor in Vascular Parkinsonism is either reduced [6, 7], or absent [8, 9]. Parkinson's Disease symptoms that occurred in Vascular Parkinsonism were bradykinesia (100%), rigidity (96%), falls (76%), pyramidal signs (54%), urinary incontinence (50%), and dementia (39%). None of them had visual hallucinations. Two thirds of them developed Vascular Parkinsonism in a seemingly harmless way but actually with grave effects, and then progression of the disability was relentless. People with Vascular Parkinsonism had an older age of onset than those people who had Parkinson's Disease. Only a minority, but a large minority, of people with Vascular Parkinsonism respond to L-dopa [10,11].

Causes of symptoms : Vascular Parkinsonism can cause Parkinson's Disease because of blockage of the blood supply to the brain region that is affected in Parkinson's Disease [1].

[1] Age and Ageing [2005] 34 (2) : 114-119 (T.Bhomraj, L.Nelson, T. Robinson)

[2] Archives of Neurology [2006] 63 (5) : 717-722 (E.D.Louis, J.A. Luchsinger)

[3] Journal of Neurology [2006] 253 (Supplement 3) : iii16-iii21 (K. Fukimoto)

[4] Journal of Neurology [2004] 251 (5) : 513-524 (I.Sibon, G.Fenelon, N.P.Quinn, F.Tison)

[5] Journal of Clinical Neuroscience [2001] 8 (3) : 268-271 (S.Peters, E.G.Eising, H.Przuntek, T.Muller)

[6] Di Yi Jun Yi Da Xue Xue Bao [2005] 25 (7) : 868-870 (D.Q.Zhao)

[7] Archives of Neurology [1999] 56 (1) : 98-102 (J.Winikates, J. Jankovic)

[8] Acta Neurologica Scandinavica [1992] 86 (6) : 588-592 (C.M. Chang, Y.L.Yu, H.K.Ng, S.Y.Leung, K.Y.Fong)

[9] Stroke [1997] 28 (5) : 965-969 (H.Yamanouchi, H.Nagura)

[10] Journal of Neurology [2005] 252 (9) : 1045-1049 (LRampello, A. Alvano, G.Battaglia, R.Raffaele, I.Vecchio, M.Malaguarnera)

[11] Journal of Neurological and Neurosurgical Psychiatry [2004] 75 (4) : 545-547 (J.C.Zijlmans, R.Katzenschlager, S.E.Daniel, A.J.Lees)

[12] Acta Neurologica Scandinavica [2001] 104 (2) : 63-67 (M. Demirkiran, H.Bozdemir, Y.Sarica)

[13] Movement Disorders [1996] 11 (5) : 501-508 (J.C.Zijlmans, P.J. Poels, J.Duysens, J.van der Straaten, T.Thien, M.A.Van't Hof, H.O. Thijssen, M.W.Horstink)

[14] Journal of Neurology, Neurosurgery and Psychiatry [2012] 83 (10) : 1027-1029 (P.G.Glass, A.J.Lees, A.Bacellar, J.Zijlmans, R. Katzenschlager, L.Silveira-Moriyama)

[15] Arquivos de Neuro-Psiquiatria [2013] 71 (10) : 757-762 (T.C. Vale, P.Caramelli, F.Cardoso)

Wilson's Disease

Pathophysiology : Wilson's Disease is a genetic disorder in which there is an abnormal accumulation of copper. Copper begins to accumulate immediately after birth. Wilson's Disease first affects the liver and can then affect the brain [1].

Symptoms : Wilson's Disease can result in hepatitis, psychiatric symptoms (including depression and aggression), neurological symptoms, jaundice, abdominal swelling, vomiting of blood, abdominal pain, tremors, difficulty in walking, talking and swallowing. Women may have menstrual irregularities, absent periods, infertility, or multiple miscarriages [1]. Symptoms of Parkinson's Disease can often occur with Wilson's Disease [2-6].

Causes of symptoms : This is because the excess copper that occurs in Wilson's Disease can cause the formation of a copper-dopamine complex, which leads to the oxidation of dopamine to aminochrome [2-6].

[1] Wilson's Disease : A Clinician's Guide to Recognition, Diagnosis, and Management [2013] (George J.Brewer)

[2] Journal of the Medical Association of Thailand [1992] 73 (3) : 141-145 (K.Phanthumchinda, S.Cheevinsiriwat)

[3] Hepatogastroenterology [2005] 52 (61) : 166-169 (J.J.Pan, C.J.Chu, F.Y.Chang, S.D.Lee)

[4] Neurological Science [2003] 23 (6) : 279-285 (W.Hermann, T. Villmann, F.Grahmann, H.J.Kuhn, A.Wagner)

[5] Parkinsonism & Related Disorders [2007] 13 (2) : 122-125 (G. Sechi, C.G.Antonio, A.Errigo, L.Deiana, G.Rosati, V.Agnetti, P.K. Stephen, P. G.Mario)

[6] European Neurology [2006] 57 (2) : 80-85 (A.Soltanzadeh, P. Soltanzadeh, S.Nafissi, A.Ghorbani, H.Sikaroodi, J.Lotfi)

X-LINKED DYSTONIA-PARKINSONISM

Pathophysiology : X-linked dystonia-parkinsonism syndrome is a rare movement disorder that is highly prevalent in Panay Island in the Philippines [1-6]. X-linked dystonia-parkinsonism syndrome is associated with sequence changes within the TAF1/DYT3 multiple transcript system. The function is related to vesicular transport, dopamine metabolism, synapse function, Ca^{2+} metabolism and oxidative stress [7].

Symptoms : X-linked dystonia-parkinsonism usually manifests itself primarly as torsion dystonia, later combined with or sometimes replaced with parkinsonism [2, 3, 4, 8]. It usually begins in adulthood [2, 8], normally in the third or fourth decade [3]. Imaging and autopsy studies have suggested involvement of the caudate and putamen in later stages [5].

Causes of symptoms : X-linked dystonia-parkinsonism can cause the symptoms of Parkinson's Disease because of the disturbance of dopamine function that it causes [7].

[1] European Journal of Human Genetics [2015] 23 (10) : 1334-1340 (A.Domingo, A.Westenberger, L.V.Lee, I.Brænne, T.Liu, I.Vater, R. Rosales, R.D.Jamora, P.M.Pasco, E.M.Cutiongco-Dela Paz, et al)

[2] International Journal of Neuroscience [2011] 121 (Supplement 1) : 3-11 (L.V.Lee, C.Rivera, R.A.Teleg, M.B.Dantes, P.M.Pasco, R.D. Jamora, J.Arancillo, R.F.Villareal-Jordan, R.L.Rosales, et al)

[3] International Journal of Neuroscience [2011] 121 (Supplement 1) : 12-17 (P.M.Pasco, C.V.Ison, E.L.Munoz, N.S.Magpusao, A.E.Cheng, K.T.Tan, R.W.Lo, R.A.Teleg, M.B.Dantes, R.Borres, E.Maranon, et al)

[4] Neuroscience Letters [2008] 448 (2) : 180-183 (H.Deng, W.D.Le, J. Jankovic)

[5] Clinical Neuropsychology [2009] 23 (1) : 100-117 (L.L.Howe, I.L. Kellison, H.H.Fernandez, M.S.Okun, D.Bowers)

[6] Journal Clinical Neuroscience [2005] 12 (8) : 945-946 (C.Plummer, J.Bradfield, A.B.Singleton, D.Hernandez, A.A.Singleton, J.O'Sullivan)

[7] Human Molecular Genetics [2013] 22 (5) : 941-951 (T.Herzfeld, D.Nolte, M.Grznarova, A.Hofmann, J.L.Schultze, U.Müller)

[8] Annals Neurology [2005] 58 (1) : 7-17 (S.Goto, L.V.Lee, E.L. Munoz, I.Tooyama, G.Tamiya, S.Makino, S.Ando, M.B.Dantes, K. Yamada, S.Matsumoto, H.Shimazu, J.Kuratsu, A.Hirano, R.Kaji)

CHAPTER 40

TREATMENTS OF PARKINSON'S DISEASE

BIOCHEMICAL TREATMENT

INCREASING DOPAMINE BIOSYNTHESIS

Parkinson's Disease is primarily due to the insufficient biosynthesis of dopamine. The primary methods of treating Parkinson's Disease are based on this fact. The biosynthesis of dopamine can be increased, without causing side effects or after effects, by taking the substrate, coenzyme precursors and cofactors that are necessary for dopamine biosynthesis.

ESSENTIAL FACTORS

The optimal biosynthesis of dopamine requires the following substances as the substrate, coenzyme precursors and cofactors : L-tyrosine, pyridoxine, folic acid, nicotinamide, ferrous iron, zinc, and manganese.

L-tyrosine : L-tyrosine is essential for the biosynthesis of L-dopa via the enzyme Tyrosine 3-Monooxygenase.

Folic acid : Folic acid is essential for the biosynthesis of the coenzyme tetrahydrofolic acid, which is essential for the biosynthesis of L-dopa from L-tyrosine.

Pyridoxine : Pyridoxine is essential for the biosynthesis of the coenzyme pyridoxal phosphate, which is essential for the formation of dopamine from L-dopa.

Nicotinamide : Nicotinamide is essential for the biosynthesis of the nicotinamide coenzymes. Dopamine biosynthesis requires coenzymes whose biosynthesis is dependent on the biosynthesis of the nicotinamide coenzymes.

Ferrous iron : The first step in the biosynthesis of dopamine requires ferrous iron as a cofactor.

Zinc : The second step in the biosynthesis of dopamine requires pyridoxal phosphate. The biosynthesis of pyridoxal phosphate requires zinc as a cofactor.

Manganese : The biosynthesis of dopamine requires the nicotinamide coenzymes. Their biosynthesis requires manganese as a cofactor.

ACTIVE FORMS

L-tyrosine : There are precursors of L-tyrosine that can substitute for L-tyrosine to some extent because of their similarity of structure. However, none are as effective as L-tyrosine [1-5].

Pyridoxine : Pyridoxine hydrochloride is the commercially available form of pyridoxine. Other forms of vitamin B6 can substitute for pyridoxine to some extent because of their similarity of structure. However, none are as effective as pyridoxine [6].

Folic acid : Other folates can substitute for folic acid to some extent because of their similarity of structure. However, none are as effective as folic acid [7-9].

Nicotinamide : Other forms of vitamin B3 can substitute for nicotinamide to some extent because of their similarity of structure. However, none are as effective as nicotinamide [10].

Ferrous iron : Ferrous sulphate is the best form of ferrous iron to administer as sulphate (1) combines with ferrous iron, (2) is natural to the body, (3) is required in large quantities, (4) and in combination with ferrous iron is well absorbed. Side effects can occur with the other forms of iron, all of which are less effective means of administering ferrous iron [11-12].

Zinc : Zinc sulphate is the best form of zinc to administer as sulphate (1) combines with zinc, (2) is natural to the body, (3) is required in large quantities, (4) in combination with zinc is well absorbed. Side effects can occur with other forms of zinc, all of which are less effective means of administering zinc [13].

Manganese : Manganese chloride is the best form of manganese to administer as chloride (1) combines with manganese, (2) is natural to the body, (3) is required in large quantities, (4) in combination with manganese is well absorbed. Side effects can occur with other forms of manganese, all of which are less effective means of administering manganese [14].

Optimal dosages

The daily requirements of those substances that are required for the action of dopamine are known from balance studies and surveys for : tyrosine [15, 16, 17], iron [18, 19], zinc [20], nicotinamide [21, 22], manganese [23], pyridoxine [24, 25, 26] and folic acid [27, 28].

From these studies, the amounts that will satisfy the daily requirements of over 99% of adults has been calculated, by using the mean and standard deviation of the given figures to give the following dosages :

2000.0 mg Tyrosine
20.0 mg Iron
20.0 mg Zinc
20.0 mg Nicotinamide
5.2 mg Manganese
2.0 mg Pyridoxine
0.4 mg Folic Acid

For some people, the requirement of these substances will be less than is stated. However, for people that have lower requirements of these substances the excess would be easily eliminated without having caused any ill effect. They are also consequently, unlike most synthetic substances, not dosage dependent once their saturation point has been reached. So a slight excess of any of these substances beyond any person's normal requirements is not actually of any biochemical significance as it would have no effect.

ACTIVE DOSAGES

It is necessary to administer these substances in their most active forms. By calculating the relative atomic weights of the above substances, and the administered substances, the dosages are adjusted accordingly to account for the extra weight of those substances, such as sulphate, chloride or hydrochloride, that are combined with them. (These figures must be recalculated if other forms of these substances are used) :

2000.0 mg L-Tyrosine
54.0 mg Ferrous sulphate (dried)
50.0 mg Zinc sulphate (dried)
20.0 mg Nicotinamide
12.0 mg Manganese chloride (dried)
2.4 mg Pyridoxine hydrochloride
0.4 mg Folic Acid

PRACTICAL DOSAGES

The above combination of substances is probably too much for any patient to take in one tablet or capsule. So it is recommended, though not essential, that the above quantities are divided into four tablets or capsules so that they can be easily consumed. Consequently, the following combination of substances is the ideal formulation for each tablet or capsule :

500.0 mg L-Tyrosine
13.5 mg Ferrous sulphate (dried)
12.5 mg Zinc sulphate (dried)
5.0 mg Nicotinamide
3.0 mg Manganese chloride (dried)
0.6 mg Pyridoxine hydrochloride
0.1 mg Folic Acid

The optimal formulation for increasing the biosynthesis of dopamine is available as Dopavite®, which is a supplement that is specifically for Parkinson's Disease. Dopavite® contains all of the constituents in the correct and optimal forms and precise dosages.

Administration

A total of four tablets or capsules should be taken orally every day. This should be done by taking two tablets or capsules twice a day at different times of the day, preferably immediately after meals. If after time this appears to be inadequate, some patients, especially very heavy adults, may benefit from taking five or six tablets or capsules per day, in three lots. The administration of tablets or capsules above these levels is not dosage dependent and so could be of no benefit. There is no recommended dosage for children as they are not usually affected by Parkinson's Disease.

Contra-indications

Hemochromatosis - The formulation should not be taken by people who have Hemochromatosis because it contains iron. People with Hemochromatosis excessively accumulate iron.

Tyrosinosis - The formulation should not be taken by people who have the rare metabolic disorder Tyrosinosis because it contains L-tyrosine, which cannot be metabolized by people with Tyrosinosis.

Drug interactions

The formulation should preferably not be taken just before or soon after the use of any product that contains L-dopa, such as Sinemet, Madopar, Rytary and Numient. This is because the L-tyrosine in the formulation, being similar in structure to L-dopa, can compete to some extent with L-dopa for absorption in to the brain, and may therefore lessen, to some extent, the effect of L-dopa.

Precautions

Preparations should be avoided that contain large amounts of any of the constituents of the present preparation. This is because in addition to the quantities of the present formulation, much higher additional quantities could lead to the dosages of those particular substances being excessive.

Side effects

There are no side effects caused by the use of any substances included in the formulation because they are all used in normal dosages, solely in order to satisfy daily requirements. At these dosages there are no side effects of L-tyrosine [29, 30], iron [31], zinc [32], nicotinamide [33], manganese [34, 35], pyridoxine [36], or folic acid [37].

Overdosage

Overdosage should not occur at the recommended rates of use, and is a very unlikely event even with overuse, as all of the constituents of the preparation are in dosages far below toxic levels. Symptoms caused by overdosage should be rapidly reduced upon withdrawal of the preparation.

Optimal levels

The administration of the constituents must enable all of the substances to reach their optimal levels in the body. The time taken for this differs greatly according to each substance, which can be anywhere from days, with L-tyrosine being the quickest, to as much as a year or much more, with ferrous iron being the slowest. The time taken will differ for each person because the degree of deficiency for each of the constituents will differ for each person, ranging from a severe deficiency to no deficiency at all.

Duration of administration

There would not be an almost immediate improvement as can occur with treatments of some medical disorders. The improvement to be expected in most cases should be gradual over anywhere between several months to well over a year. For those people with mild Parkinson's Disease it should be within several months. For those people with severe Parkinson's Disease it could be well beyond a year. Once improvement has clearly ceased for several months continuously, the biochemical treatment should be continued. However, it is unlikely that there will be any further significant improvement.

Pharmaceutical use

The improvement is very gradual and not immediate. Therefore, at the outset, the use of any existing pharmaceuticals should be maintained at their existing doses or at levels sufficient to control the symptoms.

Pharmaceutical inhibition

When a biochemical function is artificially stimulated or inhibited, via feedback inhibition, there will be an opposite after effect, as the body tries to counteract it. By this means, pharmaceuticals that initially rid the symptoms of medical disorder can eventually cause them. L-dopa very potently inhibits the formation of the body's own dopamine [38-41]. So although the use of L-dopa can initially be effective in treating Parkinson's Disease, over time its effects wear off and its long term use leads to the disorder becoming gradually and progressively worse. Dopamine agonists cause the dopamine receptors they stimulate to become progressively less sensitive, thereby eventually worsening the symptoms [42, 43, 44]. MAO inhibitors and COMT inhibitors initially help to maintain the levels of dopamine by inhibiting the enzymes that metabolize it. However, artificially inhibiting these enzymes eventually increases the concentrations of these enzymes. Even Deep Brain Stimulation has an artificial effect and so its effect eventually declines because its effect is counteracted [45].

Pharmaceutical reduction

When somebody is producing sufficient dopamine of their own they will no longer need to make use of any pharmaceutical means of artificially producing dopamine or artificially stimulating dopaminergic activity. So eventually, when there are very apparent signs of improvement, there could be a gradual reduction in the use of pharmaceuticals that increase dopaminergic activity. The most effective means of drug reduction is by reducing the drug intake very gradually, in small amounts, and infrequently. This avoids or minimises the transient symptoms of drug withdrawal that occur whilst there is an adjustment to the drug withdrawal. Generally, the longer a drug stays in the body, the longer it will take to adjust to its withdrawal.

[1] Journal of Biological Chemistry [1955] 213 : 913 (W.C.Rose, R.L.Wixom)

[2] Journal of Biological Chemistry [1969] 244 : 142 (G.Guroff, C.A.Rhoads)

[3] Journal of Biological Chemistry [1959] 234 : 2677 (S.Kaufman)

[4] Archives of Biochemistry and Biophysics [1956] 60 : 477 (C.Mitoma)

[5] Journal of Biological Chemistry [1952] 194 : 503 (S.Udenfriend, J.R.Cooper)

[6] Journal of Nutrition [1986] 116 (1) : 87 (J.F.Gregory, S.A. Litherland)

[7] British Journal of Haematology [1973] 25 : 513 (T.Tamaru, E.L.R.Stokstad)

[8] American Journal of Clinical Nutrition [1988] 47 : 80 (P.M.Keagy, B.Shane, S.M.Oace)

[9] Gut [1973] 13 : 544 (J.Perry, I.Chanarin)

[10] Nutrition Reports International [1976] 14 : 115 (D.H.Baker)

[11] Acta Medica Scandinavica [1962] 376 (Supplement) : 59 (H.Brise, L.Hallberg)

[12] American Journal of Clinical Nutrition [1989] 49 (6) : 1274 (R.F.Hurrell, D.E.Furniss, J.Burri, P.Whittaker, S.R.Lynch, J.D.Cook)

[13] Journal of Hygiene, Epiediology, Microbiology, Immunology [1988] 32 (4) : 397 (C.P.Shabalina, V.P. Spiridonova)

[14] Nutritional Bioavailability of Manganese (C.Kies) [1987] : 112-122 (C.W.Bales, J.H.Freeland-Graves, P-H.Lin, J.M.Stone, V. Dougherty)

[15] American Journal of Physiology [1990] 259 (6) : E835 (G.A.Zello, P.B.Pencharz, R.O.Ball)

[16] Journal of Biological Chemistry [1955] 217 : 95 (W.C.Rose, B.E.Leach, M.J.Coon, G.F.Lambert)

[17] The dietary and nutritional survey of British adults [1994] : 235 (J.Gregory, K.Foster, H.Tyler, M.Wiseman)

[18] American Journal of Clinical Nutrition [1991] 54 (6) : 1047 (L.Hallberg, L.Rossander- Hulten)

[19] Journal of Internal Medicine [1989] 226 : 357 (T.H.Bothwell, R.D.Baynes, B.J. MacFarlane, A.P.MacPhail)

[20] Journal of the American College of Nutrition [1985] 4 : 73 (H.H.Sandstead)

[21] Journal of Nutrition [1956] 60 (Supplement 1) : 1 (M.K.Horwitt, C.C. Harvey, W.S. Rothwell, J.L.Cutler, D.Haffron)

[22] The dietary and nutritional survey of British adults - further analysis [1994] : 25

[23] Nutritional Bioavailability of Manganese (C.Kies) [1987] : 90-104 (J.H.Freeland-Graves, C.W.Bales, F.Behmardi)

[24] Human vitamin B6 requirements [1976] : 226 (E.A.Donald), 279 (H.M.Linkswiller)

[25] American Journal of Clinical Nutrition [1995] 61 (5) : 1091 (M.J.Kretsch, H.E.Sauberlich, J.H. Skala, H.L.Johnson)

[26] The dietary and nutritional survey of British adults [1994] : Table 8.1 (J.Gregory, K.Foster, H.Tyler, M.Wiseman)

[27] American Journal of Clinical Nutrition [1983] 37 : 768 (D.B. Milne, L.K.Johnson, J.R.Mahalko, H.H. Sandstead)

[28] Journal of Nutrition [1995] : 125 (10) : 2717 (C.A.O'Keefe, L.B. Bailey, E.A.Thomas, S.A.Hofler, B.A.Davis, J.J.Cerda, J.F. Gregory)

[29] Naunyn Schmiedebergs Archiv fuer Pharmakologie [1976] 293 (1) : 15 (J.C.David)

[30] Archives of Pathology [1967] 84 : 238 (J.V.Klavins)

[31] The Lancet [1958] 2 : 489 (D.N.S.Kerr, S.Davidson)

[32] American Journal of Clinical Nutrition [1990] 51 (2) : 225 (G.J. Fosmire)

[33] Schizophrenia [1968] 2 : 3 (Hawkins)

[34] Archives of Environmental Health [1989] 44 : 175 (X.G. Kondiakis, N.Makris, M.Leotsinidis, M.Prinou, T.Papapetropoulos)

[35] Journal of Nutrition [1989] 119 : 1861 (K.M.Hambridge, N.F. Krebs)

[36] Toxicology Letters [1986] 34 : 129 (M.Cohen, A.Bendich)

[37] American Journal of Clinical Nutrition [1989] 50 : 353 (C.E. Butterworth Jnr, T.Tamura)

[38] Nature [1983] 302 : 830-832 (S.El Mestikawy, J.Glowinski, M. Hamon)

[39] Archives of Biochemistry and Biophysics [1967] 120 : 420-427 (M.Ikeda, M.Levitt, S.Udenfriend)

[40] Journal of Biological Chemistry [1964] 239 : 2910-2917 (T.Nagatsu, M.Levitt, S.Udenfriend)

[41] Comptes Rendue des Academie Sciences Series 3 [1986] 302 : 435-438 (D. Pigeon, R.Drissi-Daoudi, F.Gros, J.Thibault)

[42] Society for Neuroscience Abstracts [1979] 5 : 81 (R.L.Weir, R.E.Hruska, E.K.Silbergeld)

[43] Naunyn-Schmiedeberg's Archiv fuer Pharmacologie [1978] 304 : 141 (M.Quick, L.L.Iversen)

[44] Journal of Physiology [1977] 272 : 51P (L.L.Iversen, M.Quick)

[45] Chinese Medical Journal [2015] 128 (18) : 2433-2438 (L.L. Jiang, J.L.Liu, X.L. Fu, W.B.Xian, J.Gu, Y.M.Liu, J.Ye, J.Chen, H. Qian, S.H.Xu, Z.Pei, L.Chen)

CHAPTER 41

PHARMACOLOGICAL TREATMENTS OF PARKINSON'S DISEASE

L-DOPA

PHARMACOLOGY

Dopamine is not able to enter the brain. However, L-dopa can enter the brain and then form dopamine in the dopaminergic neurons via the enzyme aromatic-L-amino-acid decarboxylase (EC 4.1.1.28) : L-dopa >>> dopamine + CO_2. However, L-dopa reduces the formation of the body's own dopamine. Consequently, L-dopa can initially be effective in treating Parkinson's Disease, but its effects wear off and its long term use leads to the disorder becoming gradually and progressively worse.

FORMS OF L-DOPA

L-dopa is widely used to treat Parkinson's Disease. Sinemet, in immediate release [PAGE 593] and controlled release [PAGE 594] versions, is combined with the dopa decarboxylase inhibitor carbidopa in order to maintain the effect of L-dopa. Madopar, in immediate release [PAGE 598] and controlled versions [PAGE 599], is combined with the dopa decarboxylase inhibitor benserazide in order to maintain the effect of L-dopa. Rytary [PAGE 599] and Numient [PAGE 599] are versions of L-dopa and carbidopa in which the immediate release and controlled versions are combined. Other means of administering L-dopa that are available or being developed are : Duodopa [PAGE 601], which is L-dopa and carbidopa in a gel that is administered using a portable pump; LECIGON [PAGE 605], which is a gel formulation for continuous intestinal administration, Parcopa [PAGE 606], which is orally disintegrating L-dopa and carbidopa; L-dopa inhaler [PAGE 606]; a combination of ß-asarone [PAGE 608] and L-dopa as a means of improving Madopar; AcuForm [PAGE 609]; L-dopa prodrug [PAGE 610]; melevodopa [PAGE 611], which is a methyl ester of L-dopa; subcutaneous L-dopa [PAGE 612]; liquid L-dopa [PAGE 613]; mucuna pruriens [PAGE 614] and fava beans [PAGE 615] which are L-dopa containing vegetables.

Sinemet

Brand names : Sinemet, Atamet, Carbilev

Pharmacology : Sinemet is L-Dopa combined with carbidopa, which is a peripheral decarboxylase inhibitor. Carbidopa helps to maintain the levels of L-dopa until it is used, by inhibiting peripheral metabolism of L-dopa. Carbidopa is also available as Lodosyn, which is taken simultaneously with L-dopa.

Efficacy : In two-thirds of people taking Sinemet a good to very good improvement was obtained in the treatment of the symptoms of Parkinson's Disease [1]. Atamet was no different in its effects to Sinemet [2]. Patients who responded well to Sinemet were considerably younger than those who failed to respond [3]. After three years of treatment the response to Sinemet declined [3]. After seven years of treatment about 60%-65% of the patients had shown improvement even though to a lesser degree than during the first and second year of therapy [4]. Sinemet has been found to have little effect on many of the non-motor symptoms of Parkinson's Disease including fatigue, excessive sweating, insomnia, akathisia, anxiety, and constipation [5]. Protein intake can alter the efficacy because some of the amino acids in protein compete with L-dopa for entry in to the brain. A lack of protein can increase the effect of L-dopa, requiring a reduction in L-dopa intake. A high protein intake can prevent the effect of L-dopa [6]. Large quantities of pyridoxine (vitamin B6) can reduce the effect of L-dopa [7], but the interaction does not occur when taking a decarboxylase inhibitor as there is in Sinemet [8].

Adverse effects : The most troublesome side effects of Sinemet are dyskinesia, hypotonia, gastrointestinal symptoms, and also psychotic symptoms in 10% of people [1, 3]. Other common side effects are nausea (34%), postural hypotension (22%), and "on-off" phenomena in 12% of patients [3]. Patients discontinued treatment mostly because of psychoses, nausea, dyskinesia or exacerbation of urinary incontinence [3]. Sinemet worsened bladder overactivity [9].

[1] Schweizerische Medizinische Wochenschrift [1977] 107 (14) : 474-479 (J.Hayek)

[2] Movement Disorders [1996] 11 (4) : 427-430 (R.Pahwa, J. Marjama, D.McGuire, K.Lyons, F.Zwiebel, P.Silverstein, R.Ward, W. C.Koller)

[3] Clinical and Experimental Neurology [1978] 15 : 299-306 (F.J. Vajda, G.A.Donnan, P.F.Bladin)

[4] Acta Neurologica Scandinavica [1978] 57 (2) : 186-192 (L. Battistin, G.Meneghetti, S.Rigotti, A.Saia)

[5] Mymensingh Medical Journal [2014] 23 (1) : 18-23 (M.M.Rahman, M.J.Uddin, J.H. Chowdhury, T.I.Chowdhury)

[6] Archives of Neurology [1987] 44 (3) : 270-272 (J.H.Pincus, K. Barry)

[7] Archives of Neurology [1974] 30 (6) : 444-447 (H.Mars)

[8] Journal of Neurology, Neurosurgery and Psychiatry [1971] 34 (6) : 682-686 (H.L.Klawans, S.P.Ringel, D.M.Shenker)

[9] Neurology [2007] 68 (18) : 1455-1459 (L.Brusa, F.Petta, A.Pisani, V.Moschella, C.Iani, P.Stanzione, R.Miano, E.Finazzi-Agrò)

SINEMET CR

Brand names : Sinemet CR, Caramet CR

Pharmacology : Sinemet CR is a sustained release version of Sinemet. Sinemet CR is intended to release the medicine slowly and continuously over several hours in order to help provide steady blood levels of L-dopa throughout the day. The capsules must be swallowed whole and not broken or chewed in order to avoid damaging the modified release action. Treatment with Sinemet CR instead of Sinemet or L-dopa resulted in a significant increase in total L-dopa dose [1-7].

Efficacy : Of those people that changed from L-dopa to Sinemet CR, there was significant improvement in symptoms [8]. Most people changing from Sinemet to Sinemet CR improved their symptoms [2, 3, 5, 7, 9-33]. However, after 5 years, Sinemet and Sinemet CR had similar effects [34]. Sinemet CR was preferred to Sinemet and L-dopa by a clear majority of patients [2, 8, 12, 23]. Sinemet CR and Madopar CR differed little in their effect [35, 36]. Patients improved gradually whilst taking Sinemet CR, usually taking over a week to achieve maximum response. After ceasing chronic use of Sinemet CR it took about a week for the beneficial effects to wear off [37].

Adverse effects : Of those people that changed from L-dopa to Sinemet CR, two thirds experienced motor complications and one third had a stable motor response. Adverse effects were usually mild or moderate [8]. The number of drug-related adverse effects was similar in the two groups [10]. Some people ceased the use of Sinemet CR because of adverse effects [2]. The severity of dyskinesia increased when changing from L-dopa [2]. The most common drug-related effect of Sinemet CR was nausea. Other drug related effects were dizziness, insomnia, abdominal pain, dyskinesia, headache and depression. Drug related withdrawals were less than 10% of all patients, primarily due to nervous or psychiatric complaints [14]. The number of drug related adverse experiences were similar with Sinemet and Sinemet CR [16].

[1] Neurology [1993] 43 (4) : 677-681 (R.Pahwa, K.Busenbark, S.J. Huber, D.Michalek, J.P.Hubble, W.C.Koller)

[2] Neurologia [1996] 11 (1) : 1-9 (C.Leiva Santana, B.Galvan Berenguer, J.Gomez Garca, J.Cabello Lopez)

[3] Neurology [1989] 39 (11 Supplement 2) : 45-53 (P.A.LeWitt, M.V. Nelson, R.C.Berchou, M.P.Galloway, N.Kesaree, D.Kareti, P. Schlick)

[4] Neurology [1989] 39 (11 Supplement 2) : 25-38 (K.C.Yeh, T.F. August, D.F.Bush, K.C.Lasseter, D.G.Musson, S.Schwartz, M.E. Smith, D.C.Titus)

[5] Neurology [1989] 39 (11 Supplement 2) : 101-104 (D.F.Bush, C.L. Liss, A.Morton)

[6] Neurology [1989] 39 (11 Supplement 2) : 74-77 (P.Rondot, M. Ziegler, N.Aymard, A.Teinturier)

[7] Neurology [1989] 39 (11 Supplement 2) : 38-44 (J.M. Cedarbaum, H.Kutt, F.H.McDowell)

[8] Journal of Neurology [1998] 245 (Supplement 1) : S31-S33 (F. Grandas, P.Martnez-Martn, G.Linazasoro)

[9] Journal of Neurology [1998] 245 (Supplement 1) : S28-S30 (P.G. Wasielewski, W.C.Koller)

[10] Journal of Neurology [1996] 243 (3) : 235-240 (E.C.Wolters, H.J. Tesselaar)

[11] Clinical Neuropharmacology [1991] 14 (3) : 235-240 (C.W. Olanow, K.Nakano, P.Nausieda, J.A.Tetrud, B.Manyam, B.Last, G. Block, C.Liss, D.Bush)

[12] Clinical Neuropharmacology [1999] 22 (2) : 74-79 (G.Linazasoro, F.Grandas, P.Martinez Martin, J.L.Bravo)

[13] Australian and New Zealand Journal of Medicine [1991] 21 (4) : 397-400 (M.T.Bulling, L.M.Wing, R.J.Burns)

[14] European Neurology [1997] 37 (1) : 23-27 (G.Block, C.Liss, S. Reines, J.Irr, D.Nibbelink)

[15] Zhurnal Nevrologii i Psikhiatrii Imeni S.S.Korsakova [1995] 95 (5) : 31-35 (D.V.Artem'ev, I.V.Damulin, N.N.Iakhno)

[16] Journal of Neurology [1996] 243 (3) : 235-240 (E.C.Wolters, H.J. Tesselaar)

[17] European Journal of Clinical Pharmacology [1992] 43 (5) : 483-489 (S.G.Bowes, R.J.Dobbs, M.Henley, A.Charlett, C.J.O'Neill, P. W.Nicholson, A.G.Purkiss, C.Weller, S.M.Dobbs)

[18] Clinical Neurology and Neurosurgery [1992] 94 (3) : 205-211 (E. C.Wolters, M.W.Horstink, R.A.Roos, E.N.Jamsen)

[19] Canadian Journal of Neurological Sciences [1991] 18 (4) : 467-471 (J.T.Hutton, J.L.Morris)

[20] Journal of Neural Transmission [1990] 2 (3) : 205-213 (J.M. Cedarbaum, M.Silvestri, M.Clark, L.Toy, A.Harts, A.Green-Parsons, F. H.McDowell)

[21] European Neurology [1990] 30 (2) : 75-78 (A.Lieberman, G. Gopinathan, E.Miller, A.Neophytides, G.Baumann, L.Chin)

[22] Neurology [1989] 39 (11 Supplement 2) : 88-92 (D.Deleu, M. Jacques, Y.Michotte, G.Ebinger)

[23] Neurology [1989] 39 (11 Supplement 2) : 67-72 (J.T.Hutton, J.L. Morris, D.F.Bush, M.E.Smith, C.L.Liss, S.Reines)

[24] Neurology [1989] 39 (11 Supplement 2) : 92-95 (R.L.Rodnitzky, Q.S.Dickins, J.Dobson)

[25] Neurology [1989] 39 (11 Supplement 2) : 82-85 (J.A.Aarli, N.E. Gilhus)

[26] Neurology [1989] 39 (11 Supplement 2) : 63-66 (G.G.Goetz, C.M. Tanner, D.W.Gilley, H.L.Klawans)

[27] Annals of Clinical and Laboratory Science [1989] 19 (2) : 101-106 (M.H.Mark, J.I.Sage)

[28] Journal of Neurology, Neurosurgery, and Psychiatry [1989] 52 (2) : 207-212 (J.M.Cedarbaum, M.Hoey, F.H.McDowell)

[29] Clinical Neurology and Neurosurgery [1989] 91 (4) : 303-309 (D. Deleu, M.Jacques, Y.Michotte, G.Ebinger)

[30] Mayo Clinic Proceedings [1988] 63 (9) : 876-886 (J.E.Ahlskog, M.D.Muenter, P.G.McManis, G.N.Bell, P.A.Bailey)

[31] Archives of Neurology [1988] 45 (8) : 861-864 (J.T.Hutton, J.L. Morris, G.C.Román, S.C.Imke, J.W.Elias)

[32] Neurology [1988] 38 (7) : 1143-1146 (C.G.Goetz, C.M.Tanner, K. M.Shannon, V.S.Carroll, H.L.Klawans, P.M.Carvey, D.Gilley)

[33] Neurology [1987] 37 (10) : 1607-1612 (J.M.Cedarbaum, L.Breck, H.Kutt, F.H.McDowell)

[34] Neurology [1999] 53 (5) : 1012-1019 (W.C.Koller, J.T.Hutton, E. Tolosa, R.Capilldeo)

[35] Journal of Neural Transmission [1992] 4 (2) : 173-178 (B. Kleedorfer, W.Poewe)

[36] Neurology [1989] 39 (11 Supplement 2) : 78-81 (U.K.Rinne, J.O. Rinne)

[37] Clinical Neuropharmacology [1997] 20 (5) : 394-401 (L.Barbato, F.Stocchi, A.Monge, L.Vacca, S.Ruggieri, G.Nordera, C.D.Marsden)

Madopar

Brand names : Madopar, Prolopa

Pharmacology : Madopar is L-Dopa combined with benserazide, which is a peripheral decarboxylase inhibitor [1]. Benserazide helps to maintain the levels of L-dopa until it is used, by inhibiting peripheral metabolism of L-dopa. Benserazide is also marketed separately as Co-beneldopa, which is usually taken simultaneously with L-dopa. Generic versions of Madopar can differ according to their quantities of benserazide and L-dopa [2].

Efficacy : The efficacy was the same as that of Sinemet [1, 3, 4, 5]. The beneficial effects appeared equally quickly [5].

Adverse effects : The adverse effects are the same as Sinemet except that the gastrointestinal side-effects and involuntary movements are less when using Madopar [5].

[1] European Neurology [1975] 13 (2) : 65-71 (J.J.Korten, A.Keyser, E.M.Joosten, F.J.Gabrels)

[2] BMC Pharmacology and Toxicology [2013] 14 (1) : 24 (U.E. Gasser, A.Fischer, J.P.Timmermans, I.Arnet)

[3] Current Medical Research Opinions [1979] 6 (1) : 1-7 (B.O. Williams, D.Carlyle)

[4] Neurology [1978] 28 (9 Part 1) : 964-968 (A.Lieberman, E.Estey, G.Gopinathan, T.Ohashi, A.Sauter, M.Goldstein)

[5] Acta Neurologica Scandinavica [1976] 53 (5) : 376-385 (H. Pakkenberg, E.Birket-Smith, E.Dupont, E.Hansen, B.Mikkelsen, J. Presthus, I.Rautakorpi, E.Riman, U.K.Rinne)

Madopar CR

Brand names : Madopar CR

Pharmacology : Madopar CR is a sustained release version of Madopar. Madopar CR is designed to release the medicine slowly and continuously over several hours to help provide steady blood levels of the medicine throughout the day [1]. Madopar CR was bioequivalent with Sinemet CR with respect to L-dopa [2].

Efficacy : Madopar CR was usually found to be more effective than Madopar, but there had to be an increase in the dosage in order to achieve this [3, 4, 5]. However, some patients responded better to Madopar CR and some to standard Madopar [4, 5].

Adverse effects : Madopar CR caused far fewer adverse effects than regular Madopar [5].

[1] European Neurology [1987] 27 (Supplement 1) : 21-27 (W.Erni, K. Held)

[2] European Neurology [1992] 32 (6) : 343-348 (A.Grahnn, S.A. Eckerns, C.Collin, A.Ling-Andersson, G.Tiger, M.Nilsson)

[3] European Neurology [1987] 27 (Supplement 1) : 76-80 (G.P. Nordera, A.Lorizio, P.Lion, C.Durisotti, G.D'Andrea, F.Ferro-Milone)

[4] Clinical Neuropharmacology [1989] 12 (6) : 498-505

[5] Journal of Neurology, Neurosurgery and Psychiatry [1990] 53 (3) : 220-223 (D.G.MacMahon, D.Sachdev, H.G.Boddie, C.J.Ellis, B.R. Kendal, N.A.Blackburn)

Rytary and Numient

Brand names : Rytary, Numient

Pharmacology : Rytary and Numient include L-dopa and carbidopa and combine the immediate release version of L-dopa and the controlled release version of L-dopa. Rytary is marketed in the U.S.. Rytary is combined with carbidopa in a 4 : 1 ratio. Rytary was initially assessed as IPX054 and then IPX066. Numient is the same as Rytary but is marketed in the EU.

Efficacy : It improved symptoms in both early and advanced Parkinson's Disease, significantly improved Unified Parkinson Disease Rating Scale scores, and increased "on" times [1]. It is slightly more effective than conventional forms of L-dopa despite only being taken twice a day instead of throughout the day [2]. It substantially reduced variability in plasma concentrations of L-dopa [3]. The most beneficial dosages were 145mg, then 245mg, then 390mg. Reduction in "off" time was marginally better than when taking Sinemet [4, 5], or Stalevo [6], and was achieved without causing more dyskinesias [7, 8]. Around 43% of people taking IPX066 were much or very much improved in comparison to their previous treatment. Around 68% of people taking IPX066 were at least minimally improved in comparison to their previous treatment [10].

Adverse effects : The most frequently reported adverse effect is nausea [5-9], which was reported in 12% of patients [5, 9]. Other commonly reported adverse effects are : dyskinesia [5-9], insomnia [5-9], falls [6-8], confusional state [7, 8], dizziness, headache, abnormal dreams, dry mouth, anxiety, constipation, vomiting, orthostatic hypotension, which all occurred in at least 5% of patients [5, 9]. Serious adverse effects from gastrointestinal haemorrhage and allergic oedema were uncommon [5, 9].

[1] Neurology [2016] 86 (14 Supplement 1) : S13-S24 (R.Dhall, D.L. Kreitzman)

[2] Clinical Neuropharmacology [2009] 32 (4) : 189-192 (V.K.Hinson, C.G.Goetz, S.Leurgans, W.Fan, T.Nguyen, A.Hsu)

[3] Movement Disorders [2011] 26 (12) : 2246-2252 (R.A.Hauser, A.L. Ellenbogen, L.V.Metman, A.Hsu, M.J.O'Connell, N.B.Modi, H.M.Yao, S.H.Kell, S.K.Gupta)

[4] Lancet Neurology [2013] 12 (4) : 346-356 (R.A.Hauser, A.Hsu, S. Kell, A.J.Espay, K.Sethi, M.Stacy, W.Ondo, M.O'Connell, S.Gupta)

[5] Impaxlabs http://www.impaxlabs.com

[6] CNS Drugs [2016] 30 (1) :79-90 (S.L.Greig, K. McKeage)

[7] Parkinsonism & Related Disorders [2014] 20 (12) : 1335-1340 (F. Stocchi, A.Hsu, S.Khanna, A.Ellenbogen, A.Mahler, G.Liang, U. Dillmann, R.Rubens, S.Kell, S. Gupta)

[8] CNS Drugs [2015] 29 (4) : 341-350 (C.H.Waters, P.Nausieda, L. Dzyak, J.Spiegel, M.Rudzinska, D.E.Silver, E.S. Tsurkalenko, S.Kell, A.Hsu, S.Khanna, S.Gupta)

[9] Parkinsonism & Related Disorders [2014] 20 (2) : 142-148 (R. Pahwa, K.E.Lyons, R.A.Hauser, S.Fahn, J.Jankovic, E.Pourcher, A. Hsu, M.O'Connell, S.Kell, S.Gupta)

[10] Journal of Neurological Science [2017] 373 : 116-123 (J.Tetrud, P.Nausieda, D.Kreitzman, G.S.Liang, A.Nieves, A.P.Duker, R.A. Hauser, E.S.Farbman, A.Ellenbogen, A. Hsu, S.Kell, S.Khanna, et al)

Duodopa

Brand name : Duodopa

Pharmacology : Duodopa is a combination of L-dopa and carbidopa in the form of a gel. It is administered throughout the day using a portable pump directly into the small intestine through a surgically placed tube. This ensures a flow of L-dopa that can be adjusted according to the patient's individual needs [1]. It enables more consistent plasma concentrations of L-dopa [2].

Efficacy : Significant improvements in symptoms were found with its use [3 - 24, 31], and also in the quality of life [7, 10, 12, 13, 14, 25]. There was a reduction in "off" time [24, 25, 33, 34], an increase in "on" time without dyskinesia [24, 26, 33, 34], and improvements in freezing of gait, tremor, dizziness, fatigue or mood [26], and dyskinesia [31].

Adverse effects : Most people using Duodopa had adverse effects [15, 32]. Most of the side effects are similar to those observed with oral administration of L-dopa and carbidopa [2, 27, 28]. Dislocation of the intestinal tube to the stomach was the most common technical problem [2, 3, 7, 27], occurring in nearly 70% of the patients during the first year [27]. In one study adverse effects occurred in 87% of people. The most common were abdominal pain (30%), complication of device insertion (21%), procedural pain (17%), constipation (13%), nausea (13%), excessive granulation tissue (13%), falls (10%), dyskinesia (10%), insomnia (10%), post-operative wound infection (10%), and anxiety (10%). The most severe complications from surgery were : abdominal inflammation (3%), and gas or air in the peritoneal cavity (5%). Serious adverse effects occurred in 16% to 31% of people [13, 29, 33]. Procedure and device adverse effects occurred in 76% of people [29]. Most frequently reported adverse effects were complications of device insertion (41% and 8%, respectively) and abdominal pain (36% and 4%, respectively). Non-procedure and device adverse effects occurred in 92% of people. The most frequently reported were insomnia (23%) and falls (23%). 42% had non-procedure and device adverse effects with the most frequently reported being pneumonia (5%) and Parkinson's Disease symptoms (2%). Adverse events led to discontinuation in 17% to 26% of cases [29, 32], with 9% of cases occurring in the first year [32], most frequently because of complication of device insertion (2%) [29, 32]. L-dopa being reduced or increased differed according to the study [3, 5, 27]. Addition of the COMT inhibitors, entacapone or tolcapone, reduced the need for L-dopa by 20% without altering plasma L-dopa concentrations, reducing symptoms, or reducing "off" time [30]. Those adverse effects related to L-dopa, gastrostomy and technical issues were reported in 36%, 42% and 43% of patients, respectively [26].

[1] Duodopa's guide for health care givers [online]

[2] Neurological Sciences [2008] 29 (Supplement 5) : S387-S388 (P. Odin, E.Wolters, A.Antonini)

[3] Revue Neurologique (Paris) [2009] 165 (8-9) : 718-727 (A.Annic, D.Devos, D.Seguy, K.Dujardin, A.Destée, L.Defebvre)

[4] Tidsskrift for den Norske Laegeforening [2005] 125 (19) : 2638-2640 (C.Lundqvist, T.Nystedt, O.Reiertsen, R.Grotli, A.G.Beiske)

[5] Acta Neurologica Scandinavica [2001] 104 (6) : 343-348 (D. Nilsson, D.Nyholm, S.M.Aquilonius)

[6] Neurologia [2010] 25 (9) : 536-543 (D.Santos-García, M.Macías, M.Llaneza, L.Fuster-Sanjurjo, A.Echarri-Piudo, S.Belmonte, S.Blanco)

[7] Journal of Neurology [2013] 260 (1) : 105-114 (M.Zibetti, A. Merola, V.Ricchi, A.Marchisio, C.A.Artusi, L.Rizzi, E.Montanaro, D. Reggio, C.De Angelis, M.Rizzone, L.Lopiano)

[8] Parkinsonism & Related Disorders [2012] 18 (8) : 916-929 (D. Nyholm)

[9] Acta Neurologica Scandinavica [2012] 126 (6) : e29-e33 (S.E. Pålhagen, N.Dizdar, T.Hauge, B.Holmberg, R.Jansson, J.Linder, D. Nyholm, O.Sydow, M.Wainwright, H.Widner, A.Johansson)

[10] Clinical Neuropharmacology [2012] 35 (5) : 205-207 (P.Reddy, P. Martinez-Martin, A.Rizos, A.Martin, G.C.Faye, I.Forgacs, P.Odin, A. Antonini, K.R.Chaudhuri)

[11] Journal of Neural Transmission [2013] 120 (11) : 1553-1558 (A. Antonini, P.Odin, L.Opiano, V.Tomantschger, C.Pacchetti, B. Pickut, U.E.Gasser, D.Calandrella, F.Mancini, M.Zibetti, B.Minafra, et al)

[12] Journal of Neurology [2013] 260 (1) : 105-114 (M.Zibetti, A. Merola, V.Ricchi, A.Marchisio, C.A.Artusi, L.Rizzi, E.Montanaro, D. Reggio, C.De Angelis, M.Rizzone, L.Lopiano)

[13] Parkinsonism & Related Disorders [2013] 19 (3) : 339-345 (H.H. Fernandez, A.Vanagunas, P.Odin, A.J.Espay, R.A.Hauser, D.G. Standaert, K.Chatamra, J.Benesh, Y.Pritchett, S.L.Hass, R.A.Lenz)

[14] Journal of Neurology [2014] 261 (3) : 561-569 (M.T.Cáceres-Redondo, F.Carrillo, M.J.Lama, I.Huertas-Fernández, L.Vargas-González, M.Carballo, P.Mir)

[15] Lancet Neurology [2014] 13 (2) : 141-149 (C.W.Olanow, K. Kieburtz, P.Odin, A.J.Espay, D.G.Standaert, H.H.Fernandez, A. Vanagunas, A.A.Othman, K.L.Widnell, W.Z.Robieson, et al)

[16] Movement Disorders [2015] 30 (4) : 500-509 (H.H.Fernandez, D.G.Standaert, R.A.Hauser, A.E.Lang, V.S.Fung, F.Klostermann, M.F. Lew, P.Odin, M.Steiger, E.Z.Yakupov, S. Chouinard, et al)

[17] Journal of Parkinsons Disease [2015] 5 (1) : 165-174 (J.T.Slevin, H.H.Fernandez, C.Zadikoff, C.Hall, S.Eaton, J.Dubow, K.Chatamra, J. Benesh)

[18] Parkinsonism & Related Disorders [2014] 21 (3) : 317-320 (F.C. Chang, D.S.Tsui, N.Mahant, N.Wolfe, S.D.Kim, A.D.Ha, M.Drury, J. M.Griffith, V.S.Fung)

[19] Clinical Pharmacokinetics [2015] 54 (9) : 975-984 (A.A.Othman, K.Chatamra, M.E.Mohamed, S.Dutta, J.Benesh, M.Yanagawa, M. Nagai)

[20] Parkinsonism & Related Disorders [2015] 21 (3) : 231-235 (A. Antonini, A.Yegin, C.Preda, L.Bergmann, W.Poewe)

[21] European Neurology [2015] 74 (5-6) : 227-236 (S.Bohlega, H. Abou Al-Shaar, T.Alkhairallah, F.Al-Ajlan, N.Hasan, K.Alkahtani)

[22] Journal of Neural Transmission [2016] 123 (4) : 407-414 (O. Bajenaru, A.Ene, B.O.Popescu, J.A.Szász, M.Sabau, D.F.Muresan, L. Perju-Dumbrava, C.D.Popescu, A.Constantinescu, I. Buraga, M.Simu)

[23] Movement Disorders [2016] 31 (4) : 530-537 (A.Antonini, V.S.Fung, J.T.Boyd, J.T.Slevin, C.Hall, K.Chatamra, S. Eaton, J.A.Benesh)

[24] Neurological Science [2016] Jul 15 [Epub ahead of print] (L. Lopiano, N.Modugno, P.Marano, M.Sensi, G.Meco, A.Cannas, G. Gusmaroli, F.Tamma, F.Mancini, R.Quatrale, A.M.Costanz, et al)

[25] Acta Neurologica Scandinavica [2011] 125 (3) : 187-191 (D. Santos-García, L.F.Sanjurjo, M.Macías, M.Llaneza, P. Carpintero, R.de la Fuente-Fernández)

[26] Neurodegenerative Disease Management [2016] Jul 21 [Epub ahead of print] (F.Valldeoriola, F.Grandas, D.Santos-García, I.Regidor, M.J.Catalán, J.M.Arbelo, V.Puente, P.Mir, J.C.Parra)

[27] Clinical Neuropharmacology [2008] 31 (2) : 63-73 (D.Nyholm, T. Lewander, A.Johansson, P.A.Lewitt, C.Lundqvist, S.M.Aquilonius)

[28] Journal of Neurology [2012] 259 (8) : 1668-1672 (D.Santos-García, R.de la Fuente-Fernández, F.Valldeoriola, A.Palasí, F.Carrillo, M.Grande, P.Mir, O.De Fabregues, J.Casanova)

[29] Movement Disorders [2016] 31 (4) : 538-546 (A.E.Lang, R.L. Rodriguez, J.T.Boyd, S.Chouinard, C.Zadikoff, A.J.Espay, J.T.Slevin, H.H.Fernandez, M.F.Lew, D.A.Stein, P.Odin, V.S.Fung, et al)

[30] European Journal of Neurology [2011] 19 (6) : 820-826 (D. Nyholm, A.Johansson, H.Lennernäs, H.Askmark)

[31] Parkinsonism and Related Disorders [2017] Feb 3 [Epub ahead of print] (A.Juhász, Z.Aschermann, P.Ács, J.Janszky, M.Kovács, A. Makkos, M.Harmat, D.Tényi, K.Karádi, S.Komoly, A.Takáts, et al)

[32] Parkinsonism and Related Disorders [2017] Feb 21 [Epub ahead of print] (M.Sensi, G.Cossu, F.Mancini, M.Pilleri, M.Zibetti, N.Modugno, R.Quatrale, F.Tamma, A.Antonini)

[33] Zhurnal Nevrologii i Psikhiatrii Imeni S.S.Korsakova [2017] 117 (2) : 22-31 (A.A.Skoromets, M.M.Odinak, E.Z.Yakupov, I.V. Litvinenko, Z.A.Zalyalova, A.A.Timofeeva, S.Y.Kirtaev, et al)

[34] CNS Drugs [2016] 30 (5) : 381-404 (K.Wirdefeldt, P.Odin, D. Nyholm)

LECIGON

Brand name : LECIGON

Pharmacology : LECIGon is a gel formulation of L-dopa, carbidopa, and entacapone for continuous intestinal administration through a proprietary small, lightweight ambulatory pump system. Continuous intestinal delivery, tailored for the individual patient, has been shown to secure a smooth L-dopa plasma level [1]

Efficacy : The degree of efficacy did not differ from that when using Duodopa [1].

Adverse effects : It was well tolerated [1].

[1] Movement Disorders [2016] Dec 17 [Epub ahead of print] (M. Senek, E.I.Nielsen, D.Nyholm)

PARCOPA

Brand name : Parcopa

Pharmacology : Parcopa is an orally disintegrating combination of L-dopa and carbidopa, which is the same combination as Sinemet. Parcopa disintegrates in the mouth, so it shortens the time from the ingestion of the drug until the ridding or reduction of symptoms.

Efficacy : When compared to the use of Sinemet, there were no significant differences according to any means of assessment, including improvements in symptoms, preference, or the time taken for the drug to have effect. However, there was a tendency in favour of Parcopa [1].

Adverse effects : When compared to the use of Sinemet, there were no significant differences in adverse effects. However, there was a tendency in favour of Parcopa [1].

[1] Movement Disorders [2010] 25 (16) : 2724-2727 (W.G.Ondo, L.Shinawi, S. Moore)

L-DOPA INHALER

CVT-301

Brand names : none (due to being in development)

Pharmacology : CVT-301 is the name of an inhaled version of L-dopa presently being developed for the treatment of Parkinson's Disease. CVT-301 uses the ARCUS inhalation technology, which delivers a reliable and consistent drug dose with a compact, breath actuated inhaler. It uses a dry powder and inhaler combination that is unique in its ability to deliver a large, precise dose independent of inspiratory flow rate from a simple, easy-to-use device suitable for convenient self-administration. In contrast, the efficacy of oral L-dopa is significantly compromised by delayed absorption and variability in the circulating drug concentrations. Civitas has conducted preclinical studies showing CVT-301's ability to deliver more rapid and consistent systemic exposure of L-dopa compared to the oral administration of L-dopa. The inhaled version of L-dopa would be used alongside the use of oral L-dopa [1]. Among people with Parkinson's Disease inhaling CVT-301 as a single 50mg dose during an "off" period, 77% of them showed an increase in plasma L-dopa within 10 minutes [2].

Efficacy : After administration of 50mg, improvements in motor function were seen within 5 and 15 minutes, which were the earliest assessment times [2]. A clinical trial showed that patients experiencing an "off" episode, treated with either 35mg or 50mg CVT-301, had significantly greater improvements in motor function than patients treated with inhaled placebo. The difference in improvement was already apparent 10 minutes after dosing and was durable for at least an hour, the longest time point at which patients were measured. In a Phase 3 clinical trial, patients who received CVT-301 in addition to their oral carbidopa/levodopa showed a significant improvement in motor function in people with Parkinson's Disease experiencing OFF periods. Two doses of CVT-301 were assessed - 84 mg and 60 mg (equivalent to 50 mg and 35 mg fine-particle doses) [1].

Adverse effects : Both doses of CVT-301 were well tolerated, with no increase relative to placebo in troublesome or non-troublesome dyskinesias during ON periods. There were no adverse effects on cardiovascular or lung function [1]. The most common adverse effects were dizziness, headache and cough [1, 2].

[1] http://ir.acorda.com

[2] Science Translational Medicine [2016] 8 (360) : 360ra136 (M.M. Lipp, R. Batycky, J.Moore, M.Leinonen, M.I.Freed)

CYCLOPS

Brand names : none (due to being in development)

Pharmacology : A dry powder inhaler is being developed as a means of administering L-dopa. Its means of administration could enable a very quick therapeutic effect. They used an instrumented test inhaler with three different resistances to air flow. The volumes inhaled varied from 1.2 litres to 3.5 litres. Total inhalation time and the time to peak inspiratory flow rate both decreased with decreasing inhaler resistance. The data from this study indicate that patients with Parkinson's Disease will be able to use a dry powder inhaler during an off period and they provide an adequate starting point for the development of an L-dopa powder inhaler [1]. The high dose dry powder inhaler (Cyclops) used doses of 20mg, 30mg and 40mg, which are representative of those to be expected in practice. A co-micronised L-dopa formulation with 2% L-leucine appeared to yield the best aerosol properties for inhalation and the highest delivered dose reproducibility [2].

Efficacy : The efficacy has not yet been assessed [1, 2].

Adverse effects : The adverse effects have not yet been assessed [1, 2].

[1] PLoS One [2015] 10 (7) : e0132714 (M.Luinstra, A.W.Rutgers, H.Dijkstra, F.Grasmeijer, P.Hagedoorn, J.M.Vogelzang, H.W.Frijlink, A.H.de Boer)

[2] European Journal of Pharmaceutics and Biopharmaceutics [2015] 97 (Part A) : 22-29 (M.Luinstra, F.Grasmeijer, P.Hagedoorn, J.R. Moes, H.W.Frijlink, A.H.Boer)

ß-ASARONE

Brand names : none (due to being in development)

Pharmacology : The co-administration of ß-asarone and L-dopa is being developed as a means of improving the effect of Madopar. ß-asarone is found in the flowering plant acorus and also in asarum, which is known as wild ginger.

Efficacy : In animal studies the use of L-dopa with ß-asarone increased dopamine levels in the striatum and in blood plasma. The co-administration of ß-asarone and L-dopa could also increase the levels in blood plasma of tyrosine hydroxylase, which is the enzyme that is responsible for the biosynthesis of L-dopa from L-tyrosine [1].

Adverse effects : The adverse effects of ß-asarone have not yet been assessed [1].

[1] Clinical and Experimental Pharmacology and Physiology [2014] 41 (9) : 685-690 (L.Huang, M.Deng, S.Zhang, Y.Fang, L.Li)

AcuForm

Brand names : none (due to being in development)

Pharmacology : Depomed are developing a new drug called DM-1992. Just like Sinemet, DM-1992 is a combination of L-dopa and carbidopa. DM-1992 also includes AcuForm [1]. Acuform is a polymer-based technology designed to optimize drug delivery. Acuform's unique swelling polymers allow the tablet to be retained in the stomach for approximately eight to ten hours. During this time the tablet's active ingredients are steadily delivered to the upper GI tract at the desired rate and time. This gradual and extended release of the active ingredients allows for more of the drug to be absorbed in the upper GI tract, offering the potential for greater treatment efficacy and increased treatment tolerability [2].

Efficacy : DM-1992 was able to extend the therapeutic duration of L-dopa to nine hours compared to Sinemet CR's seven hours. The time taken to reach peak blood levels was extended to four hours compared to 2 hours for Sinemet CR [1]. DM-1992 also reduced the "off" time [3].

Adverse effects : More people taking DM-1992 had adverse effects than those people who were taking immediate release L-dopa/carbidopa [3].

[1] Morningstar Document Research, Form 10-Q, Depomed Inc - Depo [2009] : 24

[2] Depomed - http://www.depomed.com/technology

[3] Movement Disorders [2015] 30 (9) : 1222-1228 (L.Verhagen Metman, N.Stover, C.Chen, V.E.Cowles, M.Sweeney)

L-DOPA PRODRUG

Brand names : none (due to being in development)

Pharmacology : XP21279 is a new chemical entity being developed for the treatment of Parkinson's Disease. It uses naturally occurring, high capacity nutrient transporters in the gastrointestinal tract to generate active and efficient absorption into the body. Once absorbed it is rapidly converted into L-dopa. In a clinical trial, patients with Parkinson's Disease were given XP21279 with carbidopa, or L-dopa with carbidopa. With the use of XP21279 there was significantly less variability in the concentration of L-dopa. XP21279 may therefore provide better control of motor fluctuations [1].

Efficacy : Overall, there was a reduction in daily "off" time. There was also more "on" time without troublesome dyskinesia. The average time to "on" time was not delayed when using XP21279 [1]. In another clinical trial the average daily off time was reduced more when using XP21279 with carbidopa but only by 18 minutes. There was little difference between the two in their effect on dyskinesia. However, XP21279 significantly reduced the variability of L-dopa concentration that occurs when using Sinemet. This was achieved by taking XP21279 only three times per day, instead of the four to five times a day that the L-dopa with carbidopa was taken [2].

Adverse effects : The adverse effects have not yet been assessed. [1, 2].

[1] Clinical Neuropharmacology [2012] 35 (3) : 103-110 (P.A.Lewitt, A.Ellenbogen, D.Chen, R.Lal, K.McGuire, K.Zomorodi, W.Luo, F.J. Huff)

[2] Movement Disorders [2014] 29 (1) : 75-82 (P.A.Lewitt, F.J.Huff, R. A.Hauser, D.Chen, D.Lissin, K.Zomorodi, K.C. Cundy)

MELEVODOPA

Brand names : none (due to being in development)

Pharmacology : Melevodopa is the methyl ester of L-dopa. Continuous intravenous infusions of L-Dopa are limited by the insolubility and acidity of L-Dopa. The methyl ester of L-dopa overcomes this as it is a soluble neutral derivative [1]. It is a highly water soluble derivative produced by esterification of the carboxilic acid moiety of the L-Dopa molecule that is rapidly hydrolyzed to L-Dopa and can be administered orally in an easily dosable liquid form [2].

Efficacy : Melevodopa infusions demonstrated efficacy in Parkinson's Disease [2]. Compared with oral L-dopa, melevodopa infusions resulted in marked reductions of plasma L-dopa variations and motor response fluctuations in patients with either wearing-off or on-off phenomena [3]. Melevodopa led to a significantly more rapid reversal of "off" periods [4], and reduction in "off" time [5], and more readily led to "on" periods [6-8]. When people switched from Sinemet to melevodopa they improved regarding their "on-time". The benefit of melevodopa was greater in people with "delayed-on", and especially in those people who had both "delayed-on" and "wearing-off". Most patients showed improvement in their PDQ-39 total score [9].

Adverse effects : No significant adverse effects were reported with its use [10, 11]

[1] Clinical Neuropharmacology [1984] 7 (1) : 89-98 (D.R.Cooper, C. V.Marrel, B.Testa, H.van de Waterbeemd, N.Quinn, P.Jenner, C.D. Marsden)

[2] Functional Neurology [1994] 9 (5) : 259-264 (F.Stocchi, L.Barbato, L.Bramante, A.Bonamartini, S.Ruggieri)

[3] Neurology [1987] 37 (7) : 1242-1245 (J.L.Juncos, M.M. Mouradian, G.Fabbrini, C.Serrati, T.N.Chase)

[4] Clinical Neuropharmacology [1991] 14 (3) : 241-244 (M.J. Steiger, F.Stocchi, A.Carta, S.Ruggieri, A.Agnoli, N.P.Quinn, C.D.Marsden)

[5] Movement Disorders [2010] 25 (12) : 1881-1887 (F.Stocchi, M. Zappia, V.Dall'armi, J.Kulisevsky, P.Lamberti, J.A.Obeso)

[6] Journal of Neurology [1996] 243 (5) : 377-380 (F.Stocchi, L. Barbato, L.Bramante, G.Nordera, L.Vacca, S.Ruggieri)

[7] Clinical Neuropharmacology [2007] 30 (1) : 18-24 (F.Stocchi, L. Fabbri, L.Vecsei, A.Krygowska-Wajs, P.A.Monici Preti, S.A.Ruggieri)

[8] Clinical Neuropharmacology [2010] 33 (2) : 61-66 (R.Zangaglia, F. Stocchi, M.Sciarretta, A.Antonini, F.Mancini, M.Guidi, E.Martignoni, C.Pacchetti)

[9] Minerva Medica [2011] 102 (2) : 125-132 (D.Bosco, M.Plastino, F. Bosco, A.Fava, A.Rotondo)

[10] Movement Disorders [2010] 25 (12) : 1881-1887 (F.Stocchi, M. Zappia, V.Dall'Armi, J.Kulisevsky, P.Lamberti, J.A.Obeso)

[11] Clinical Neuropharmacology [2010] 33 (2) : 61-66 (R.Zangaglia, F.Stocchi, M.Sciarretti, A.Antonini, F.Mancini, M.Guidi, E. Martignoni, C.Pacchetti)

SUBCUTANEOUS L-DOPA

Brand names : none (due to being in development)

Pharmacology : ND0612 is a combination of L-dopa and carbidopa in a liquid formula administered continuously sub-cutaneously through a patch pump. It is designed to provide steady L-dopa blood levels for the reduction of motor complications in Parkinson's Disease.

Efficacy : In a controlled, dose-escalation trial in young, healthy volunteers, ND0612 was shown to be safe and tolerable in the tested doses. Clinically meaningful L-dopa concentrations were reached. L-dopa plasma levels were proportionate to the dose. ND0612H achieved maximum concentrations of 1,436ng/ml, which with oral entacapone were even higher, at 1,807ng/ml. ND0612L achieved lower maximum concentrations of 528ng/ml. With oral entacapone the L-dopa levels were slightly higher, at 596ng/ml. Fluctuations in L-dopa plasma levels were reduced when compared with the use of oral L-dopa [1].

Adverse effects : Treatment with ND0612L and ND0612H did not raise safety and tolerability concerns, causing only minimal and transient local reactions at the infusion site [1].

[1] Neuroderm - http://www.neuroderm.com

LIQUID L-DOPA

Brand names :

Pharmacology : Liquid L-dopa is usually combined as L-dopa, carbidopa, and ascorbic acid (vitamin C) in a solution called LCAS [1].

Efficacy : Around 37% of people maintained the LCAS treatment after 12 months. In those people, on time without dyskinesia significantly increased from 33% to 57% after the initiation of LCAS treatment. Around 31% of patients were still receiving LCAS treatment after 30 months [1]. LCAS reduced bradykinesia, decreased dyskinesia, and increased functional "on" time when compared with the previous use of L-dopa / carbidopa in tablet form [2].

Adverse effects : The main reasons for discontinuation of LCAS treatment were worsening of wearing-off, persistent dyskinesia, and poor drug adherence. There were a small number of each of these [1].

[1] Journal of Neurological Science [2017] 377 : 6-11 (H.J.Yang, G. Ehm, Y.E.Kim, J.Y.Yun, W.W.Lee, A.Kim, H.J.Kim, B.Jeon)

[2] Neurology [1993] 43 (5) : 1036-1039 (M.C.Kurth, J.W.Tetrud, I. Irwin, W.H.Lyness, J.W.Langston)

Mucuna Pruriens

Common names : Mucuna pruriens

Pharmacology : Mucuna pruriens is a tropical legume whose seeds are a natural source of high quantities of L-dopa. Immature seeds contain maximum L-dopa content [1]. About 5% of dried mucuna pruriens seeds is L-dopa [2]. Boiling reduces the L-dopa content of mucuna pruriens by about 70% [2]. Mucuna Pruriens is mild source of L-dopa. Its mildness lessens the problem of excessive dosage that often occurs with the use of L-dopa in its pharmaceutical form. Mucuna Pruriens is more adjustable in its dosages because there are no precise quantities as there are when taking tablets [3].

Efficacy : Mucuna Pruriens acts more quickly than L-dopa, and its effects on Parkinson's Disease symptoms last longer [4], and can be better [7]. The quantity of L-dopa in Mucuna Pruriens has to be about 3.5 times the quantity of L-dopa in drug form when L-dopa is accompanied by a dopa decarboxylase inhibitor [2]. Mucuna Pruriens has anti-oxidant qualities, and has metal chelating activity, which helps to protect against excessive quantities of metals [5].

Adverse effects : There are no major differences between Mucuna Pruriens and L-dopa regarding their adverse effects [4]. However, Mucuna Pruriens can cause fewer adverse effects [7]. The adverse effects of Mucuna pruriens are mild and mainly gastrointestinal [6].

[1] Panta [2010] 231 (6) : 1361-1369 (P.M.Luthra, S.Singh)

[2] Journal of Neurological Science [2016] 365 : 175-180 (E.Cassani, R.Cilia, J.Laguna, M.Barichella, M.Contin, E.Cereda, I.U.Isaias, F. Sparvoli, A.Akpalu, K.O.Budu, M.T.Scarpa, G.Pezzoli)

[3] Neurotoxicity Research [2009] 15 (2) : 111-122 (S.Kasture, S. Pontis, A.Pinna, N.Schintu, L.Spina, R.Longoni, N.Simola, M.Ballero, M.Morelli)

[4] Journal of Neurology, Neurosurgery and Psychiatry [2004] 75 (12) : 1672-1677 (R.Katzenschlager, A.Evans, A.Manson, P.N.Patsalos, N. Ratnaraj, H.Watt, L.Timmermann, R.Van der Giessen, A.J.Lees)

[5] Phytotherapy Research [2008] 22 (1) : 6-11 (M.Dhanasekaran, B. Tharakan, B.V.Manyam)

[6] Journal of Alternative and Complementary Medicine [1995] 1 (3) : 249-255

[7] Neurology [2017] Jul 5 [Epub ahead of print] (R.Cilia, J.Laguna, E.Cassani, E.Cereda, N.G.Pozzi, I.U.Isaias, M.Contin, M.Barichella, G.Pezzoli)

Fava beans

Common names : Fava beans, broad beans

Brand names : Atremorine

Pharmacology : Cooked fava beans are a natural source of L-dopa that can enable both a substantial increase in plasma levels of L-dopa [1], and a therapeutic effect [2,3].

Efficacy : The therapeutic effect can be similar to the use of L-dopa [2]. The quantity of cooked fava beans used to obtain therapeutic effects in clinical trials was 250g [2,4]. The therapeutic effect lasted about four hours [4]. Fava beans are not a practical means of treating Parkinson's Disease, because the therapeutic use of fava beans would mean having to eat fava beans several times a day.

Adverse effects : In higher doses, in some cases, fava beans caused dyskinesia [4].

[1] European Journal of Neurology [2009] 16 (10) : e171 (L.Raguthu, S.Varanese, L.Flancbaum, E.Tayler, A.Di Rocco)

[2] Advances in Neurology [1993] 60 : 681-684 (J.M.Rabey, Y.Vered, H.Shabtai, E.Graff, A.Harsat, A.D.Korczyn)

[3] Movement Disorders [2000] 15 (1) : 164-166 (H.Apaydin, S.Ertan, S.Ozekmeki)

[4] Journal of Neurology, Neurosurgery and Psychiatry [1992] 55 (8) : 725- 727 (J.M.Rabey, Y.Vered, H.Shabtai, E.Graff, A.D.Korczyn)

CHAPTER 42

PHARMACOLOGICAL TREATMENTS OF PARKINSON'S DISEASE

DOPAMINE AGONISTS

PHARMACOLOGY

Dopamine agonists are drugs that mimic dopamine by stimulating the dopamine receptors (D1, D2, D3, D4, D5) via translation. Although there are five dopamine receptors, dopamine agonists only significantly stimulate some of them. Besides the side effects they cause, dopamine agonists cause the dopamine receptors to become progressively less sensitive, thereby eventually increasing the symptoms.

TYPES OF DOPAMINE AGONISTS

Those dopamine agonists that are presently being used for the treatment of Parkinson's Disease are apomorphine [PAGE 617], bromocriptine [PAGE 622], cabergoline [PAGE 630], lisuride [PAGE 633], pardoprunox [PAGE 636], pergolide [PAGE 637], piribedil [PAGE 644], pramipexole [PAGE 646], ropinirole [PAGE 652] and rotigotine [PAGE 657]. Some of these dopamine agonists are taken by different means of administration, including orally, subcutaneous, intranasally, and sublingually.

APOMORPHINE

Brand names : Apokyn, Uprima, APO-Go, APO-Go Pen

Pharmacology : Apomorphine is a non-specific dopamine agonist with a strong action on D2, D3, D4 receptors [1, 2]. It has weaker action on D1 and D5 receptors [1, 2]. Apomorphine is administered in single subcutaneous injection, or in continuous subcutaneous infusion if more than 7 to 9 single injections are required daily [1]. The subcutaneous administration of apomorphine has effect within 10 minutes [1, 3, 4] but wears off within 40 to 90 minutes [1, 3] or within 2 hours [4].

Apomorphine may also be administered intranasally and sublingually. Intranasal apomorphine is more quickly and completely absorbed. Other routes of administration, including rectally, are not well absorbed but may also be used effectively [5].

Efficacy : Apomorphine significantly improved Parkinson's Disease symptoms [6-14], reduced "off" time [10, 12-26] by 36% to 59% [27, 28], even in more advanced stages of Parkinson's Disease [29]. Apomorphine reduced the L-dopa dose [9, 14, 20, 22, 25, 27], improved dyskinesia [10, 30, 31], but not in all cases [32], reduced tremor [33], improved male sexual function [34], enabled a small improvement in some aspects of visual perception [35], greatly reduced nocturnal awakenings, nocturia, and nocturnal off periods [36], and increased walking speed [37]. Intranasal apomorphine caused a significant improvement in Parkinson's Disease symptoms [38, 39] but intranasal apomorphine did not significantly reduce the daily "off" periods [38, 40]. All patients responded favourably to intranasal apomorphine [41]. The effect of subcutaneous apomorphine was quicker and longer lasting than the use of sublingual apomorphine [42].

Adverse effects : Common adverse effects are nausea [6-9], dyskinesia [3, 6, 43, 44, 45], somnolence [6, 43, 44], orthostatic hypotension [3, 37, 44], vomiting [43, 44], hallucinations [3, 43], yawning [6, 43], drowsiness [44], dizziness [42], psychiatric side effects [15, 48], disagreeable taste [37], impulse-control disorder (10%) [46], decreased blood pressure [6], injection site bruising [43], infusion site inflammation [15], nodular skin lesions when continuous apomorphine infusions were used [16], nasal irritation when apomorphine spray was used [47]. Adverse events were often benign [32].

[1] Neurologia i Neurochirurgia Polska [1999] 33 (6) : 1297-1303 (B. Zaleska, T.Domzal)

[2] Journal of Neural Transmission (Supplementum) [1995] 45 : 133-136 (R.Maggio, P.Barbier, G.U.Corsini)

[3] Neurology [2004] 62 (6 Supplement 4) : S18-S21 (M.Stacy)

[4] Neurology [2004] 62 (6 Supplement 4) : S12-S17 (S.A.Factor)

[5] Journal of Neural Transmission (Supplementum) [1995] 45 : 137-141 (S.Gancher)

[6] Parkinsonism & Related Disorders [2014] 20 (8) : 819-823 (N. Hattori, M.Nomoto)

[7] Drugs & Aging [2004] 21 (11) : 687-709 (D.Deleu, T.Hanssens, M.G.Northway)

[8] CNS Drugs [2008] 22 (6) : 519-527 (R.M.Trosch, D.Silver, P.B. Bottini)

[9] Journal of Parkinson's Disease [2011] 1 (2) : 197-203 (P.Martinez -Martin, P.Reddy, A.Antonini, T.Henriksen, R.Katzenschlager, P. Odin, A.Todorova, Y.Naidu, S.Tluk, C. Chandiramani, A.Martin, et al)

[10] Movement Disorders [2008] 23 (8) : 1130-1136 (P.J.García Ruiz, A.Sesar Ignacio, B.Ares Pensado, A.Castro García, F.Alonso Frech, M.Alvarez López, J.Arbelo González, J.Baiges Octavio, et al)

[11] Journal of the Neurological Sciences [2007] 258 (1-2) : 137-143 (R.Pahwa, W.C.Koller, R.M.Trosch, J.H.Sherry)

[12] Neurological Sciences [2002] 23 (Supplement 2) : S99-S100 (L. Priano, G.Albani, S.Calderoni, S.Baudo, L.Lopiano, M.Rizzone, V. Astolfi, R.Cavalli, M.R.Gasco, F.Fraschini, B.Bergamasco, A.Mauro)

[13] Archives of Neurology [2001] 58 (9) : 1385-1392 (R.B. Jr. Dewey, J.T.Hutton, P.A.LeWitt, S.A.Factor)

[14] Lancet [1988] 1 (8582) : 403-406 (C.M.Stibe, A.J.Lees, P.A. Kempster, G.M.Stern)

[15] Journal of Neurology, Neurosurgery, and Psychiatry [1998] 65 (5) : 709-716 (K.Pietz, P.Hagell, P.Odin)

[16] Clinical Neuropharmacology [1994] 17 (3) : 243-259 (C. Colosimo, M.Merello, A.Albanese)

[17] Clinical Neuropharmacology [2003] 26 (3) : 151-155 (F.Stocchi, A.Berardelli, L.Vacca, L.Barbato, A.Monge, G.Nordera, S.Ruggieri)

[18] Acta Neurologica Scandinavica [2009] 119 (5) : 345-348 (D. Nyholm, R.Constantinescu, B.Holmberg, N.Dizdar, H.Askmark)

[19] Clinical Therapeutics [2005] 27 (11) : 1710-1724 (J.J.Chen, C. Obering)

[20] Neurological Sciences [2003] 24 (3) : 174-175 (A.E.Di Rosa, A.Epifanio, A.Antonini, F.Stocchi, G.Martino, L.Di Blasi, A.Tetto, G.Basile, D.Imbesi, P.La Spina, G.Di Raimondo, L.Morgante)

[21] Harefuah [1999] 137 (10) : 444-446, 512, 511 (J.Zoldan, D. Merims, A.Kuritzky, I.Ziv, E.Melamed)

[22] Movement Disorders [1995] 10 (1) : 37-43 (S.T.Gancher, J.G. Nutt, W.R.Woodward)

[23] Medical Journal of Australia [1991] 155 (6) : 371-374 (P.K. Panegyres, S.J.Graham, B.K.Williams, B.M.Higgins, J.G.Morris)

[24] Arquivos de Neuro-Psiquiatria [1995] 53 (2) : 245-251 (H.B. Ferraz, S.M.Azevedo Silva, V.Borges, M.S.Rocha, L.A.Andrade)

[25] Annals of Pharmacotherapy [1995] 29 (3) : 282-288 (D.L. Corboy, M.L.Wagner, J.I.Sage)

[26] Clinical Neurology and Neurosurgery [1993] 95 (3) : 231-235 (T.van Laar, E.N.Jansen, A.W.Essink, C.Neef, S.Oosterloo, R.A.Roos)

[27] Parkinsonism & Related Disorders [2012] 18 (1) : 40-44 (S. Drapier, A.S.Gillioz, E.Leray, J.Péron, T.Rouaud, A.Marchand, M. Vérin)

[28] Movement Disorders [2000] 15 (5) : 789-794 (W.Poewe, G.K. Wenning)

[29] Praxis [2001] 90 (23) : 1024-1034 (C.Gutknecht)

[30] Movement Disorders [2005] 20 (2) : 151-157 (R.Katzenschlager, A.Hughes, A.Evans, A.J.Manson, M.Hoffman, L.Swinn, H.Watt, K. Bhatia, N.Quinn, A.J.Lees)

[31] Movement Disorders [2002] 17 (6) : 1235-1241 (A.J.Manson, K. Turner, A.J.Lees)

[32] Revue Neurologique [2014] 170 (3) : 205-215 (M.Rambour, C. Moreau, J.Salleron, D.Devos, A.Kreisler, E.Mutez, C.Simonin, A. Annic, K.Dujardin, A.Destée, L.Defebvre)

[33] Biomedicine & Pharmacotherapy [2008] 62 (4) : 250-252 (M.A. Hellmann, T.Sabach, E.Melamed, R.Djaldetti)

[34] Movement Disorders [1998] 13 (3) : 536-539 (J.D.O'Sullivan, A.J.Hughes)

[35] Journal of Neural Transmission [2000] 107 (1) : 87-94 (T.Büttner, T.Müller, W.Kuhn)

[36] Acta Neurologica Scandinavica [1999] 100 (3) : 163-167 (I. Reuter, C.M.Ellis, K.Ray Chaudhuri)

[37] Clinical Neuropharmacology [1999] 22 (1) : 1-4 (W.Ondo, C. Hunter, M.Almaguer, S.Gancher, J.Jankovic)

[38] Journal of Parkinson's Disease [2013] 3 (1) : 31-37 (K.A.Grosset, N.Malek, F.Morgan, D.G.Grosset)

[39] Acta Neurologica Scandinavica [2013] 128 (3) : 166-171 (K.A. Grosset, N.Malek, F.Morgan, D.G.Grosset)

[40] European Journal of Neurology [2013] 20 (11) : 1445-1450 (K.A. Grosset, N.Malek, F.Morgan, D.G.Grosset)

[41] Archives of Neurology [1992] 49 (5) : 482-484 (T.van Laar, E.N. Jansen, A.W.Essink, C.Neef)

[42] Journal of Neurology, Neurosurgery, and Psychiatry [1993] 56 (1) : 101-103 (D.Deffond, F.Durif, M.Tournilhac)

[43] Clinical Neuropharmacology [2009] 32 (2) : 89-93 (P.A.LeWitt, W.G.Ondo, B.Van Lunen, P.B.Bottini)

[44] The Medical Letter on Drugs and Therapeutics [2005] 47 (1200) : 7-8 (No authors listed)

[45] Movement Disorders [1993] 8 (2) : 165-170 (A.J.Hughes, S. Bishop, B.Kleedorfer, N.Turjanski, W.Fernandez, A.J.Lees, G.M. Stern)

[46] Synapse [2015] 69 (4) : 183-189 (P.Seeman)

[47] Movement Disorders [1998] 13 (5) : 782-787 (R.B.Jr. Dewey, D.M.Maraganore, J.E.Ahlskog, J.Y.Matsumoto)

[48] Journal of Neurology [2017] Mar 31 [Epub ahead of print] (A.Sesar, G.Fernández-Pajarín, B.Ares, M.T.Rivas, A.Castro)

BROMOCRIPTINE

Brand names : Parlodel, Cycloset, Brotin

Pharmacology : Bromocriptine is a dopamine receptor agonist that primarily stimulates the D2 dopamine receptor [1, 2].

Efficacy : Bromocriptine reduced Parkinson's Disease symptoms in most people [2-33]. The least disabled patients showed the greatest response [2, 10, 34]. The effectiveness of bromocriptine may persist for at least one to two years [7, 11, 18, 20, 26, 35, 36], in some cases three years or more [15, 20, 37], and even four years or more [33]. Results of more prolonged treatment are not available [35]. However, bromocriptine is ineffective in the very advanced stages of Parkinson's Disease [38]. The optimal daily requirement of bromocriptine was correlated to the severity and duration of the illness but not to the age of the patient [39]. Some people were able to stop taking L-dopa [8, 9, 12], reduce their L-dopa dose [21, 23, 40-43], or reduce end of dose deterioration [13], but a reduction in L-dopa dose could also result in an increased bromocriptine requirement [44]. Neurological deficits improved by almost 20% in severely disabled patients [45]. Amelioration of mildly affected patients was about 10% [45]. There was a modest but significant improvement, which was most evident in the improvement in tremor [46]. Bromocriptine therapy improved neurologic manifestations and reduced both supine and standing systolic blood pressures and standing diastolic blood pressure with no consistent change in heart rate [47].

Adverse effects : Adverse reactions were similar to those observed with the use of L-dopa [6, 8, 12] except that, in individual patients, abnormal involuntary movements and diurnal oscillations in performance (the on-off effect) were decreased, but orthostatic hypotension and mental changes were increased [12]. Adverse reactions were dose dependent and usually reversible [8]. Adverse effects were common [46], and occur in as many as 70% of people [25] thereby limiting the usefulness of bromocriptine, but they were generally mild in severity [46] or in some cases could be transient [4]. Only 15% of patients had adverse reactions severe enough to necessitate discontinuation of bromocriptine [10]. However, a lot of people discontinued bromocriptine anyway because of the dyskinesia it caused [27]. No serious adverse reactions were noted with the gradually increasing dosage regimen [3]. High cost and severe psychosis are the main disadvantages of bromocriptine [48]. The main adverse effect was a confusional state [49]. Other adverse effects include nausea [13, 21, 40, 50], dyskinesia [21, 27, 50], hallucinations [41, 50], alopecia (which is uncommon) [51], impulse-control disorder (in 6%) [52], delusions [41], substantial confusion [41], dizziness [40], acute myocardial infarction [41], active peptic ulceration [41], hyperkinesia [5], pleuroplumonary disease (which is uncommon) [41, 53-56], vomiting and epigastric discomfort [24], mental changes [21, 27], valvular heart disease [57], erythromelalgia [40], and psychiatric disturbances [40].

Comparison : Comparisons were made between the use of bromocriptine and other dopamine agonists or L-dopa. When added to the use of L-dopa, bromocriptine had no additional effect [58-66], or there was a beneficial effect but at the expense of unacceptable adverse effects [67]. However, in another study adding bromocriptine was beneficial [7]. The effect of bromocriptine on its own was less [68, 69, 70] or similar [71-74] to the effect of L-dopa. Pergolide was more effective than bromocriptine [75-80] or was similar in effect to bromocriptine [81, 82], and caused fewer [79] or similar adverse effects [77, 78]. Ropinirole was more effective than bromocriptine [83, 84, 85] or was little different in effect [86]. Cabergoline was slightly more effective than bromocriptine and the adverse effects were similar [87]. Lisuride had similar efficacy to bromocriptine [82, 88-91] but caused fewer adverse effects [91]. Pramipexole was little different in effect to bromocriptine [92, 93], or was more effective [94], and caused similar adverse effects [94].

[1] Progress in Neuro-Psychopharmacology and Biological Psychiatry [1995] 19 (7) : 1147-1154 (J.De Keyser, J.P.De Backer, N.Wilczak, L.Herroelen)

[2] Journal of Neurology, Neurosurgery, and Psychiatry [1976] 39 (2) : 184-193 (J.D.Parkes, C.D.Marsden, I.Donaldson, A.Galea-Debono, J. Walters, G.Kennedy, P.Asselman)

[3] Clinical Neuropharmacology [1984] 7 (3) : 231-237 (G.Devathasan, P.N.Chong, K.Puvanendran, K.C.Lun, P.K.Wong)

[4] Clinical Neuropharmacology [1987] 10 (2) : 168-174 (E.Tolosa, R. Blesa, A.Bayes, F.Forcadell)

[5] Acta Neurologica Scandinavica [1977] 56 (3) : 269-273 (U.Gron)

[6] Lancet [1976] 2 (7980) : 272-275 (R.Kartzinel, P.Teychenne, M.M. Gillespie, M.Perlow, A.C.Gielen, D.A.Sadowsky, D.B.Calne)

[7] Clinical Neuropharmacology [1986] 9 (2) : 138-145 (P.F. Teychenne, D.Bergsrud, R.L.Elton, A.Racy)

[8] Lancet [1975] 2 (7933) : 473-476 (P.F.Teychenne, P.N.Leigh, J.L. Reid, D.B.Calne, J.K.Greenacre, A.Petrie, A.N.Bamji)

[9] Medical Journal of Australia [1978] 2 (3 Supplement) : 28-31 (J. Wodak, R.Stark, B.Gilligan)

[10] Neurology [1985] 35 (2) : 199-206 (M.M.Hoehn, R.L.Elton)

[11] Advances in Neurology [1983] 37 : 17-21 (G.M.Stern, A.J.Lees)

[12] New England Journal of Medicine [1976] 295 (25) : 1400- 1404 (A.Lieberman, M.Kupersmith, E.Estey, M.Goldstein)

[13] Canadian Journal of Neurological Sciences [1984] 11 (4) : 452-456 (J.D.Grimes, D.B.King, O.S.Kofman, P.Molina-Negro, A.F. Wilson, S.Bouchard)

[14] European Neurology [1982] 21 (4) : 217-226 (G.Gauthier, A. Martins da Silva)

[15] European Neurology [1990] 30 (Supplement 1) : 3-8 (T.Nakanishi, I.Kanazawa, I.Goto, M.Iwata, H.Kowa, T.Mannen, Y.Mizuno, H. Nishitani, N.Ogawa, A.Takahashi)

[16] Clinical Neuropharmacology [1994] 17 (5) : 435-444 (S.Giménez-Roldán, D.Mateo)

[17] Revue Neurologique [1982] 138 (5) : 401-408 (A.Rascol, J.L. Montastruc, B.Guiraud-Chaumeil, M.Clanet)

[18] Journal of Neurology, Neurosurgery, and Psychiatry [1976] 39 (11) : 1101-1108 (J.D.Parkes, A.G.Debono, C.D.Marsden)

[19] Clinical Neuropharmacology [1985] 8 (1) : 73-77 (J.D.Grimes, M.R.Delgado)

[20] Journal of Neurology, Neurosurgery, and Psychiatry [1981] 44 (11) : 1020-1023 (A.J.Lees, G.M.Stern)

[21] Canadian Journal of Neurological Sciences [1984] 11 (1 Supplement) : 233-237 (A.N.Lieberman, G.Gopinathan, H.Hassouri, A.Neophytides, M.Goldstein)

[22] Acta Neurologica Scandinavica [1985] 72 (2) : 157-170 (Y. Toyokura, Y.Mizuno, M.Kase, I.Sobue, Y.Kuroiwa, H.Narabayashi, M. Uono, T.Nakanishi, M.Kameyama, H.Ito)

[23] Journal of Neurology [1982] 228 (4) : 249-258 (E.Schneider, P.A.Fischer)

[24] Neurology [1991] 41 (10) : 1598-1602 (T.Mannen, Y.Mizuno, M.Iwata, I.Goto, I.Kanazawa, H.Kowa, H.Nishitani, N.Ogawa, A. Takahashi, K.Tashiro)

[25] Neurology [1979] 29 (8) : 1077-1083 (S.Fahn, L.J.Cote, S.R. Snider, R.E.Barrett, W.P.Isgreen)

[26] Neurology [1980] 30 (5) : 518-523 (A.Lieberman, M.Kupersmith, A.Neophytides, I.Casson, R.Durso, S.H.Foo, M.Khayali, G.Bear, M. Goldstein)

[27] Neurology [1979] 29 (3) : 363-369 (A.N.Lieberman, M. Kupersmith, G.Gopinathan, E.Estey, A.Goodgold, M.Goldstein)

[28] Neurology [1982] 32 (6) : 577-583 (P.F.Teychenne, D.Bergsrud, A.Racy, R.L.Elton, B.Vern)

[29] Srpski Arhiv za Celokupno Lekarstvo [1992] 120 (1-2) : 1-5 (N. Sternic, V.Kostic)

[30] Journal of Neurology, Neurosurgery, and Psychiatry [1979] 42 (2) : 143-150 (A.Rascol, B.Guiraud, J.L.Montastruc, J.David, M.Clanet)

[31] European Neurology [1997] 38 (Supplement 2) : 37-49 (N.Ogawa, I.Kanazawa, H.Kowa, S.Kuno, Y.Mizuno, K.Tashiro, N.Yanagisawa)

[32] Pharmacological Reviews [1985] 37 (2) : 217-227 (A.N. Lieberman, M.Goldstein)

[33] Journal of Neurology, Neurosurgery, and Psychiatry [1994] 57 (9) : 1034-1038 (J.L.Montastruc, O.Rascol, J.M.Senard, A.Rascol)

[34] European Neurology [1996] 36 (3) : 164-170 (H.Fukuyama, J. Kawamura, I.Akiguchi, J.Kimura, T.Imai)

[35] Journal of the American Geriatrics Society [1981] 29 (6) : 251-258 (M.M.Hoehn)

[36] Acta Neurologica Scandinavica [1990] 81 (5) : 383-387 (B. Bergamasco, P.Benna, L.Scarzella)

[37] European Neurology [1991] 31 (Supplement 1) : 3-16 (T. Nakanishi, Y.Mizuno, I.Goto, M.Iwata, I.Kanazawa, H.Kowa, T. Mannen, H. Nishitani, N.Ogawa, A.Takahashi)

[38] Canadian Journal of Neurological Sciences [1984] 11 (1 Supplement) : 229-232 (A.Rascol, J.L.Montastruc, O.Rascol)

[39] Neurology [1984] 34 (6) : 795-797 (T.A.Larsen, R.Newman, P.LeWitt, D.B.Calne)

[40] Lancet [1978] 1 (8067) : 735-738 (D.B.Calne, C.Plotkin, A.C. Williams, J.G.Nutt, A.Neophytides, P.F.Teychenne)

[41] Journal of Neural Transmission [1981] 51 (1-2) : 175-184 (P.A.Le Witt, D.B.Calne)

[42] European Neurology [1990] 30 (2) : 108-111 (A.M.Bakheit, L.M. Henderson, A.P.Moore, J.A.Simpson, M.Thomas)

[43] South African Medical Journal [1990] 78 (11) : 680-685 (J.A. Temlett, A.Ming, M.Saling, V.U.Fritz, A.Blumenfeld, T.R.Bilchik, A.L.Becker, P.B.Fourie, H.E.Reef)

[44] Canadian Journal of Neurological Sciences [1984] 11 (1 Supplement) : 225-228 (J.D.Grimes)

[45] British Medical Journal [1974] 4 (5942) : 442-444 (D.B.Calne, P.F.Teychenne, L.E.Claveria, R.Eastman, J.K.Greenacre, A.Petrie)

[46] Archives of Neurology [1985] 42 (6) : 586-588 (R.F.Pfeiffer, K. Wilken, C.Glaeske, A.S.Lorenzo)

[47] Neurology [1985] 35 (11) : 1644-1647 (J.L.Montastruc, B. Chamontin, A.Rascol)

[48] British Medical Journal [1978] 1 (6124) : 1402-1404 (I.Pearce, J.M.Pearce)

[49] Canadian Journal of Neurological Sciences [1983] 10 (2) : 86-90 (J.D.Grimes, M.N.Hassan)

[50] Medical Journal of Australia [1978] 2 (3 Supplement) : 27-28 (R.A.Mackenzie, J.W.Lance)

[51] Clinical Neuropharmacology [1993] 16 (3) : 266-268 (N.Fabre, J.L.Montastruc, O.Rascol)

[52] Synapse [2015] 69 (4) : 183-189 (P.Seeman)

[53] Clinical and Experimental Neurology [1990] 27 : 79-82 (D.H. Todman, W.A.Oliver, R.L.Edwards)

[54] Archives of Internal Medicine [1988] 148 (10) : 2231-2236 (N.G. McElvaney, P.G.Wilcox, A.Churg, J.A.Fleetham)

[55] Chest [1988] 94 (5) : 1034-1036 (E.Kinnunen, A.Viljanen)

[56] La Semaine des Hopitaux [1984] 60 (11) : 741-744 (J.Vergeret, M.Barat, A.Taytard, P.Bellvert, P.Domblides, J.J.Douvier, P.Fréour)

[57] Movement Disorders [2009] 24 (3) : 344-349 (L.C.Tan, K.K.Ng, W.L.Au, R.K.Lee, Y.H.Chan, N.C.Tan)

[58] European Journal of Neurology [1998] 5 (3) : 255-263 (F.Alarcon, N.Cevallos, A.J.Lees)

[59] Journal of Clinical and Experimental Neuropsychology [1978] 15 : 228-236 (R.A.Mackenzie, J.W.Lance)

[60] Clinical Neuropharmacology [1997] 20 (1) : 67-76 (S. Giménez-Roldán, E.Tolosa, J.A.Burguera, J.Chacón, H.Liaño, F. Forcadell)

[61] European Neurology [1996] 36 (Supplement 1) : 32-37 (K. Tashiro, I.Goto, I.Kanazawa, H.Kowa, S.Kuno, Y.Mizuno, N.Ogawa, N.Yanagisawa)

[62] Clinical and Experimental Neurology [1989] 26 : 129-139 (G. Selby)

[63] European Neurology [1994] 34 (Supplement 3) : 29-35 (N. Yanagisawa, I.Kanazawa, I.Goto, H.Kowa, S.Kuno, Y.Mizuno, K. Tashiro, N.Ogawa)

[64] European Neurology [1992] 32 (Supplement 1) : 9-22 (T. Nakanishi, M.Iwata, I.Goto, I.Kanazawa, H.Kowa, T.Mannen, Y. Mizuno, H. Nishitani, N.Ogawa, A.Takahashi)

[65] Journal of Neurology, Neurosurgery, and Psychiatry [1999] 67 (3) : 300-307 (M.A.Hely, J.G.Morris, R.Traficante, W.G.Reid, D.J. O'Sullivan, P.M.Williamson)

[66] Cochrane Database of Systematic Reviews [2002] (2) : CD003634 (C.Ramaker, J.J.Hilten)

[67] Archives of Neurology [1978] 35 (8) : 503-505 (A.J.Lees, S. Haddad, K.M.Shaw, L.J.Kohout, G.M.Stern)

[68] Journal of Neurology, Neurosurgery, and Psychiatry [1989] 52 (3) : 324-328 (M.A.Hely, J.G.Morris, D.Rail, W.G.Reid, D.J.O'Sullivan, P.M.Williamson, S.Genge, G.A.Broe)

[69] Rivista di Patologia Nervosa e Mentale [1978] 99 (3) : 150-163 (A.Quattrini, A.Paggi, M.Del Pesce, P.Di Bella)

[70] BMJ [1993] 307 (6902) : 469-472 (No authors listed)

[71] Archives of Neurology [1978] 35 (8) : 503-505 (A.J.Lees, S. Haddad, K.M.Shaw, L.J.Kohout, G.M.Stern)

[72] European Neurology [1988] 28 (Supplement 1) : 11-14 (R.J. Riopelle, M.J.Gawel, I.Libman, D.B.King, D.R.McLean, R.Paulseth, B. Raphy, S.Bouchard)

[73] Canadian Journal of Neurological Sciences [1987] 14 (4) : 576-580 (I.Libman, M.J.Gawel, R.J.Riopelle, S.Bouchard)

[74] Neurology [1987] 37 (5) : 826-828 (U.K.Rinne)

[75] Value in Health [2001] 4 (4) : 308-315 (P.Davey, N.Rajan, M. Lees, M.Aristides)

[76] Cochrane Database of Systematic Reviews [2000] (2) : CD000236 (C.E.Clarke, J.M.Speller)

[77] Neurology [1995] 45 (3 Supplement 3) : S22-S27 (G.Pezzoli, E. Martignoni, C.Pacchetti, V.Angeleri, P.Lamberti, A.Muratorio, U. Bonuccelli, M.De Mari, N.Foschi, E.Cossutta)

[78] Revista de Neurología (1997) 25 (145) : 1343-1345 (J.G.de Yébenes, P.J.García-Ruiz, R.Sánchez-Pernaute)

[79] Movement Disorders [1994] 9 (4) : 431-436 (G.Pezzoli, E.Martignoni, C.Pacchetti, V.A.Angeleri, P.Lamberti, A.Muratorio, U. Bonuccelli, M.De Mari, N.Foschi, E.Cossutta)

[80] Advances in Neurology [1983] 37 : 95-108 (A.N.Lieberman, A. Neophytides, M.Leibowitz, G.Gopinathan, V.Pact, R.Walker, A. Goodgold, M.Goldstein)

[81] Cleveland Clinic Journal of Medicine [1995] 62 (4) : 212-217 (R. Pahwa, W.C.Koller)

[82] Neurology [1983] 33 (8) : 1009-1014 (P.A.LeWitt, C.D.Ward, T.A.Larsen, M.I.Raphaelson, R.P.Newman, N.Foster, J.M.Dambrosia, D.B.Calne)

[83] Clinical Neuropharmacology [2001] 24 (6) : 346-351 (S. Giménez-Roldán, E.M.Esteban, D.Mateo)

[84] American Journal of Health-System Pharmacy [1999] 56 (3) : 217-224 (M.D.Kuzel)

[85] Movement Disorders [1998] 13 (1) : 46-51 (A.D.Korczyn, D.J. Brooks, E.R.Brunt, W.H.Poewe, O.Rascol, F.Stocchi)

[86] Cochrane Database of Systematic Reviews [2000] (3) : CD001517 (C.E.Clarke, K.H.Deane)

[87] Neurology [1996] 47 (3) : 785-788 (R.Inzelberg, P.Nisipeanu, J.M. Rabey, E.Orlov, T.Catz, S.Kippervasser, E.Schechtman, A.D. Korczyn)

[88] Cochrane Database of Systematic Reviews [2000] (2) : CD001514 (C.E.Clarke, J.M.Speller)

[89] Acta Neurologica Scandinavica [1992] 86 (6) : 593-595 (A. Laihinen, U.K.Rinne, I.Suchy)

[90] Neurology [1982] 32 (1) : 69-72 (P.A.LeWitt, G.Gopinathan, C. D.Ward, J.N.Sanes, J.M.Dambrosia, R.Durso, D.B.Calne)

[91] Annals of Neurology [1983] 13 (1) : 44-47 (A.N.Lieberman, G. Gopinathan, A.Neophytides, M.Leibowitz, R.Walker, E.Hiesiger)

[92] Cochrane Database of Systematic Reviews [2000] (3) : CD002259 (C.E.Clarke, J.M.Speller, J.A.Clarke)

[93] Neurology [1999] 52 (6) : 1227-1229 (C.G.Goetz, L.Blasucci, G. T.Stebbins)

[94] Neurology [1997] 49 (4) : 1060-1065 (M.Guttman)

CABERGOLINE

Brand names : Cabaser, Dostinex

Pharmacology : Cabergoline is a dopamine agonist that primarily stimulates the D2 receptor activity and has a very long half-life [1]. Besides being used for the treatment of Parkinson's Disease, cabergoline is also used for the treatment of hyperprolactinemia, and exerts anti-depressant effects [2].

Efficacy : When cabergoline was compared to the use of L-dopa : motor complications, such as dyskinesia occurred less frequently [3], symptoms overall were worse [4], some symptom scores apart from motor disability were better [3], off time was reduced [5,6], there were greater side effects [3,4,7], including nausea, vomiting, dyspepsia, gastritis, dizziness, postural hypotension, and peripheral oedema [8]. When cabergoline was added to the use of L-dopa : symptoms improved [9-14] but not by much [13], there was a small reduction in off time [3,12,13,15,16], the L-dopa dose was reduced [3,5], and side effects increased [10,11,13].

Adverse effects : Cabergoline is associated with the risk of valvular heart disease [17, 18], valvular regurgitation [18-25], and worsens contrast sensitivity [26].

Comparison : Cabergoline was found to be slightly more effective or similar in effect to the use of bromocriptine [15, 27].

[1] Clinical Neuropharmacology [2008] 31 (1) : 19-24 (G.Linazasoro)

[2] Psychopharmacology [2010] 211 (3) : 291-301 (S.Chiba, T. Numakawa, M.Ninomiya, H.S.Yoon, H.Kunugi)

[3] Cochrane Database Systematic Reviews [2001] (1) : CD001518 (C.E.Clarke, K.H.Deane)

[4] Neurology [1997] 48 (2) : 363-368 (U.K.Rinne, F.Bracco, C. Chouza, E.Dupont, O.Gershanik, J.F.MartiMasso, J.L.Montastruc, C.D. Marsden, A.Dubini, N.Orlando, R.Grimaldi)

[5] Journal of Neurology [1996] 243 (1) : 68-72 (M.J.Steiger, T. El-Debas, T.Anderson, L.J.Findley, C.D.Marsden)

[6] Neurology [1993] 43 (12) : 2587-2590 (G.Lera, J.Vaamonde, M. Rodriguez, J.A.Obeso)

[7] Neurology [1993] 43 (3 Part 1) : 613-616 (J.T.Hutton, J.L.Morris, M.A.Brewer)

[8] CNS Drugs [2004] 18 (11) : 733-746 (F.Bracco, A.Battaglia, C. Chouza, E.Dupont, O.Gershanik, J.F.Marti Masso, J.L.Montastruc)

[9] European Neurology [2001] 46 (Supplement 1) : 18-23 (H.K.Baas, P.Schueler)

[10] Clinical Neuropharmacology [1996] 19 (3) : 202-212 (J.E. Ahlskog, K.F.Wright, M.D.Muenter, C.H.Adler)

[11] Neurology [1996] 46 (4) : 1062-1065 (J.T.Hutton, W.C.Koller, J. E.Ahlskog, R.Pahwa, H.I.Hurtig, M.B.Stern, B.C.Hiner, A.Lieberman, R.F.Pfeiffer, R.L.Rodnitzky, C.H.Waters, M.D.Muenter, et al)

[12] Neurology [1993] 43 (10) : 1981-1984 (A.Lieberman, S.Imke, M. Muenter, K.Wheeler, J.E.Ahlskog, J.Y.Matsumoto, D.M.Maraganore, K.F.Wright, J.Schoenfelder)

[13] Clinical Neuropharmacology [1994] 17 (3) : 286-293 (J.M.Rabey, P.Nissipeanu, R.Inzelberg, A.D.Korczyn)

[14] Archives of Neurology [1994] 51 (12) : 1236-1241 (J.E.Ahlskog, M.D.Muenter, D.M.Maraganore, J.Y.Matsumoto, A.Lieberman, K.F. Wright, K.Wheeler)

[15] Movement Disorders [1995] 10 (5) : 604-607 (R.Inzelberg, P. Nisipeanu, M.J.Rabey, A.D.Korczyn)

[16] Drugs [1998] 55 (Supplement 1) : 17-22 (C.D.Marsden)

[17] Journal of Neural Transmission [2009] 116 (2) : 179-191 (M. Steiger, W.Jost, F.Grandas, G.Van Camp)

[18] CNS Drugs [2015] 29 (12) : 985-998 (T.Tran, J.M.Brophy, S. Suissa, C.Renoux)

[19] Journal of Neural Transmission [2009] 116 (2) : 171-178 (T.Oeda, M.Masaki, K.Yamamoto, E.Mizuta, N.Kitagawa, T.Isono, S.Taniguchi, K.Doi, H.Yaku, C.Yutani, T.Kawamura, S.Kuno, H.Sawada)

[20] Movement Disorders [2008] 23 (7) : 935-941 (K.Yamashiro, M. Komine-Kobayashi, T.Hatano, T.Urabe, H.Mochizuki, N.Hattori, Y. Iwama, H.Daida, M.Sakai, T.Nakayama, Y.Mizuno)

[21] Clinical Neurology and Neurosurgery [2007] 109 (4) : 350-353 (G. Kenangil, S.Ozekmekçi, L.Koldas, T.Sahin, E.Erginöz)

[22] New England Journal of Medicine [2007] 356 (1) : 39-46 (R. Zanettini, A.Antonini, G.Gatto, R.Gentile, S.Tesei, G.Pezzoli)

[23] New England Journal of Medicine [2007] 356 (1) : 29-38 (R. Schade, F.Andersohn, S.Suissa, W.Haverkamp, E.Garbe)

[24] Movement Disorders [2007] 22 (2) : 234-238 (S.Junghanns, J.T. Fuhrmann, G.Simonis, C.Oelwein, R.Koch, R.H.Strasser, H. Reichmann, A.Storch)

[25] Movement Disorders [2011] 26 (5) : 801-806 (V.G.Rasmussen, K.Østergaard, E.Dupont, S.H.Poulsen)

[26] Parkinsonism & Related Disorders [1999] 5 (3) : 87-91 (J.T.Hutton, J.L.Morris, J.W.Elias)

[27] Neurology [1996] 47 (3) : 785-788 (R.Inzelberg, P.Nisipeanu, J. M.Rabey, E.Orlov, T.Catz, S.Kippervasser, E.Schechtman, A.D. Korczyn)

LISURIDE

Brand names : Dopergin, Proclacam, Revanil

Pharmacology : Lisuride is primarily a Dopamine D2 receptor agonist. There is also lesser stimulation of the D3 Dopamine receptor [1]. Lisuride is also a serotonin agonist [2]. Subcutaneous lisuride can be administered using a portable infusion pump [3].

Efficacy : Lisuride improved Parkinson's Disease symptoms [2-18], including an increase in "on" time [2, 7] and a reduction in "off" periods [7, 12, 19]. Lisuride resulted in 34% to 56% improvement in disability scores and 47% in relief in Activities of Daily Living [12, 16, 20]. Multiple doses of lisuride achieved better results than its usual schedule of only 3 to 4 times a day [21]. Lisuride enabled a reduction in L-dopa dosage in half or more patients [3, 11, 16, 20, 22]. The initiation of L-dopa could be postponed in 60% of patients for over a year [23]. There was a slight decrease in the efficacy of lisuride after three months [24]. After 18 to 24 months there was a slight increase in symptoms [16], and even more so after 45 months [25], but not in all cases [7].

Adverse effects : Psychiatric symptoms were commonly reported [3, 12, 13, 14, 17, 18, 24, 25, 26]. Most people with adverse effects of psychiatric symptoms withdrew treatment [13]. Dry mouth, nausea, weakness, postural hypotension, and headache were the other most frequently encountered side effects of lisuride [20]. Less commonly reported were chorea and orofacial dyskinesia [9]. Discontinuation of lisuride due to adverse effects was necessary in 17% of people [16]. When lisuride was administered as an infusion via an externally worn pump the most common side effect was the presence of subcutaneous nodules appearing at the injection site. Other patients reported mild hemorrhagic complications or nausea [18]. The long term use of lisuride led to dyskinesias or "off" periods, or both in most people taking it [17].

Comparison : Lisuride could not replace the use of L-dopa in all patients [27, 28, 29], but it was more effective than L-dopa in some people [25]. After four years of use, lisuride resulted in significantly fewer end-of-dose disturbances and peak-dose dyskinesias, but also caused less improvement in Parkinson's Disease symptoms than with L-dopa [30]. Lisuride and pergolide are equally useful in advanced Parkinson's Disease [31]. Lisuride is similar in efficacy and adverse effects to bromocriptine [32, 33, 34]. The only significant differences were slightly better control of akinesia with bromocriptine [35]. With lisuride there was more control [8], and also gastro-intestinal and neuropsychiatric side effects [27].

[1] Progress in Neuro-Psychopharmacology & Biological Psychiatry [1995] 19 (7) : 1147-1154 (J.De Keyser, J.P.De Backer, N.Wilczak, L.Herroelen)

[2] Neurology [1981] 31 (11) : 1466-1469 (A.N.Lieberman, M. Goldstein, M.Leibowitz, A.Neophytides, G.Gopinathan, R.Walker, V. Pact)

[3] Journal of Neural Transmission (Supplementum) [1988] 27 : 17-25 (J.A.Obeso, M.R.Luquin, J.Vaamonde, J.M.Martînez Lage)

[4] Movement Disorders [2001] 16 (2) : 301-305 (F.Stocchi, L.Vacca, A.Berardelli, F.De Pandis, S.Ruggieri)

[5] Internal Medicine [1998] 37 (5) : 444-448 (R.Hayashi, K.Tako, H. Makishita, J.Koyama, N.Yanagisawa)

[6] Acta Neurologica Scandinavica [1992] 86 (6) : 593-595 (A. Laihinen, U.K.Rinne, I.Suchy)

[7] Brain [2002] 125 (Part 9) : 2058-2066 (F.Stocchi, S.Ruggieri, L. Vacca, C.W.Olanow)

[8] Neurology [1981] 31 (4) : 371-376 (G.Gopinathan, H.Teräväinen, J.M.Dambrosia, C.D.Ward, J.N.Sanes, W.K.Stuart, E.V.Evarts, D.B. Calne)

[9] Annals of Neurology [1981] 9 (1) : 48-52 (J.D.Parkes, M.Schachter, C.D.Marsden, B.Smith, A.Wilson)

[10] Therapie [1991] 46 (6) : 481-486 (P.Vermersch, J.Fondarai, H. Petit)

[11] European Neurology [1983] 22 (4) : 240-255 (R.J.McDonald, R. Horowski)

[12] European Neurology [1983] 22 (2) : 119-123 (A.N.Lieberman, M. Goldstein, G.Gopinathan, M.Leibowitz, A.Neophytides, R.Walker, E. Hiesiger)

[13] Journal of Neural Transmission (Supplementum) [1988] 27 : 55-60 (P.H.Critchley, F.Grandas Perez, N.P.Quinn, J.D.Parkes, C.D.Marsden)

[14] Journal of Neural Transmission (Supplementum) [1988] 27 : 85-90 (O.S.Gershanik, O.Scipioni, S.García)

[15] Progress in Neuro-Psychopharmacology & Biological Psychiatry [1989] 13 (1-2) : 173-183 (S.Ruggieri, F.Stocchi, A.Carta, M.Bragoni, C.Agostini, L.Barbato, A.Agnoli)

[16] Wiener Medizinische Wochenschrift [1987] 137 (7-8) : 155-159 (K.Jellinger)

[17] Brain [1991] 114 (Part 1B) : 601-617 (J.Vaamonde, M.R.Luquin, J.A.Obeso)

[18] Journal of Neural Transmission (Supplementum) [1988] 27 : 75-84 (M.Fernandez Pardal, F.Micheli, M.Gatto, N.Perez y Gonzalez)

[19] Journal of Neural Transmission. Parkinson's Disease and Dementia Section [1992] 4 : 291-301 (A.Heinz, I.Suchy, I.Klewin, W. Kuhn, P. Klotz, H.Przuntek)

[20] Advances in Neurology [1996] 69 : 519-530 (K.Bayülkem, K. Erisir, A.Tuncel, B.Bayülkem)

[21] Neurologia [1989] 4 (7) : 229-232 (M.R.Luquín, J.A.Obeso, J. Vaamonde, J.M.Martínez Lage)

[22] European Neurology [2000] 44 (1) : 22-30 (H.Allain, A.Destée, H. Petit, M.Patay, S.Schück, D.Bentué-Ferrer, P.Le Cavorzin)

[23] Journal of Neural Transmission. Parkinson's Disease and Dementia Section [1991] 3 (4) : 273-283 (I.Runge, R.Horowski)

[24] European Neurology [1986] 25 (1) : 74-80 (G.Meneghetti, F. Bracco, B.Giometto, S.Ferla, E.Schergna)

[25] Neurology [1981] 31 (8) : 961-965 (A.Lieberman, M.Goldstein, A. Neophytides, M.Kupersmith, M.Leibowitz, N.Zasorin, R.Walker, D. Kleinberg)

[26] Clinical and Experimental Neurology [1986] 22 : 63-69 (D.Chin, Y.L.Yu, C.Y.Huang)

[27] Acta Neurologica Scandinavica [1980] 62 (6) : 382-385 (M. Schachter, M.P.Sheehy, J.D.Parkes, C.D.Marsden)

[28] Journal of Neural Transmission (Supplementum) [1988] 27 : 27-33 (F.Stocchi, S.Ruggieri, A.Antonini, F.Baronti, G.Brughitta, P. Bellantuono, D.Bravi, A.Agnoli)

[29] Movement Disorders [1988] 3 (4) : 313-319 (S.Ruggieri, F. Stocchi, A.Carta, D.Bravi, M.Bragoni, L.Giorgi, A.Agnoli)

[30] Neurology [1989] 39 (3) : 336-339 (U.K.Rinne)

[31] American Journal of the Medical Sciences [1985] 290 (3) : 102-106 (A.N.Lieberman, M.Leibowitz, G.Gopinathan, R.Walker, E. Hiesiger, J.Nelson, M.Goldstein)

[32] Advances in Neurology [1983] 37 : 131-140 (P.A.LeWitt, R.S. Burns, D.B.Calne)

[33] Annals of Neurology [1983] 13 (1) : 44-47 (A.N.Lieberman, G. Gopinathan, A.Neophytides, M.Leibowitz, R.Walker, E.Hiesiger)

[34] Cochrane Database of Systematic Reviews [2000] (2) : CD001514 (C.E.Clarke, J.M.Speller)

[35] Neurology [1982] 32 (1) : 69-72 (P.A.LeWitt, G.Gopinathan, C.D. Ward, J.N.Sanes, J.M.Dambrosia, R.Durso, D.B.Calne)

PARDOPRUNOX

Brand names : none (due to being in development)

Pharmacology : Pardoprunox is a partial dopamine agonist being assessed for its use in Parkinson's Disease. It partially stimulates dopamine and fully stimulates serotonin. It is thought that Pardoprunox could avoid some severe side effects that dopamine agonists cause by reducing the effect of dopamine when dopaminergic activity is high [1].

Efficacy : Pardoprunox significantly reduced Parkinson's Disease symptoms. In one study 6mg was better than 12mg or 12mg to 42mg [2]. When Pardoprunox was taken in dosages of up to 42mg per day Pardoprunox reduced "off" time by 1 hour 37 minutes per day, but even a placebo reduced the "off" time by 55 minutes per day. So the benefit beyond that of a placebo was a reduction in "off" time of only 42 minutes per day. Pardoprunox made no significant difference to scores on the PDQ-39, which assesses Parkinson's Disease symptoms [3].

Adverse effects : Pardoprunox tolerability was dose related. The higher dosages showed the highest drop out rate due to adverse effects, which occurred in about half of patients. The main problems caused were nausea, somnolence, and dizziness. Observations suggest that the 12mg to 42mg per day dose range was higher than therapeutically required [2]. There was a high drop-out rate (37% of people) due to adverse effects suggesting that the selected dose range may have been too high, or that the increase in dose may have been too rapid [3].

Comparison : Pardoprunox was not quite as effective as the dopamine agonist pramipexole [2].

[1] Movement Disorders [2010] 25 (6) : 738-746 (J.Bronzova, C. Sampaio, R.A.Hauser, A.E.Lang, O.Rascol, A.Theeuwes, S.V.van de Witte, G.van Scharrenburg)

[2] Movement Disorders [2011] 26 (8) : 1464-1476 (C.Sampaio, J. Bronzova, R.A.Hauser, A.E.Lang, O.Rascol, S.V.van de Witte, A.A. Theeuwes)

[3] Parkinsonism & Related Disorders [2012] 18 (4) : 370-376 (O. Rascol, J.Bronzova, R.A.Hauser, A.E.Lang, C.Sampaio, A.Theeuwes, S.V.van de Witte)

Pergolide

Brand names : Permax, Prascend

Pharmacology : Pergolide is a D1, D2 and D3 dopamine receptor agonist. Pergolide has been withdrawn from use in the U.S.A. since 2007 because of safety concerns.

Efficacy : Pergolide improved Parkinson's Disease symptoms [1-18], including on-off phenomena [5, 7, 8, 11, 13, 17, 19, 20, 21], motor fluctuations [2, 3, 22, 23, 24], gait [3, 25], rest tremor [18, 26], fatigue [27], rigidity [1, 25], speech [25], bradykinesia [1], motor symptoms [8, 22], dyskinesia [5, 24, 28], posture [25], and all sexual functions in younger males [29], but did not enable improvement in all people [30]. A mild symptomatic effect was even possible at subtherapeutic doses [30]. The improvement in Parkinson's Disease symptoms enabled a reduction in L-dopa dosage [5, 6, 7, 15, 19, 20, 22, 31, 32], and a reduction in L-dopa frequency [19]. The improvements in response to pergolide gradually declined over time, and lasted only 1 to 4 years [13, 14, 16, 18,, 33, 34].

Adverse effects : The most widely reported and serious adverse effect is an increased risk of cardiac valve regurgitation [35-49, 74], which was highly enhanced by comorbid hypertension or aging [37]. The risk was reduced [50] or not apparent [51] when using lower dosages. The side effect profile of pergolide is otherwise similar to that of other dopamine agonists [52]. Significant adverse effects were otherwise not usually encountered [17, 53]. The adverse effects of pergolide were fairly frequent but they were relatively mild and reversible [5, 15]. Adverse events led to discontinuation of therapy in 17% of patients [24]. Other adverse effects are : nausea [21, 25, 53, 54], vomiting [21, 25], hallucinations [8, 21, 54], impulse-control disorder in 16% of people [55], dyskinesia [8, 14, 23], lowering of blood pressure [8], an organic confusional syndrome [14], repetitive ventricular rhythms [56], myocardial infarction or ventricular ectopy [34]. There is also worsened sleep [25, 57] and increased irresistible daytime sleepiness (IDS) [21, 53, 58, 59].

Comparison : Pergolide was similar to L-dopa regarding efficacy and side effects in the short term treatment of newly diagnosed Parkinson's Disease [60]. However, generally, L-dopa was more effective than pergolide [24]. Pergolide was more effective than ropinirole in the very elderly [61], and was more effective than lisuride [62]. Pergolide is little better [61], or no better [63] than pramipexole but is significantly more likely than pramipexole to cause nausea or vomiting [26]. Otherwise, pergolide was no better than other dopamine agonists [64]. A comparison of the outcomes regarding response and toxicity revealed that bromocriptine and pergolide act differently in individual patients [65]. In comparison to bromocriptine, pergolide caused fewer adverse effects [66, 67], and be more effective than bromocriptine [28, 66-72], but to be no more effective in some other studies [9, 73].

[1] Neurology [1981] 31 (6) : 675-682 (A.Lieberman, M.Goldstein, M. Leibowitz, A.Neophytides, M.Kupersmith, V.Pact, D.Kleinberg)

[2] Parkinsonism & Related Disorders [2005] 11 (6) : 393-398 (A. Storch, C.Trenkwalder, C.Oehlwein, J.Winkelmann, U.Polzer, H.P. Hundemer, J.Schwarz)

[3] Clinical Neuropharmacology [1985] 8 (3) : 260-265 (J.I.Sage, R.C. Duvoisin)

[4] Movement Disorders [2000] 15 (4) : 613-626 (J.Kulisevsky, C. García-Sánchez, M.L.Berthier, M.Barbanoj, B.Pascual-Sedano, A. Gironell, A.Estévez-González)

[5] Presse Medicale [1985] 14 (26) : 1409-1411 (M.Gonce, P.J. Delwaide)

[6] Cleveland Clinic Journal of Medicine [1995] 62 (4) : 212-217 (R. Pahwa, W.C.Koller)

[7] Neurology [1983] 33 (4) : 505-507 (J.Jankovic)

[8] Zhonghua Yi Xue Za Zhi [1995] 56 (5) : 312-318 (D.E.Shan, S.I. Yeh)

[9] Neurology [1995] 45 (3 Supplement 3) : S13-S21 (Y.Mizuno, T. Kondo, H.Narabayashi)

[10] Neurology [1984] 34 (7) : 983-986 (J.Y.Mear, G.Barroche, Y.de Smet, M.Weber, F.Lhermitte, Y.Agid)

[11] Clinical Pharmacology and Therapeutics [1982] 32 (1) : 70-75 (A. N.Lieberman, M.Goldstein, A.Neophytides, M.Leibowitz, G. Gopinathan, R.Walker, V.Pact)

[12] Neurology [1985] 35 (3) : 291-295 (S.G.Diamond, C.H.Markham, L.J.Treciokas)

[13] Neurology [1984] 34 (2) : 223-226 (A.N.Lieberman, M.Goldstein, M.Leibowitz, G.Gopinathan, A.Neophytides, E.Hiesiger, J.Nelson, R. Walker)

[14] Neurology [1982] 32 (10) : 1181-1184 (A.N.Lieberman, M. Goldstein, G.Gopinathan, M.Leibowitz, A.Neophytides, R.Walker, E. Hiesiger, J.Nelson)

[15] Movement Disorders [1994] 9 (1) : 40-47 (C.W.Olanow, S.Fahn, M.Muenter, H.Klawans, H.Hurtig, M.Stern, I.Shoulson, R.Kurlan, J.D. Grimes, J.Jankovic)

[16] Clinical Neuropharmacology [1986] 9 (2) : 160-164 (J.I.Sage, R. C.Duvoisin)

[17] Neurology [1982] 32 (10) : 1175-1179 (C.M.Tanner, C.G.Goetz, R.H.Glantz, S.L.Glatt, H.L.Klawans)

[18] Clinical Neurophysiology [2000] 111 (7) : 1198-1202 (A.P. Strafella, F.Valzania, S.A.Nassetti, A.Tropeani, A.Bisulli, M. Santangelo, C.A.Tassinari)

[19] Mayo Clinic Proceedings [1988] 63 (10) : 969-978 (J.E.Ahlskog, M.D.Muenter)

[20] Cochrane Database of Systematic Reviews [2000] (2) : CD000235 (C.E.Clarke, J.M.Speller)

[21] Annals of Neurology [1982] 12 (3) : 243-247 (A.E.Lang, N.Quinn, S.Brincat, C.D.Marsden, J.D.Parkes)

[22] Neurology [1985] 35 (3) : 296-299 (J.Jankovic)

[23] The American Journal of the Medical Sciences [1985] 290 (3) : 102-106 (A.N.Lieberman, M.Leibowitz, G.Gopinathan, R.Walker, E.Hiesiger, J.Nelson, M.Goldstein)

[24] Movement Disorders [2006] 21 (3) : 343-353 (W.H.Oertel, E. Wolters, C.Sampaio, S.Gimenez-Roldan, B.Bergamasco, M.Dujardin, D.G.Grosset, G.Arnold, K.L.Leenders, H.P.Hundemer, A.Lledó, et al)

[25] Journal of Neurology [1984] 231 (3) : 148-152 (P.Jeanty, M.Van den Kerchove, A.Lowenthal, H.De Bruyne)

[26] Movement Disorders [2003] 18 (2) : 176-180 (P.Navan, L.J. Findley, J.A.Jeffs, R.K.Pearce, P.G.Bain)

[27] Behavioural Neurology [2001-2002] 13 (3-4) : 117-121 (K.Abe, M.Takanashi, T.Yanagihara, S.Sakoda)

[28] Movement Disorders [1995] 10 (5) : 668-671 (A.M.Bonnet, I. Serre, R.Marconi, Y.Agid, B.Dubois)

[29] Parkinsonism & Related Disorders [2005] 11 (8) : 509-512 (M. Pohanka, P.Kanovský, M.Bares, J.Pulkrábek, I.Rektor)

[30] Movement Disorders [2005] 20 (3) : 363-366 (K.Grosset, D. Grosset, A.Lees)

[31] Drugs [1990] 39 (3) : 491-506 (H.D.Langtry, S.P.Clissold)

[32] Neurology [1999] 53 (3) : 573-579 (P.Barone, D.Bravi, F. Bermejo-Pareja, R.Marconi, J.Kulisevsky, S.Malagù, R.Weiser, N. Rost)

[33] Mayo Clinic Proceedings [1988] 63 (10) : 979-987 (J.E.Ahlskog, M.D.Muenter)

[34] Neurology [1985] 35 (5) : 738-742 (R.Kurlan, C.Miller, R.Levy, B.Macik, R.Hamill, I.Shoulson)

[35] Neurology [2004] 63 (2) : 301-304 (D.G.Baseman, P.E. O'Suilleabhain, S.C.Reimold, S.R.Laskar, J.G.Baseman, R.B. Jr. Dewey)

[36] Journal of Cardiothoracic Surgery [2009] 4 : 65 (E.E.Apostolakis, N.G.Baikoussis, D.Tselikos, I.Koniari, C.Prokakis, E.Fokaeas, M. Karanikolas)

[37] Journal of Neural Transmission [2009] 116 (2) : 171-178 (T.Oeda, M.Masaki, K.Yamamoto, E.Mizuta, N.Kitagawa, T.Isono, S.Taniguchi, K.Doi, H.Yaku, C.Yutani, T.Kawamura, S.Kuno, H.Sawada)

[38] Canadian Journal of Neurological Sciences [2008] 35 (2) : 173-178 (C.Zadikoff, M.Duong-Hua, K.Sykora, C.Marras, A.Lang, P. Rochon)

[39] Journal of Neurology [2008] 255 (7) : 1045-1048 (D.Dupuy, J.P. Lesbre, P.Gérard, M.Andrejak, O.Godefroy)

[40] Archives of Neurology [2007] 64 (12) : 1721-1726 (J.C.Corvol, J. B.Anzouan-Kacou, E.Fauveau, A.M.Bonnet, B.Lebrun-Vignes, C. Girault, Y.Agid, P.Lechat, R.Isnard, L.Lacomblez)

[41] Lancet [2004] 363 (9416) : 1179-1183 (G.Van Camp, A.Flamez, B.Cosyns, C.Weytjens, L.Muyldermans, M.Van Zandijcke, J.De Sutter, P.Santens, P.Decoodt, C.Moerman, D.Schoors)

[42] Archives of Neurology [2007] 64 (3) : 377-380 (R.B.Dewey, S.C. Reimold, P.E.O'Suilleabhain)

[43] New England Journal of Medicine [2007] 356 (1) : 39-46 (R. Zanettini, A.Antonini, G.Gatto, R.Gentile, S.Tesei, G.Pezzoli)

[44] New England Journal of Medicine [2007] 356 (1) : 29-38 (R.Schade, F.Andersohn, S.Suissa, W.Haverkamp, E.Garbe)

[45] Neurology [2006] 67 (7) : 1225-1229 (M.Yamamoto, T.Uesugi, T. Nakayama)

[46] Movement Disorders [2006] 21 (8) : 1109-1113 (C.Peralta, E. Wolf, H.Alber, K.Seppi, S.Müller, S.Bösch, G.K.Wenning, O. Pachinger, W.Poewe)

[47] Mayo Clinic Proceedings [2005] 80 (8) : 1016-1020 (E.A.Waller, J.Kaplan, M.G.Heckman)

[48] Canadian Journal of Neurological Sciences [2006] 33 (1) : 27-33 (C.Zadikoff, P.Rochon, A.Lang)

[49] Cardiovascular Therapeutics [2011] 29 (6) : 404-410 (R.Zanettini, A.Antonini, G.Gatto, R.Gentile, S.Tesei, G.Pezzoli)

[50] Journal of Neurology [2007] 254 (11) : 1575-1578 (E.Ruzicka, H. Línková, M.Penicka, O.Ulmanová, L.Nováková, J.Roth)

[51] Journal of Clinical Neuroscience [2009] 16 (1) : 83-87 (F.Ozer, R. Tiras, S.Cetin, O.Ozturk, T.Aydemir, S.Ozben, H.Meral, S.Kizkin, H. Bader, B.Ozben)

[52] Clinical Neuropharmacology [2002] 25 (1) : 1-10 (U.Bonuccelli, A.Colzi, P.Del Dotto)

[53] Journal of the Medical Association of Thailand [1996] 79 (4) : 205-209 (N.Poungvarin, N.Prayoonwiwat, V.Devahasatin, et al)

[54] Drug Safety [2010] 33 (2) : 147-161 (J.Kulisevsky, J. Pagonabarraga)

[55] Synapse [2015] 69 (4) :183-189 (P.Seeman)

[56] Advances in Neurology [1983] 37 : 121-130 (M.Leibowitz, A.N. Lieberman, A.Neophytides, G.Gopinathan, M.Goldstein)

[57] Neurology [2005] 64 (8) : 1450-1451 (C.L.Comella, M.Morrissey, K.Janko)

[58] Archives of Neurology [2005] 62 (8) : 1242-1248 (J.Avorn, S. Schneeweiss, L.R.Sudarsky, J.Benner, Y.Kiyota, R.Levin, R.J.Glynn)

[59] European Neurology [2003] 49 (1) : 30-33 (I.Schlesinger, P.D. Ravin)

[60] Clinical Neuropharmacology [1998] 21 (6) : 358-362 (J. Kulisevsky, D.López Villegas, C.García-Sánchez, M.Barbanoj, A. Gironell, B.Pascual-Sedano)

[61] Movement Disorders [2000] 15 (4) : 664-668 (L.M.Shulman, A.Minagar, A.Rabinstein, W.J.Weiner)

[62] Advances in Neurology [1984] 40 : 503-507 (A.N.Lieberman, G. Gopinathan, A.Neophytides, M.Leibowitz, M.Goldstein)

[63] Movement Disorders [2003] 18 (11) : 1324-1331 (P.Navan, L.J. Findley, J.A.Jeffs, R.K.Pearce, P.G.Bain)

[64] Journal of Neural Transmission [2001] 108 (1) : 63-70 (P.A. Hanna, L.Ratkos, W.G.Ondo, J.Jankovic)

[65] Journal of Neurology, Neurosurgery, and Psychiatry [1988] 51 (4) : 529-533 (S.A.Factor, J.R.Sanchez-Ramos, W.J.Weiner)

[66] Neurology [1995] 45 (3 Supplement 3) : S22-S27 (G.Pezzoli, E. Martignoni, C.Pacchetti, V.A.Angeleri, P.Lamberti, A.Muratorio, U. Bonuccelli, M.De Mari, N.Foschi, E.Cossutta)

[67] Movement Disorders [1994] 9 (4) : 431-436 (G.Pezzoli, E. Martignoni, C.Pacchetti, V.A.Angeleri, P.Lamberti, A.Muratorio, U. Bonuccelli, M.De Mari, N.Foschi, E.Cossutta)

[68] The Cochrane Database of Systematic Reviews [2000] (2) : CD000236 (C.E.Clarke, J.M.Speller)

[69] Revista de Neurología [1997] 25 (145) : 1343-1345 (J.G.de Yébenes, P.J.García-Ruiz, R.Sánchez-Pernaute)

[70] Neurology [1985] 35 (5) : 749-751 (C.G.Goetz, C.M.Tanner, R.H. Glantz, H.L.Klawans)

[71] Value in Health [2001] 4 (4) : 308-315 (P.Davey, N.Rajan, M. Lees, M.Aristides)

[72] Advances in Neurology [1983] 37 : 95-108 (A.N.Lieberman, A. Neophytides, M.Leibowitz, G.Gopinathan, V.Pact, R.Walker, A. Goodgold, M.Goldstein)

[73] Prescrire International [2000] 9 (50) : 177-179 (No authors listed)

[74] CNS Drugs [2015] 29 (12) : 985-998 (T.Tran, J.M.Brophy, S. Suissa, C.Renoux)

PIRIBEDIL

Brand names : Pronoran, Trivastal Retard, Trastal, Trivastan, Clarium

Pharmacology : Piribedil is a D2 and D3 dopamine receptor agonist. It also has a significant antagonist action on alpha2A and alpha2C adrenergic receptors [1-4]. It is not available in all countries [5].

Efficacy : Piribedil reduced daytime sleepiness [6], moderately reduced apathy [7], moderately reduced depression [7], improved quality of life [7], reduced anhedonia [7], reduced impulse control disorders [8], moderately improved Parkinson's Disease symptoms [2, 3, 4, 9-13], improved activities of daily living [10], reduced L-dopa dose [10], increased duration of L-dopa dose [10]. Among the cardinal symptoms of parkinsonism, tremor responded the best of all of them. Depression also appeared to respond favourably to piribidel [11]. There was an improvement in most people in bradykinesia, tremor and rigidity [14]. Transdermal piribedil did not demonstrate any significant clinical efficacy [15].

Adverse effects : The most common side effects were hallucinations (20%) [10, 16], dyskinesias (20%) [10], nausea (11%) [15, 16], dizziness (8%) [10], vomiting (7%) [15], malaise (7%) [15] and sleep attacks [10, 16-19]. Other adverse effects can include pathological gambling [5], gastrointestinal side effects [9], giddiness [16] and lethargy [16].

[1] Pharmacology and Therapeutics [2010] 128 (2) : 229-273 (M.J. Millan)

[2] Movement Disorders [2006] 21 (4) : 500-509 (A.Castro-Caldas, P. Delwaide, W.Jost, M.Merello, A.Williams, P.Lamberti, M.Aguilar, S. Del Signore, P.Cesaro)

[3] Journal of Medical Association Thailand [2004] 87 (11) : 1293-1300 (J.Suwantamee, S.Nidhinandana, S.Srisuwananukorn, S. Laptikultham, A.Pisarnpong, S.Chankrachang, A.Bundhukul)

[4] Movement Disorders [2003] 18 (4) : 418-425 (M.Ziegler, A. Castro-Caldas, S.Del Signore, O.Rascol)

[5] Arquivos de Neuro-Psiquiatria [2015] 73 (2) : 115-118 (F.E. Micheli, J.C.Giugni, M.E.Espinosa, D.S.Calvo, G.B.Raina)

[6] Clinical Neuropharmacology [2014] 37 (4) : 116-122 (K.Eggert, C. Öhlwein, J.Kassubek, M.Wolz, A.Kupsch, A.Ceballos-Baumann, R. Ehret, U.Polzer, F.Klostermann, J.Schwarz, G.Fuchs, W.Jost, et al)

[7] Brain [2013] 136 (Part 5) : 1568-1577 (S.Thobois, E.Lhommée, H.Klinger, C.Ardouin, E.Schmitt, A.Bichon, A.Kistner, A.Castrioto, J.Xie, V.Fraix, P.Pelissier, S.Chabardes, P.Mertens, J.L.Quesada, et al)

[8] Clinical Neuropharmacology [2010] 33 (1) : 11-13 (LTschopp, Z.Salazar, M.T.Gomez Botello, C.U.Roca, F.Micheli)

[9] Movement Disorders [2006] 21 (12) : 2110-2115 (O.Rascol, B. Dubois, A.C.Caldas, S.Senn, S.Del Signore, A.Lees)

[10] Parkinsonism & Related Disorders [2003] 10 (2) : 117-121 (V.G. Evidente, R.P.Esteban, F.M.Domingo, L.O.Carbajal, M.A.Parazo)

[11] Clinical Neuropharmacology [1989] 12 (1) : 23-28 (G. Mentenopoulos, Z.Katsarou, S.Bostantjopoulou, J.Logothetis)

[12] Revue Neurologique [2004] 38 (8) : 715-719 (G.Salazar Tortolero, R.Wix Ramos, P.Salazar Aladrén, J.C.Jiménez León)

[13] Movement Disorders [2005] 20 (7) : 803-809 (N.Simon, J. Micallef, J.C.Reynier, M.Lesourd, T.Witjas, A.Alicherif, J.P.Azulay, O.Blin)

[14] Zhurnal Nevrologii Psikhiatrii Imeni S S Korsakova [2003] 103 (9) : 54-58 (A.N.Boiko, T.T.Batysheva, E.S.Chikina, Ilu Artemova, T.V.Vdovichenko, A.M.Ismailov, N.A.Obydenova, et al)

[15] Movement Disorders [1999] 14 (2) : 336-341 (J.L.Montastruc, M. Ziegler, O.Rascol, M.Malbezin)

[16] Acta Neurologica Scandinavica [2003] 107 (3) : 202-206 (E.K. Tan, P.Ratnagopal, S.Y.Han, M.C.Wong)

[17] Prescrire International [2013] 22 (143) : 265 (No authors listed)

[18] Clinical Neuropharmacology [2011] 34 (3) : 104-107 (A.Gouraud, A.Millaret, J.Descotes, T.Vial)

[19] Fundamental and Clinical Pharmacology [2003] 17 (1) : 117-119 (E.K.Tan)

Pramipexole

Brand names : Mirapex, Mirapexin, Pexola, Sifrol

Pharmacology : Pramipexole is a dopamine agonist indicated for treating early-stage Parkinson's Disease and restless legs syndrome (RLS). Pramipexole has a preference for the D3 dopamine receptor [1]. It has affinity for the D2 receptor types (D2, D3, D4) but does not have affinity for the D1 and D5 dopamine receptors [2].

Efficacy : Pramipexole reduced Parkinson's Disease symptoms [3-18], even more so in advanced Parkinson's Disease [5, 10]. Pramipexole reduced fatigue [19], reduced "off" time [11, 13, 18], improved motor function [20], reduced tremor [20, 21, 22], including resting tremor in 54% of people [23], postural tremor in 50% of people [23], and kinetic tremor in 15% of people [23]; reduced depression [20, 21, 23-26], reduced anhedonia [26], reduced motor fluctuations [23], reduced dyskinesias [23, 27], reduced motor and non-motor symptoms (in 83% of patients) [23], improved mood and motivation [16, 28], improved sleep [29], reduced akinesia [21], reduced rigidity [21]. Fifteen months of use showed no benefit when compared to the use of pramipexole being delayed for 6 to 9 months [30].

Adverse effects : Over 80% of people who took pramipexole reported adverse effects. Serious adverse effects were reported by 10% of people who took pramipexole [30]. Those adverse effects that were most commonly reported were : nausea [7, 8, 12, 14, 30, 31], constipation [7, 12, 14], fatigue [7, 11, 14], peripheral edema [5, 7, 32, 33], insomnia [9, 12], somnolence [5, 7, 12, 14, 15] in as many as 15% of people [5], back pain in 10% of people [5], vomiting [31], higher heart failure risk [34], vivid dreams [11], hallucinations [9] including auditory hallucinations [35] and visual hallucinations [12], dyskinesia [5, 11, 35]; impairment of short term verbal memory, attentional-executive functions and verbal fluency [37]; impuse-control disorders [5, 38] including gambling [39, 40, 41], hypersexuality [41, 42], and compulsive eating [43]; increased risk of heart failure [59], that increases considerably with age [44]. In those people with early Parkinson's Disease the most reported side effects were somnolence (15%), peripheral edema (11%) and back pain (10%). Higher risks of dizziness, somnolence, constipation, vomiting, and insomnia were more commonly found in early Parkinson's Disease [8]. Higher risks of dyskinesia and hallucination were usually only found in advanced Parkinson's Disease [8]. In those people with advanced Parkinson's Disease the most reported side effects were dyskinesia (27%), somnolence (13%), and impulse control disorders (1%) [5].

Comparison : Initial pramipexole treatment resulted in significantly less development of wearing off, dyskinesias, or on-off motor fluctuations compared with L-dopa [45]. Somnolence was more common with pramipexole than L-dopa. L-dopa was more effective than pramipexole [45]. The adverse effects of pramipexole are similar, in general, to those of other dopamine agonists [46], but are less than those of ropinirole [47]. Prampipexole was found to be similar in its efficacy to pergolide [48, 49], bromocriptine [50], and slightly better than rotigotine [51]. Cabergoline, pramipexole and ropinirole are similarly effective in reducing the risk for dyskinesia relative to L-dopa [52]. Switching from bromocriptine, pergolide or ropinirole to pramipexole in an overnight schedule is safe [53]. Immediate release pramipexole was slightly more effective than extended-release pramipexole, but otherwise, extended-release pramipexole could be readily substituted for immediate-release pramipexole [3, 4, 5, 54, 60]. Patients can change overnight from IR pramipexole to ER pramipexole without any loss in efficacy [54-58]. There was no significant difference in the adverse effects between extended-release and immediate-release pramipexole [60].

[1] European Journal of Neurology [2000] 7 (Supplement 1) : 21-25 (J.C.Möller, W.H.Oertel)

[2] Nihon Yakurigaku Zasshi. Folia Pharmacologica Japonica [2004] 123 (6) : 429-440 (Y.Kohno, S.Takeuchi)

[3] Neurology [2011] 77 (8) : 759-766 (W.Poewe, O. Rascol, P.Barone, R.A.Hauser, Y.Mizuno, M.Haaksma, L.Salin, N. Juhel, A.H.Schapira)

[4] Neurology [2011] 77 (8) : 767-774 (A.H.Schapira, P. Barone, R.A. Hauser, Y.Mizuno, O.Rascol, M.Busse, L.Salin, N.Juhel, W.Poewe)

[5] European Journal of Neurology [2014] 21 (5) : 736-743 (R.A. Hauser, A.H.Schapira, P.Barone, Y.Mizuno, O.Rascol, M.Busse, C. Debieuvre, M.Fraessdorf, W.Poewe)

[6] Parkinson's Disease [2014] 467131 (R.A.Hauser, M.F.Gordon, Y. Mizuno, W.Poewe, P.Barone, A.H.Schapira, O.Rascol, C.Debieuvre, M.Fräßdorf)

[7] Movement Disorders [2011] 26 (1) : 37-44 (K.Kieburtz)

[8] Journal of Clinical Neuroscience [2014] 21 (7) : 1094-1101 (C.Q. Zhou, J.W.Zhang, M.Wang, G.G.Peng)

[9] Clinical Neuropharmacology [2007] 30 (2) : 72-85 (Parkinson Study Group)

[10] JAMA [1997] 278 (2) : 125-130 (No authors listed)

[11] Journal of Neurology, Neurosurgery, and Psychiatry [1999] 66 (4) : 436-441 (M.M.Pinter, O.Pogarell, W.H.Oertel)

[12] Neurology [1997] 49 (3) : 724-728 (K.M.Shannon, J.P.Bennett Jr, J.H.Friedman)

[13] CNS Drugs [2010] 24 (4) : 327-336 (C.M.Chwieduk, M.P.Curran)

[14] Movement Disorders [2010] 25 (15) : 2542-2549 (R.A.Hauser, A. H.Schapira, O.Rascol, P.Barone, Y.Mizuno, L.Salin, M.Haaksma M, N.Juhel, W.Poewe)

[15] Archives of Neurology [2009] 66 (5) : 563-570 (Parkinson Study Group CALM Cohort Investigators)

[16] Movement Disorders [2005] 20 (5) : 602-610 (J.C.Möller, W.H. Oertel, J.Köster, G.Pezzoli, L.Provinciali)

[17] Journal of the Neurological Sciences [2003] 216 (1) : 81-87 (K.S. Wong, C.S.Lu, D.E.Shan, C.C.Yang, T.H.Tsoi, V.Mok)

[18] Archives of Neurology [2004] 61 (7) : 1044-1053 (R.G.Holloway, I.Shoulson, S.Fahn, K.Kieburtz, A.Lang, K.Marek, M.McDermott, J. Seibyl, W.Weiner, B.Musch, C.Kamp, M.Welsh, A.Shinaman, et al)

[19] Internal Medicine [2011] 50 (19) : 2163-2168 (A.Morita, Y. Okuma, S.Kamei, F.Yoshii, T.Yamamoto, S.Hashimoto, H.Utsumi, T. Hatano, N.Hattori, M.Matsumura, K.Takahashi, S.Nogawa, et al)

[20] Der Nervenarzt [2002] 73 (8) : 745-750 (H.Reichmann, H.M. Brecht, P.H.Kraus, M.R.Lemke)

[21] CNS Drugs [2003] 17 (13) : 965-973 (H.Reichmann, M.H.Brecht, J.Köster, P.H.Kraus, M.R.Lemke)

[22] Journal of Neurology, Neurosurgery, and Psychiatry [2002] 72 (6) : 713-720 (O.Pogarell, T.Gasser, J.J.van Hilten, S.Spieker, S.Pollentier, D.Meier, W.H.Oertel)

[23] Zhurnal Nevrologii i Psikhiatrii imeni S.S.Korsakova [2010] 110 (2) : 39-44 (O.S.Levin, A.N. Boiko, O.S.Nesterova, O.V.Otcheskaia, E.I.Zhuravleva, I.I.Artemova, A.A. Khozova, A.M.Ismailov, et al)

[24] Kobe Journal of Medical Sciences [2011] 56 (5) : E214-E219 (N. Yasui, K.Sekiguchi, H.Hamaguchi, F.Kanda)

[25] Lancet Neurology [2010] 9 (6) : 573-580 (P.Barone, W.Poewe, S. Albrecht, C.Debieuvre, D.Massey, O.Rascol, E.Tolosa, D. Weintraub)

[26] Journal of the Neurological Sciences [2006] 248 (1-2) : 266-270 (M.R.Lemke, H.M.Brecht, J.Koester, H.Reichmann)

[27] Internal Medicine [2013] 52 (3) : 325-332 (H.Utsumi, Y.Okuma, O.Kano, Y.Suzuki, M.Iijima, H.Tomimitsu, H.Hashida, S.Kubo, M. Suzuki K.Nanri, M.Matsumura, H.Murakami, N.Hattori)

[28] Clinical Therapeutics [2009] 31 (1) : 89-98 (A.F.Leentjens, J. Koester, B.Fruh, D.T.Shephard, P.Barone, J.J.Houben)

[29] British Journal of Clinical Pharmacology [2009] 67 (3) : 333-340 (J.Micallef, M.Rey, A.Eusebio, C.Audebert, F.Rouby, E.Jouve, S. Tardieu, O.Blin)

[30] Lancet Neurology [2013] 12 (8) : 747-755 (A.H.Schapira, M.P. McDermott, P.Barone, C.L.Comella, S.Albrecht, H.H. Hsu, D.H. Massey, Y.Mizuno, W.Poewe, O.Rascol, K.Marek)

[31] Movement Disorders [2003] 18 (2) : 176-180 (P.Navan, L.J. Findley, J.A.Jeffs, P.K.Pearce, P.G.Bain)

[32] Archives of Neurology [2000] 57 (5) : 729-732 (E.K.Tan, W. Ondo)

[33] Archives of Neurology [2007] 64 (6) : 820-824 (G. Kleiner-Fisman, D.N.Fisman)

[34] Expert Opinion on Drug Safety [2014] 13 (3) : 351-360 (S. Perez-Lloret, M.V.Rey, J.Crispo, D.Krewski, M.Lapeyre-Mestre, J.L. Montastruc, O.Rascol)

[35] Medicine [2014] 93 (27) : e251 (H.Kataoka, S.Ueno)

[36] Archives of Neurology [2010] 67 (1) : 27-32 (M.A.Brodsky, B.S. Park, J.G.Nutt)

[37] Journal of Neural Transmission [2003] 110 (4) : 373-380 (L.Brusa, A.Bassi, A.Stefani, M.Pierantozzi, A.Peppe, M.D.Caramia, L.Boffa, S. Ruggieri, P.Stanzione)

[38] Synapse [2015] 69 (4) : 183-189 (P.Seeman)

[39] European Journal of Neurology [2008] 15 (4) : 350-354 (A. Imamura, Y.E.Geda, J.Slowinski, Z.K.Wszolek, L.A.Brown, R.J.Uitti)

[40] Clinical Neuropharmacology [2007] 30 (5) : 249-255 (E.D. Driver-Dunckley, B.N.Noble, J.G.Hentz, V.G.Evidente, J.N.Caviness, J.Parish, L.Krahn, C.H.Adler)

[41] Mayo Clinic Proceedings [2009] 84 (4) : 310-316 (J.M.Bostwick, K.A.Hecksel, S.R.Stevens, J.H.Bower, J.E.Ahlskog)

[42] Journal of Sexual Medicine [2009] 6 (4) : 1177-1180 (R.P. Munhoz, G.Fabiani, N.Becker, H.A.Teive)

[43] Movement Disorders [2006] 21 (4) : 524-529 (M.J.Nirenberg, C. Waters)

[44] Pharmacological Research [2011] 65 (3) : 358-64 (M.M.Mokhles, G.Trifirò, J.P.Dieleman, M.D.Haag, E.M.van Soest, K.M.Verhamme, G.Mazzaglia, R.Herings, C.de Luise, D.Ross, G.Brusselle, et al)

[45] JAMA [2000] 284 (15) : 1931-1938 (Parkinson Study Group)

[46] Clinical Neuropharmacology [1995] 18 (4) : 338-347 (J.P.Hubble, W.C.Koller, N.R.Cutler, J.J.Sramek, J.Friedman, C.Goetz, A. Ranhosky, D.Korts, A.Elvin)

[47] Drug Safety [2003] 26 (6) : 439-444 (M.Etminan, S.Gill, A.Samii)

[48] Journal of Neural Transmission [2001] 108 (1) : 63-70 (P.A. Hanna, L.Ratkos, W.G.Ondo, J.Jankovic)

[49] Movement Disorders [2003] 18 (11) : 1324-1331 (P.Navan, L.J. Findley, J.A.Jeffs, R.K.Pearce, P.G.Bain)

[50] Cochrane Database of Systematic Reviews [2000] (3) : CD002259 (C.E.Clarke, J.M.Speller, J.A.Clarke)

[51] Lancet Neurology [2007] 6 (6) : 513-520 (W.H.Poewe, O. Rascol, N.Quinn, E.Tolosa, W.H.Oertel, E.Martignoni, M.Rupp, B. Boroojerdi)

[52] Drugs & Aging [2003] 20 (11) : 847-855 (R.Inzelberg, E. Schechtman, P.Nisipeanu)

[53] Journal of Neurology [2004] 251 (3) : 335-339 (G.Linazasoro)

[54] Clinical Neuropharmacology [2012] 35 (4) : 174-181 (Y.Mizuno, M.Yamamoto, S.Kuno, K.Hasegawa, N.Hattori, T.Kagimura, A. Sarashina, O.Rascol, A.H.Schapira, P.Barone, R.A. Hauser, W.Poewe)

[55] Movement Disorders [2010] 25 (14) : 2326-2332 (O.Rascol, P. Barone, R.A.Hauser, Y.Mizuno, W.Poewe, A.H.Schapira, L.Salin, M. Sohr, C.Debieuvre)

[56] European Journal of Neurology [2013] 20 (1) : 180-187 (A.H. Schapira, P.Barone, R.A.Hauser, Y.Mizuno, O.Rascol, M.Busse, C. Debieuvre, M.Fraessdorf, W.Poewe)

[57] Journal of Clinical Interventions in Aging [2012] 7 : 83-88 (E.M. Hametner, K.Seppi, W.Poewe)

[58] Expert Review of Neurotherapeutics [2011] 11 (9) : 1229-1234 (E. M.Hametner, K.Seppi, W.Poewe)

[59] CNS Drugs [2015] 29 (12) : 985-998 (T.Tran, J.M.Brophy, S. Suissa, C.Renoux)

[60] European Journal of Neurology [2017] May 8 [Epub ahead of print] (T.Shen, R.Ye, B.Zhang)

Ropinirole

Brand names : Requip, Repreve, Ronirol, Adartrel

Pharmacology : Ropinirole hydrochloride is a dopamine receptor agonist, with a non-ergot alkaloid structure, that is highly selective for the dopamine D2 and D3 receptors [1]. When taken as oral tablets, ropinirole is rapidly and almost completely absorbed, and it is extensively distributed from the vascular compartment [2]. A prolonged release version allows the drug to be released slowly and continuously so that it only has to be given once daily [3]. Ropinirole 24-hour prolonged release provided continuous delivery of ropinirole over 24 hours, resulting in a smooth plasma concentration-time profile. Food had no effect on its absorption [4]. Switching from ropinirole immediate release (ropinirole IR) to prolonged release (ropinirole PR) at the nearest equivalent total daily dose can take place overnight. The acceptance and tolerability are good [3]. A nasal gel is being developed that can increase the bioavailability of ropinirole in the brain by five times when compared to intravenous administration of ropinirole [5].

Efficacy : Ropinirole improved Parkinson's Disease symptoms [6-16], enabled a reduction in the dose of L-dopa [10, 13, 16-24], reduced "off" time [5, 8, 19, 25, 26, 27], improved nocturnal symptoms [28], reduced dyskinesia [18, 21, 23, 25, 27, 29, 30, 31], and enabled improvements in resting [22, 32]. Doses of ropinirole have to gradually increase [33]. Ropinirole once daily, twice daily and three times daily were not significantly different in their effects [24, 34] apart from an improvement in sleep [35]. High dose ropinirole was not more advantageous [54].

Adverse effects : The most common adverse effects are nausea [1, 13, 29, 36-40], somnolence [1, 11, 13, 29, 37, 39, 40, 41], impulse-control disorder [42-45], orthostatic hypotension [11, 13, 36, 37], dyskinesia [11, 13, 25, 40, 41], dizziness [13, 29, 36, 38, 40, 41], back pain [29, 38], insomnia [29, 36], hallucinations [1, 13, 40, 41], psychotic features [40], constipation [1], nasopharyngitis [1], upper abdominal discomfort [36], palpitation [36], arthralgia [29], fatigue [29], pain [29], abdominal pain or discomfort [13], nausea [41], vertigo [37], dyspepsia [37], oedema [37, 38], headache [38], gastrointestinal symptoms [11], decreased weight [40, 41]. Using ropinirole XL/PR 87% of people reported at least one adverse event [53]. The most common adverse events were back pain (14%), hallucinations (13%), somnolence (11%) and peripheral edema (11%) [53].

Comparison : Ropinirole was more effective than bromocriptine [36, 46-50], but not in another study except for causing less nausea than with bromocriptine [51]. Ropinirole was less effective than L-dopa [52].

[1] Journal of Clinical Pharmacy and Therapeutics [2012] 37 (5) : 571-577 (N.Hattori, K. Hasegawa, T.Sakamoto)

[2] Clinical Pharmacokinetics [2000] 39 (4) : 243-254 (C.M.Kaye, B. Nicholls)

[3] Journal of Neurology [2008] 255 (Supplement 5) : 60-63 (W.H.Jost, C.Buhmann, G.Fuchs, W.Greulich, S.Hummel, A.Korchounov, M. Müngersdorf, M.Schwarz, M.Spiegel Meixensberger)

[4] Clinical Therapeutics [2007] 29 (12) : 2654-2666 (D.J.Tompson, D. Vearer)

[5] Drug Development and Industrial Pharmacy [2016] Aug 17 :1-34 [Epub ahead of print] (M.Rao, D.K.Agrawal, C.Shirsath)

[6] Movement Disorders [2010] 25 (7) : 927-931 (B.P.Hersh, N.L.Earl, R.A.Hauser, M.Stacy)

[7] Clinical Neuropharmacology [2009] 32 (3) : 140-148 (D.Tompson, R.Oliver Willwong)

[8] Neurology [2007] 68 (14) : 1108-1115 (R.Pahwa, M.A.Stacy, S.A. Factor, K.E.Lyons, F.Stocchi, B.P.Hersh, L.W.Elmer, D.D.Truong, N. L.Earl)

[9] Neurology [1997] 49 (2) : 393-399 (C.H.Adler, K.D.Sethi, R.A. Hauser, T.L.Davis, J.P.Hammerstad, J.Bertoni, R.L.Taylor, J.Sanchez-Ramos, C.F.O'Brien)

[10] Clinical Neuropharmacology [2008] 31 (5) : 261-266 (I. Rektorova, M.Balaz, J.Svatova, K.Zarubova, I.Honig, V.Dostal, S. Sedlackova, I. Nestrasil, J.Mastik, M.Bares, J.Veliskova, L.Dusek)

[11] Clinical Neurology and Neurosurgery [2009] 111 (9) : 742-747 (F.Valldeoriola, S.Cobaleda, J.Lahuerta)

[12] Fortschritte der Neurologie-Psychiatrie [2007] 75 (4) : 236-241 (B. Buchwald, D.Angersbach, W.H.Jost)

[13] Clinical Interventions in Aging [2009] 4 : 179-186 (M.M. Nashatizadeh, K.E.Lyons, R.Pahwa)

[14] Movement Disorders [2007] 22 (13) : 1860-1865 (Y.Mizuno, T. Abe, K.Hasegawa, S.Kuno, T.Kondo, M.Yamamoto, M.Nakashima, I. Kanazawa)

[15] Movement Disorders [2007] 22 (4) : 483-489 (P.Barone, J.Lamb, A.Ellis, Z.Clarke)

[16] Journal of Neural Transmission (Supplementum) [1995] 45 : 231-238 (D.J.Brooks, N.Torjanski, D.J.Burn)

[17] Fortschritte der Neurologie-Psychiatrie [2010] 78 (Supplement 1) : S20-S24 (W.H.Jost, L.Bergmann)

[18] Parkinsonism & Related Disorders [2009] 15 (Supplement 4) : S85-S92 (M.Onofrj, L.Bonanni, M.V.De Angelis, F.Anzellotti, F. Ciccocioppo, A.Thomas)

[19] Neurology [1998] 51 (4) : 1057-1062 (A.Lieberman, C.W.Olanow, K.Sethi, P.Swanson, C.H.Waters, S.Fahn, H.Hurtig, M.Yahr)

[20] Archives of Neurology [1998] 55 (9) : 1211-1216 (K.D.Sethi, C.F. O'Brien, J.P.Hammerstad, C.H.Adler, T.L.Davis, R.L.Taylor, J. Sanchez-Ramos, J.M.Bertoni, R.A.Hauser)

[21] New England Journal of Medicine [2000] 342 (20) : 1484- 1491 (O.Rascol, D.J.Brooks, A.D.Korczyn, P.P.De Deyn, C.E.Clarke, A.E. Lang)

[22] Der Nervenarzt [2005] 76 (10) : 1239-1240 (H.Reichmann, D. Angersbach, B.Buchwald)

[23] Clinical Neuropharmacology [2003] 26 (3) : 146-150 (S.Cristina, R.Zangaglia, F.Mancini, E.Martignoni, G.Nappi, C.Pacchetti)

[24] Current Medical Research and Opinion [2008] 24 (10) : 2883-2895 (F.Stocchi, B.P.Hersh, B.L.Scott, P.A.Nausieda, L.Giorgi)

[25] Parkinsonism & Related Disorders [2013] 19 (11) : 1022-1026 (Z.Zhang, J.Wang, X.Zhang, S,Chen, Z.Wang, B.Zhang, C.Liu, Q.Qu, Y.Cheng, J.Li, H.Cao, M.Cai, R.Zhu)

[26] CNS Drugs [2009] 23 (1) : 81-90 (J.Weber, G.M.Keating)

[27] Movement Disorders [2007] 22 (16) : 2409-2417 (R.A.Hauser, O. Rascol, A.D.Korczyn, A.Jon Stoessl, R.L.Watts, W.Poewe, P.P.De Deyn, A.E.Lang)

[28] European Journal of Neurology [2012] 19 (1) : 105-113 (K.Ray Chaudhuri, P.Martinez-Martin, K.A.Rolfe, J.Cooper, C.B.Rockett, L. Giorgi, W.G.Ondo)

[29] Movement Disorders [2010] 25 (7) : 858-366 (R.L.Watts, K.E. Lyons, R.Pahwa, K.Sethi, M.Stern, R.A.Hauser, W.Olanow, A.M.Gray, B.Adams, N.L.Earl)

[30] Clinical Neuropharmacology [1998] 21 (3) : 169-175 (A.E. Schrag, D.J.Brooks, E.Brunt, D.Fuell, A.Korczyn, W.Poewe, N.P. Quinn, O.Rascol, F.Stocchi)

[31] Movement Disorders [2006] 21 (11) : 1844-1850 (O.Rascol, D.J. Brooks, A.D.Korczyn, P.P.De Deyn, C.E.Clarke, A.E.Lang, M. Abdalla)

[32] European Journal of Neurology [2002] 9 (3) : 253-257 (A.Schrag, J.Keens, J.Warner)

[33] Acta Neurologica Scandinavica [2002] 106 (4) : 200-204 (A.D. Korczyn, C.Thalamas, C.H.Adler)

[34] BMC Neurology [2013] 13 : 113 (J.Y.Yun, H.J.Kim, J.Y.Lee, Y. E.Kim, J.S.Kim, J.M.Kim, B.S.Jeon)

[35] Clinical Neuropharmacology [2010] 33 (4) : 186-190 (P.Dusek, J.Busková, E.Ruzicka, V.Majerová, A.Srp, R.Jech, J.Roth, K.Sonka)

[36] Zhonghua Yi Xue Za Zhi [2013] 93 (25) : 1952-1957 (S.H.Li, H.B.Chen, Z.F.Wang, R.H.Tang, X.Y.Zhang, J.S.Yang, W.Q.Zhao, X. R.Sun, J.Ma)

[37] Bratislavské Lekárske Listy [2008] 109 (6) : 273-275 (M.Titlic, A. Tonkic, I.Jukic, I.Lusic, M.Dikanovic)

[38] International Journal of Neuroscience [2011] 121 (5) : 246- 253 (R.A.Hauser, H.Reichmann, M.Lew, A.Asgharian, C.Makumi, K.J. Shulman)

[39] Movement Disorders [2007] 22 (16) : 2398-2404 (N.Giladi, B. Boroojerdi, A.D.Korczyn, D.J.Burn, C.E.Clarke, A.H.Schapira)

[40] Annals of Pharmacotherapy [2009] 43 (9) : 1426-1432 (S.C. Stoner, M.M.Dahmen, M.Makos, J.W.Lea, L.J.Carver, R.S.Rasu)

[41] Current Medical Research Opinions [2015] 31 (4) : 723-730 (Z. Zhang, J.Wang, X.Zhang, S,Chen, Z.Wang, B.Zhang, C.Liu, Q.Qu, Y.Cheng, R.Zhu, J.Li, J.Hu, M.Cai)

[42] Synapse [2015] Jan 22 [Epub ahead of print] (P.Seeman)

[43] JAMA Internal Medicine [2014] 174 (12) : 1930-1933 (T.J.Moore, J.Glenmullen, D.R.Mattison)

[44] Journal of Neurology, Neurosurgery, and Psychiatry [2014] 85 (8) : 840-844 (P.J.Garcia-Ruiz, J.C.Martinez Castrillo, A.Alonso-Canovas, A.Herranz Barcenas, L.Vela, P.Sanchez Alonso, M.Mata, et al)

[45] Journal of Clinical Psychopharmacology [2013] 33 (5) : 691-694 (M.Poletti, C.Logi, C.Lucetti, P.Del Dotto, F.Baldacci, A.Vergallo, M. Ulivi, S.Del Sarto, G.Rossi, R.Ceravolo, U.Bonuccelli)

[46] Neurology [1999] 53 (2) : 364-370 (A.D.Korczyn, E.R.Brunt, J.P. Larsen, Z.Nagy, W.H.Poewe, S.Ruggieri)

[47] Drugs & Aging [2003] 20 (11) : 847-855 (R.Inzelberg, E. Schechtman, P.Nisipeanu)

[48] Neurologia [2007] 22 (10) : 882-894 (J.Chacon)

[49] Journal of Neurology [2003] 250 (1) : 90-96 (J.H.Im, J.H.Ha, I.S. Cho, M.C.Lee)

[50] Drugs [2000] 60 (1) : 115-137 (A.J.Matheson, C.M.Spencer)

[51] Cochrane Database of Systematic Reviews [2000] (3) : CD001517 (C.E.Clarke, K.H.Deane)

[52] Movement Disorders [1998] 13 (1) : 39-45 (O.Rascol, D.J.Brooks, E.R.Brunt, A.D.Korczyn, W.H.Poewe, F.Stocchi)

[53] International Journal of Neuroscience [2016] 126 (1) : 30-38 (C.W.Makumi, AAsgharian, J.Ellis, S.Shaikh, T.Jimenez, S.VanMeter)

[54] Parkinsonism and Related Disorders [2017] Apr 13 [Epub ahead of print] (N.Hattori, K.Hasegawa, K.Sato, E.Mitsuyama, Y.Numachi)

Rotigotine

Brand names : Neupro

Pharmacology : Rotigotine is a high-potency agonist at dopamine D1, D2 and D3 receptors with a lower potency at D4 and D5 receptors [1,

2]. Neupro is a transdermal system that provides continuous delivery of rotigotine for 24 hours following application to intact skin [2-6]. Rotigotine is indicated for the treatment of Parkinson's Disease and moderate to severe restless legs syndrome [7].

Efficacy : Rotigotine reduced Parkinson's Disease symptoms [3, 8-27, 64], without increasing behavioural disturbances [28], reduced "off" time [9, 23, 27, 64], by 0.8 hours to 1.8 hours per day [29, 30, 31], reduced non-motor symptoms [25, 32], reduced L-dopa intake in less than half of people [6, 33], improved swallowing [34], reduced drooling [65], reduced pain [35], reduced daytime sleepiness [36], improved sleep (sleep disturbances, nocturnal motor symptoms, and nocturnal symptoms) [37, 38, 39], improved gastro-intestinal symptoms [40], improved walking ability [41], improved anxiety [42], reduced restless legs syndrome [43], improved mood and reduced depression [44], and improved dysphagia [63].

Adverse effects : The most commonly reported adverse effects are nausea [10, 11, 12, 16, 19, 20, 25-29, 37, 45-50], application site reactions [12, 14, 19, 20, 22, 25, 26, 27, 29, 33, 48, 49, 51-54], dyskinesia [3, 9, 10, 22, 24, 29, 46, 49, 53, 55, 56], dizziness [9, 12, 14, 21, 37, 45, 46, 50], somnolence [12, 14, 16, 19, 24, 25, 26, 49, 50, 53], vomiting [3, 11, 12, 22, 28, 47, 50], impulse-control disorder [49, 57, 58, 59]. Other less commonly reported adverse effects are drowsiness [11, 28, 55], tachycardia [11, 28], dystonia [11, 28], nail dyschromia [60], anxiety [37], orthostatic hypotension [11, 28], erythema [9, 50], application site pruritus [9, 46, 50], nasopharyngitis [46], insomnia [12, 24], headache [25, 45], hallucinations [24], fatigue [12], visual hallucinations [10], dry mouth [29], peripheral edema [49, 53].

Comparison : The effects of transdermal rotigotine are similar to those of ropinirole and pramipexole [17, 26, 61, 62].

[1] British Journal of Pharmacology [2015] 172 (4) : 1124-1135 (M. Wood, V.Dubois, D.Scheller, M.Gillard)

[2] Drugs [2015] 75 (5) : 487-501 (J.P.Elshoff, W.Cawello, J.O. Andreas, F.X.Mathy, M.Braun)

[3] PLoS One [2013] 8 (7) : e69738 (C.Q.Zhou, S.S.Li, Z.M.Chen, F.Q. Li, P.Lei, G.G.Peng)

[4] Drugs of Today [2010] 46 (7) : 483-505 (B.Boroojerdi, H.M.Wolff, M.Braun, D.K.Scheller)

[5] IDrugs [2003] 6 (9) : 894-899 (H.A.Mucke)

[6] Movement Disorders [2001] 16 (3) : 459-463 (J.T.Hutton, L.V. Metman, T.N.Chase, J.L.Juncos, W.C.Koller, R.Pahwa, P.A.LeWitt, A.Samii, J.K.Tsui, D.B.Calne, C.H.Waters, V.P.Calabrese, et al)

[7] European Journal of Drug Metabolism and Pharmacokinetics [2016] 41 (4) : 353-362 (W.Cawello, S.R.Kim, M.Braun, J.P.Elshoff, T.Masahiro, J.Ikeda, T.Funaki)

[8] Movement Disorders [2013] 28 (10) : 1447-1450 (Y.Mizuno, M. Nomoto, T.Kondo, K.Hasegawa, M.Murata, M.Takeuchi, J.Ikeda, T. Tomida, N.Hattori)

[9] Expert Opinion on Pharmacotherapy [2015] 16 (7) : 961-970 (S.J. Chung, J.M.Kim, J.W.Kim, B.S.Jeon, P.Singh, S.Thierfelder, J.Ikeda, L.Bauer)

[10] Clinical Neuropharmacology [2009] 32 (4) : 193-198 (I.Rektor, T.Babic, B.Boothmann, J.Polivka, B.Boroojerdi, O.Randerath)

[11] Neuropsychiatric Disease and Treatment [2014] 10 : 1003-1009 (D.Moretti, G.Binetti, O.Zanetti, G.B.Frisoni)

[12] Archives of Neurology [2003] 60 (12) : 1721-1728 (Parkinson Study Group)

[13] Clinical Neuropharmacology [2005] 28 (3) : 106-110 (W.M. Güldenpfennig, K.H.Poole, K.W.Sommerville, B.Boroojerdi)

[14] Neurology [2007] 68 (4) : 272-276 (R.L.Watts, J.Jankovic, C. Waters, A.Rajput, B.Boroojerdi, J.Rao)

[15] Annals of Pharmacotherapy [2007] 41 (2) : 285-295 (M.Y. Splinter)

[16] Archives of Neurology [2007] 64 (5) : 676-682 (J.Jankovic, R.L. Watts, W.Martin, B.Boroojerdi)

[17] CNS Drugs [2007] 21 (12) : 1039-1055 (C.M.Baldwin, G.M. Keating)

[18] Zhurnal Nevrologii i Psikhiatrii imeni S.S.Korsakova [2015] 115 (5) : 34-40 (E.A.Katunina, N.V.Titova, Y.N.Bezdolny, R.K. Shykkerimov, M.G.Gasanov, S.G.Burd, A.V.Lebedeva, A.N.Boiko)

[19] Clinical Neuropharmacology [2007] 30 (5) : 256-265 (P.A.LeWitt, B.Boroojerdi, D.MacMahon, J.Patton, J.Jankovic)

[20] Movement Disorders [2011] 26 (1) : 90-99 (C.Trenkwalder, B. Kies, M.Rudzinska, J.Fine, J.Nikl, K.Honczarenko, P.Dioszeghy, D. Hill, T.Anderson, V.Myllyla, J.Kassubek, M.Steiger, M.Zucconi, et al)

[21] Journal of Neural Transmission [2010] 117 (12) : 1395-1399 (N. Giladi, A.Fichtner, W.Poewe, B.Boroojerdi)

[22] PLoS One [2013] 8 (7) : e69738 (C.Q.Zhou, S.S.Li, Z.M.Chen, F.Q.Li, P.Lei, G.G.Peng)

[23] Journal of Neurology [2014] 261 (10) : 1887-1893 (M.Nomoto, Y.Mizuno, T.Kondo, K.Hasegawa, M.Murata, M.Takeuchi, J.Ikeda, T.Tomida, N.Hattori)

[24] Journal of Neural Transmission [2013] 120 (7) : 1069-1081 (P.A. LeWitt, B.Boroojerdi, E.Surmann, W.Poewe)

[25] European Journal of Neurology [2015] 22 (10) : 1400-1407 (A. Antonini, L.Bauer, E.Dohin, W.H.Oertel, O.Rascol, H.Reichmann, M. Schmid, P.Singh, E.Tolosa, K.R.Chaudhuri)

[26] Movement Disorders [2007] 22 (16) : 2398-2404 (N.Giladi, B.Boroojerdi, A.D.Korczyn, D.J.Burn, C.E.Clarke, A.H.Schapira)

[27] Clinical Therapeutics [2008] 30 (5) : 813-824 (D.Q.Pham, A. Nogid)

[28] Neuropharmacology [2014] 85 : 284-289 (D.V.Moretti, G.Binetti, O.Zanetti, G.B.Frisoni)

[29] Journal of Parkinson's Disease [2014] 4 (3) : 361-373 (A.P. Nicholas, R.Borgohain, P.Chaná, E.Surmann, E.L.Thompson, L.Bauer, J.Whitesides, L.W.Elmer)

[30] Neurology [2007] 68 (16) : 1262-1267 (P.A.LeWitt, K.E.Lyons, R.Pahwa)

[31] Lancet Neurology [2007] 6 (6) : 513-520 (W.H.Poewe, O.Rascol, N.Quinn, E.Tolosa, W.H.Oertel, E.Martignoni, M.Rupp, B.Boroojerdi)

[32] BMC Neurology [2011] 11 : 100 (H.J.Kim, B.S.Jeon, W.Y.Lee, M.C.Lee, J.W.Kim, J.M.Kim, T.B.Ahn, J.Cho, S.J.Chung, F.Grieger, J. Whitesides, B.Boroojerdi)

[33] Current Medical Research and Opinion [2011] 27 (10) : 1899-1905 (A.Ceballos-Baumann, H.J.Häck)

[34] Dysphagia [2015] 30 (4) : 452-456 (M.Hirano, C.Isono, H. Sakamoto, S.Ueno, S.Kusunoki, Y.Nakamura)

[35] BMC Neurology [2014] 14 : 42 (J.Kassubek, K.R.Chaudhuri, T.Zesiewicz, E.Surmann, B.Boroojerdi, K.Moran, L.Ghys, C. Trenkwalder)

[36] Clinical Neuropharmacology [2015] 38 (6) : 231-235 (K.Ohta K, T.Osada)

[37] Parkinson's Disease [2015] : 475630 (F.Vallderiola, Y.Compta, J.Aparicio, J.Tarradellas, G.Salazar, J.M. Oliver, A.Callén, T.Delgado, F.Nobbe)

[38] Functional Neurology [2010] 25 (4) : 201-204 (M.Canesi, C.B. Mariani, J.U.Isaias, G.Pezzoli)

[39] Parkinson's Disease [2015] : 131508 (J.Pagonabarraga, G.Piñol, A. Cardozo, P.Sanz, V.Puente, P.Otermín, I. Legarda, T.Delgado, C. Serrano, E.Balaguer, et al)

[40] Parkinsonism & Related Disorders [2015] 21 (3) : 199-204 (D. Woitalla, J.Kassubek, L.Timmermann, T.Lauterbach, R.Berkels, F. Grieger, T.Müller)

[41] Journal of Neurology [2015] 262 (11) : 2539-2547 (M.Serrao, A. Ranavolo, C.Conte, C.Davassi, S.Mari, A.Fasano, G.Chini, G.Coppola, F.Draicchio, F.Pierelli)

[42] Aging Clinical and Experimental Research [2013] 25 (5) : 601-603 (A.Fanciulli, F.Assogna, C.Caltagirone, G.Spalletta, F.E.Pontieri)

[43] Expert Opinion on Pharmacotherapy [2010] 11 (4) : 649-656 (F. Sixel-Döring, C.Trenkwalder)

[44] Parkinsonism & Related Disorders [2013] 19 (7) : 660-665 (K.Ray Chaudhuri, P.Martinez-Martin, A.Antonini, R.G.Brown, J.H.Friedman, M.Onofrj, E.Surmann, L.Ghys, C.Trenkwalder)

[45] Parkinsonism & Related Disorders [2013] 19 (1) : 37-42 (W. Oertel, P.LeWitt, N.Giladi, L.Ghys, F.Grieger, B.Boroojerdi)

[46] BMC Neurology [2015] 15 : 17 (J.M.Kim, S.J.Chung, J.W.Kim, B.S.Jeon, P.Singh, S.Thierfelder, J.Ikeda, L.Bauer)

[47] Clinical Neuropharmacology [2006] 29 (4) : 238-242 (T.Babic, B. Boothmann, J.Polivka, I.Rektor, B.Boroojerdi, H.J.Häck, O.Randerath)

[48] Parkinsonism & Related Disorders [2010] 16 (8) : 513-516 (A. Schnitzler, K.W.Leffers, H.J.Häck)

[49] Journal of Neural Transmission [2013] 120 (9) : 1321-1329 (N. Giladi, B.Boroojerdi, E.Surmann)

[50] Parkinsonism & Related Disorders [2016] 28 : 49-55 (Z.X.Zhang, H.F.Shang, X.Hu, S.Chen, Z.Zhao, X.Du, E.Surmann, L.Bauer, M.Asgharnejad)

[51] CNS Drugs [2011] 25 (8) : 699-719 (M.Sanford, L.J.Scott)

[52] Parkinsonism & Related Disorders [2014] 20 (12) : 1388-1393 (Y.Mizuno, M.Nomoto, K.Hasegawa, N.Hattori, T.Kondo, M.Murata, M.Takeuchi, M.Takahashi, T.Tomida)

[53] Parkinsonism & Related Disorders [2012] 18 (5) : 488-493 (L.W. Elmer, E.Surmann, B.Boroojerdi, J.Jankovic)

[54] Revista de Neurología [2013] 56 (7) : 359-362 (P.E.Bermejo, M.A.Zea, L.Alba-Alcántara, C.Ruiz-Huete)

[55] Revista de Neurología [2008] 46 (5) : 257-260 (C.Ruiz-Huete, P.E.Bermejo, C.Terrón, B.Anciones)

[56] Parkinsonism & Related Disorders [2014] 20 (12) : 1345-1351 (N.Giladi, L.Ghys, E.Surmann, B.Boroojerdi, J.Jankovic)

[57] Synapse [2015] 69 (4) : 183-189 (P.Seeman)

[58] Journal of Neurology, Neurosurgery, and Psychiatry [2014] 85 (8) : 840-844 (P.J.Garcia-Ruiz, J.C.Martinez Castrillo, A.Alonso-Canovas, A.Herranz Barcenas, L.Vela, P.Sanchez Alonso, M.Mata, et al)

[59] Clinical Neuropharmacology [2009] 32 (2) : 59-62 (T.S.Wingo, M.Evatt, B.Scott, A.Freeman, M.Stacy)

[60] Neurology [2011] 76 (18) : 1605 (H.A.Teive, R.P.Munhoz)

[61] Neuropsychiatric Disease and Treatment [2014] 10 : 767-776 (K. Thorlund, P.Wu, E.Druyts, S.Eapen, E.J.Mills)

[62] Prescrire International [2008] 17 (94) : 60 [No authors listed]

[63] Dysphagia [2015] 30 (4) : 452-456 (M.Hirano, C.Isono, H. Sakamoto, S.Ueno, S.Kusunoki, Y.Nakamura)

[64] Neurodegenerative Disease Management [2017] 7 (1) : 61-72 (A. Zesiewicz, S.Chriscoe, T.Jimenez, J.Upward, M.Davy, S.VanMeter)

[65] Clinical Neurology and Neurosurgery [2017] 156 : 63-65 (T. Schirinzi, P.Imbriani, A.D'Elia, G.Di Lazzaro, N.B.Mercuri, A.Pisani)

CHAPTER 43

PHARMACOLOGICAL TREATMENTS OF PARKINSON'S DISEASE

MAO INHIBITORS

Pharmacology

MAO inhibitors help to maintain dopamine levels by inhibiting the enzyme Monoamine Oxidase (EC 1.4.3.4), which has two forms : MAO-A and MAO-B. Monoamine oxidase metabolizes dopamine : Dopamine + H_2O + O_2 >>> Dihydroxyphenylacetic acid + H_2O_2

Types of Mao inhibitor

The main MAO inhibitors in use are selegiline [PAGE 664], rasagiline [PAGE 669] and Safinamide [PAGE 673]. Zelapar [PAGE 667] is a form of Selegiline designed for absorption in the mouth. P2B001 is a combination of rasagiline and pramipexole [PAGE 672]. Safinamide is believed to have both dopaminergic and non-dopaminergic actions, including the inhibition of monoamine oxidase B (MAO-B) and inhibition of glutamate release.

Selegiline

Common brand names : Selegiline, Selegilin, Deprenyl, Eldepryl, Jumex, Jumexil, Sefmex, Elepril, Niar, Antiparkin, Selegelina

Pharmacology : Selegiline is a MAO-B inhibitor [1]. To some extent Selegiline is also a MAO-A inhibitor [2].

Efficacy : Selegiline caused a significant improvement in Parkinson's Disease symptoms [3-14], and a reduced need for L-dopa [1, 4, 5, 6, 8, 12, 13, 15, 16]. However, the improvement was only moderate or minimal [17]. When added to the use of L-dopa, selegiline was not impressive with regard to preventing the future progression of

Parkinson's Disease [1, 18]. Consequently, selegiline is sufficient on its own in very few people. Selegiline causes more fluctuations than dopamine agonists. Withdrawals due to side effects are far less common with selegiline than with dopamine agonists [19, 20]. Daily dosages of 5 mg are indistinguishable in their effect from daily dosages of 10 mg [21]. Higher doses of selegiline, of up to 40mg a day produce additional therapeutic benefits above those of the conventional dose of 10 mg a day [22]. Selegiline use for up to three years or more was associated with a slower progression of Parkinson's Disease [18, 23]. However, the improvement rate declined in the course of the therapy [8]. The effect started to decline after three years [18, 24] or earlier [14], and there was subsequent worsening [10], which was greater in people with fluctuating symptoms [25], and in people whose Parkinson's Disease was worse [26]. L-Dopa treated patients who received Selegiline within five years from the onset of Parkinson's Disease compared better than those who took Selegiline approximately ten years from the onset [27]. Fewer people worsen when selegiline is added earlier to L-dopa than when it is added later [25]. After three years there was no difference between rasagiline and selegiline on their effect on clinical progression [31].

Adverse effects : Selegiline causes many side effects [28], and long term side effects [5]. Notable side effects can include cardiovascular problems including postural hypotension, atrial fibrillation, and arterial hypertension [1]. Selegiline may also be related to the incidence of hallucination [29]. Those with a recorded diagnosis of Parkinson's Disease taking selegiline alone had an increased death rate [1, 30].

[1] Prescrire International [2002] 11 (60) : 108-111 (No authors listed)

[2] Neuropsychopharmacology [2014] 40 (3) : 650-657 (J.S. Fowler, J.Logan, N.D.Volkow, E.Shumay, F.McCall-Perez, M. Jayne, G.J.Wang, D.L.Alexoff, K.Apelskog-Torres, et al)

[3] Journal of the Association of Physicians of India [1999] 47 (8) : 784-786 (S.N.Dixit, M.Behari, G.K.Ahuja)

[4] European Journal of Neurology [1999] 6 (5) : 539-547 (J.P.Larsen, J.Boas, J.E.Erdal)

[5] European Journal of Neurology [1999] 6 (2) : 141-150 (H. Przuntek, B.Conrad, J.Dichgans, P.H.Kraus, P.Krauseneck, G. Pergande, U.Rinne, K.Schimrigk, J.Schnitker, H.P.Vogel)

[6] Neurology [1998] 51 (2) : 520-525 (S.Pålhagen, E.H. Heinonen, J. Hägglund, T.Kaugesaar, H.Kontants, O.Mäki-Ikola, R.Palm, J. Turunen)

[7] Zhonghua Yi Xue Za Zhi [1996] 58 (4) : 264-268 (D.E.Shan, S.I. Yeh)

[8] No To Shinkei [1994] 46 (5) : 465-471 (Y. Mizuno, T.Kondo, H. Takubo, F.Yokochi)

[9] Folia Phoniatrica [1993] 45 (1) : 40-46 (B.R.Shea, S.S.Drummond, W.S.Metzer, K.M.Krueger)

[10] Journal of the Association of Physicians of India [1994] 42 (1) : 30-32 (M.Bhatia, S.Jain, M.C.Maheshwari)

[11] Movement Disorders [1993] 8 (Supplement 1) : S36-S40 (H. Allain, P.Pollak, H.C.Neukirch)

[12] Acta Neurologica Scandinavica (Supplementum) [1989] 126 : 147-152 (B.Sivertsen, E.Dupont, B.Mikkelsen, P.Mogensen, C. Rasmussen, F.Boesen, E.Heinonen)

[13] Journal of Neural Transmission (Supplementum) [1987] 25 : 149-155 (U.K.Rinne)

[14] Journal of Neural Transmission (Supplementum) [1987] 25 : 131-135 (W.Poewe, F.Gerstenbrand, G.Ransmayr)

[15] Acta Neurologica Scandinavica [1997] 95 (4) : 211-218 (V.V. Myllylä, K.A.Sotaniemi, P.Hakulinen, O.Mäki-Ikola, E.H.Heinonen)

[16] Acta Neurologica Scandinavica [1995] 91 (3) : 177-182 (V.V. Myllylä, E.H. Heinonen, J.A.Vuorinen, O.L.Kilkku, K.A.Sotaniemi)

[17] Acta Neurologica Scandinavica (Supplementum) [1983] 95 : 107-111 (U.K.Rinne)

[18] Archives of Neurology [1989] 46 (12) : 1280-1283 (T.S.Elizan, M. D.Yahr, D.A.Moros, M.R.Mendoza, S.Pang, C.A.Bodian)

[19] Cochrane Database of Systematic Reviews [2009] 4 : CD006661 (R.Caslake, A.Macleod, N.Ives, R.Stowe, C.Counsell)

[20] Cochrane Database of Systematic Reviews [2005] 20 (3) : CD004898 (A.D.Macleod, C.E.Counsell, N.Ives, R.Stowe)

[21] Clinical Neuropharmacology [1993] 16 (1) : 83-87 (J.P.Hubble, W.C.Koller, C.Waters)

[22] Acta Neurologica Scandinavica (Supplementum) [1989] 126 : 139-145 (A.J.Lees, J.Frankel, V.Eatough, G.M.Stern)

[23] Parkinsonism & Related Disorders [2011] 17 (3) : 194-197 (Y.J. Zhao, H.L.Wee, W.L.Au, S.H.Seah, N.Luo, S.C.Li, L.C.Tan)

[24] No To Shinkei [2002] 54 (12) : 1041-1048 (T.Kondo, H.Takubo, F.Yokochi, Y.Okuma, Y. Mizuno)

[25] Neurology [1992] 42 (Supplement 4) : 32-36; discussion 41-48 (A.Lieberman)

[26] Acta Neurologica Scandinavica (Supplementum) [1991] 136 : 66-69 (A.Lieberman, E.Fazzini)

[27] Clinical Neuropharmacology [2010] 33 (1) : 1-4 (Y.Mizuno, T. Kondo, S.Kuno, M.Nomoto, N.Yanagisawa)

[28] Journal of Geriatric Psychiatry and Neurology [1992] 5 (1) : 31-34 (C.H.Waters)

[29] Parkinsonism & Related Disorders [2004] 10 (4) : 235-242 (K. Kamakura, H.Mochizuki, K.Kaida, A.Hirata, M.Kanzaki, T.Masaki, R. Nakamura, K.Motoyoshi)

[30] BMJ [1998] 317 (7153) : 252-254 (M.Thorogood, B.Armstrong, T.Nichols, J.Hollowell)

[31] Journal of Neurology [2017] May 26 [Epub ahead of print] (E.Cereda, R.Cilia, M.Canesi, S.Tesei, C.B.Mariani, A.L.Zecchinelli, G.Pezzoli)

ZELAPAR

Brand names : Zelapar

Pharmacology : Zelapar is a transmucosal preparation that is used for the administration of selegiline. Zydis is the technology used to manufacture the orally disintegrating tablets. A lozenge is placed between the cheek and gum. The tablets dissolve within seconds in the mouth. The medication then enters the bloodstream directly. Almost a third of the selegiline is absorbed inside the mouth within a minute. The active drug then moves into the bloodstream to the brain [1].

Efficacy : In clinical trials, the orally disintegrating form of selegiline demonstrated moderate efficacy [2], or very limited efficacy [3, 4]. Plasma concentrations of metabolites were significantly lower than following conventional selegiline. There was a much higher variability of plasma selegiline concentrations after using conventional selegiline. The absorption of selegiline from Zydis selegiline was more efficient and less variable than from conventional selegiline tablets. So lower doses could be used whilst still having the same effect [1]. Doses of 1.25mg and 10mg were shown to be therapeutically equivalent to conventional 10mg selegiline based on a comparison of the Unified Parkinson's Disease Rating Scale (UPDRS) scores and when compared to the motor sub scores of the UPDRS. The 1.25mg dose was slightly more advantageous. People who were taking regular selegiline slightly improved when they changed over to the 1.25mg Zydis selegiline [5]. Zydis selegiline in doses of 2.5mg reduced off time by 2.2 hours in comparison to 0.6 hours with a placebo. The average number of hours free of dyskinesia increased by 1.8 hours [2]. Overall, people preferred Zydis selegiline to selegiline when they changed over to Zydis selegiline. They improved according to clinician global impressions, fluctuations, and the "on" scores of the UPDRS improved [6]. Most of the patients (65%) preferred taking Zydis selegiline to their usual medication.

Adverse effects : Because the digestive system is bypassed, there are fewer metabolites [1], and fewer side effects than with conventional selegiline. There were no apparent differences in the occurrence of drug related adverse effects between the Zydis selegiline group and placebo treated groups [2]. Most patients preferred Zydis selegiline to selegiline and found it easy to take [5]. Zydis selegiline did not potentiate the tyramine effect. This was in contrast to conventional selegiline whose threshold soon lowered for eliciting the tyramine effect [5].

[1] Journal of Neural Transmission [2003] 110 (11) : 1241-1255 (A. Clarke, F.Brewer, E.S.Johnson, N.Mallard, F.Hartig, S.Taylor, T.H. Corn)

[2] Movement Disorders [2004] 19 (4) : 426-432 (C.H.Waters, K.D. Sethi, R.A.Hauser, E.Molho, J.M.Bertoni)

[3] Clinical Neuropharmacology [2007] 30 (5) : 295-300 (W.G.Ondo, K.D.Sethi, G.Kricorian)

[4] Current Medical Research and Opinion [2007] 23 (4) : 741-750 (M. F.Lew, R.Pahwa, M.Leehey, J.Bertoni, G.Kricorian)

[5] Journal of Neural Transmission [2003] 110 (11) : 1257-1271 (A. Clarke, E.S.Johnson, N.Mallard, T.H.Corn, A.Johnston, M.Boyce, S. Warrington, D.G.MacMahon)

[6] Parkinsonism & Related Disorders [2011] 17 (2) : 117-118 (W.G. Ondo, C.Hunter, S.H.Isaacson, D.E.Silver, R.M.Stewart, J.W.Tetrud, A.Davidson)

Rasagiline

Brand name : Azilect

Pharmacology : Rasagiline is a MAO-B inhibitor. It is used as either monotherapy or adjunct therapy [1].

Efficacy : Rasagiline caused a moderate reduction in Parkinson's Disease symptoms [2-22, 28], and reduced "off" time [8-12, 17, 23]. The effect was still evident six weeks after drug discontinuation [13]. Rasagiline was found to be more effective than selegiline [14]. Rasagiline significantly improves tremor on its own and when added to optimal dopaminergic treatment [18]. Fatigue is moderately improved [24]. The quality of sleep is improved [27]. However, rasagiline does not slow down

Parkinson's Disease progression [14, 25]. Starting treatment early or delaying the start of treatment made no difference [25]. After three years there was no difference between rasagiline and selegiline on their effect on clinical progression [29]

Adverse effects : Rasagiline causes infrequent cardiovascular or psychiatric side effects [26].

[1] Drugs [2007] 67 (12) : 1725-1747 (V.Oldfield, G.M.Keating, C.M. Perry)

[2] Movement Disorders [2009] 24 (4) : 564-573 (R.A.Hauser, M.F. Lew, H.I.Hurtig, W.G.Ondo, J.Wojcieszek, C.J.Fitzer-Attas)

[3] International Journal of Neuroscience [2010] 120 (6) : 404-408 (M. F.Lew, R.A.Hauser, H.I.Hurtig, W.G.Ondo, J.Wojcieszek, T.Goren, C. J.Fitzer-Attas)

[4] Movement Disorders [2004] 19 (8) : 916-923 (M.B.Stern, K.L. Marek, J.Friedman, R.A.Hauser, P.A.LeWitt, D.Tarsy, C.W. Olanow)

[5] Archives of Neurology [2004] 61 (4) : 561-566 (Parkinson Study Group)

[6] Archives of Neurology [2002] 59 (12) : 1937-1943 (Parkinson Study Group)

[7] New England Journal of Medicine [2009] 361 (13) : 1268-1278 (C. W.Olanow, O.Rascol, R.Hauser, P.D.Feigin, J.Jankovic, A.Lang, W. Langston, E.Melamed, W.Poewe, F.Stocchi, E.Tolosa)

[8] Fortschritte der Neurologie Psychiatrie [2008] 76 (10) : 594-599 (W.H.Jost, M.Klasser, H.Reichmann)

[9] European Journal of Neurology [2010] 17 (9) : 1164-1171 (H. Reichmann, W.H.Jost)

[10] Lancet [2005] 365 (9463) : 947-954 (O.Rascol, D.J.Brooks, E. Melamed, W.Oertel, W.Poewe, F.Stocchi, E.Tolosa, LARGO study group)

[11] Archives of Neurology [2005] 62 (2) : 241-248 (Parkinson Study Group)

[12] Drugs and Aging [2005] 22 (1) : 83-91 (M.A.Siddiqui, G.L. Plosker)

[13] Clinical Neuropharmacology [2000] 23 (6) : 324-330 (J.M. Rabey, I.Sagi, M.Huberman, E.Melamed, A.Korczyn, N.Giladi, R.Inzelberg, R.Djaldetti, C.Klein, G.Berecz)

[14] Clinical Therapeutics [2007] 29 (9) : 1825-1849 (J.J.Chen, D.M. Swope, K.Dashtipour)

[15] Lancet Neurology [2011] 10 (5) : 415-423 (O.Rascol, C.J. Fitzer-Attas, R.Hauser, J.JankovicJ, A.Lang, J.W.Langston, E.Melamed, W. Poewe, F.Stocchi, E.Tolosa, E.Eyal, Y.M.Weiss, C.W.Olanow)

[16] Nederlands Tijdschrift voor Geneeskunde [2009] 154 (38) : A2496 (T.van Laar, A.J.Boon, B.R.Bloem)

[17] European Journal of Neurology [2011] 19 (2) : 258-264 (E.Tolosa, M.B.Stern)

[18] International Journal of Neuroscience [2013] 123 (12) : 859- 865 (M.F.Lew)

[19] Neurologist [2011] 17 (6) : 318-324 (R.E.Wilson, L.C.Seeberger, D.Silver, A.Griffith, J.B.Conner, P.M.Salzman)

[20] Neurological Science [2013] 34 (11) : 2007-2013 (S.Zambito Marsala, R.Vitaliani, D.Volpe, F.Capozzoli, L.Baroni, E.Belgrado, C. Borsato, M.Gioulis, C.Marchini, A.Antonini)

[21] Parkinsonism & Related Disorders [2014] 20 (6) : 640-643 (J. Jankovic, E.Berkovich, E.Eyal, E.Tolosa)

[22] Movement Disorders [2014] 29 (8) : 1028-1034 (R.A.Hauser, D. Silver, A.Choudhry, E.Eyal, S.Isaacson)

[23] European Neurology [2015] 73 (1-2) : 5-12 (J.P.Cai, W.J.Chen, Y.Lin, B.Cai, N.Wang)

[24] Movement Disorders [2015] 30 (13) : 1825-1830 (T.T.Lim, B.M. Kluger, R.L.Rodriguez, I.A.Malaty, R.Palacio Jr, O.O.Ojo, S.Patel, Y.Gujrati, B.Nutter, C.Swartz, C.Hennessy, H.H.Fernandez)

[25] Movement Disorders [2016] Jul 19 [Epub ahead of print] (O. Rascol, R.A.Hauser, F.Stocchi, C.J.Fitzer-Attas, Y.Sidi, V.Abler, C.W. Olanow)

[26] Journal of Clinical Pharmacology [2005] 45 (8) : 878-894 (J.J. Chen, D.M.Swope)

[27] Canadian Journal of Neurologocal Sciences [2016] 43 (6) : 809-814 (M.Panisset, J.L.Stril, M.Bélanger, G.Lehoux, D.Coffin, S. Chouinard)

[28] Annals of Medicine [2017] 15 : 1-14 [Epub ahead of print] (Y.Chang, L.B.Wang, D.Li, K.Lei, S.Y.Liu)

[29] Journal of Neurology [2017] May 26 [Epub ahead of print] (E.Cereda, R.Cilia, M.Canesi, S.Tesei, C.B.Mariani, A.L.Zecchinelli, G.Pezzoli)

P2B001

Brand name : none (due to being in development)

Pharmacology : P2B001 is a novel combination of slow release and low dose rasagiline and pramipexole for synergistic use in early Parkinson's Disease that is presently in development. Rasagiline is a MAO inhibitor for use in treating Parkinson's Disease. Pramipexole is a dopamine agonist that is also for use in Parkinson's Disease [1].

Efficacy : People with early Parkinson's Disease were assessed when taking : P2B001 (0.3mg pramipexole / 0.75mg rasagiline), P2B001 (0.6mg pramipexole / 0.75mg rasagiline) or a placebo. The most effective of these was P2B001 with a higher dose of pramipexole, followed by P2B001 with a lower dose of pramipexole. Significant benefits were observed for both doses in : Parkinson Disease Quality of Life Scale-39 scores, the UPDRS motor score, and activities of daily living [1].

Adverse effects : The adverse effects of P2B001 were comparable to the use of a placebo apart from transient nausea and somnolence, which were more common with P2B001 [1].

[1] Movement Disorders [2017] Apr 3 [Epub ahead of print] (C.W. Olanow, K. Kieburtz, M.Leinonen, L.Elmer, N.Giladi, R.A.Hauser, O.S.Klepiskaya, D.L.Kreitzman, M. F.Lew, D.S.Russell, et al)

SAFINAMIDE

Brand name : Xadago

Pharmacology : Safinamide has both dopaminergic properties (highly selective and reversible inhibition of monoamine oxidase-B) and non-dopaminergic properties (selective sodium channel blockade and calcium channel modulation, with consequent inhibition of excessive glutamate release) [1]. It is usually added to the use of L-dopa or dopamine agonists.

Efficacy : In once daily dosages of 50mg to 100mg, after six months, Safinamide improved Parkinson's Disease symptoms and reduced "off" time when added to existing Parkinson's Disease treatments. The reduction in "off" time in comparison to a placebo was minimal. The increase in "on" time beyond that of a placebo was only 40 minutes for 50mg safinamide, and 50 minutes for 100mg safinamide. Higher dosages had no beneficial effects [2, 3, 4, 6]. People taking 100 mg daily dosages had a lower need for increased dopamine agonists [5].

Adverse effects : The side effects of safinamide were not disclosed. After 24 months, the improvement in dyskinesia was not statistically significant [2, 3]. The most frequently reported adverse event was dyskinesia (14%], and as a severe event (2%) [6].

[1] Drugs [2015] 75 (6) : 705-711 (E.D.Deeks)

[2] Movement Disorders [2012] 27 (1) : 106-112 (F.Stocchi, R. Borgohain, M.Onofrj, A.H.Schapira, M.Bhatt, V.Lucini, R.Giuliani, R. Anand)

[3] Movement Disorders [2014] 29 (10) : 1273-1280 (R.Borgohain, J. Szasz, P.Stanzione, C.Meshram, M.H.Bhatt, D.Chirilineau, F.Stocchi, V.Lucini, R.Giuliani, E.Forrest, P.Rice, R.Anand)

[4] Journal of Parkinsons Disease [2016] 6 (1) : 165-173 (C.Cattaneo, M.Sardina, E.Bonizzoni)

[5] European Journal of Neurology [2013] 20 (2) : 271-280 (A.H. Schapira, F.Stocchi, R.Borgohain, M.Onofrj, M.Bhatt, P.Lorenzana, V. Lucini, R.Giuliani, R.Anand)

[6] JAMA Neurology [2017] 74 (2) : 216-224 (A.H.Schapira, S.H.Fox, R.A.Hauser, J.Jankovic, W.H.Jost, C.Kenney, J.Kulisevsky, R.Pahwa, W.Poewe, R.Anand)

CHAPTER 44

PHARMACOLOGICAL TREATMENTS OF PARKINSON'S DISEASE

COMT INHIBITORS

PHARMACOLOGY

COMT inhibitors help to maintain dopamine levels by inhibiting Catechol-O-methyl transferase (COMT) (EC 2.1.1.6), which is an enzyme that metabolizes dopamine : Dopamine + S-adenosyl-L-methionine >>> S-adenosyl-L-homocysteine + 3-Methoxytyramine.

TYPES OF COMT INHIBITOR

The most commonly used COMT inhibitor is Entacapone [PAGE 675]. Entacapone is often taken as Stalevo [PAGE 679], which combines L-dopa, carbidopa and entacapone. A new format of Stalevo, ODM-101 [PAGE 681], is being developed. Other COMT inhibitors being used or assessed for the treatment of Parkinson's Disease are tolcapone [PAGE 682], opicapone [PAGE 685], and nebicapone [PAGE 686].

ENTACAPONE

Brand names : Comtan, Stalevo (combined with L-dopa and carbidopa)

Pharmacology : Entacapone is a COMT inhibitor.

Efficacy : Entacapone efficacy was considered by physicians to be "very good" or "good" in 77% of patients [1]. Entacapone moderately increases "on" time [2-18], moderately improves Activities of Daily Living [18], moderately improved Clinical Global Impression of Change (CGIC) [19-21] and Quality of Life [19, 20], led to a moderate reduction in the L-dopa dose [1, 4, 7, 8, 17, 20, 22-25], led to a moderate reduction in dyskinesia [1], led to a moderate improvement in Parkinson's Disease symptom scores and motor fluctuations [25, 26], and led to a moderate improvement in Parkinson's Disease symptom scores [6, 12, 16, 18, 23, 24, 27-31]. The increase in efficacy when taken with L-dopa did not differ according to whether carbidopa or benserazide was the decarboxylase inhibitor used [32]. Adding entacapone did not improve motor symptoms in Parkinson's Disease treated with L-dopa without motor fluctuations [33].

Adverse effects : Entacapone is generally well tolerated [2, 14, 20, 22, 23, 24, 27, 34, 35]. The tolerability of entacapone was considered by physicians to be "very good" or "good" in 92% of patients [1]. However, there are a number of adverse effects with its use, the most common of which are : dyskinesia [2, 6, 16, 20, 23, 36, 37], which occurred in 10% to 52% of people [6, 16, 37], and was common in those taking dopamine agonists [38]; nausea [16, 23, 28, 37, 39], which occurs in 1% to 14% of people [16, 37, 39]; diarrhea [24, 28, 37, 39], which occurs in 2% to 8% of people [36, 38]; and in some people : urine discoloration [22, 40], an increase in liver enzymes [39], insomnia [4], dizziness [4], and hallucinations [4]. Reasons for discontinuation of entacapone included lack of efficacy (46%), worsening symptoms (28%), worse cognition (20%), dyskinesia (17%), nausea (11%), diarrhea (9%), cost (4%), other side effects (8%), other non-medication related reasons (19%). Presence of wearing off at the time of initial treatment and male gender were associated with decreased dropout rates, while the presence of orthostatic hypotension increased the likelihood of discontinuation [41].

[1] Current Medical Research and Opinion [2004] 20 (1) : 115-120 (A. Kupsch, T.Trottenberg, D.Bremen)

[2] Movement Disorders [2007] 22 (1) : 75-80 (Y.Mizuno, I. Kanazawa, S.Kuno, N.Yanagisawa, M.Yamamoto, T.Kondo)

[3] Journal of Neurology, Neurosurgery and Psychiatry [2003] 74 (8) : 1071-1079 (D.J.Brooks, H.Sagar)

[4] European Journal of Neurology [2003] 10 (2) : 137-146 (J.P. Larsen, J.Worm-Petersen, A.Sidén, A.Gordin, K.Reinikainen, M. Leinonen)

[5] Annals of Neurology [1997] 42 (5) : 747-755 [No authors listed]

[6] European Neurology [2001] 45 (2) : 111-118 (F.Durif, I.Devaux, J. J.Pere, J.C.Delumeau, I.Bourdeix)

[7] Journal of Neurology, Neurosurgery and Psychiatry [1996] 60 (1) : 36-40 (H.M.Ruottinen, U.K.Rinne)

[8] Neurology [1994] 44 (5) : 913-919 (J.G.Nutt, W.R.Woodward, R. M.Beckner, C.K.Stone, K.Berggren, J.H.Carter, S.T.Gancher, J.P. Hammerstad, A.Gordin)

[9] Revista de Neurologica [1999] 28 (8) : 817-834 (J.A.Burguera, F.Grandas, J.F.Horga de la Parte, R.Luquin, F.Martí, J.Matías-Guiu, J. A.Obeso, J.Kulisevsky)

[10] Neurological Research [2009] 31 (1) : 74-76 (C.Pellicano, D. Benincasa, M.Giovannelli, F.R.Buttarelli, S.Ruggieri, F.E.Pontieri)

[11] Journal of Neural Transmission [2004] 111 (2) : 173-180 (F. Stocchi, L.Barbato, G.Nordera, A.Bolner, T.Caraceni)

[12] European Journal of Neurology [2007] 14 (3) : 282-289 (F. Grandas, B.Hernández)

[13] Movement Disorders [2009] 24 (9) : 1319-1324 (P.A.LeWitt, D. Jennings, K.E.Lyons, R.Pahwa, A.L.Rabinowicz, J.Wang, M. Guarnieri, J.P.Hubble, H.Murck)

[14] Clinical Neuropharmacology [2001] 24 (3) : 150-157 (H. Heikkinen, J.G.Nutt, P.A.LeWitt, W.C.Koller, A.Gordin)

[15] Journal of Neurology, Neurosurgery and Psychiatry [2000] 68 (5) : 589-594 (P.Piccini, D.J.Brooks, K.Korpela, N.Pavese, M. Karlsson, A. Gordin)

[16] Acta Neurologica Scandinavica [2014] 130 (4) : 239-247 (M. Kuoppamäki, M.Vahteristo, J.Ellmén, K.Kieburtz)

[17] Neurological Science [2008] 29 (Supplement 5) : S380-S382 (M. Canesi, A.L.Zecchinelli, G.Pezzoli, A.Antonini)

[18] Acta Neurologica Scandinavica [2005] 111 (1) : 21-28 (H. Reichmann, J.Boas, D.Macmahon, V.Myllyla, A.Hakala, K. Reinikainen)

[19] Journal of Neural Transmission [2004] 111 (8) : 1053-1063 (M. Onofrj, A.Thomas, F.Vingerhoets, W.Martin, S.Giménez-Roldán, J.P. Azulay, G.Bernhard, W.Schmidt, S.Markabi)

[20] Journal of Neural Transmission [2003] 110 (3) : 239-251 (G. Fénelon, S.Giménez-Roldán, J.L.Montastruc, F.Bermejo, F.Durif, I. Bourdeix, J.J.Péré, L.Galiano, J.Schadrack)

[21] Journal of Clinical Neurology [2007] 3 (2) : 82-85 (T.B.Ahn, J.H. Im, M.C.Lee, J.W.Kim, W.Y.Lee, B.S.Jeon)

[22] European Journal of Neurology [2001] 8 (1) : 53-60 (V.V. Myllylä, E.R.Kultalahti, H.Haapaniemi, M.Leinonen)

[23] Clinical Therapeutics [2001] 23 (6) : 802-832 (J.Najib)

[24] Neurology [1998] 51 (5) : 1309-1314 (J.P.Larsen, A.Siden, J. Worm-Petersen)

[25] European Journal of Neurology [2008] 15 (7) : 643-648 (P. Damier, F.Viallet, M.Ziegler, I.Bourdeix, K.Rerat)

[26] Neurological Sciences [2003] 24 (3) : 197-198 (C.Paci, S. Sanguigni, T.Carboni, R.Gobbato, L.Curatola)

[27] Progress in Neuropsychopharmacology and Biological Psychiatry [2003] 27 (6) : 963-971 (O.Gershanik, M.Emre, G. Bernhard, D.Sauer)

[28] Movement Disorders [2009] 24 (4) : 541-550 (R.A.Hauser, M. Panisset, G.Abbruzzese, L.Mancione, N.Dronamraju, A.Kakarieka)

[29] Current Medical Research and Opinion [2008] 24 (11) : 3207-3215 (M.Jog, M.Panisset, O.Suchowersky, B.Réhel, R. Schecter)

[30] Journal of Neural Transmission [2010] 117 (3) : 333-342 (K. Eggert, O.Skogar, K.Amar, L.Luotonen, M.Kuoppamk, M.Leinonen, H.Nissinen, W.Oertel)

[31] European Journal of Neurology [2009] 16 (12) : 1305-1311 (H. Nissinen, M.Kuoppamki, M.Leinonen, A.H.Schapira)

[32] Journal of Neural Transmission [2015] 122 (12) : 1709-1714 (M. Kuoppamäki, M.Leinonen, W.Poewe)

[33] Archives of Neurology [2004] 61 (10) : 1563-1568 (C.W. Olanow, K.Kieburtz, M.Stern, R.Watts, J.W.Langston, M.Guarnieri, J.Hubble)

[34] CNS Neuroscience and Therapeutics [2008] 14 (1) : 83-93 (A.J. Lees)

[35] Journal of Neural Transmission [2008] 115 (6) : 843-849 (D.J. Brooks, M.Leinonen, M.Kuoppamäki, H.Nissinen)

[36] Nature Reviews Neurology [2010] 6 (11) : 590-591 (C.Sampaio, J. J.Ferreira)

[37] Acta Neurologica Scandinavica [2002] 105 (4) : 245-255 (W.H. Poewe, G.Deuschl, A.Gordin, E.R.Kultalahti, M.Leinonen)

[38] Annals of Neurology [2010] 68 (1) : 18-27 (F.Stocchi, O.Rascol, K.Kieburtz, W.Poewe, J.Jankovic, E.Tolosa, P.Barone, A.E.Lang, C.W. Olanow)

[39] Clinical Neuropharmacology [2014] 37 (1) : 1-5 (K.Eggert, W.H. Oertel, A.J.Lees)

[40] Drugs [1999] 58 (1) : 159-177 (K.J.Holm, C.M.Spencer)

[41] Clinical Neuropharmacology [2004] 27 (3) : 119-123 (S.A. Parashos, C.L.Wielinski, J.A.Kern)

STALEVO

Brand name : Stalevo

Pharmacology : Stalevo is a combination of L-dopa, carbidopa and entacapone, which is the same as Sinemet plus entacapone. The therapeutic constituent is L-dopa. Carbidopa is a dopa-decarboxylase inhibitor, which helps to prevent the breakdown of the L-dopa. Entacapone is able to slow down the degradation of L-dopa. Stalevo is intended for the treatment of people with Parkinson's Disease who experience signs and symptoms of end-of-dose "wearing off" [1].

Efficacy : Stalevo resulted in an improvement in Parkinson's Disease symptoms [2-6]. There was also an improvement in "on" time [7, 8].

Patients found Stalevo simpler to dose, more convenient to use, easier to remember and easier to swallow [9]. Most patients preferred Stalevo to L-dopa and carbidopa in a sustained release form and improved their symptoms when they changed over to it [10]. Pharmacokinetic studies demonstrated bioequivalence between Stalevo and the corresponding dosages of L-dopa with carbidopa plus entacapone [11]. Patients can take one Stalevo tablet rather than two or more tablets [11]. Over 70% of those who added entacapone to their L-dopa and a dopa decarboxylase inhibitor, or who switched to Stalevo, felt that they clinically improved. Over 80% of them experienced a reduction in fluctuations [12].

Adverse effects : About 8% of people that changed to Stalevo discontinued treatment mostly because of adverse effects. There was also a tendency for Stalevo to initiate or worsen dyskinesia [2]. The U.S. Food and Drug Administration (FDA) evaluated clinical trial data that might suggest that Stalevo increases the risk of developing prostate cancer. The number of people taking Stalevo with prostate cancer was small but was four times what would be expected. They suggested that "Patients should not stop taking their medication unless directed to do so by their healthcare professional" [13].

[1] Drugs in R & D [2003] 4 (5) : 310-311

[2] Journal of Neural Transmission [2005] 112 (2) : 221-230 (W. Koller, M.Guarnieri, J.Hubble, A.L.Rabinowicz, D.Silver)

[3] Zhurnal Nevrologii i Psikhiatrii Imeni S S Korsakova [2006] 106 (9) : 39-46 (N.V.Fedorova, O.S.Levin, I.G.Smolentseva, T.K. Kulua)

[4] Zhurnal Nevrologii i Psikhiatrii Imeni S S Korsakova [2008] 108 (7) : 27-34 (O.S.Levin, I.G.Smolentseva, N.V.Fedorova, I.P.Chigir, L. V.Dokadina, S.O.Makhnev)

[5] Movement Disorders [2009] 24 (4) : 541-550 (R.A.Hauser, M. Panisset, G.Abbruzzese, L.Mancione, N.Dronamraju, A.Kakarieka)

[6] Journal of Neural Transmission [2014] 121 (4) : 357-366 (E. Tolosa, B.Hernández, G.Linazasoro, J.J.López-Lozano, P.Mir, J. Marey, J.Kulisevsky)

[7] European Journal of Neurology [2008] 15 (3) : 257-261 (G. Linazasoro, J.Kulisevsky, B.Hernndez, Spanish Stalevo Study Group)

[8] Neuroscience and Behavioral Physiology [2008] 38 (9) : 933-936 (A.N.Boiko, T.T.Batysheva, N.G.Minaeva, L.A.Babina, T.V. Vdovichenko, E.Y.Zhuravleva, R.K.Shikhkerimov, et al)

[9] Acta Neurologica Scandinavica [2006] 114 (3) : 181-186 (V. Myllyl, T.Haapaniemi, S.Kaakkola, E.Kinnunen, P.Hartikainen, J. Nuutinen, A.Rissanen, A.M.Kuopio, T.Jolma, O.Satomaa, et al)

[10] Clinical Neuropharmacology [2006] 29 (2) : 73-76 (K.E.Lyons, R. Pahwa)

[11] Neurology [2004] 62 (Supplement 1) : S64-S71 (R.A.Hauser)

[12] European Neurology [2005] 53 (4) : 197-202 (D.J.Brooks, Y.Agid, K.Eggert, H.Widner, K.Ostergaard, A.Holopainen)

[13] FDA Drug Safety Communication : Ongoing Safety Review of Stalevo (entacapone / carbidopa / levodopa) and possible development of Prostate Cancer

ODM-101

Brand name : none (due to being in development)

Pharmacology : Stalevo contains three active substances in one tablet : L-dopa, plus carbidopa and entacapone. ODM-101, which is being developed, has the same components as Stalevo but has a higher and fixed amount of carbidopa (either 65mg or 105 mg) regardless of the L-dopa dosage. As it is made by the same manufacturers it is effectively an improved form of Stalevo.

Effcacy : People with Parkinson's Disease were given two forms of ODM-101 with two different amounts of carbidopa : ODM-101/65mg and ODM-101/105mg. Both of them reduced daily OFF-time more than Stalevo. ODM-101/105mg was marginally better than ODM-101/ 65mg. Both ODM-101 combinations increased on-time without troublesome dyskinesia significantly more than Stalevo. There were no significant differences between the treatments in on-time, with troublesome dyskinesia, or in UPDRS symptom scores.

Adverse effects : The tolerability and safety of ODM-101 was comparable to that of Stalevo [1].

[1] http://www.orion.fi/en/

TOLCAPONE

Brand name : Tasmar

Pharmacology : Tolcapone is a COMT inhibitor. COMT inhibitors inhibit the enzyme catechol-O-methyl transferase (COMT), which is involved in degrading neurotransmitters such as dopamine.

Efficacy : Tolcapone reduces Parkinson's Disease symptoms [1-8], and reduces off time [4, 5, 9-17] by 26% to 40% and as much as or more than 2 hours per day [13, 17]. It increased on time in most people [1, 4, 11, 12, 14, 17, 18] by 25% in some cases [19], and by as much as or more than 2 hours per day [13], and modestly improved motor impairments and disability [10, 16]. Tolcapone improves sleep [20] and Quality of Life [2, 4, 21, 22]. Tolcapone reduces L-dopa requirements [2-5, 9-12, 13, 16, 19, 23, 24, 25], and it improves L-dopa induced motor fluctuations [11, 23]. Switching from entacapone to tolcapone slightly improved efficacy [14, 26].

Adverse effects : The main adverse effects of taking tolcapone are dyskinesias [2, 4, 10, 13, 16, 18, 25], nausea [2, 10, 13, 25, 27, 28], diarrhea [2, 3, 5, 6, 10, 11, 16, 17, 27, 28, 29], vomiting [10], urine discoloration [28], dizziness [28], headaches [28], abdominal pain [11, 28], dystonia [25], cramps [25], and raised liver enzyme levels [9, 10, 22, 27, 29, 30, 31, 32]. Regular monitoring of liver function can be required in case of raised liver enzyme levels resulting from taking tolcapone [30]. Around 95% of those people with Parkinson's Disease who took tolcapone experienced good tolerability of it in the first four weeks [28].

[1] Clinical Neuropharmacology [2010] 33 (3) : 142-150 (V.Ries, R. Selzer, T.Eichhorn, W.H.Oertel, K.Eggert)

[2] Clinical Neuropharmacology [2001] 24 (4) : 214-220 (O. Suchowersky, P.Bailey, E.Pourcher, L.Bulger, G.Facciponte)

[3] Neurology [1998] 50 (Supplement 5) : S39-S45 (C.H.Waters, M. Kurth, P.Bailey, L.M.Shulman, P.LeWitt, E.Dorflinger, D.Deptula, S. Pedder)

[4] Journal of Neurology, Neurosurgery, and Psychiatry [1997] 63 (4) : 421-428 (H.Baas, A.G.Beiske, J.Ghika, M.Jackson, W.H.Oertel, W. Poewe, G.Ransmayr)

[5] Neurology [1997] 49 (4) : 1066-1071 (A.H.Rajput, W.Martin, M.H. Saint-Hilaire, E.Dorflinger, S.Pedder)

[6] Neurology [1997] 49 (3) : 665-671 (C.H.Waters, M.Kurth, P. Bailey, L.M.Shulman, P.LeWitt, E.Dorflinger, D.Deptula, S.Pedder)

[7] Journal of Neural Transmission [1997] 104 (2-3) : 229-236 (M. Yamamoto, M.Yokochi, S.Kuno, Y.Hattori, Y.Tsukamoto, H. Narabayashi, H.Tohgi, Y.Mizuno, N.Kowa, N.Yanagisawa, et al)

[8] CNS Spectrums [2010] 15 (1) : 27-32 (K.Sethi, S.Factor, R.Watts)

[9] Neurological Sciences [2008] 29 (Supplement 5) : S380-S382 (M. Canesi, A.L.Zecchinelli, G.Pezzoli, A.Antonini)

[10] The Cochrane Database of Systematic Reviews [2004] (4) : CD004554 (K.H.Deane, S.Spieker, C.E.Clarke)

[11] Journal of Neural Transmission [2004] 111 (10-11) : 1343-1363 (A.Gordin, S.Kaakkola, H.Teräväinen)

[12] European Neurology [2001] 46 (1) : 11-16 (M.Onofrj, A.Thomas, D.Iacono, A.Di Iorio, L.Bonanni)

[13] Archives of Neurology [1998] 55 (8) : 1089-1095 (C.H.Adler, C. Singer, C.O'Brien, R.A.Hauser, M.F.Lew, K.L.Marek, E.Dorflinger, S. Pedder, D.Deptula, K.Yoo)

[14] CNS Neuroscience and Therapeutics [2008] 14 (1) : 83-93 (A.J. Lees)

[15] Drugs and Aging [2000] 16 (1) : 55-65 (D.Lambert, C.H.Waters)

[16] Neurology [1998] 50 (Supplement 5) : S54-S59 (A.H.Rajput, W. Martin, M.H.Saint-Hilaire, E.Dorflinger, S.Pedder)

[17] Neurology [1998] 50 (Supplement 5) : S46-S53 (H.Baas, A.G. Beiske, J.Ghika, M.Jackson, W.H.Oertel, W.Poewe, G.Ransmayr)

[18] Movement Disorders [2007] 22 (1) : 14-19 (Entacapone to Tolcapone Switch Study Investigators)

[19] Neurology [1997] 48 (1) : 81-87 (M.C.Kurth, C.H.Adler, M.S. Hilaire, C.Singer, C.Waters, P.LeWitt, D.A.Chernik, E.E.Dorflinger, K. Yoo)

[20] Archives of Gerontology and Geriatrics [2010] 51 (3) : e125-e128 (G.Ebersbach, K.Hahn, M.Lorrain, A.Storch)

[21] CNS Spectrums [2010] 15 (1) : 27-32 (K.Sethi, S.Factor, R.Watts)

[22] Archives of Gerontology and Geriatrics [2009] 49 (1) : e40-e44 (G.Ebersbach, A.Storch)

[23] CNS Drugs [2005] 19 (2) : 165-184 (G.M.Keating, K.A. Lyseng-Williamson)

[24] Clinical Pharmacology and Therapeutics [2000] 67 (6) : 610-620 (K.Jorga, L.Banken, B.Fotteler, P.Snell, J.L.Steimer)

[25] Movement Disorders [1997] 12 (6) : 928-934 (E.Dupont, J.M. Burgunder, L.J.Findley, J.E.Olsson, E.Dorflinger)

[26] Movement Disorders [2007] 22 (1) : 14-19 (Entacapone to Tolcapone Switch Study Investigators)

[27] Clinical Neuropharmacology [2014] 37 (1) : 1-5 (K.Eggert, W.H. Oertel, A.J.Lees)

[28] Movement Disorders [1998] 13 (4) : 643-647 (R.A.Hauser, E. Molho, H.Shale, S.Pedder, E.E.Dorflinger)

[29] Journal of Neurology, Neurosurgery, and Psychiatry [2007] 78 (9) : 944-948 (A.J.Lees, V.Ratziu, E.Tolosa, W.H.Oertel)

[30] Clinical Neuropharmacology [2007] 30 (5) : 287-394 (C.W. Olanow, P.B.Watkins)

[31] Clinical Neuropharmacology [2007] 30 (5) : 281-286 (M.F.Lew, G.Kricorian)

[32] Neurology [2000] 55 (11 Supplement 4) : S51-S52; discussion S53-S56 (P.Watkins)

Opicapone

Brand name : Ongentys

Pharmacology : Opicapone is a novel COMT inhibitor for use as an adjuvant for the treatment of Parkinson's Disease.

Efficacy : A comparison was made in people with Parkinson's Disease between the use of a placebo, oral treatment with opicapone (5 mg, 25 mg, or 50 mg once daily), or entacapone (200 mg with every L-dopa intake). The reductions in off times were 56 minutes for a placebo, 96 minutes for entacapone, 91 minutes for 5mg opicapone, 86 minutes for 25mg opicapone, and best of all, 116 minutes for 50mg opicapone [1]. In another study the change in off time was a reduction of 64 minutes for those taking a placebo, 101 minutes for those taking 25mg opicapone, and 118 minutes for those people taking 50mg opicapone [3].

Adverse effects : Adverse effects were reported in 50% of people taking a placebo, 57% taking entacapone, 52% taking 5mg opicapone, 55% taking 25mg opicapone, and 54% taking 50mg opicapone. The most common adverse effects were dyskinesia, insomnia and constipation. There was little difference in this respect between entacapone and certain dosages of opicapone [1]. Opicapone was otherwise well tolerated at all the doses tested, which were 10mg, 25mg, 50mg, 100mg, 200mg, 400mg, 800mg and 1200 mg [2]. In another study assessing 25mg and 50mg opicapone, the most common adverse effects were dyskinesia, constipation, and a dry mouth [3].

[1] Lancet Neurology [2015] Dec 22 [Epub ahead of print] (J.J.Ferreira, A.Lees, J.F.Rocha, W.Poewe, O.Rascol, P.Soares-da-Silva)

[2] Clinical Pharmacokinetics [2013] 52 (2) : 139-151 (L.Almeida, J.F. Rocha, A.Falcão, P.N.Palma, A.I.Loureiro, R.Pinto, M.J.Bonifácio, L. C.Wright, T.Nunes, P.Soares-da-Silva)

[3] JAMA Neurology [2016] Dec 27 [Epub ahead of print] (A.J.Lees, J. Ferreira, O.Rascol, W.Poewe, J.F.Rocha, M.McCrory, P.Soares-da-Silva)

NEBICAPONE

Brand name : none (due to being in development)

Pharmacology : Nebicapone is a novel COMT inhibitor presently being developed as an adjuvant for the treatment of Parkinson's Disease.

Efficacy : A clinical trial compared the use in people with Parkinson's Disease of 50 mg, 100 mg, and 150 mg doses of nebicapone with the use of entacapone (200mg), which is another COMT inhibitor or a placebo administered with levodopa/carbidopa (Sinemet) or levodopa/ benserazide (Madopar). The 150mg dosage of nebicapone was found to be more effective than the existing COMT inhibitors, by decreasing the off time by 81 minutes in comparison to entacapone, and by 106 minutes in comparison to the placebo. The 50mg and 100mg dosages of nebicapone failed to have a significant effect in reducing off time [1].

Adverse effects : Treatment-emergent adverse effects were reported by 32% to 49% of patients in any treatment group with no observed dose relationship in the nebicapone groups. Adverse events were mild or moderate. Liver transaminases were elevated in 8% of the 150mg nebicapone group [1].

[1] CNS Neuroscience & Therapeutics [2010] 16 (6) : 337-347 (J.J. Ferreira, O.Rascol, W.Poewe, C.Sampaio, J.F.Rocha, T.Nunes, L. Almeida, P.Soares-da-Silva)

CHAPTER 45

PHARMACOLOGICAL TREATMENTS OF PARKINSON'S DISEASE

ANTI-CHOLINERGICS

PHARMACOLOGY

Anticholinergics are classified according to the receptors they affect. Antimuscarinic agents affect the muscarinic acetylcholine receptors. Antinicotinic agents affect the nicotinic acetylcholine receptors. Most anticholinergic drugs are anti-muscarinics.

Acetylcholine affects muscle contraction via the five muscarinic receptors : m1, m2, m3, m4, and m5. The receptors m1, m3 and m5 are stimulatory. The receptors m2 and m4 are inhibitory. The combined stimulatory effect of m1, m3 and m5 is more powerful in total than the combined inhibitory effect of m2 and m4. So the overall effect of acetylcholine is to stimulate muscle contraction.

The excessive muscle contraction in Parkinson's Disease is caused when the cholinergic function, which increases muscle contraction, is more powerful than dopaminergic function, which decreases muscle contraction.

Instead of increasing dopaminergic effect which is what most pharmacological treatments of Parkinson's Disease aim at achieving, anti-muscarinics increase dopaminergic effect by reducing cholinergic function. Anticholinergics are now uncommonly used because of their limited efficacy and widespread adverse effects.

TYPES OF ANTI-CHOLINERGIC

The anti-cholinergics used for Parkinson's Disease include benztropine, which is anti-muscarinic and anti-histaminergic [PAGE 688], and biperiden [PAGE 689], procyclidine [PAGE 690], and trihexyphenidyl [PAGE 690], which are all anti muscarinic.

Benztropine

Brand names : Cogentin

Pharmacology : Benzatropine is anti-muscarinic and anti-histaminergic [1]. It is a selective m1 and m3 muscarinic receptor antagonist [2].

Efficacy : Benztropine, which is injectable, is also known and sold as benztropine mesylate. Benztropine has been used in the treatment of Parkinson's Disease [3-7], but it has limited efficacy. Benztropine can improve Parkinson's Disease symptoms [5-8], including tremor [9].

Adverse effects : Anti-muscarinics can cause neuropsychiatric and cognitive side effects [5], including a reduction in memory [10], a significant increase in tardive dyskinesia [7], and more anxiety and depression [7]. The psychotoxic, cognitive and autonomic adverse effects make it inappropriate for the treatment of the elderly [8].

[1] Journal of Pharmacological and Experimental Therapeutics [2005] 315 (2) : 631-640 (V.C.Campbell, T.A.Kopajtic, A.H.Newman, J.L. Katz)

[2] Nature [2013] 502 (7471) : 327-332 (V.A.Deshmukh, V.Tardif, C.A.Lyssiotis, C.C.Green, B.Kerman, H.J.Kim, K.Padmanabhan, J.G. Swoboda, I.Ahmad, T.Kondo, F.H.Gage, A.N.Theofilopoulos, et al)

[3] International Journal of Pharmaceutics [2008] 357 (1-2) : 55-60 (N.T.Hai, J.Kim, E.S.Park, S.C.Chi)

[4] Wiener Klinische Wochenschrift [1963] 75 : 924-926 (H.J. Avenarius, F.Gerstenbrand)

[5] Cochrane Database of Systematic Reviews [2003] (2) : CD003735 (R.Katzenschlager, C.Sampaio, J.Costa, A.Lees)

[6] Progress in Neuropsychopharmacology and Biological Psychiatry [1982] 6 (1) : 51-55 (W.W.Tourtellotte, A.R.Potvin, K.Syndulko, S.B. Hirsch, E.R.Gilden, J.H.Potvin, E.C.Hansch)

[7] Journal of Clinical Psychiatry [1979] 40 (3) : 147-152 (G. Chouinard, L.Annable, A.Ross-Chouinard, M.L.Kropsky)

[8] Drugs and Aging [2005] 22 (9) : 731-740 (A.Lees)

[9] Neurology [1997] 48 (4) : 1077-1081 (J.H.Friedman, W.C.Koller, M.C.Lannon, K.Busenbark, E.Swanson-Hyland, D.Smith)

[10] International Journal of Neuroscience [1981] 14 (1-2) : 61-66 (K.Syndulko, E.R.Gilden, E.C.Hansch, A.R.Potvin, W.W.Tourtellotte, J.H.Potvin)

Biperiden

Brand names : Akineton

Pharmacology : Biperiden is a muscarinic receptor antagonist.

Efficacy : Biperiden has been used in the treatment of Parkinson's Disease [1-6], but it has limited efficacy.

Adverse effects : Anti-muscarinics have a significant adverse effect on cognitive and physical functions [7]. Their adverse effects can be quite widespread.

[1] Arquivos de Neuro-Psiquiatria [1989] 47 (1) : 31-38 (J.C.Villares)

[2] Archiv fur Psychiatrie und Nervenkrankheiten [1975] 221 (1) : 15-28 (E.Schneider, P.Jacobi, H.Maxion, P-A.Fischer)

[3] Current Therapeutic Research, Clinical and Experimental [1974] 16 (8) : 838-843 (N.S.Kline, B.T.Mason, L.Winick)

[4] Diseases of the Nervous System [1967] 28 (3) : 191-193 (R.R. Strang)

[5] Archives of Neurology [1961] 560-564 (W.H.Timberlake, R.S. Schwab, A.C.England Jnr)

[6] Southern Medical Journal [1960] 53 : 465-467 (P.F.Lerner)

[7] Age and Ageing [2014] 43 (5) : 604-615 (C.Fox, T.Smith, I. Maidment, W.Y.Chan, N.Bua, P.K.Myint, M.Boustani, C.S.Kwok, M. Glover, I.Koopmans, N.Campbell)

PROCYCLIDINE

Brand names : Kemadrin

Pharmacology : Procyclidine is a muscarinic receptor antagonist.

Efficacy : Procyclidine has been used in the treatment of Parkinson's Disease [1-4], but it has limited efficacy.

Adverse effects : Anti-muscarinics have a significant adverse effect on cognitive and physical functions [5]. Their adverse effects can be quite widespread.

[1] Journal of Pharmacy and Pharmaceutical Sciences [1999] 2 (2) : 39-46 (D.R.Brocks)

[2] Neurology [1970] 20 (12) : 31-35 (W.H.Timberlake)

[3] Wiener Klinische Wochenschrift [1962] 74 : 569-570 (H.Gross, E. Langner)

[4] Neurology [1957] 7 (7) : 485-489 (A.Zier, L.J.Doshay)

[5] Age and Ageing [2014] 43 (5) : 604-615 (C.Fox, T.Smith, I. Maidment, W.Y.Chan, N.Bua, P.K.Myint, M.Boustani, C.S.Kwok, M. Glover, I.Koopmans, N.Campbell)

TRIHEXYPHENIDYL

Brand names : Artane, Trihexane

Pharmacology : Trihexyphenidyl is a muscarinic receptor antagonist.

Efficacy : Trihexyphenidyl has been used in the treatment of Parkinson's Disease [1-4]. It has improved axial symptoms [4]. However, otherwise it has limited efficacy.

Adverse effects : Anti-muscarinics have a significant adverse effect on cognitive and physical function [5]. Their adverse effects can be quite widespread.

[1] Shinkei Kenkyu No Shimpo [1971] 15 (1) : 267-285 (K.Hirayama, M.Uono, T.Nakanishi, N.Kato, Y.Nagao)

[2] Journal of Neural Transmission (Supplement) [1991] 33 : 125-132 (L.Schelosky, T.Benke, W.H.Poewe)

[3] Journal of Clinical Psychopharmacology [1989] 9 (6) : 407-411 (W.C.Wirshing, D.L.Freidenberg, J.L.Cummings, G.Bartzokis)

[4] Clinical Neurology and Neurosurgery [2012] 114 (10) : 1308- 1311 (Y.Baba, M.A.Higuchi, H.Abe, K.Fukuyama, R.Onozawa, Y. Uehara, T.Inoue, T.Yamada)

[5] Age and Ageing [2014] 43 (5) : 604-615 (C.Fox, T.Smith, I. Maidment, W.Y.Chan, N.Bua, P.K.Myint, M.Boustani, C.S.Kwok, M. Glover, I.Koopmans, N.Campbell)

CHAPTER 46

PHARMACOLOGICAL TREATMENTS OF PARKINSON'S DISEASE

NON-DOPAMINERGIC

PHARMACOLOGY

There are drugs being used for Parkinson's Disease or being developed for Parkinson's Disease that do not act by directly increasing the activity of dopamine. They are intended for use either in the treatment of Parkinson's Disease by other biochemical means [PAGE 692], or are normally used for other medical disorders [PAGE 708], or are for use in medical disorders that are associated with Parkinson's Disease [PAGE 718].

NON-DOPAMINERGIC DRUGS
PART 1 : THOSE USED FOR PARKINSON'S DISEASE

Those drugs being used or assessed for the treatment of Parkinson's Disease that do not act by directly increasing the activity of dopamine are : adenosine receptor antagonists (tozadenant, preladenant, istradefylline, caffeine) [PAGE 692], calcium channel blockers (isradipine) [PAGE 698], glutamate antagonists (perampanel, amantadine, dipraglurant, mavoglurant) [PAGE 699], neurotrophic factors (cogane) [PAGE 703], nicotine agonists (nicotine) [PAGE 704], and noradrenaline precursors (droxidopa) [PAGE 706].

ADENOSINE RECEPTOR ANTAGONISTS

Adenosine receptor antagonists are drugs that act as an antagonist of one or more adenosine receptors. Those adenosine antagonists that are presently being assessed for their use in the treatment of Parkinson's Disease include tozadenant, preladenant, istradefylline and caffeine.

TOZADENANT

Trade names : none (due to being in development)

Pharmacology : Tozadenant (SYN115) is an inhibitor of the adenosine 2a (A2a) receptor that is being developed for the treatment of Parkinson's Disease.

Efficacy : SYN115 caused a decrease in 'off' time, an increase in 'on' time, an improved score on UPDRS part III and UPDRS parts I-III combined symptom scores, as well as improvements on clinician and patient assessed global impression scores [1]. Clinical trials assessed the use of 60mg, 120mg, 180mg, or 240mg, Daily off-time was reduced by more than an hour when taking either 120mg or 180mg tozadenant. Tozadenant, 60 mg twice daily, was not associated with a reduction in off-time [2].

Adverse effects : The most common adverse effects were dyskinesia (16% of people taking 120mg, 20% of people taking 180mg), nausea (11% of people taking 120mg, 12% of people taking 180mg), dizziness (5% of people taking 120mg, 13% of people taking 180mg) [2]. Tozadenant, 240 mg twice daily, was associated with an increased rate of discontinuation because of adverse effects that occurred in 20% of people taking that dosage [2].

[1] Biotie Therapies - http://www.biotie.com - Tozadenant (SYN115)

[2] Lancet Neurology [2014] 13 (8) : 767-776 (R.A.Hauser, C.W. Olanow, K.D.Kieburtz, E. Pourcher, A.Docu-Axelerad, M.Lew, O. Kozyolkin, A.Neale, C.Resburg, U.Meya, C.Kenney, S.Bandak)

PRELADENANT

Trade names : none (due to being in development)

Pharmacology : Preladenant is a novel adenosine A2A receptor antagonist that is presently being developed for the treatment of Parkinson's Disease.

Efficacy : Doses of 5mg Preladenant twice a day reduced off time provided by 1.4-1.9 hours per day and increased on time by 1.2-1.5 hours per day [1]. Doses of 2mg, 5mg or 10mg preladenant for 12 weeks caused reductions in off time of 42 minutes for 2mg, 30 minutes for 5mg, and 18 minutes for 10mg preladenant [1, 6]. When twice 1mg, 2mg, 5mg and 10mg daily doses were taken, 1mg and 2mg had no significant effect, 5mg reduced off time by 1 hour, and 10mg reduced off time by 1.2 hours [1]. In other studies, 2mg, 5mg and 10mg daily doses had no effect on off time [2, 7]. Merck ceased developing preladenant because it failed to show any benefit in Parkinson's Disease in three studies.

Adverse effects : Some people had increased dyskinesia or constipation [1]. Phase I and II clinical trials indicated that preladenant was well tolerated [3]. The adverse effects were not much different from those of a placebo [4]. When the doses were increased from 5mg or 10mg to 200mg daily preladenant was generally well tolerated [5].

[1] Movement Disorders [2013] 28 (6) : 817-820 (S.A.Factor, K. Wolski, D.M.Togasaki, S.Huyck, M.Cantillon, T.W.Ho, R.A.Hauser, E.Pourcher)

[2] JAMA Neurology [2015] 72 (12) : 1491-1500 (R.A.Hauser, F.Stocchi, O.Rascol, S.B.Huyck, R.Capece, T.W.Ho, P.Sklar, C.Lines, D.Michelson, D.Hewitt)

[3] Drugs [2010] 13 (10) : 723-731 (J.D.Salamone)

[4] Lancet Neurology [2011] 10 (3) : 221-229 (R.A.Hauser, M. Cantillon, E.Pourcher, F.Micheli, V.Mok, M.Onofrj, S.Huyck, K. Wolski)

[5] Journal of Clinical Pharmacy and Therapeutics [2012] 37 (5) : 578-587 (D.L.Cutler, A.Tendolkar, I.D.Grachev)

[6] Parkinsonism & Related Disorders [2016] Aug 27 [Epub ahead of print] (N.Hattori, M.Kikuchi, N.Adachi, D.Hewitt, S.Huyck, T.Saito)

[7] JAMA Neurology [2017] May 10 [Epub ahead of print] (F.Stocchi, O.Rascol, R.A.Hauser, S.B.Huyck, A.Tzontcheva, R.Capece, T.W.Ho, P.Sklar, C.Lines, D.Michelson, D.J.Hewitt)

ISTRADEFYLLINE

Trade names : none (due to being in development)

Pharmacology : Istradefylline is an A(2A) adenosine receptor antagonist, and so does not act by increasing the activity of dopamine.

Efficacy : In some clinical trials, istradefylline was ineffective in reducing Parkinson's Disease symptoms [1]. In another clinical trial istradefylline in dosages of 20mg and 40mg reduced "off" time from between 39 and 95 minutes [2-7], but in another study, istradefylline in dosages of 10mg, 20mg and 40mg did not reduce "off" time [8]. An analysis of randomised controlled trials showed a significant reduction in "off" time and improvement in the UPDRS score. There was no significant difference between the 20mg and 40mg istradefylline. There was a significant difference in the effect of istradefylline on dyskinesia [9].

Adverse effects : They included : nasopharyngitis, dyskinesia, tremor, constipation, light headedness, hallucinations, weight decrease, nausea, dizziness [2-7].

[1] Parkinsonism & Related Disordes [2010] 16 (1) : 16-20 (H.H. Fernandez, D.R.Greeley, R.M.Zweig, J.Wojcieszek, A.Mori, N.M. Sussman)

[2] Movement Disorders [2010] 25 (10) : 1437-1443 (Y.Mizuno, K. Hasegawa, T.Kondo, S.Kuno, M.Yamamoto)

[3] Movement Disorders [2008] 23 (15) : 2177-2185 (R.A.Hauser, L. M.Shulman, J.M.Trugman, J.W.Roberts, A.Mori, R.Ballerini, N.M. Sussman)

[4] Neurology [2008] 70 (23) : 2233-2240 (M.Stacy, D.Silver, T. Mendis, J.Sutton, A.Mori, P.Chaikin, N.M.Sussman)

[5] Annals of Neurology [2008] 63 (3) : 295-302 (P.A.LeWitt, M. Guttman, J.W.Tetrud, P.J.Tuite, A.Mori, P.Chaikin, N.M.Sussman)

[6] Neurology [2003] 61 (3) : 297-303 (R.A.Hauser, J.P.Hubble, D.D. Truong)

[7] Clinical Neuropharmacology [2015] 38 (2) : 41-46 (T.Kondo, Y. Mizuno)

[8] Parkinsonism & Related Disorders [2012] 18 (2) : 178-184 (E. Pourcher, H.H.Fernandez, M.Stacy, A.Mori, R.Ballerini, P. Chaikin)

[9] Journal of Neurological Science [2012] 324 (1-2) : 21-28 (W. Chen, H.Wang, H.Wei, S.Gu, H.Wei)

CAFFEINE

Trade names : Caffeine

Pharmacology : Caffeine is a naturally occurring adenosine antagonist that is commonly found in coffee, and to a lesser extent in tea, yerba mate, cola drinks, cocoa, and chocolate.

Efficacy : Caffeine modestly reduces Parkinson's Disease symptoms [1-7, 15] or lessens the likelihood of developing Parkinson's Disease [8, 9]. This was true whether the source of caffeine was coffee, tea [10], or yerba mate [9], but not with chocolate [11]. Caffeine is associated with a lower rate of starting L-dopa treatment, down to 63% of normal [15]. The effect of caffeine is accentuated by smoking and the use of NSAIDs [5]. However, women who take hormones had a fourfold higher risk of Parkinson's Disease when they consumed 6 or more cups of coffee per day [12]. Caffeine was associated with a reduced risk of developing dyskinesia. Those people who consumed 12 ounces of coffee per day (about two cups) reduced their likelihood of developing dyskinesia to 61%. Those people who consumed 4 to 12 ounces of coffee per day (less than two cups), reduced their likelihood of developing dyskinesia to 73% [13].

Adverse effects : Caffeine can cause indigestion, palpitations, tremor, headache and insomnia, all of which increase significantly with caffeine intake [14].

[1] Neurology [2012] 79 (7) : 651-658 (R.B.Postuma, A.E. Lang, R.P. Munhoz, K.Charland, A.Pelletier, M.Moscovich, L.Filla, D. Zanatta, S. R.Romenets, R.Altman, R.Chuang, B.Shah)

[2] Movement Disorders [2012] 27 (10) : 1276-1282 (N.Palacios, X. Gao, M.L.McCullough, M.A.Schwarzschild, R.Shah, S.Gapstur, A. Ascherio)

[3] Neurology [2012] 79 (7) : 651-658 (R.B.Postuma, A.E.Lang, R.P. Munhoz, K.Charland, A.Pelletier, M.Moscovich, L.Filla, D.Zanatta, S. Rios Romenets, R.Altman, R.Chuang, B.Shah)

[4] Movement Disorders [2011] 26 (13) : 2427-2431 (R.D.Altman, A. E.Lang, R.B.Postuma)

[5] Movement Disorders [2008] 23 (1) : 88-95 (K.M.Powers, D.M. Kay, S.A.Factor, C.P.Zabetian, D.S.Higgins, A.Samii, J.G.Nutt, A. Griffith, B.Leis, J.W.Roberts, E.D.Martinez, J.S.Montimurro, et al)

[6] American Journal of Epidemiology [2015] 181 (10) : 808-816 (L. Kenborg, C.F.Lassen, B.Ritz, K.K.Andersen, J.Christensen, E.S. Schernhammer, J.Hansen, L.Wermuth, N.H.Rod, J.H.Olsen)

[7] Parkinsonism & Related Disorders [2016] Aug 4 [Epub ahead of print] (M.Moccia, R.Erro, M.Picillo, C.Vitale, K.Longo, M.Amboni, M.T.Pellecchia, P.Barone)

[8] Functional Neurology [2013] 28 (2) : 107-113 (N.Hosseini Tabatabaei, B.Babakhani, A.Hosseini Tabatabaei, Z.Vahabi, A. Soltanzadeh)

[9] Journal of Neurological Science [2015] 356 (1-2) : 163-167 (E.M. Gatto, C.Melcon, V.L.Parisi, L.Bartoloni, C.D.Gonzalez)

[10] Geriatrics and Gerontology International [2013] 14 (2) : 430-439 (H.Qi, S.Li)

[11] Journal of Neurology [2012] 259 (11) : 2447-2451 (M.Wolz, C. Schleiffer, L.Klingelhöfer, C.Schneider, F.Proft, U.Schwanebeck, H. Reichmann, P.Riederer, A.Storch)

[12] Neurology [2003] 60 (5) : 790-795 (A.Ascherio, H.Chen, M.A. Schwarzschild, S.M.Zhang, G.A.Colditz, F.E.Speizer)

[13] Movement Disorders [2013] 28 (3) : 380-383 (A.M.Wills, S. Eberly, M.Tennis, A.E.Lang, S.Messing, D.Togasaki, C.M.Tanner, C. Kamp, J.F.Chen, D.Oakes, M.P.McDermott, M.A.Schwarzschild)

[14] International Journal of Epidemiology [1985] 14 (2) : 239-248 (M. J.Shirlow, C.D.Mathers)

[15] Parkinsonism and Related Disorders [2016] 32 : 116-119 (M. Moccia, R.Erro, M.Picillo, C.Vitale, K. Longo, M.Amboni, M.T. Pellecchia, P.Barone

Calcium channel blockers

In some studies, the use of calcium channel blockers was associated with a 22% to 30% reduction in the risk of having Parkinson's Disease. [1-4]. However, in other studies there was no evidence of the use of calcium channel blockers causing a reduction in the risk of having Parkinson's Disease [5-8].

ISRADIPINE

Trade names : none (due to being in development)

Pharmacology : Isradipine is a dihydropyridine calcium channel blocker that is usually prescribed to treat high blood pressure in order to reduce the risk of stroke and heart attack.

Efficacy : Isradipine had no significant effect on Parkinson's Disease [9]. A Phase III clinical trial is assessing the effect of 10mg on efficacy in Parkinson's Disease [10]. Varying the dosage did not affect the efficacy [11].

Adverse effects : The tolerability of isradipine CR for people with Parkinson's Disease is dose dependent : 94% of people with 5 mg, 87% with 10 mg, 68% with 15 mg, and 52% with 20 mg [9]. In another study the tolerability was : 83% of people with 5mg, 73% with 10mg, and 37% with 20mg [11]. The most common reasons for dose reduction were leg edema and dizziness [9].

[1] Neurology [2008] 70 (16 Part 2) : 1438-1444 (C.Becker, Jick SS, C. R.Meier)

[2] American Journal of Epidemiology [2012] 175 (7) : 627-635 (B. Pasternak, H.Svanström, N.M.Nielsen, L.Fugger, M.Melbye, A.Hviid)

[3] Annals of Neurology [2010] 67 (5) : 600-606 (B.Ritz, S.L. Rhodes, L.Qian, E.Schernhammer, J.H.Olsen, S.Friis)

[4] International Journal of Chronic Disorders [2015] : 697404 (K. Gudala, R.Kanukula, D.Bansal)

[5] Annals of Neurology [2012] 71 (3) : 362-369 (C.Marras, A. Gruneir, P.Rochon, X.Wang, G.Anderson, J.Brotchie, C.M.Bell, S.Fox P.C.Austin)

[6] Movement Disorders [2010] 25 (12) : 1818-1822 (K.C.Simon, X. Gao, H.Chen, M.A.Schwarzschild, A.Ascherio)

[7] Cochrane Database Systematic Reviews [2011] (11) : CD008535 (K.Rees, R.Stowe, S.Patel, N.Ives, K.Breen, Y.Ben-Shlomo, C.E. Clarke)

[8] Parkinsonism & Related Disorders [2007] 13 (3) : 165-169 (T.G. Ton, S.R.Heckbert, W.T.Longstreth Jr, M.A.Rossing, W.A.Kukull, G.M.Franklin, P.D.Swanson, T.Smith-Weller, H.Checkoway)

[9] Movement Disorders [2010] 25 (16) : 2863-2866 (T.Simuni, E. Borushko, M.J.Avram, S.Miskevics, A.Martel, C.Zadikoff, A. Videnovic, F.M.Weaver, K.Williams, D.J.Surmeier)

[10] The Michael J.Fox Foundation - https://www.michaeljfox.org/foundation/news-detail.php?podcast-drug-that-may-slow-parkinson-progression-granted-23-million-from-nih-for-phase-iii

[11] Movement Disorders [2013] 28 (13) : 1823-1831 (T.Simuni, K. Biglan, D.Oakes, G.Bakris, R.A.Hauser, A.Lang, J.D.Surmeier, et al)

Glutamate antagonists

Glutamate antagonists act as antagonists of one or more of the glutamate receptors. Those glutamate antagonists that are presently being assessed for their use in the treatment of Parkinson's Disease include perampanel, amantadine, dipraglurant, and mavoglurant.

PERAMPANEL

Trade names : none (due to being in development)

Pharmacology : Perampanel is a non-competitive AMPA-type glutamate receptor antagonist, being assessed for use in Parkinson's Disease.

Efficacy : Perampanel failed to demonstrate efficacy in Parkinson's Disease using daily doses of 0.5mg [1], 1mg [1], 2mg [1, 2], and 4mg [2, 3].

Adverse effects : Adverse event related study withdrawals were associated with daily doses of 4m and 12mg. Adverse events included dizziness, ataxia, somnolence, irritability and weight increase [4].

[1] Movement Disorders [2010] 25 (7) : 896-905 (K.Eggert, D. Squillacote, P.Barone, R.Dodel, R.Katzenschlager, M.Emre, A.J.Lees, O.Rascol, W.Poewe, E.Tolosa, C.Trenkwalder, M.Onofrj, et al)

[2] Movement Disorders [2012] 27 (2) : 284-288 (A.Lees, S.Fahn, K. M.Eggert, J.Jankovic, A.Lang, F.Micheli, M.M.Mouradian, W.H. Oertel, C.W.Olanow, W.Poewe, O.Rascol, E.Tolosa, et al)

[3] Clinical Neuropharmacology [2012] 35 (1) : 15-20 (O.Rascol, P. Barone, M.Behari, M.Emre, N.Giladi, C.W.Olanow, E.Ruzicka, F. Bibbiani, D.Squillacote, A.Patten, E.Tolosa)

[4] European Journal of Neurology [2013] 20 (8) : 1204-1211 (G. Zaccara, F.Giovannelli, M.Cincotta, A.Verrotti, E.Grillo)

AMANTADINE

Trade names : Symmetrel

Pharmacology : Amantadine is a weak antagonist of the NMDA type glutamate receptor, increases dopamine release, and blocks dopamine reuptake. ADS-5102 is a long-acting, extended-release capsule of amantadine HCl. It is administered once daily at bedtime [5].

Efficacy : A clinical trial was carried out using 300mg per day of amantadine. Using the Rush Dyskinesia Rating Scale (RDRS) 64% of those people taking amantadine improved but only 16% of those people taking the placebo improved. Some Parkinson's Disease symptoms improved but others did not. Results from the study demonstrated that amantadine exhibited beneficial effects against dyskinesias in 60% to 70% of people with Parkinson's Disease. However, the study did not indicate the side effects [1]. Ten of eleven patients reported improvement in freezing of gait after initiation of an average dosage of 100mg amantadine. Four of the patients reported a reduction in benefit after 4 months [2]. ADS-5102 340mg significantly reduced dyskinesia by 27% [5, 6]. ADS-5102 significantly increased ON time without troublesome dyskinesia, at 260 mg, 340 mg, and 420mg [5, 6].

Adverse effects : Three patients reported adverse effects, including blurred vision, visual hallucinations, and peripheral edema [2]. Another study showed that intravenous amantadine was not beneficial for freezing of gait [3]. Amantadine doubled the likelihood of corneal edema, and increased the likelihood even further when taking high doses [4]. Constipation, hallucinations, dizziness, and dry mouth were the most frequent adverse effects of ADS-5102 [5, 6]. Study withdrawal rates using ADS-5102 were 9%, 15%, 14%, and 40% for the placebo, 260-mg, 340-mg, and 420-mg groups, respectively. All study withdrawals in the active treatment groups were attributable to adverse effects [5].

[1] BasedPLoS One [2010] 5 (12) : e15298 (H.Sawada, T.Oeda, S. Kuno, M.Nomoto, K.Yamamoto, M.Yamamoto, K.Hisanaga, T. Kawamura)

[2] Clinical Neuropharmacology [2012] 35 (6) : 266-268 (R.Malkani, C.Zadikoff, O.Melen, A.Videnovic, E.Borushko, T.Simuni)

[3] Journal of Neurology [2013] 260 (12) : 3030-3038 (J.Y.Lee, S.Oh, J.M.Kim, J.S.Kim, E.Oh, H.T.Kim, B.S.Jeon, J.W.Cho)

[4] American Journal of Ophthalmology [2016] Sep 1 [Epub ahead of print] (P.Y.Lee, H.P.Tu, C.P.Lin, C.H.Chang, K.C.Cheng, C.C.Lin, S.L.Hsu)

[5] Movement Disorders [2015] 30 (6) : 788-795 (R.Pahwa, C.M. Tanner, R.A.Hauser, K.Sethi, S.Isaacson, D.Truong)

[6] JAMA Neurology [2017] Jun 12 [Epub ahead of print] (R.Pahwa, C.M.Tanner, R.A.Hauser, S.H.Isaacson, P.A.Nausieda, D.D.Truong, P.Agarwal, K.L.Hull, K.E.Lyons, R.Johnson, M.J.Stempien)

DIPRAGLURANT

Brand names : none (due to being in development)

Pharmacology : Dipraglurant is an orally taken drug being developed for use in Parkinson's Disease that inhibits the glutamate receptor 5.

Efficacy : Exploratory efficacy data showed an anti-dyskinetic effect. People taking dipraglurant had up to 70 minutes more on-time without dyskinesia than people who were taking a placebo. After 4 weeks of taking dipraglurant patients reported reduced daily off-time of 50 minutes [1]. Dipraglurant reduced peak dose dyskinesia on day 1 and on day 14. There was no worsening of the symptoms of Parkinson's Disease [2].

Adverse effects : The incidence of adverse effects was slightly higher in those taking dipraglurant (88%) than in those taking a placebo (75%). Adverse events such as vertigo, visual disturbances, and feeling drunk, were seen in less than 10% of people taking dipraglurant but were not severe [1]. The most frequent adverse effects included dyskinesia, dizziness, nausea, and fatigue [2].

[1] http://www.addextherapeutics.com

[2] Movement Disorders [2016] May 23 [Epub ahead of print] (F. Tison, C.Keywood, M.Wakefield, F.Durif, J.C.Corvol, K.Eggert, M. Lew, S.Isaacson, E.Bezard, S.M.Poli, C.G.Goetz, C.Trenkwalder, et al)

MAVOGLURANT

Trade names : none (due to being in development)

Pharmacology : Mavoglurant (AFQ056) is a metabotropic glutamate receptor 5 antagonist.

Efficacy : Mavoglurant dose was increased from 25mg twice daily to 100mg, then up to 300mg per day. Off time reduced by more than two hours. On time without troublesome dyskinesia increased by more than 4 hours [1]. People with Parkinson's Disease and L-dopa induced dyskinesia took AFQ056 in daily doses of either 20mg, 50mg, 100mg, 150mg, or 200mg. The greatest improvements in dyskinesia were with 200mg AFQ056. There were also improvements in Parkinson's Disease symptoms. However, no significant changes were observed on the 26-item Parkinson's Disease Dyskinesia Scale and UPDRS (part III) scores were not significantly changed [2]. Further clinical trials were discontinued due to the lack of efficacy [3].

Adverse effects : The most common adverse effects are dizziness, hallucination, fatigue, diarrhea, and insomnia [2].

[1] International Journal of Neuroscience [2016] 126 (1) : 20-24 (R. Kumar, R.A.Hauser, J.Mostillo, N.Dronamraju, A.Graf, M. Merschhemke, C.Kenney)

[2] Movement Disorders [2013] 28 (13) : 1838-1846 (F.Stocchi, O. Rascol, A.Destee, N.Hattori, R.A.Hauser, A.E.Lang, W.Poewe, M. Stacy, E.Tolosa, H.Gao, J.Nagel, M.Merschhemke, A.Graf, et al)

[3] Expert Opinion on Investigational drugs [2014] 23 (8) : 1165-1179 (D.Petrov, I.Pedros, M.L.de Lemos, M.Pallàs, A.M.Canudas, A. Lazarowski, C.Beas-Zarate, C.Auladell, J.Folch, A.Camins)

Neurotrophic factors

COGANE

Trade names : none

Pharmacology : Cogane, which can be taken orally, readily crosses the blood-brain barrier and has been shown to stimulate the release of the trophic factor GDNF [1].

Efficacy : Cogane had been claimed to reduce the effects of Parkinson's Disease. However, the study was only short term and carried out on animals who did not actually have Parkinson's Disease [2]. Cogane did not have any beneficial effect in people with Parkinson's Disease [3]. Consequently, all research and development of cogane was suspended.

Adverse effects : No adverse effects were reported [3].

[1] The FASEB Journal [2008] 22 (7) : 2488-2497 (N.P.Visanji, A. Orsi, T.H.Johnston, P.A.Howson, K.Dixon, N.Callizot, J.M.Brotchie, D.D.Rees)

[2] Phytopharm http://www.phytopharm.com/assets/REL-155.pdf

[3] Phytopharm http://www.phytopharm.co.uk/images/stories/Rel_190_Final_130117.pdf

NICOTINE AGONISTS

NICOTINE

Trade names : Nicotine

Pharmacology : Nicotine is thought to activate the nigrostriatal dopaminergic pathway and consequently to increase the release of dopamine [1]. Nicotine is found in large concentrations in tobacco and also to a lesser extent in vegetables from the same botanical family as tobacco, Solanaceae, which includes peppers, tomatoes, and potatoes. Nicotine is also found in Swedish moist smokeless tobacco (snus) [18].

Efficacy : People that ate more peppers, tomatoes, tomato juice, and potatoes during adulthood were only 81% as likely to develop Parkinson's Disease. The association was intensified when the nicotine concentration of the vegetables was higher [2]. Smoking reduced the risk of Parkinson's Disease [1, 3, 4, 5], by 20% to 50% [4, 6-10, 19].

Heavy smokers reduced the risk of developing Parkinson's Disease by more than 60% [5, 9, 11]. After chronic use of intravenous nicotine, improvements were seen in several motor measures [12]. The use of transdermal nicotine improved motor scores and reduced the use of dopaminergic drugs of people who had Parkinson's Disease [13]. In another study the use of transdermal nicotine had no effect on the symptoms of people with Parkinson's Disease [14]. The use of nicotine gum made no difference to Parkinson's Disease symptoms in one study [15], but improved Parkinson's Disease symptoms in another study [16]. The use of moist smokeless tobacco (snus) in ever-snus users had a lower Parkinson's Disease risk compared with never-snus users. The risk reduced even more when more snus was used [18, 19].

Adverse effects : The use of transdermal nicotine in people with Parkinson's Disease caused frequent but moderate nausea, and vomiting and dizziness in most people taking it [13, 17].

[1] Journal of the Neurological Sciences [1993] 117 (1-2) : 28-32 (A. Ishikawa, T.Miyatake)

[2] Annals of Neurology [2013] 74 (3) : 472-477 (S.S.Nielsen, G.M. Franklin, W.T.Longstreth, P.D.Swanson, H.Checkoway)

[3] Neurology [1986] 36 (11) : 1490-1496 (J.A.Baron)

[4] American Journal of Epidemiology [2015] 181 (10) : 808-816 (L. Kenborg, C.F.Lassen, B.Ritz, K.K.Andersen, J.Christensen, E.S. Schernhammer, J.Hansen, L.Wermuth, N.H.Rod, J.H.Olsen)

[5] Archives of Gerontology and Geriatrics [2015] 61 (3) : 510-516 (X.Li, W.Li, G.Liu, X.Shen, Y.Tang)

[6] Movement Disorders [2008] 23 (1) : 88-95 (K.M.Powers, D.M.Kay, S.A.Factor, C.P.Zabetian, D.S.Higgins, A.Samii, J.G.Nutt, A.Griffith, B.Leis, J.W.Roberts, E.D.Martinez, J.S.Montimurro, et al)

[7] Movement Disorders [2004] 19 (9) : 1087-1092 (G.Alves, M.Kurz, S.A.Lie, J.P.Larsen)

[8] Reviews on Environmental Health [1991] 9 (3) : 123-136 (G.S. Shahi, S.M.Moochhala)

[9] Neurology [1999] 52 (1) : 115-119 (J.M.Gorell, B.A.Rybicki, C.C. Johnson, E.L.Peterson)

[10] Parkinsonism & Related Disorders [2015] 21 (3) : 216-220 (M. Moccia, R.Erro, M.Picillo, E.Vassallo, C.Vitale, K.Longo, M.Amboni, G.Santangelo, R.Palladino, A.Nardone, M.Triassi, P.Barone, et al)

[11] Journal of Neurological Science [2003] 216 (1) : 163-167 (E.K.Tan, C.Tan, S.M.Fook-Chong, S.Y.Lum, A.Chai, H.Chung, H. Shen, Y.Zhao, M.L.Teoh, Y.Yih, R.Pavanni, V.R.Chandran, et al)

[12] Brain and Cognition [2000] 43 (1-3) : 274-282 (M.C.Kelton, H.J. Kahn, C.L.Conrath, P.A.Newhouse)

[13] European Journal of Neurology [2007] 14 (12) : 1313-1316 (G. Villafane, P.Cesaro, A.Rialland, S.Baloul, S.Azimi, C.Bourdet, J.Le Houezec, I.Macquin-Mavier I, P.Maison)

[14] Neurology [2001] 57 (6) : 1032-1035 (A.Vieregge, M.Sieberer, H. Jacobs, J.M.Hagenah, P.Vieregge)

[15] Psychopharmacology [1995] 117 (2) : 253-256 (P.Clemens, J.A.Baron, D.Coffey, A.Reeves)

[16] Psychopharmacology [1994] 116 (1) : 117-119 (K.O.Fagerström, O.Pomerleau, B.Giordani, F.Stelson)

[17] Clinical Neuropharmacology [2003] 26 (5) : 227-229 (S.Lemay, P. Blanchet, S.Chouinard, H.Masson, V.Soland, M.A.Bédard)

[18] International Journal of Epidemiology [2016] Dec 10 [Epub ahead of print] (F.Yang, N.L.Pedersen, W.Ye, Z.Liu, M.Norberg, L.Forsgren, Y.Trolle Lagerros, R.Bellocco, L.Alfredsson, A.Knutsson, et al)

[19] American Journal of Epidemiology [2017] Mar 9 : 1-8 [Epub ahead of print] (Z.Liu, A.Roosaar, T.Axéll, W.Ye)

Noradrenaline precursors

DROXIDOPA

Brand name : Northera

Pharmacology : Droxidopa is a synthetic amino acid precursor of noradrenaline. Droxidopa can pass the blood brain barrier and then form noradrenaline and adrenaline, which are derivatives of dopamine. Droxidopa is also known as L-threo-dihydroxyphenylserine [1].

Efficacy : The use of droxidopa was compared to the use of a placebo. With droxidopa Parkinson's Disease symptom scores were significantly better from the outset. Individual symptoms such as stiffness, resting tremor, and alternate hand motion were also significantly improved with the use of droxidopa, suggesting that droxidopa is effective in improving rigidity, tremor and alternate motion of hand [1]. It also improves freezing [2, 3, 4], and reduces falls [5]. Improvement was obtained in about two thirds of the cases on freezing in gait, difficulty of postural control, depressive mood and bradyphrenia [6].

Adverse effects : Those adverse effects reported were headache (7%) and dizziness (3%). Treatment was not discontinued because of adverse effects [7].

[1] Parkinsonism & Related Disorders [2015] 21 (10) : 1214-1218 (S. Zhao, R.Cheng, J.Zheng, Q.Li, J.Wang, W.Fan, L.Zhang, Y.Zhang, H. Li, S.Liu)

[2] Acta Medica Okayama [1984] 38 (3) : 301-304 (N.Ogawa, H. Kuroda, M.Yamamoto, I.Nukina, Z.Ota)

[3] Journal of Medicine [1985] 16 (5-6) : 525-534 (N.Ogawa, M. Yamamoto, H.Takayama)

[4] Neuroscience Letters [1990] 116 (1-2) : 194-197 (H.Tohgi, T.Abe, S.Takahashi, J.Takahashi, M.Ueno, Y.Nozaki)

[5] Clinical Neuropharmacology [2016] Jun 21 [Epub ahead of print] (R.A.Hauser, S.Heritier, G.J.Rowse, L.A.Hewitt, S.H.Isaacson)

[6] No To Shinkei [1991] 43 (3) : 263-268 (H.Narabayashi, F. Yokochi, T.Ogawa, T.Igakura)

[7] Neurology [2014] 83 (4) : 328-335 (H.Kaufmann, R.Freeman, I.Biaggioni, P.Low, S.Pedder, L.A.Hewitt, J.Mauney, M.Feirtag, C.J.Mathias)

Non-dopaminergic drugs

PART 2 : THOSE NORMALLY USED FOR OTHER DISORDERS

Those drugs that are normally used for other purposes but are being assessed for use in Parkinson's Disease are : anti-cancer drugs (nilotinib) [PAGE 708], anti-diabetics (exenatide, glitazones) [PAGE 709], anti-epileptics (zonisamide) [PAGE 711], CNS stimulants (methylphenidate) [PAGE 712], NSAIDs (Non-steroidal anti-inflammatory drugs) [PAGE 713], statins (for lowering cholesterol) [PAGE 715], vaccines (PD01A, PRX002) [PAGE 716].

Anticancer drugs

NILOTINIB

Trade names : Tasigna (when used for cancer)

Pharmacology : Nilotinib is a cAbl tyrosine kinase inhibitor that is normally used for the treatment of cancer [1, 2]. It is claimed to facilitate the degradation of alpha-synuclein [3, 4, 5].

Efficacy : Efficacy has only been assessed concerning motor function in animals that did not have Parkinson's Disease [6]. The weakness in the theory on which the method is reliant is that a lot of people with Parkinson's Disease do not accumulate alpha-Synuclein. So there is none to get rid of.

Adverse effects : Doses of 150mg or 300mg for 6 months were claimed to be safe and well tolerated despite some side effects including one serious side effect [1, 2].

[1] Journal of Parkinsons Disease [2016] Jul 12 [Epub ahead of print] (R.K.Wyse, P.Brundin, T.B.Sherer)

[2] Journal of Parkinsons Disease [2016] Jul 11 [Epub ahead of print] (F.Pagan, M.Hebron, E.H.Valadez, Y.Tores-Yaghi, X.Huang, R.R. Mills, B.M.Wilmarth, H.Howard, C.Dunn, A.Carlson, et al)

[3] Human Molecular Genetics [2014] 23 (11) : 2858-2879 (A.L.Mahul-Mellier, B.Fauvet, A.Gysbers, I.Dikiy, A.Oueslati, S. Georgeon, A.J.Lamontanara, A.Bisquertt, D.Eliezer, E.Masliah, et al)

[4] Autophagy [2013] 9 (8) : 1249-1250 (M.L.Hebron, I.Lonskaya, C.E.Moussa)

[5] Human Molecular Genetics [2013] 22 (16) : 3315-3328 (M.L. Hebron, I.Lonskaya, C.E.Moussa)

[6] Frontiers in Cellular Neuroscience [2014] 8 : 50 (A.Tanabe, Y. Yamamura, J.Kasahara, R.Morigaki, R.Kaji, S.Goto)

ANTI-DIABETICS

EXENATIDE

Trade names : Byetta, Bydureon

Pharmacology : Exenatide is a type 2 diabetes treatment that differs in its pharmacological action and structure from insulin. Exenatide is an injected glucagon-like peptide-1 agonist. The possible means of how it might affect Parkinson's Disease is not known.

Efficacy : When people with moderate Parkinson's Disease received subcutaneous injections of exenatide for a year there were clinically relevant improvements in Parkinson's Disease motor and cognitive measures. They had a mean improvement after one year on the UPDRS of 2.7 compared with a mean decline of 2.2 points in controls [1]. Using the MDS-UPDRS, which is a means of assessing the extent of Parkinson's Disease symptoms, people with Parkinson's Disease were assessed who had previously taken exenatide. People with Parkinson's Disease had an advantage of 5.6 points (with a range of 2.2 to 9.0) on the symptom assessment. They also had a better score when assessed concerning dementia. Unusually, the effects of exenatide on Parkinson's Disease had continued beyond its use [2].

Adverse effects : Exenatide was well tolerated but weight loss was common [1]. Other adverse effects of the use of exenatide are nausea, injection-site induration, dyslipidemia, vomiting, diarrhoea, headache and hypoglycaemia [3, 4].

[1] Journal of Clinical Investigation [2013] 123 (6) : 2730-2736 (I. Aviles-Olmos, J.Dickson, Z.Kefalopoulou, A.Djamshidian, P.Ell, T. Soderlund, P.Whitton, R.Wyse, T.Isaacs, A.Lees, P.Limousin, et al)

[2] Journal of Parkinson's Disease [2014] 4 (3) : 337-344 (I.Aviles-Olmos, J.Dickson, Z.Kefalopoulou, A.Djamshidian, J.Kahan, P.E. Fmedsci, P.Whitton, R.Wyse, T. Isaacs, A.Lees, P.Limousin, et al)

[3] Journal of Diabetes Investigation [2013] 4 (1) : 53-61 (L.Ji, Y. Onishi, C.W.Ahn, P.Agarwal, C.W.Chou, H.Haber, K.Guerrettaz, M.K. Boardman)

[4] Diabetes Obesity and Metabolism [2009] 11 (6) : 544-556 (R. Gentilella, C.Bianchi, A.Rossi, C.M.Rotella)

GLITAZONES

Trade names : Various (when used for diabetes)

Pharmacology : Glitazones are peroxisome proliferation-activated receptor gamma agonists that are used for the treatment of diabetes.

Efficacy : Pioglitazone failed to have any effect in Parkinson's Disease [1]. Diabetics, who did not have Parkinson's Disease, who were prescribed the glitazones reduced their incidence of Parkinson's Disease by 28% [2].

Adverse effects : Glitazones have been associated with some serious side effects [2].

[1] Lancet Neurology [2015] 14 (8) : 795-803 (T.Simuni, K.Kieburtz, B.Tilley, J.Elm, B.Ravina, D.Babcock, M.Emborg, R.Hauser, C.Kamp, J.C.Morgan, G.W.Ross, D.K.Simon, J.Bainbridge, L.Baker, et al)

[2] PLoS Medicine [2015] 12 (7) : e1001854 (R.Brauer, K.Bhaskaran, N.Chaturvedi, D.T.Dexter, L.Smeeth, I.Douglas)

ANTI-EPILEPTICS

ZONISAMIDE

Trade names : Zonegran

Pharmacology : Zonisamide is a widely available anti-epileptic drug [1]. It is an oral 1,2-benzisoxazole-3-methanesulfonamide [1]. It activates dopamine biosynthesis by increasing the level of mRNA of tyrosine hydroxylase. Zonisamide also moderately inhibits monoamine oxidase B [2]. Therapeutic doses of zonisamide for Parkinson's Disease are considerably lower than those for the treatment of epilepsy [3].

Efficacy : The addition of zonisamide in dosages of 25mg [1], 25mg to 50mg [4], 50mg [2, 5], or 25mg to 100mg [6] to the use of existing Parkinson's Disease drugs reduced Parkinson's Disease symptoms. Zonisamide reduced Parkiinson's Disease symptoms [9]. It significantly reduced the wearing off time [9].

Adverse effects : The incidence of adverse effects was similar between the 25mg, 50mg, and placebo groups but higher in the 100mg group [5, 6]. Adverse effects involved nausea and vomiting (9%) or drowsiness (6.3%) [7], somnolence and weight decrease [8].

[1] CNS Drugs [2009] 23 (8) : 703-711 (L.P.Yang, C.M.Perry)

[2] Current Pharmaceutical Design [2004] 10 (6) : 687-693 (M. Murata)

[3] Expert Review of Neurotherapeutics [2007] 7 (9) : 1077-1083 (H. Miwa)

[4] Drugs Today [2010] 46 (4) : 251-258 (M.Murata)

[5] Movement Disorders [2015] 30 (10) : 1343-1350 (M.Murata, K. Hasegawa, I.Kanazawa, J.Fukasaka, K.Kochi, R.Shimazu)

[6] Neurology [2007] 68 (1) : 45-50 (M.Murata, K.Hasegawa, I. Kanazawa)

[7] Seizure [2015] 32 : 69-71 (A.C.Jongeling, R.J.Richins, C.W.Bazil)

[8] Expert Review of Neurotherapeutics [2015] 15 (8) : 857-865 (A. Schulze-Bonhage)

[9] Journal of Alzheimers Disease [2017] Feb 1 [Epub ahead of print] (S.Matsunaga, T.Kishi, N.Iwata)

CNS STIMULANTS

METHYLPHENIDATE

Trade names : Ritalin

Pharmacology : Methylphenidate is a central nervous system stimulant that is normally used in the treatment of ADHD and narcolepsy.

Efficacy : In response to 10 mg methylphenidate, total walking time, total freezing time, number of freezing episodes and the non-freezing walking time significantly improved [1]. In response to 10 mg methylphenidate (three times per day), there was a reduction in fatigue [2]. In response to 20mg methylphenidate, attention significantly improved but memory and visual-spatial performance were unchanged. Gait speed, stride time variability, and demonstrated measures of fall risk, significantly improved [3]. In response to up to 80mg methylphenidate, freezing and shuffling improved, and depression marginally improved. There was no improvement in gait. Freezing of gait, sleepiness and overall Parkinson's Disease symptoms worsened [4]. In response to an intake of 0.2mg methylphenidate per kg followed by intravenous L-dopa for several days, dyskinesia increased. Methylphenidate increased the motor effects of L-dopa with minimal effects on cognitive or affective functions [5]. In response to 0.4mg methylphenidate per kg (three times per day), the effect on the motor response to L-dopa was small and variable and clinically insignificant [6]. In response to chronic, high doses of methylphenidate, there was improved gait and motor symptoms without L-dopa, and an increased in the intensity of the response of these symptoms to L-dopa [7].

Adverse effects : The frequency of the following side effects increased

: insomnia, appetite disturbance, stomach ache, headache, and dizziness. The frequency of the following side effects decreased : staring and daydreaming, irritability, anxiety, and nail biting [8].

[1] Journal of Neural Transmission [2007] (Supplementum) (72) : 145-148 (L.Pollak, Y.Dobronevsky, T.Prohorov, S.Bahunker, J.M. Rabey)

[2] Movement Disorders [2007] 22 (14) : 2070-2076 (D.A.Mendonça, K.Menezes, M.S.Jog)

[3] Clinical Neuropharmacology [2006] 29 (1) : 15-17 (E.Auriel, J.M. Hausdorff, T.Herman, E.S.Simon, N.Giladi)

[4] Neurology [2011] 76 (14) : 1256-1262 (A.J.Espay, A.K.Dwivedi, M.Payne, L.Gaines, J.E.Vaughan, B.N.Maddux, J.T.Slevin, M.Gartner, A.Sahay, F.J.Revilla, A.P.Duker, R.Shukla)

[5] Clinical Neuropharmacology [2001] 24 (4) : 208-213 (R.Camicioli, E.Lea, J.G.Nutt, G.Sexton, B.S.Oken)

[6] Archives of Neurology [2007] 64 (3) : 319-323 (J.G.Nutt, J.H. Carter, N.E.Carlson)

[7] Journal of Neurology, Neurosurgery amd Psychiatry [2007] 78 (5) : 470-475 (D.Devos, P.Krystkowiak, F.Clement, K.Dujardin, O. Cottencin, N.Waucquier, K.Ajebbar, B.Thielemans, et al)

[8] Pediatrics [1993] 91 (6) : 1101-1106 (P.A.Ahmann, S.J.Waltonen, K.A.Olson, F.W.Theye, A.J.Van Erem, R.J.LaPlant)

NSAIDs

Trade names : none (due to being in development)

Pharmacology : NSAIDs (Non-steroidal anti-inflammatory drugs) are drugs with analgesic, antipyretic and in higher doses, anti-inflammatory effects.

Efficacy : NSAIDs use mostly had little or no effect on Parkinson's Disease [1-13]. The prior use of NSAIDs had no effect [11]. Long term use of NSAIDs slightly lowered the risk of Parkinson's Disease [11, 14, 15]. There was little or no effect on Parkinson's Disease with the use of aspirin [2, 5, 11-15], aectamonophen [5, 14, 15], or ibuprofen [1, 2, 5].

Adverse effects : They mainly increase the risk of gastrointestinal (GI) and cardiovascular complications compared with non-NSAID users [16].

[1] Cochrane Database of Systematic Reviews [2011] (11) : CD008454 (K.Rees, R.Stowe, S.Patel, N.Ives, K.Breen, C.E.Clarke, Y. Ben-Shlomo)

[2] Neuroepidemiology [2011] 36 (3) : 155-161 (A.D.Manthripragada, E.S.Schernhammer, J.Qiu, S,Friis, L.Wermuth, J.H.Olsen, B.Ritz)

[3] BMJ [2011] 342 : d198 (J.A.Driver, G.Logroscino, L.Lu, J.M. Gaziano, T.Kurth)

[4] Neurology [2006] 66 (7) : 1097-1099 (M.A.Hernán, G.Logroscino, L.A.García Rodríguez)

[5] Neurology [2011] 76 (10) : 863-869 (X.Gao, H.Chen, M.A. Schwarzschild, A.Ascherio)

[6] Neuroepidemiology [2007] 28 (4) : 193-196 (M.Bornebroek, L.M. de Lau, M.D.Haag, P.J.Koudstaal, A.Hofman, B.H.Stricker, M.M. Breteler)

[7] Journal of Clinical Neuroscience [2008] 15 (5) : 576-577 (M. Etminan, B.C.Carleton, A.Samii)

[8] Movement Disorders [2008] 23 (1) : 88-95 (K.M.Powers, D.M.Kay, S.A.Factor, C.P.Zabetian, D.S.Higgins, A.Samii, J.G.Nutt, A.Griffith, B.Leis, J.W.Roberts, E.D.Martinez, J.S.Montimurro, et al).

[9] Current Drug Safety [2006] 1 (3) : 223-225 (M.Etminan, S.Suissa)

[10] Archives of Neurology [2007] 64 (4) : 576-580 (D.B.Hancock, E. R.Martin, J.M.Stajich, R.Jewett, M.A.Stacy, B.L.Scott, J.M.Vance, W.K.Scott)

[11] European Journal of Neurology [2011] 18 (11) : 1336-1342 (C. Becker, S.S.Jick, C.R.Meier)

[12] Neurology [2007] 69 (19) : 1836-1842 (AD.Wahner, J.M. Bronstein, Y.M.Bordelon, B.Ritz)

[13] Movement Disorders [2006] 21 (7) : 964-969 (T.G.Ton, S.R. Heckbert, W.T.Longstreth Jr, M.A.Rossing, W.A.Kukull, G.M. Franklin, P.D.Swanson, T.Smith-Weller, H.Checkoway)

[14] Neurology [2010] 74 (12) : 995-1002 (J.J.Gagne, M.C.Power)

[15] Drugs and Aging [2009] 26 (9) : 769-779 (A.Samii, M.Etminan, M.O.Wiens, S.Jafari)

[16] Best Practice and Research : Clinical Gastroenterology [2010] 24 (2) : 121-132 (C.Sostres, C.J.Gargallo, M.T.Arroyo, A.Lanas)

STATINS

Trade names : none (due to being in development)

Pharmacology : Statins (HMG-CoA reductase inhibitors) are used to lower cholesterol levels by inhibiting the enzyme HMG-CoA reductase, which has a key role in cholesterol biosynthesis in the liver.

Efficacy : Statins are not usually used to treat Parkinson's Disease but can reduce its incidence down to between 42% and 98% [1-9]. In by far the largest assessment the risk was reduce to 81% [10]. The age of onset of Parkinson's Disease was delayed by 9 years [11]. The long term risk of Parkinson's Disease is unaffected by the use of statins [3]. Statin use can also moderately increase Parkinson's Disease symptoms [12, 13].

Adverse effects : Muscle adverse effects are the most reported problem. The destruction of striated muscle cells is the most feared. Risk is amplified by drug interactions that functionally increase statin potency. Additional adverse effects are cognitive loss, neuropathy, pancreatic, hepatic dysfunction, and sexual dysfunction [14].

[1] American Journal of Management Care [2013] 19 (8) : 626-632 (B. Friedman, A.Lahad, Y.Dresner, S.Vinker)

[2] Neurology [2013] 81 (5) : 410-416 (Y.C.Lee, C.H.Lin, R.M.Wu, M.S.Lin, J.W.Lin, C.H.Chang, M.S.Lai)

[3] Journal of Neurology [2013] 260 (1) : 158-165 (K.Undela, K. Gudala, S.Malla, D.Bansal)

[4] Archives of Neurology [2012] 69 (3) : 380-384 (X.Gao, K.C.Simon, M.A.Schwarzschild, A.Ascherio)

[5] Journal of Clinical Neuroscience [2008] 15 (11) : 1272-1273 (A. Samii, B.C.Carleton, M.Etminan)

[6] Drug Safety [2008] 31 (5) : 399-407 (C.Becker, S.S.Jick, C.R. Meier)

[7] Neurology [2008] 70 (16 Part 2) : 1418-1422 (A.D.Wahner, J.M. Bronstein, Y.M.Bordelon, B.Ritz)

[8] Behavioral Brain Research [2016] Apr 27 [Epub ahead of print] (Z.Sheng, X.Jia, M.Kang)

[9] Annals of Neurology [2016] Jul 29 [Epub ahead of print] (K.D. Lin, C.Y.Yang, M.Y.Lee, S.C.Ho, C.K.Liu, S.J.Shin)

[10] PLoS One [2016] 11 (3) : e0152564 (S.Bai, Y.Song, X.Huang, L. Peng, J.Jia, Y.Liu, H.Lu)

[11] Pharmacological Research [2009] 60 (1) : 41-45 (E.Mutez, A. Duhamel, L.Defebvre, R.Bordet, A.Destée, A.Kreisler)

[12] Expert Opinions on Drug Safety [2009] 8 (3) : 261-271 (C.Becker, C.R.Meier)

[13] Movement Disorders [2015] 30 (4) : 552-559 (X.Huang, A. Alonso, X.Guo, D.M.Umbach, M.L.Lichtenstein, C.M.Ballantyne, R.B. Mailman, T.H.Mosley, H.Chen)

[14] American Journal of Cardiovascular Drugs [2008] 8 (6) : 373-418 (B.A.Golomb, M.A.Evans)

VACCINES

Vaccines stimulate the body's immune system to recognize disease causing agents so that the immune system can more easily recognize and destroy any of these agents that it later encounters. The vaccine PD01A is presently being assessed for the treatment of Parkinson's Disease. It is directed against alpha-Synuclein.

PD01A

Trade names : none (due to being in development)

Pharmacology : PD01A is a vaccine directed against an accumulation of alpha-Synuclein. Vaccination aims to educate the immune system to generate antibodies that are directed against alpha-Synuclein.

Efficacy : They believe that a reduction of the brain's alpha-Synuclein aggregates will have a beneficial impact on the progress of Parkinson's Disease. The vaccine is being tested on people with Parkinson's Disease. The primary purpose is to assess the safety and tolerability of PD01A. The weakness in the theory on which the method is reliant is that a lot of people with Parkinson's Disease do not accumulate alpha-Synuclein. So there is none to get rid of. Most people that have an accumulation of alpha-Synuclein in the brain do not have Parkinson's Disease either, thereby proving that alpha-Synuclein is not the cause of Parkinson's Disease [1].

Adverse effects : The adverse effects of PD01A have not yet been assessed.

[1] AFFiRis : http://www.affiris.com/html/en/presse_medien/pressemel dungen.html

PRX002

Trade names : none (due to being in development)

Pharmacology : PRX002 is a new protein immunotherapy being developed for Parkinson's Disease [1].

Efficacy : Prothena Corporation have reported a reduction of alpha-synuclein by up to 96% after a single dose of PRX002. Five doses were used. Only healthy volunteers were involved. However, the clinical trial did not involve people with Parkinson's Disease and no efficacy was demonstrated in Parkinson's Disease [1]. The weakness in the theory on which the method is reliant is that a lot of people with Parkinson's Disease do not accumulate alpha-Synuclein. So there is none to get rid of. Most people that have an accumulation of alpha-Synuclein in the brain do not have Parkinson's Disease either, thereby proving that alpha-Synuclein is not the cause of Parkinson's Disease [1].

Adverse effects : There were mild adverse effects in 5% to 10% of subjects [1].

[1] http://ir.prothena.com/releasedetail.cfm?ReleaseID=902569

NON-DOPAMINERGIC DRUGS

PART 3 : THOSE USED FOR RELATED DISORDERS

Those drugs that are used for problems that can occur in Parkinson's Disease are : sialhorrhea (glycopyrrolate) [PAGE 718], dementia (rivastigmine) [PAGE 719], dyskinesia (tetrabenazine, fipamezole, AFQ056, levetiracetam, eltoprazine, memantine, dextromethorphan) [PAGE 721], fatigue (modafinil) [PAGE 726], anti-psychotics (pimavanserin, clozapine, quetiapine) [PAGE 727].

SIALHORRHEA

Sialorrhea (drooling or excessive salivation) often occurs in Parkinson's Disease, especially in the later stages. However, it is not entirely due to Parkinson's Disease. A means of treating sialorrhea in Parkinson's Disease that is presently being used is Glycopyrrolate.

GLYCOPYRROLATE

Trade names : none (due to being in development)

Pharmacology : Sialorrhea is often treated with anticholinergics but the side effects caused by anticholinergics limit their usefulness. Glycopyrrolate (glycopyrronium bromide) is an anticholinergic drug that is not able to cross the blood-brain barrier in considerable amounts. Therefore, glycopyrrolate exhibit minimal central nervous system side effects, which may be an advantage in dealing with Parkinson's Disease [1].

Efficacy : When clinically tested, around 39% of people taking glycopyrrolate had a clinically relevant improvement in sialorrhea of at least 30%, without causing any side effects. 1 mg 3 times daily was suggested as an effective and safe therapy for sialorrhea in Parkinson disease [1].

Adverse effects : There were no significant differences in adverse effects between glycopyrrolate and placebo treatment [1].

[1] Neurology [2010] 74 (15) : 1203-1207 (M.E.Arbouw, K.L.Movig, M.Koopmann, P.J.Poels, H.J.Guchelaar, T.C.Egberts, C.Neef, J.P.van Vugt)

DEMENTIA

Dementia commonly occurs in Parkinson's Disease, especially in the later stages of Parkinson's Disease. However, it is not actually a Parkinson's Disease symptom. A method of treating dementia in Parkinson's Disease presently being used is rivastigmine.

RIVASTIGMINE

Trade names : Exelon

Pharmacology : Rivastigmine is an inhibitor of cholinesterase, which is an enzyme that facilitates the breakdown of the neurotransmitter acetylcholine [1].

Efficacy : In people with Parkinson's Disease Dementia, rivastigmine treatment is associated with improvement in memory and language [2], ADL (actvities of daily living) [3], and moderate improvements in dementia [4]. It modestly improves cognition, function, global outcome and neuropsychiatric symptoms [1]. It improves word recall, following commands, ideational praxis, remembering test instructions, and comprehension of spoken language, memory, language, and praxis. Overall, rivastigmine was associated with improvements on individual cognitive items and general cognitive domains [5]. Rivastigmine was also associated with significant improvements in tests that evaluated the flexibility of thinking, problem solving and planning in patients [6].

Adverse effects : In people with Parkinson's Disease Dementia using rivastigmine there were adverse effects in 36% who took capsules and 32% who used a patch. Rivastigmine was discontinued in 4% of people taking capsules and 2% of people using a patch. The most common adverse effects were nausea (capsules 40%, patch 8%), tremor (capsules 24%, patch 9%), falls (capsules 17%, patch 20%), vomiting (capsules 15%, patch 2%), application site erythema (capsules 0% patch 14%) [7]. Emerging or worsening of tremor occurred in 10% of people. Incidences of worsening parkinsonism, bradykinesia and rigidity were all less than 5% [8]. The most frequent adverse effects were nausea (29%), vomiting (16%), and tremor (10%) [4].

[1] Drugs and Aging [2011] 28 (10) : 769-777 (C.Ballard, Z.Kahn, A. Corbett)

[2] American Journal of Alzheimer's Disease and other Dementias [2011] 26 (6) : 443-449 (D.Weintraub, M.Somogyi, X.Meng)

[3] Dementia and Geriatric Cognitive Disorders [2010] 29 (6) : 510-515 (J.T.Olin, D.Aarsland, X.Meng)

[4] New England Journal of Medicine [2004] 35 (24) : 2509-2518 (M. Emre, D.Aarsland, A.Albanese, E.J.Byrne, G.Deuschl, P.P.De Deyn, F.Durif, J.Kulisevsky, T.van Laar, A.Lees, W.Poewe, et al)

[5] American Journal of Alzheimer's Disease and other Dementias [2010] 25 (5) : 407-413 (F.A.Schmitt, D.Aarsland, K.S.Brønnick, X. Meng, S.Tekin, J.T.Olin)

[6] CNS Neuroscience and Therapeutics [2010] 16 (6) : 330-336 (F.A. Schmitt, M.R.Farlow, X.Meng, S.Tekin, J.T.Olin)

[7] Clinical Neuropharmacology [2014] 37 (1) : 9-16 (M.Emre, W. Poewe, P.P.De Deyn, P. Barone, J.Kulisevsky, E.Pourcher, T.van Laar, A.Storch, F.Micheli, D.Burn, F.Durif, R.Pahwa, F.Callegari, et al)

[8] Drug Safety [2008] 31 (1) : 79-94 (W.Oertel, W.Poewe, E.Wolters, P.P.De Deyn, M.Emre, C.Kirsch, C.Hsu, S.Tekin, R.Lane)

DYSKINESIA

Dyskinesia commonly occurs in Parkinson's Disease, especially in the later stages of Parkinson's Disease. However, it is not a Parkinson's Disease symptom. It is normally due to the effect of dopaminergic drugs. Those methods of treating dyskinesia in Parkinson's Disease presently being used or assessed include tetrabenazine, fipamezole, AFQ056, levetiracetam, and eltoprazine.

TETRABENAZINE

Trade names : none (due to being in development)

Pharmacology : Tetrabenazine (TBZ) is a monoamine-depleting agent that is used for the treatment of chorea in Huntington's disease. Tetrabenazine acts by depletion of the monoamines serotonin, norepinephrine, and dopamine in the central nervous system. Tetrabenazine does this by reversibly inhibiting vesicle monoamine transporter type 2 and thereby prevents monoamine uptake into presynaptic neurons [1].

Efficacy : Taking up to 50mg tetrabenazine daily resulted in an improvement in L-dopa induced peak dyskinesias (LIDs) by as much as 45%. The patients experienced a clear benefit in terms of their quality of life [2].

Adverse effects : The most adverse effects caused by tetrabenazine included drowsiness (36%), parkinsonism (28%), depression (15%), insomnia (11%), nervousness or anxiety (10%), and akathisia (9%). The adverse effects were controlled with reduction in the dose of tetrabenazine [3].

[1] The American Journal of Geriatric Pharmacotherapy [2010] 8 (4) : 331-373 (D.R.Guay)

[2] Functional Neurology [2013] 28 (2) : 101-105 (L.Brusa, A. Orlacchio, A.Stefani, S.Galati, M.Pierantozzi, C.Iani, N.B.Mercuri)

[3] Neurology [1997] 48 (2) : 358-362 (J.Jankovic, J.Beach)

FIPAMEZOLE

Trade names : none (due to being in development)

Pharmacology : Fipamezole is an alpha (2)-adrenergic receptor antagonist being assessed for its use in treating the dyskinesia that can occur in Parkinson's Disease.

Efficacy : The study was carried out in the U.S.A. and India. The total study population showed no statistically significant difference. However, a prespecified subgroup analysis of U.S. subjects was conducted, showing that fipamezole at 90 mg moderately reduced dyskinesia that was due to L-dopa. The response was shown to be according to the dose used when assessing the different dosages (30mg, 60mg, and 90 mg fipamezole) [1].

Adverse effects : Fipamezole induced mild and transient blood pressure elevation and was associated with what the authors describe as "an acceptable profile of adverse effects." [1].

[1] Neurology [2012] 79 (2) : 163-169 (P.A.Lewitt, R.A.Hauser, M.Lu, Nicholas AP, Weiner W, Coppard N, Leinonen M, Savola JM.)

AFQ056

Trade names : none (due to being in development)

Pharmacology : AFQ056 is a glutamate receptor 5 antagonist being assessed for the treatment of dyskinesia.

Efficacy : Using doses of 20 mg to 200mg AFQ056 caused significant dose related improvements in dyskinesia with 200mg having the greatest effect. There were no major reductions in Parkinson's Disease symptoms [1]. Using doses of 25 mg to 150mg AFQ056 caused significant improvements in dyskinesia without reducing Parkinson's Disease symptoms [2].

Adverse effects : Dizziness was the most reported adverse event [2]. Hallucination, fatigue, nasopharyngitis, diarrhea, and insomnia were the other most common adverse effects [1].

[1] Movement Disorders [2013] 28 (13) : 1838-1846 (F. Stocchi, O. Rascol, A.Destee, N.Hattori, R.A.Hauser, A.E.Lang, W. Poewe, M. Stacy, E.Tolosa, H.Gao, J.Nagel, M.Merschhemke, A.Graf, et al)

[2] Movement Disorders [2011] 26 (7) : 1243-1250 (D.Berg, J.Godau, C.Trenkwalder, K.Eggert, I.Csoti, A.Storch, H.Huber, M.Morelli-Canelo, M.Stamelou, V.Ries, M.Wolz, C.Schneider, T.Di Paolo, et al)

LEVETIRACETAM

Trade names : none (due to being in development)

Pharmacology : The precise action of levetiracetam, which is an anti-epileptic is unknown. However, it has been shown to bind to synaptic vesicle protein SV2A, which has been related to modulation of synaptic vesicle exocytosis and neurotransmitter release [1].

Efficacy : Levetiracetam was assessed for the ability to treat L-dopa induced dyskinesias (LID) in Parkinson's Disease. On with LID time decreased 37 minutes at 500 mg/day and 75 minutes at 1,000 mg/day. On without LID time increased by 46 minutes at 500 mg/day and 55 minutes at 1,000 mg/day. The Parkinson's Disease symptom score UPDRS 32 showed a decreased dyskinesia duration mean change of 0.35 at 1,000 mg/day. However, there was no comparison made with a placebo. Patient diaries and UPDRS scores showed no increase in off time [2]. Doses up to 2000mg had little [3], or no [4] effect [3] on dyskinesias.

Adverse effects : The most frequent adverse effects were sleepiness, difficulty concentrating, tiredness, and memory problems. It can also cause anger and aggression, nervousness and agitation, upset stomach, depression, and sleep disturbance [5].

[1] Frontiers in Neurology [2013] 4 : 192 (C.Wright, J.Downing, D. Mingall, O.Khan, A.Williams, E.Fonkem, D.Garrett, J.Aceves, B. Kirmani)

[2] Movement Disorders [2011] 26 (2) : 264-270 (P.Stathis, S. Konitsiotis, G.Tagaris, D.Peterson)

[3] Journal of Neural Transmission [2010] 117 (11) : 1279-1286 (M. Wolz, M.Löhle, K.Strecker, U.Schwanebeck, C.Schneider, H. Reichmann, X.Grählert, J.Schwarz, A.Storch)

[4] Movement Disorders [2011] 26 (8) : 1552-1555 (K.K.Wong, J.E. Alty, A.G.Goy, S.Raghav, D.C.Reutens, P.A.Kempster)

[5] Epilepsy Behavior [2015] 54 : 150-157 (A.B.Kowski, F.Weissinger, V.Gaus, P.Fidzinski, F.Losch, M.Holtkamp)

ELTOPRAZINE

Trade names : none (due to being in development)

Pharmacology : Eltoprazine is a 5HT partial agonist being developed for the treatment of L-dopa induced dyskinesias in people with Parkinson's Disease.

Efficacy : A clinical trial was conducted using 2.5mg, 5.0mg and 7.5mg eltoprazine in combination with Sinemet in people with Parkinson's Disease who had L-dopa induced dyskinesias. They found that 5mg eltoprazine significantly reduced L-dopa induced dyskinesias, and had an anti-dyskinetic effect with the use of 7.5mg eltoprazine. Parkinson's Disease symptoms scores did not otherwise alter [1].

Adverse effects : The most frequent adverse effects were nausea and dizziness [1].

[1] Brain [2015] 138 (Part 4) : 963-973 (P.Svenningsson, C.Rosenblad, K.AfEdholm Arvidsson, K.Wictorin, C.Keywood, B.Shankar, D.A. Lowe, A.Björklund, H.Widner)

MEMANTINE

Trade names : none (due to being in development)

Pharmacology : Memantine is a glutamate antagonist that is being assessed for possible use in the reduction of dyskinesia as a side effect of L-dopa in people being treated for Parkinson's Disease.

Efficacy : The primary outcome measure, a change in observed dyskinesia ratings, did not reach significance. However, data from the self-administered diaries, as a secondary outcome measure, did show a significant (35%) reduction in the amount of the day spent with dyskinesia, from 25% (placebo) to 16% (memantine) [1].

Adverse effects : Memantine was well tolerated, without any serious adverse effects, or worsening in the parkinsonian motor score [1].

[1] Acta Neurologica Scandinavica [2016] 133 (5) : 355-360 (K. Wictorin, H.Widner)

DEXTROMETHORPHAN

Trade names : Nuedexta (when used for PseudoBulbar Affect (PBA))

Pharmacology : Dextromethorphan is a sigma-1 receptor-agonist and glutamatergic/monoaminergic modulator. Dextromethorphan/quinidine is a combination drug containing dextromethorphan and the antiarrhythmic agent quinidine. Quinidine is included to inhibit dextromeththorphan metabolism [1].

Efficacy : A pilot study (NCT01767129) examined the efficacy of dextromethorphan plus quinidine for treating L-dopa induced dyskinesia. People with Parkinson's Disease were randomised to 45mg dextromethorphan and 10mg twice daily, alternated with a placebo. Dyskinesia severity was a bit lower with dextromethorphan and quinidine than with a placebo, and subsequently significantly lower. Most of the patients rated their dyskinesia "much or very much improved" when taking dextromethorphan and quinidine [1].

Adverse effects : Dextromethorphan and quinidine was generally well tolerated, but was associated with more frequent adverse effects. [1].

[1] Movement Disorders [2017] Mar 30 [Epub ahead of print] (S.H. Fox, L.V. Metman, J.G.Nutt, M.Brodsky, S.A.Factor, A.E.Lang, L.E. Pope, N.Knowles, J.Siffert)

FATIGUE

Fatigue commonly occurs in Parkinson's Disease, especially in the later stages of Parkinson's Disease. A method of treating fatigue in Parkinson's Disease presently being used is modafinil.

MODAFINIL

Trade names : none (due to being in development)

Pharmacology : Modafinil is a psychostimulant that is approved for use in narcolepsy. It is often used to treat a variety of somnolent conditions. Modafinil appears to inhibit the actions of the dopamine transporter thereby also leading to an increase in concentrations of dopamine [1].

Efficacy : A daily dose of 100mg modafinil caused a reduction in Parkinson's Disease severity and in Clinical Global Impression (CGI) [2]. Modafinil also caused a statistically significant improvement on the Epworth Sleepiness Scale (ESS) using daily doses of 100mg [2], 172mg [3], 200mg [4] and 400mg [5]. Besides being modestly effective for treating excessive daytime sleepiness, daily use of 200mg modafinil caused few side effects [6]. However, in another study the daily use of

200mg-400mg modafinil failed to improve the Epworth Sleepiness Scale and failed to improve Parkinson's Disease motor symptoms [7].

Adverse effects : Most adverse effects were mild to moderate in severity, and the majority resolved during treatment. The most commonly reported adverse effects were insomnia (29%), headache (20%), and decreased appetite (16%) [8].

[1] Journal of Pharmacology and Experimental Therapeutics [2009] 329 (2) : 738-746 (D.Zolkowska, R.Jain, R.B.Rothman, J.S.Partilla, B. L.Roth, V.Setola, T.E.Prisinzano, M.H.Baumann)

[2] Neuropsychiatric Disease and Treatment [2010] 6 : 93-97 (J. Lökk)

[3] Clinical Neuropharmacology [2002] 25 (2) : 111-114 (A.V. Nieves, A.E.Lang)

[4] Sleep [2002] 25 (8) : 905-909 (B.Högl, M.Saletu, E.Brandauer, S. Glatzl, B.Frauscher, K.Seppi, H.Ulmer, G.Wenning, W.Poewe)

[5] Journal of Neurology [2010] 257 (3) : 452-456 (H.L.Tyne, J. Taylor, G.A.Baker, M.J.Steiger)

[6] Movement Disorders [2003] 18 (3) : 287-293 (C.H.Adler, J.N. Caviness, J.G.Hentz, M.Lind, J.Tiede)

[7] Journal of Neurology, Neurosurgery and Psychiatry [2005] 76 (12) : 1636-1639 (W.G.Ondo, R.Fayle, F.Atassi, J.Jankovic)

[8] Pediatrics [2005] 116 (6) : e777-e784 (J.Biederman, J.M.Swanson, S. B.Wigal, C.J.Kratochvil, S.W.Boellner, C.Q.Earl, J.Jiang, L.Greenhill)

Psychosis

Psychosis often occurs in Parkinson's Disease, especially in the later stages of Parkinson's Disease. Psychosis is not a Parkinson's Disease symptom. It is normally due to the effect of dopaminergic drugs. Those methods of treating psychosis in Parkinson's Disease presently being used or assessed include pimavanserin, clozapine, and quetiapine.

PIMAVANSERIN

Trade names : Nuplazid

Pharmacology : Pimavanserin is used for treating psychosis related to Parkinson's Disease. It is a 5-HT 2A receptor inverse agonist.

Efficacy : In one assessment it failed to have any beneficial effect in clinical trials [1]. In a 28 day study pimavanserin did not differentiate from placebo with regard to motor impairment, sedation, hypotension, or other side effects. The principal measure of efficacy of antipsychotic response to pimavanserin, the SAPS total domain score, only showed a trend. However, the pimavanserin treated patients showed significantly greater improvement in some but not all measures of psychosis, including SAPS global measures of hallucinations and delusions, persecutory delusions, and the UPDRS measure of delusions and hallucinations. Pimavanserin showed significantly greater improvement in psychosis in people with Parkinson's Disease at a dose that did not impair motor function, or cause sedation or hypotension [2]. Doses of 34mg pimavanserin improved hallucinations and delusions in 80% of patients and in 58% of those taking a placebo [6]. Doses of 40mg per day over 6 weeks reduced SAPS scores more than a placebo [3]. In another study pimavanserin significantly reduced hallucinations and delusions [4]. The psychosis sometimes experienced in Parkinson's Disease is normally due to the excessive use of dopaminergic drugs. So a reduction in the use of those drugs is a more rational approach than using an additional drug to combat the effects of dopaminergic drugs.

Adverse effects : There was a significant increase in the mortality rate, antipsychotic-related events, cognition-related events, infections and edema. The risk of falls, stroke, sedation, orthostatic hypotension, and thromboembolic events was increased but this was not significant [5].

[1] Parkinsonism & Related Disorders [2009] 15 (Supplement 4) : S105- S110 (J.M.Rabey)

[2] Neuropsychopharmacology [2010] 35 (4) : 881-892 (H.Y.Meltzer, R.Mills, S.Revell, H.Williams, A.Johnson, D.Bahr, J.H.Friedman)

[3] Lancet [2014] 383 (9916) : 533-540 (J.Cummings, S.Isaacson, R. Mills, H.Williams, K.Chi-Burris, A.Corbett, R.Dhall, C.Ballard)

[4] Journal of Alzheimers Disease [2015] 50 (3) : 733-740 (I.Yasue, S.Matsunaga, T.Kishi, K.Fujita, N.Iwata)

[5] Journal of the American Medical Directors Association [2015] 16 (10) : 898.e1-7 (C.Ballard, S.Isaacson, R.Mills, H.Williams, A.Corbett, B.Coate, R.Pahwa, O.Rascol, D.J.Burn)

[6] Journal of Clinical Psychiatry [2017] May 9 [Epub ahead of print] (M.V.Mathis, B.M.Muoio, P.Andreason, A.M.Avila, T.Farchione, A.Atrakchi, R.J.Temple)

CLOZAPINE

Trade names : Clozaril

Pharmacology : The antipsychotic basis of clozapine is to transiently occupy dopamine D2 receptors in the human striatum. The chemical structure of clozapine facilitates a relatively rapid dissociation from D2 receptors [1].

Efficacy : Clozapine significantly improved psychiatric symptoms in most people [2-14] without worsening Parkinsonism [3, 4, 6, 11]. Clozapine also significantly reduced dyskinesias [15, 16, 17], and tremor [18]. Clozapine and quetiapine appeared to be equally effective for the treatment of psychosis in people with Parkinson's Disease [19]. Clozapine was slightly more advantageous over quetiapine in controlling the frequency of hallucinations and in reducing delusions [20].

Adverse effects : The most common adverse effects of clozapine in Parkinson's Disease are sedation, orthostatic hypotension and sialorrhoea [21]. Clozapine also has the potential to cause agranulocytosis, which is idiosyncratic and is not related to the dose [18, 21].

[1] ACS Chemical Neuroscience [2014] 5 (1) : 24-29 (P.Seeman)

[2] Clinical Neuropharmacology [2006] 29 (4) : 215-219 (C.Klein, T. Prokhorov, A.Miniovich, E.Dobronevsky, J.M.Rabey)

[3] Journal of Neurology, Neurosurgery, and Psychiatry [2004] 75 (5) : 689-695 (P.Pollak, F.Tison, O.Rascol, A.Destée, J.J.Péré, J.M.Senard, F.Durif, L.Bourdeix)

[4] New England Journal of Medicine [1999] 340 (10) : 757-763

[5] American Journal of Psychiatry [1999] 156 (2) : 294-298 (A. F.Breier, A.K.Malhotra, D.A.Su TP, Pinals, I.Elman, C.M.Adler, R.T. Lafargue, A.Clifton, D.Pickar)

[6] Acta Neurologica Scandinavica [1996] 94 (5) : 329-336 (P.Auzou, C.Ozsancak, D.Hannequin, N.Moore, P.Augustin)

[7] Journal of Neuropsychiatry and Clinical Neurosciences [1996] 8 (3) : 276-280 (M.L.Wagner, J.L.Defilippi, M.A.Menza, J.I.Sage)

[8] Revue Neurologique [1995] 151 (4) : 251-257 (N.Diederich, M. Keipes, M.Graas, H.Metz)

[9] Neurology [1995] 45 (3 Part 1) : 432-434 (J.M.Rabey, T.A.Treves, M.Y.Neufeld, E.Orlov, A.D.Korczyn)

[10] Neurology [1994] 44 (3 Part 1) : 544-546 (S.A.Factor, D.Brown, E.S.Molho, G.D.Podskalny)

[11] Journal of Clinical Psychiatry [1992] 53 (10) : 373-376 (S.L.Wolk, C.J.Douglas)

[12] Movement Disorders [1992] 7 (2) : 125-131 (S.A.Factor, D. Brown)

[13] Neurology [1990] 40 (5) : 832-834 (E.C.Wolters, T.A.Hurwitz, E. Mak, P.Teal, F.R.Peppard , R.Remick, S.Calne, D.B.Calne)

[14] Neurology [1989] 39 (9) : 1219-1221 (J.H.Friedman, M.C. Lannon)

[15] Neurology [2004] 62 (3) : 381-388 (F.Durif, B.Debilly, M. Galitzky, D.Morand, F.Viallet, M.Borg, S.Thobois, E.Broussolle, O.Rascol)

[16] Acta Neurologica Scandinavica [1998] 97 (5) : 295-299 (F. Pierelli, A.Adipietro, G.Soldati, F.Fattapposta, G.Pozzessere, C. Scoppetta)

[17] Neurology [1997] 48 (3) : 658-662 (F.Durif, M.Vidailhet, F.Assal, C.Roche, A.M.Bonnet, Y.Agid)

[18] Acta Neurologica Scandinavica [1994] 89 (4) : 262-265 (E.N. Jansen)

[19] Clinical Neuropharmacology [2004] 27 (4) : 153-156 (L. Morgante, A.Epifanio, E.Spina, M.Zappia, A.E.Di Rosa, R.Marconi, G. Basile, G.Di Raimondo, P.La Spina, A.Quattrone)

[20] Clinical Neuropharmacology [2006] 29 (6) : 331-337 (D.Merims, M.Balas, C.Peretz, H.Shabtai, N.Giladi)

[21] Drug Safety [2003] 26 (9) : 643-659 (H.H.Fernandez, M.E. Trieschmann, J.H.Friedman)

QUETIAPINE

Trade names : Seroquel

Pharmacology : It has been proposed that the efficacy of quetiapine is mediated through a combination of dopamine type 2 (D2) and serotonin type 2 (5HT2) antagonism. Antagonism at receptors other than dopamine and 5HT2 with similar receptor affinities may explain some of its other effects [1].

Efficacy : Quetiapine improved psychosis symptoms [2-6], visual hallucinations in most people [7], and behaviour [8], but had less effect on paranoia [7] and delusions [7, 9]. A partial to complete ridding of psychosis occurred in around 80% to 90% of people [10-13]. In over half the patients, effectiveness was scored as very good or good both by examiners and caregivers [14], but in some cases quetiapine was not beneficial [12, 15, 16, 17] or the results were conflicting [18, 19]. Quetiapine had effect without causing a decline in motor function [2] or increase in Parkinsonism [8, 13, 19, 20, 21]. However, over time there was still a slow, gradual worsening of motor function [7]. Motor worsening was noted in 13% to 32% of patients [10, 11]. No overall differences in effect were found between the use of clozapine and the use of quetiapine [21, 22] but clozapine was slightly better in controlling frequency of hallucinations and in reducing delusions [20].

Adverse effects : The adverse effects most commonly associated with quetiapine are : somnolence, dizziness, postural hypotension, headache, dry mouth, asthenia, constipation, tachycardia, orthostatic hypotension, dyspepsia, and weight gain. Furthermore, weight gain, syncopal episodes, leucopenias, neutropenias, and peripheral angioedema are sporadically associated with quetiapine treatment [23, 24].

[1] International Journal of Neuropsychopharmacology [2013] 16 (10) : 2235-2244 (S.Nyberg, A.Jucaite, A.Takano, M.Kågedal, Z.Cselényi, C.Halldin, L.Farde)

[2] Movement Disorders [1999] 14 (3) : 484-487 (H.H.Fernandez, J.H. Friedman, C.Jacques, M.Rosenfeld)

[3] Movement Disorders [2004] 19 (1) : 29-35 (J.L.Juncos, V.J. Roberts, M.L.Evatt, R.D.Jewart, C.D.Wood, L.S.Potter, H.C. Jou, P.P. Yeung)

[4] Revista de Neurología [2004] 39 (7) : 661-667 (L.J.López del Val, S.Santos)

[5] Clinical Neuropharmacology [2004] 27 (1) : 33-37 (F.Mancini, C. Tassorelli, E.Martignoni, A.Moglia, G.Nappi, S.Cristina, C. Pacchetti)

[6] Journal of Neurology [2006] 253 (2) : 171-175 (T.Prohorov, C. Klein, A.Miniovitz, E.Dobronevsky, J.M.Rabey)

[7] Journal of Clinical Psychopharmacology [2000] 20 (1) : 54-60 (S.D. Targum, J.L.Abbott)

[8] Annals of Clinical Psychiatry [1999] 11 (3) : 141-144 (M.M. Menza, B.Palermo, M.Mark)

[9] No To Shinkei [2005] 57 (6) : 491-494 (M.Ito, N.Atsuta, H. Watanabe, M.Hirayama, G.Sobue)

[10] Journal of Clinical Psychiatry [2002] 63 (6) : 513-515 (H.H. Fernandez, M.E.Trieschmann, M.A.Burke, J.H.Friedman)

[11] Movement Disorders [2002] 17 (4) : 676-681 (S.Reddy, S.A. Factor, B.S.Molho, P.J.Feustel)

[12] Movement Disorders [2003] 18 (5) : 510-514 (H.H.Fernandez, M. E.Trieschmann, M.A. Burke, C.Jacques, J.H.Friedman)

[13] No To Shinkei [2002] 54 (6) : 489-492 (J.Kohmoto, T.Kihira, H. Miwa, T.Kondo)

[14] Revista de Neurología [2003] 36 (5) : 401-404 (S.Giménez-Roldán, E.Navarro, D.Mateo)

[15] Movement Disorders [2007] 22 (3) : 313-318 (J.M.Rabey, T. Prokhorov, A.Miniovitz, E.Dobronevsky, C.Klein)

[16] Movement Disorders [2005] 20 (8) : 958-963 (W.G.Ondo, R. Tintner, K.D.Voung, D.Lai, G.Ringholz)

[17] Journal of Geriatric Psychiatry and Neurology [2016] 29 (4) : 227 -236 (P.Desmarais, F.Massoud, J.Filion, Q.D.Nguyen, P.Bajsarowicz)

[18] The American Journal of Geriatric Pharmacotherapy [2010] 8 (4) : 316-330 (M.L.Eng, T.E.Welty)

[19] Neurology [2007] 68 (17) : 1356-1363 (R.Kurlan, J.Cummings, R.Raman, L.Thal)

[20] Clinical Neuropharmacology [2006] 29 (6) : 331-337 (D.Merims, M.Balas, C.Peretz, H.Shabtai, N.Giladi)

[21] Neurological Sciences [2002] 23 (Supplement 2) : S89-S90 (L. Morgante, A.Epifanio, E.Spina, A.E.Di Rosa, M.Zappia, G. Basile, P. La Spina, A.Quattrone)

[22] Clinical Neuropharmacology [2004] 27 (4) : 153-156 (L. Morgante, A.Epifanio, E.Spina, M.Zappia, A.E.Di Rosa, R.Marconi, G. Basile, G.Di Raimondo, P.La Spina, A.Quattrone)

[23] Neuropsychiatric Disease and Treatment [2007] 3 (2) : 219-235 (M.Riedel, N.Müller, M.Strassnig, I.Spellmann, E.Severus, H-J. Möller)

[24] Journal of Clinical Pharmacy and Therapeutics [2016] 41 (1) : 7-18 (N.El-Saifi, W.Moyle, C.Jones, H.Tuffaha)

CHAPTER 47

SURGICAL TREATMENTS OF PARKINSON'S DISEASE

BIOCHEMISTRY

Surgical methods of treating Parkinson's Disease aim to have effect by different means. These include : stimulating the dopaminergic neurons, inserting new dopamine containing cells, delivering genes for the formation of dopamine, repairing damaged dopaminergic neurons, destroying certain parts of the brain by surgery or radiation, and increasing the levels of GABA.

SURGICAL TREATMENTS

Deep Brain Stimulation is the most effective surgical treatment for Parkinson's Disease [PAGE 734]. Other forms of treating Parkinson's Disease involving surgery are Acupucture [PAGE 744], Extradural cortical stimulation (ECS) [PAGE 745], GDNF [PAGE 746], Gene Therapy [PAGE 747], Magnetic brain stimulation [PAGE 748], Neurturin [PAGE 749], NTCELL [PAGE 749], Pallidotomy [PAGE 750], ProSavin [PAGE 755], Retinal Cell Therapy [PAGE 756], Spinal cord stimulation [PAGE 757], Stem cell therapy [PAGE 758], and Stereotactic radio surgery (SRS) [PAGE 760], Subthalamotomy [PAGE 760], and Thalamotomy [PAGE 762].

DEEP BRAIN STIMULATION (DBS)

Method : Deep Brain Stimulation (DBS) involves the use of electrodes that are implanted into the brain and connected to a small electrical device called a pulse generator that can be externally programmed. DBS uses a surgically implanted, battery-operated medical device called a neurostimulator, which is similar to a heart pacemaker and approximately the size of a stopwatch. It delivers electrical stimulation to targeted areas in the brain that control movement, blocking the abnormal nerve signals that cause tremor and Parkinson's Disease symptoms. The two main targets in the brain are the subthalamic nucleus (STN) and the globus pallidus internus (GPi). The most common method is bilateral stimulation of the subthalamic nucleus (STN). Before the procedure, a neurosurgeon uses magnetic resonance imaging (MRI) or computed tomography (CT) scanning to identify and locate the exact target within the brain where electrical nerve signals generate the Parkinson's Disease symptoms. Some surgeons may use microelectrode recording, which involves a small wire that monitors the activity of nerve cells in the target area, to more specifically identify the precise brain target that will be stimulated. Generally, these targets are the thalamus, subthalamic nucleus, and globus pallidus. The DBS system consists of three components : the lead, the extension, and the neurostimulator. The lead (also called an electrode), which is a thin, insulated wire, is inserted through a small opening in the skull and implanted in the brain. The tip of the electrode is positioned within the targeted brain area. The extension is an insulated wire that is passed under the skin of the head, neck, and shoulder, connecting the lead to the neurostimulator. The neurostimulator ("battery pack") is the third component and is usually implanted under the skin near the collarbone. In some cases it may be implanted lower in the chest or under the skin over the abdomen. Once the system is in place, electrical impulses are sent from the neurostimulator up along the extension wire and the lead and into the brain. These impulses interfere with and block the electrical signals that cause Parkinson's Disease symptoms [1-4]. The effects of Deep Brain Stimulation depend strongly on the stimulation frequency : high frequencies (>90 Hz) improve motor symptoms, while low frequencies (<50 Hz) are ineffective or exacerbate symptoms [5].

Method (comparison) : STN DBS is more effective than GPi DBS in improving Unified Parkinson's Disease Rating Scale motor scores [6], bradykinesia [6], dyskinesia [6], attention, working memory and processing speed, phonemic fluency, learning and memory, and cognition [7], and is far more effective in reducing L-dopa dosage [6]. There were no significant differences in neuropsychological outcome between GPi DBS and STN DBS [8]. Tremor dominant patients had greater mean overall motor improvement after GPi DBS, compared to STN DBS [9].

Efficacy (general symptoms) : Decreased efficacy started to occur after one year [10], and deteriorated further after five years [11]. However, prior to then, Deep Brain Stimulation improves Parkinson's Disease symptom scores generally. DBS improves the PDQ39 [12-15]. It improves the UPDRS score [11, 13, 16-21] but sometimes only for parts II-IV [18]. The improvements in the UPDRS score were 25% to 70% [14, 23-29]. The improvements changed little over the first seven years [16], but reduced after seven years. DBS enabled a reduction in the L-dopa dosage by 15% to 63% [14, 21, 23, 24, 27, 28, 30, 31, 32]. Reductions in L-dopa dosage were still as much as 52% or more after five years [29]. Some people were even able to cease all dopaminergic drugs [32]. However, in one study, Deep Brain Stimulation made no difference to Parkinson's Disease symptoms generally beyond the use of Parkinson's Disease drugs [29].

Efficacy (specific symptoms) : Deep Brain Stimulation improved the following symptoms : rigidity [33-36] by 58% to 95% [30, 37], bradykinesia [23, 34, 36] by 23% to 37% [23, 30], tremor [23, 34, 36, 38, 39, 40] by 74% to 93% [23, 30, 37], akinesia [28, 35], motor function by 78% initially and by 66% after 5 years [41], motor symptoms [42] by 40% and 44% [31], by 35% after 5 years and even after 11 years [29, 43], mobility [19], pain (substantial improvement) [44, 45], axial signs [36] by 42% [30], dyskinesia [18, 23, 25, 39, 46] by 61% to 84% [21, 24, 26, 28, 43], dystonia [37] by 39% [39], balance [19], speech by 13% [30], gait initiation [47] by 44% [30], psychomotor speed [48], non-motor symptoms [49, 50], depression [19], bladder dysfunction [36, 51], motor fluctuations [23] by 65% after 11 years [43], facial expression [36], perception of most facial expressions [52], Quality of Life [21, 23, 25] by 25% to 58% [29, 39] but declined afterwards [29, 43], off time reduced by 68% to 74% [14, 21, 46]. Deep Brain Stimulation did not prevent further deterioration in speech, walking, and postural instability, including falling and freezing [23].

Adverse effects (symptoms) : After DBS there can be a significant worsening of mood (25%) [53], including depression [36, 54, 55], in as many as 18% of patients [26], and anxiety in as many as 12% of patients [55]. However, as many as 20% of patients improved their mood and 23% reduced anxiety [55]. Adverse effects that occurred in a smaller proportion of patients in different studies were : cognitive decline [54] in as many as 7% of patients [26], speech impairment [54, 56], hypophonia [36], worsening of verbal fluency [57], fatigue [58, 59], seizures (1% to 3%) [60], weight gain [61], dysarthria [59], dyskinesia [36, 59], confusion [36], gait problems [54, 59], disequilibrium [59], falls [59], increased impulsivity [62], psychosis more rarely [55], and increased likelihood of carpal tunnel syndrome [63].

Adverse effects (surgical) : Adverse effects that occurred due to the surgery itself occurred in 20% to 54% of patients [11, 64], with very serious adverse effects occurring in 1% to 2% [65]. The two main targets for DBS, the subthalamic nucleus (STN) and the globus pallidus interus (GPi), did not differ in the extent of their adverse effects [66]. Most patients do not sustain any long term complications from the surgery [67]. The adverse effects that occurred due to the surgery were : hardware complications (7% to 25%) [65, 39], skin complications (24%) [68], infection (2% to 9%) [26, 39, 59, 60, 65, 69, 70], intracranial hemorrhage (1% to 4%) [21, 37, 59, 60, 70, 71], electrode migration (2%) [69], electrode fracture [26], in 2% of cases [69], decreased consciousness (2%) [71], incorrect lead placement [26, 71], in 2% of patients [72], hardware discomfort (1%) [71], component fracture (1%) [71], symptomatic ICH (1%) [71], pulmonary embolism (0.5% to 1%) [70], severe intraoperativevasovagal response (0.8%) [71], component malfunction (0.5%) [71], ischemic infarction (0.4%) [71], hypotension (0.3%) [71], seizures (0.3%) [71], intracerebral hematoma [26], intracranial abscess [60], paraesthesias [59], oedema [59, 72], persistent neurological sequelae [73], venous air embolism [74], and on rare occasions, asphyxia [75]. Chronic DBS does not cause damage to adjacent brain tissue [76].

[1] Deep Brain Stimulation Management [2015] (William J.Marks Jr)

[2] DBS A Patient Guide to Deep Brain Stimulation [2013] (Sierra M. Farris, Monique L.Giroux)

[3] Deep Brain Stimulation: A New Life for People with Parkinson's, Dystonia, and Essential Tremor [2011] (Kelvin L.Chou, Susan Grube)

[4] Life With A Battery-Operated Brain: A Patient's Guide to Deep Brain Stimulation Surgery for Parkinson's Disease [2012] (Jackie Hunt Christensen, Alex Christensen)

[5] Journal of Neuroscience [2012] 32 (45) : 15657-15668 (G.C. McConnell, R.G.So, J.D.Hilliard, P.Lopomo, W.M.Grill)

[6] Archives of Neurology [2005] 62 (4) : 554-560 (V.C.Anderson, K.J.Burchiel, P.Hogarth, J.Favre, J.P.Hammerstad)

[7] World Neurosurgery [2016] Jun 10 [Epub ahead of print] (M. Mathkour, J.Garces, T.Scullen, J.Hanna, E.Valle-Giler, L.Kahn, T. Arrington, D.Houghton, G.Lea, E.Biro, C.J.Bui, O.A.Sulaiman, et al)

[8] Neurology [2015] 84 (13) : 1355-1361 (V.J.Odekerken, J.A.Boel, G.J.Geurtsen, B.A.Schmand, I.P.Dekker, R.J.de Haan, P.R.Schuurman, R.M.de Bie)

[9] Annals of Neurology [2015] 77 (4) : 710-719 (M.Katz, M.S. Luciano, K.Carlson, P.Luo, W.J. Jr.Marks, P.S.Larson, P.A.Starr, K.A. Follett, F.M.Weaver, M.B.Stern, D.J.Reda, J.L.Ostrem)

[10] Journal of Neurosurgery [1998] 89 (5) : 713-718 (J.Ghika, J.G. Villemure, H.Fankhauser, J.Favre, G.Assal, F.Ghika-Schmid)

[11] Journal of the Formosan Medical Association [2013] Oct 5 [Epub ahead of print] (J.L.Jiang, S.Y.Chen, T.C.Hsieh, C.W.Lee, S.H.Lin, S.T.Tsai)

[12] Journal of Parkinson's Disease [2015] 5 (2) : 361-368 (G.Deli, Z.Aschermann, P.Ács, E.Bosnyák, J.Janszky, B.Faludi, A.Makkos, M. Kovács, S.Komoly, I.Balás, T.Dóczi, N.Kovács)

[13] Turkish Neurosurgery [2013] 23 (3) : 379-384 (T.Tykocki, K. Szalecki, H.Koziara, P.Nauman, T.Mandat)

[14] World Neurosurgery [2016] Jun 10 [Epub ahead of print] (D.T. Chan, C.X.Zhu, C.K.Lau, T.L.Poon, F.C.Cheung, M.Lee, B.Taw, K.N. Hung, P.Choi, M.AuYeung, G.Chan, Y.F.Cheung, et al)

[15] Lancet Neurology [2010] 9 (6) : 581-591 (A.Williams, S.Gill, T. Varma, C.Jenkinson, N.Quinn, R.Mitchell, R.Scott, N.Ives, C.Rick, J.Daniels, S.Patel, K.Wheatley)

[16] Journal of Neurosurgery [2012] 116 (1) : 107-113 (A.M.Harries, J.Kausar, S.A.Roberts, A.P.Mocroft, J.A.Hodson, H.S.Pall, R.D. Mitchell)

[17] Movement Disorders [2009] 24 (11) : 1688-1692 (J.M.Hausdorff, L.Gruendlinger, L.Scollins, S.O'Herron, D.Tarsy)

[18] Parkinsonism & Related Disorders [2008] 14 (2) : 114-119 (C. Wider, C.Pollo, J.Bloch, P.R.Burkhard, F.J.Vingerhoets)

[19] Turkish Neurosurgery [2011] 21 (2) : 140-146 (F.Altug, F.Acar, G.Acar, U.Cavlak)

[20] Neurological Sciences [2001] 22 (1) : 87-88 (A.E.Scotto di Luzio, F.Ammannati, P.Marini, S.Sorbi, P.Mennonna)

[21] Movement Disorders [2006] 21 (Supplement 14) : S290-S304 (G.Kleiner-Fisman, J.Herzog, D.N.Fisman, F.Tamma, K.E.Lyons, R. Pahwa, A.E.Lang, G.Deuschl)

[22] Journal of the Formosan Medical Association (Taiwan yi zhi) [2015] 114 (9) : 835-841 (J.L.Jiang, S.Y.Chen, T.C.Hsieh, C.W.Lee, S.H.Lin, S.T.Tsai)

[23] Archives of Neurology [2011] 68 (12) : 1550-1556 (A.Castrioto, A.M.Lozano, Yu-Yan Poon, A.E.Lang, M.Fallis, E.Moro)

[24] Acta Neurochirurgica [2006] 148 (4) : 389-394 (T.Erola, E.R. Heikkinen, T.Haapaniemi, J.Tuominen, A.Juolasmaa, V.V.Myllylä)

[25] Journal of Neurology, Neurosurgery and Psychiatry [2011] 82 (4) : 358-363 (T.Foltynie, L.Zrinzo, I.Martinez-Torres, E.Tripoliti, E. Petersen, E.Holl, I.Aviles-Olmos, M.Jahanshahi, M.Hariz, P.Limousin)

[26] Neurosurgery [2007] 61 (2) : 297-305 (M.Tir, D.Devos, S.Blond, G.Touzet, N.Reyns, A.Duhamel, O.Cottencin, K.Dujardin, F.Cassim, A.Destée, L.Defebvre, P.Krystkowiak)

[27] European Neurology [2006] 56 (2) : 127-132 (S.J.Chung, S.R. Jeon, S.R.Kim, Y.H.Sung, M.C.Lee)

[28] Ideggyogyaszati Szemle [2013] 66 (3-4) : 115-120 (G.Tamás, A.Takáts, P.Radics, I.Rózsa, E.Csibri, G.Rudas, P.Golopencza, L.Entz, D.Fabó, L.Eross)

[29] Chinese Medical Journal [2015] 128 (18) : 2433-2438 (L.L.Jiang, J.L.Liu, X.L.Fu, W.B.Xian, J.Gu, Y.M.Liu, J.Ye, J.Chen, H.Qian, S.H.Xu, Z.Pei, L.Chen)

[30] Neurosurgery [2007] 61 (3 Supplement) : 119-129 (S.D.Tabbal, F. J.Revilla, J.W.Mink, P.Schneider-Gibson, A.R.Wernle, G.A.de Erausquin, J.S.Perlmutter, K.M.Rich, J.L.Dowling)

[31] Journal of Neurological Sciences [2004] 219 (1-2) : 119-124 (M.Krause, W.Fogel, P.Mayer, M.Kloss, V.Tronnier)

[32] Parkinsonism & Related Disorders [2008] 14 (8) : 608-612 (M.Zibetti, M.Pesare, A.Cinquepalmi, M.Rosso, B.Bergamasco, A.Ducati, M.Lanotte, L.Lopiano)

[33] IEEE Transactions on Neural Systems and Rehabilitation Engineering [2007] 15 (2) : 173-181 (M.B.Shapiro, D.E.Vaillancourt, M.M.Sturman, L.V.Metman, R.A.Bakay, D.M.Corcos)

[34] Zhonghua Yi Xue Za Zhi [2007] 87 (47) : 3321-3324 (S.Tian, P. Zhuang, Y.Li)

[35] Stereotactic and Functional Neurosurgery [2001] 77 (1-4) : 61-67 (T.Yokoyama, K.Sugiyama, S.Nishizawa, N.Yokota, S.Ohta, S. Akamine, H.Namba)

[36] Acta Neurochirurgica (Supplement) [2006] 99 : 43-47 (J.G.Zhang, K.Zhang, Y.Ma, W.H.Hu, A.C.Yang, J.S.Chu, S.T.Wu, M. Ge, Y. Zhang, Z.C.Wang)

[37] Casopis Lekaru Ceskych [2011] 150 (4-5) : 223-228 (D.Urgosík, R.Jech, E.Ruzicka, F.Ruzicka, R.Liscák, V.Vladyka)

[38] Neurosurgery [2010] 67 (3) : 626-632 (H.J.Kim, B.S.Jeon, S.H. Paek, J.Y.Lee, H.J.Kim, C.K.Kim, D.G.Kim)

[39] Deutsches Ärzteblatt International [2015] 112 (31-32) : 519-526 (V.A.Coenen, F.Amtage, J.Volkmann, T.E.Schläpfer)

[40] Movement Disorders [2007] 22 (8) : 1157-1163 (M.M.Sturman, D.E.Vaillancourt, L.V.Metman, D.K.Sierens, R.A.Bakay, D.M.Corcos)

[41] Revista de Neurología [2014] 58 (10) : 433-439 (A.Monteiro, C. Andrade, M.J.Rosas, P.Linhares, J.Massano, R.Vaz, C.Garrett)

[42] Neurological Sciences [2002] 23 (Supplement 2) : S111-S112 (A. Tavella, B.Bergamasco, E.Bosticco, M.Lanotte, P.Perozzo, M.Rizzone, E.Torre, L.Lopiano)

[43] Parkinsonism & Related Disorders [2014] 20 (4) : 376-381 (M.G. Rizzone, A. Fasano, A.Daniele, M.Zibetti, A.Merola, L.Rizzi, C.Piano, C.Piccininni, L.M.Romito, L. Lopiano, A.Albanese)

[44] Parkinsonism & Related Disorders [2014] 20 (6) : 662-664 (J. Pellaprat, F.Ory-Magne, C.Canivet, M.Simonetta-Moreau, J.A. Lotterie, F.Radji, C.Arbus, A.Gerdelat, P.Chaynes, C.Brefel-Courbon)

[45] Neurology [2014] 83 (16) : 1403-1409 (R.G.Cury, R.Galhardoni, E.T.Fonoff, M.G.Dos Santos Ghilardi, F.Fonoff, D.Arnaut, M.L. Myczkowski, M.A.Marcolin, E.Bor-Seng-Shu, E.R.Barbosa, et al)

[46] Neurology [2000] 55 (12 Supplement 6) : S45-S51 (M.C. Rodriguez-Oroz, A.Gorospe, J.Guridi, E.Ramos, G.Linazasoro, M. Rodriguez-Palmero, J.A.Obeso)

[47] Gait & Posture [2006] 23 (4) : 492-498 (W.Liu, K.McIntire, S.H.Kim, J.Zhang, S.Dascalos, K.E.Lyons, R.Pahwa)

[48] Neurology [2000] 55 (3) : 411-418 (B.Pillon, C.Ardouin, P. Damier, P.Krack, J.L.Houeto, H.Klinger, A.M.Bonnet, P.Pollak, A.L. Benabid, Y.Agid)

[49] Brain Stimulation [2015] Aug 19 [Epub ahead of print] (H.S. Dafsari, P.Reddy, C.Herchenbach, S.Wawro, J.N.Petry- Schmelzer, V.Visser-Vandewalle, A.Rizos, M.Silverdale, K.Ashkan, et al)

[50] Parkinsonism & Related Disorders [2013] 19 (5) : 543-547 (S.Ortega-Cubero, P.Clavero, C.Irurzun, R.Gonzalez-Redondo, J. Guridi, J.A.Obeso, M.C.Rodriguez-Oroz)

[51] Brain [2006] 129 (Part 12) : 3366-3375 (J.Herzog, P.H.Weiss, A. Assmus, B.Wefer, C.Seif, P.M.Braun, H.Herzog, J.Volkmann, G. Deuschl, G.R.Fink)

[52] Journal of Neurology, Neurosurgery and Psychiatry [2004] 75 (4) : 648-650 (U.Schroeder, A.Kuehler, A.Hennenlotter, B.Haslinger, V.M. Tronnier, M.Krause, R.Pfister, R.Sprengelmeyer, et al)

[53] Neurology [2002] 59 (9) : 1427-1429 (A.Berney, F.Vingerhoets, A.Perrin, P.Guex, J.G.Villemure, P.R.Burkhard, C.Benkelfat, J.Ghika)

[54] Brain [2005] 128 (Part 10) : 2240-2249 (M.C.Rodriguez-Oroz, J. A.Obeso, A.E.Lang, J.L.Houeto, P.Pollak, S.Rehncrona, J. Kulisevsky, A.Albanese, J.Volkmann, M.I.Hariz, N.P.Quinn, J.D.Speel)

[55] European Neurology [2006] 55 (3) : 136-144 (L.Castelli, P. Perozzo, M.Zibetti, B.Crivelli, U.Morabito, M.Lanotte, F.Cossa, B. Bergamasco, L.Lopiano)

[56] Journal of Neurology, Neurosurgery and Psychiatry [2008] 79 (5) : 522-529 (K.Klostermann, F.Ehlen, J.Vesper, K.Nubel, M.Gross, F. Marzinzik, G.Curio, T.Sappok)

[57] Movement Disorders [2009] 24 (11) : 1621-1628 (R.Zangaglia, C.Pacchetti, C.Pasotti, F.Mancini, D.Servello, E.Sinforiani, S.Cristina, M.Sassi, G.Nappi)

[58] Acta Neurologica Scandinavica [2015] 132 (4) : 251-258 (B. Lilleeng, M.Gjerstad, R.Baardsen, I.Dalen, J.P.Larsen)

[59] Lancet Neurology [2012] 11 (2) : 140-149 (M.S.Okun, B.W.Gallo, G.Mandybur, J.Jagid, K.D.Foote, F.J.Revilla, R.Alterman, J.Jankovic, R.Simpson, F.Junn, L.Verhagen, J.E.Arle, B.Ford, R.R.Goodman)

[60] Neurocirugia [2013] 24 (1) : 33-36 (E.Brandão, M.J.Rosas, P. Abreu, P.Linhares, R.Vaz)

[61] Journal of Neurology [2010] 257 (8) : 1293-1297 (R.E.Strowd, M. S.Cartwright, L.V.Passmore, T.L.Ellis, S.B.Tatter, M.S.Siddiqui)

[62] Parkinson's Disease [2015] Jan 29 [Epub ahead of print] (U. Pham, A.K.Solbakk, I.M.Skogseid, M.Toft, A.H.Pripp, A.E. Konglund, S.Andersson, I.R.Haraldsen, D.Aarsland, E.Dietrichs, U.F.Malt)

[63] Journal of Neurology [2016] Sep 13 [Epub ahead of print] (M. Loizon, C.Laurencin, C.Vial, T.Danaila, S.Thobois)

[64] New England Journal of Medicine [2013] 368 (7) : 610-622 (W.M. Schuepbach, J.Rau, K.Knudsen, J.Volkmann, P.Krack, L.Timmermann, T.D.Hälbig, H.Hesekamp, S.M.Navarro, et al)

[65] Current Neurology and Neuroscience Reports [2004] 4 (4) : 290-295 (K.E.Lyons, R.Pahwa)

[66] Neurology [2016] 86 (8) : 755-761 (V.J.Odekerken, J.A.Boel, B.A.Schmand, R.J.de Haan, M.Figee, P.van den Munckhof, P.R. Schuurman, R.M.de Bie)

[67] Journal of Neurology, Neurosurgery and Psychiatry [2012] 83 (2) : 164-170 (E.Kahn, P.F.D'Haese, B.Dawant, L.Allen, C.Kao, P.D. Charles, P,Konrad)

[68] Acta Neurochirurgica [2010] 152 (2) : 195-200 (F.Sixel-Döring, C.Trenkwalder, C.Kappus, D.Hellwig)

[69] Stereotactic and Functional Neurosurgery [2012] 90 (5) : 300-306 (J.F.Baizabal Carvallo, G.Mostile, M.Almaguer, A.Davidson, R. Simpson, J.Jankovic)

[70] Neuromodulation [2015] Nov 16 [Epub ahead of print] (F.W. Petraglia, S.H.Farber, J.L.Han, T.Verla, J.Gallis, Y.Lokhnygina, B. Parente, P.Hickey, D.A.Turner, S.P.Lad)

[71] Journal of Neurosurgery [2014] 120 (1) : 132-139 (A.J.Fenoy, R.K.Simpson)

[72] Parkinsonism & Related Disorders [2016] 32 : 108-115 (C.M.de Cuba, A.Albanese, A.Antonini, G.Cossu, G.Deuschl, R.Eleopra, A. Galati, C.F.Hoffmann, K.Knudsen, A.Landi, M.M.Lanotte, et al)

[73] Stereotactic and Functional Neurosurgery [2001] 77 (1-4) : 73-78 (A.Beric, P.J.Kelly, A.Rezai, D.Sterio, A.Mogilner, M.Zonenshayn, B. Kopell)

[74] Stereotactic and Functional Neurosurgery [2009] 87 (1) : 25-30 (A.K.Hooper, M.S.Okun, K.D.Foote, I.U.Haq, H.H.Fernandez, D. Hegland, S.A.Robicsek)

[75] BMC Neurology [2016] 16 (1) : 216 (K.L.von Eckardstein, F. Sixel-Döring, S.Kazmaier, C.Trenkwalder, J.M.Hoover, V.Rohde)

[76] Annals of Neurology [2000] 48 (3) : 372-376 (C.Haberler, F. Alesch, P.R.Mazal, P.Pilz, K.Jellinger, M.M.Pinter, J.A.Hainfellner, H. Budka)

ACUPUNCTURE

Method : Acupuncture is a technique of inserting and manipulating needles into specific points on the body for therapeutic purposes. Acupuncture needles are typically made of stainless steel, making them flexible and preventing them from rusting or breaking [1].

Efficacy : In an assessment of the medical literature for clinical trials of acupuncture for the treatment of Parkinson's Disease, three clinical trials showed no effect. Six studies compared the use of acupuncture and conventional drugs against the use of only drugs. Only two out of six of these studies suggested a positive effect of scalp acupuncture. Two further clinical trials that tested acupuncture versus no treatment suggested beneficial effects of acupuncture. However, the results of the latter two types of trial failed to adequately control for non-specific effects. Consequently, there is a lack of evidence for the effectiveness of acupuncture in treating Parkinson's Disease [2]. The effect of scalp acupuncture on Parkinson's Disease was not conclusive [3]. In another assessment of the medical literature eleven suitable studies were identified. Two randomised clinical trials failed to show any benefit. The other study did not show beneficial effects of needle acupuncture. Three randomised clinical trials that assessed effects of acupuncture in addition to conventional drugs reported beneficial effects of acupuncture. However, there was no control acupuncture group in those studies. Two uncontrolled studies showed significant positive effects while two other uncontrolled clinical trials failed. Safety and tolerability were reported only in five clinical trials. No studies evaluated the long lasting effects of acupuncture following cessation of the treatment [4]. Electroacupuncture improved some of the symptoms of Parkinson's Disease [5, 6, 7]. A combination of acupuncture and bee venom acupuncture (BVA) showed significant improvements in gait speed, PDQL score, and Parkinson's Disease symptom scores [8].

Adverse effects : There were no adverse effects when acupuncture was used in treating people with Parkinson's Disease [9, 10].

[1] A Manual of Acupuncture [2007] (Peter Deadman, Mazin Al-Khafaji, Kevin Baker)

[2] Movement Disorders [2008] 23 (11) : 1505-1515 (M.S.Lee, B.C. Shin, J.C.Kong, E.Ernst)

[3] Chinese Journal of Integrative Medicine [2013] 19 (4) : 297-306 (H.S.Lee, H.L.Park, S.J.Lee, B.C.Shin, J.Y.Choi, M.S.Lee)

[4] Journal of Neurological Science [2014] Apr 24 [Epub ahead of print] (H.J.Kim, B.S.Jeon)

[5] Gerontology [2015] 61 (1) : 3-14 (N.Toosizadeh, H.Lei, M. Schwenk, S.J.Sherman, E.Sternberg, J.Mohler, B.Najafi)

[6] Acupuncture Medicine [2013] 31 (2) : 235-238 (D.V.Arankalle, P.M.Nair)

[7] Nan Fang Yi Ke Da Xue Xue Bao [2006] 26 (1) : 114-116 (X.M. Jiang, Y.Huang, Y.Zhuo, Y.P.Gao)

[8] Journal of Alternative and Complementary Medicine [2015] 21 (10) : 598-603 (K.H.Doo, J.H.Lee, S.Y.Cho, W.S.Jung, S.K.Moon, J.M. Park, C.N.Ko, H.Kim, H.J.Park, S.U.Park)

[9] Journal of Alternative and Complementary Medicine [2006] 12 (4) : 395-399 (M.L.Eng, K.E.Lyons, M.S.Greene, R.Pahwa)

[10] Movement Disorders [2002] 17 (4) : 799-802 (L.M.Shulman, X. Wen, W.J.Weiner, D.Bateman, A.Minagar, R.Duncan, J.Konefal)

Extradural cortical stimulation (ECS)

Method : Extradural cortical stimulation (ECS) is a surgical means of neuromodulation that has been used in Parkinson's Disease. Motor cortex stimulation is offered by positioning a stimulating plate extradurally on the primary motor cortex. With the aid of functional MRI and somato-sensory evoked potentials monitoring, the motor cortex projection over the scalp was drawn. Finally, under local anesthesia a stimulation lead was placed in the epidural space overlying the central sulcus [1].

Efficacy : The effect of Extradural cortical stimulation (ECS) on Parkinson's Disease was found to be very mild [2].

Adverse effects : No surgical complications or adverse effects occurred [3].

[1] Acta Neurochirurgica (Supplement) [2007] 97 (2) : 223-232 (S. Canavero, V.Bonicalzi)

[2] Clinical Neurology and Neurosurgery [2009] 111 (8) : 703-707 (J.C.Gutiérrez, F.J.Seijo, M.A.Alvarez Vega, F.Fernández González, B. Lozano Aragoneses, M.Blázquez)

[3] Neurosurgery [2012] 71 (4) : 815-825 (A.R.Bentivoglio, A.Fasano, C.Piano, F.Soleti, A.Daniele, M.Zinno, C.Piccininni, C.De Simone, D.Policicchio, T.Tufo, M.Meglio, B.Cioni)

GDNF

Method : GDNF (Glial cell-derived neurotrophic factor) is a type of neurotrophic factor, which is a protein that regulates neuronal survival, differentiation, growth and regeneration. GDNF is claimed to represent an alternative for treating dopaminergic neurons in Parkinson's Disease by supporting the survival of dopaminergic neurons. However, it is difficult to administer clinically because it does not pass through the blood-brain barrier. Consequently, GDNF is administered by the intraparenchymal unilateral infusion of GDNF continuously into the posterior putamen in the brain [1, 2, 3].

Efficacy : Continuous GDNF infusion in five patients showed clinical benefit within 3 months of treatment. The clinical improvement was sustained and progressive [1]. A second clinical trial in ten patients also showed a greater than 30% bilateral benefit in both on and off-medication score at 24 weeks [2, 3]. A clinical trial was conducted to confirm the previous clinical trial results. In those people undergoing chronic intracerebral GDNF infusion there was a lack of evidence of cerebellar dysfunction on clinical examination and no imaging evidence of cerebellar injury [4]. However, in randomised controlled clinical trials, people with Parkinson's Disease receiving GDNF infusion did not significantly improve their Parkinson's Disease symptoms [5, 6].

Adverse effects : Continuous GDNF infusion in five patients showed good tolerance, and few side effects [1].

[1] Annals of Neurology [2005] 57 (2) : 298-302 (N.K.Patel, M. Bunnage, P.Plaha, C.N.Svendsen, P.Heywood, S.S.Gill)

[2] Acta Neurochirurgica Supplement [2007] 97 (Part 2) : 135-154 (N. K.Patel, S.S.Gill)

[3] Journal of Neurosurgery [2007] 106 (4) : 614-620 (J.T.Slevin, D.M. Gash, C.D.Smith, G.A.Gerhardt, R.Kryscio, H.Chebrolu, A.Walton, R. Wagner, A.B.Young)

[4] Experimental Neurology [2006] 198 (2) : 450-456 (H.Chebrolu, J.T. Slevin, D.A.Gash, G.A.Gerhardt, B.Young, C.A.Given, C.D.Smith)

[5] Annals of Neurology [2006] 59 (3) : 459-466 (A.E.Lang, S.Gill, N. K.Patel, A.Lozano, J.G.Nutt, R.Penn, D.J.Brooks, G.Hotton, E.Moro, P.Heywood, M.A.Brodsky, K.Burchiel, P.Kelly, A.Dalvi, et al)

[6] Neurology [2003] 60 (1) : 69-73 (J.G.Nutt, K.J.Burchiel, C.L. Comella, J.Jankovic, A.E.Lang, E.R.Laws Jr, A.M.Lozano, R.D.Penn, R.K.Simpson Jr, M.Stacy, G.F.Wooten)

Gene therapy

Method : A surgical method of increasing the levels of GABA, which is a substance involved in muscular movement, has resulted in claims of the method being beneficial for Parkinson's Disease. AAV2-GAD, which is called NLX-P101, was delivered surgically in to the subthalamic nucleus of the brains of people with Parkinson's Disease. GAD is the enzyme that biosynthesizes GABA naturally in the brain [1].

Efficacy : There was a 23% reduction in Parkinson's Disease symptoms in the third of patients that were treated. However, even those that were not treated at all reduced their symptoms by nearly 13%. So the actual benefit of the surgical method used was only a 10% reduction in symptoms in those patients that were treated. A phase II clinical trial of

NLX-P101 is being carried out in order to try to establish the clinical efficacy of the method [1]. Improvements in symptoms persisted after 12 months [2].

Adverse effects : Of the adverse effects experienced, the most common were headache and nausea [1].

[1] Lancet Neurology [2011] 10 (4) : 309-319 (P.A.LeWitt, A.R. Rezai, M.A.Leehey, S.G.Ojemann, A.W.Flaherty, E.N.Eskandar, S.K. Kostyk, K.Thomas, A.Sarkar, M.S.Siddiqui, S.B. Tatter, et al)

[2] JCI Insight [2017] 2 (7) : e90133 (M.Niethammer, C.C.Tang, P.A. LeWitt, A.R.Rezai, M.A.Leehey, S.G.Ojemann, A.W.Flaherty, E.N. Eskandar, S.K.Kostyk, A.Sarkar, M.S.Siddiqui, S.B.Tatter, et al)

Magnetic brain stimulation

Method : Magnetic brain stimulation is novel wireless method of administering brain stimulation that requires no implants or external connections. By injecting magnetic nanoparticles into the brain, neurons can be manipulated by applying external magnetic fields. These particles are capable of deep penetration of brain tissue and can stimulate nerve cells [1].

Efficacy : Outcome measures included analysis of Unified Parkinson's Disease Rating Scale (UPDRS) scores, duration of "on" periods, and equivalent doses of L-dopa. Three months after surgery, there had been a very significant decrease in the UPDRS (Parkinson's Disease) motor scores [1].

Adverse effects : Bilateral wireless programming STN-DBS was found to be safe [1].

[1] Stereotactic and Functional Neurosurgery [2017] 95 (3) : 174-182 [Epub ahead of print] (D.Li, C.Zhang, J.Gault, W.Wang, J.Liu, M.Shao, Y.Zhao, K.Zeljic, G.Gao, B.Sun)

NEURTURIN

Method : Neurturin, is a naturally occurring neurotrophic factor. Neurturin is a member of the same protein family as GDNF. Neurturin is thought to repair damaged dopaminergic neurons by restoring their function [1]. Neurturin is administered using CERE-120, which is composed of a harmless adeno-associated virus (AAV) vector, which carries the gene for neurturin. CERE-120 is delivered by injection in to the brain [1].

Efficacy : Neurturin has failed to demonstrate any effect in Parkinson's Disease [1, 2, 3].

Adverse effects : Safety data for all subjects suggested the procedures were well tolerated with no serious adverse effects [4], including in the long term [5].

[1] Ceregene - http://www.ceregene.com/press_041913.asp

[2] Neurobiology of Disease [2012] 48 (2) : 153-178 (R.T.Bartus)

[3] Annals of Neurology [2015] 78 (2) : 248-257 (C.Warren Olanow, R.T.Bartus, T.L.Baumann, S.Factor, N.Boulis, M. Stacy, D.A.Turner, W.Marks, P.Larson, P.A.Starr, J.Jankovic, R. Simpson, R.Watts, et al)

[4] Neurology [2013] 80 (18) : 1698-1701 (R.T.Bartus, T.L.Baumann, J.Siffert, C.D.Herzog, R.Alterman, N.Boulis, D.A.Turner, M.Stacy, A. E.Lang, A.M.Lozano, C.W.Olanow)

[5] Human Gene Therapy [2015] Dec 29 [Epub ahead of print] (W.J. Marks Jr, T.L.Baumann, R.T.Bartus)

NTCELL

Method : NTCELL is an alginate coated capsule containing clusters of neonatal porcine choroid plexus cells that are sourced from a herd of designated pathogen-free pigs. Choroid plexus cells are naturally occurring support cells for the brain and secrete cerebrospinal fluid (CSF), which contains a range of factors that support nerve cell functions and protective enzymes that are crucial for nerve growth and healthy functioning. In NTCELL, the porcine choroid plexus cells are coated with LCT's propriety technology IMMUPEL in order to protect them from attack by the immune system [1]. Following the implantation of NTCELL into a damaged site within the brain, NTCELL aims to produce CSF (cerebrospinal fluid) and secreting multiple nerve growth factors while potentially removing waste products such as amyloids and proteins [1].

Efficacy : A small Phase I/IIa clinical trial of people with Parkinson's Disease was carried out in which the UPDRS scores gradually reduced. A Phase IIb study is being carried out in order to confirm the most effective dose of NTCELL [1].

Adverse effects : In a small Phase I/IIa clinical trial of people with Parkinson's Disease no adverse effects related to NTCELL were reported [1].

[1] LCT : http://www.lctglobal.com/products/ntcell

Pallidotomy

Method : In a pallidotomy, the surgeon destroys a tiny part of the globus pallidus by creating a scar. This reduces the brain activity in that area, which may help relieve movement symptoms such as tremor and rigidity. Before surgery, detailed brain scans using MRI are done to identify the precise location for treatment. The person is awake during the surgery but the scalp area where instruments are inserted is numbed with a local anesthetic. The surgeon inserts a hollow probe through a small hole drilled in the skull to the target location. An extremely cold substance, liquid nitrogen, is circulated inside the probe. The probe destroys the targeted brain tissue. The probe is then removed and the wound is closed. Surgery usually requires a two day stay in hospital. Most people recover from surgery within about six weeks [1].

Efficacy : Pallidotomy improved Parkinson's Disease symptoms [2-18], considerably in some cases [19, 20, 21]. However, some people showed little or no improvement [10, 22, 23]. Pallidotomy significantly improved the "off" state [2, 6, 9, 13, 15, 16, 24-36] and in some cases this was long term [24]. Pallidotomy improved dyskinesia [8, 10, 14, 15, 23, 24, 27, 29, 33, 34, 37, 38, 39, 40], considerably in some cases [19, 21, 29, 30, 40, 41], and almost entirely in others [26, 32]. Improvement was maintained for up to a year [40], after which it could be significantly lower [6, 13, 26], or up to two years [42], but in some people the improvement could be long term [25, 43]. Other symptoms that improved were : walking [44, 45, 46], reaching [44], pain [47], akinesia [21, 40], rigidity [15, 22, 29, 40], quality of life [30], tremor [15, 37, 39, 45], repetitive hand movements [48], postural stability [12], bradykinesia [15, 29, 39, 46, 49], postural instability [39, 46], freezing [46], cardinal motor symptoms [30]. In some studies the effects of pallidotomy lasted for only a year [7, 26], or mostly disappeared after 2 or 3 years [37, 42], or 3 or 4 years apart from improvements in tremor and akinesia [50].

Adverse effects : After Pallidotomy, 30% of the patients had adverse effects [51], and 13% to 19% of them had permanent adverse effects [31, 51]. Complications caused were mild and transient [32]. Adverse effects that occurred in a small number of patients were : hemorrhage [8, 15, 51], frequency of stroke [51], speech problems [51], facial paresis [51], contralateral weakness [8], visual field defects [8], drowsiness [52], confusion [52], mental deterioration [52], memory deficit [52], dysphasia [52], dysarthria [33, 40], facial weakness [40].

[1] Pallidotomy for the Treatment of Parkinson's Disease and Movement Disorders [1998] (Joachim K.Krauss, Robert G.Grossman, Joseph Jankovic)

[2] Parkinsonism and Related Disorders [2003] 10 (1) : 35-40 (K. Yamada, S.Goto, Y.Ushio)

[3] Journal of Neurology [2002] 249 (12) : 1671-1677 (F.Valldeoriola, J.Martínez Rodríguez, E.Tolosa, J.Rumià, M.Alegret, M.Pilleri, E. Ferrer)

[4] Movement Disorders [2002] 17 (3) : 533-538 (R.M.De Bie, P.R. Schuurman, R.A.Esselink, D.A.Bosch, J.D.Speelman)

[5] Zhonghua Wai Ke Za Zhi [2000] 38 (6) : 422-425 (Y.Li, L.Cai, M. Shao, Y.Ding)

[6] Chang Gung Medical Journal [2001] 24 (7) : 409-417 (C.S.Lu, Y.H. Weng, T.Wu, C.H.Tsai, R.S.Chen, J.D.Lee, S.T.Lee)

[7] Journal of Neurology, Neurosurgery, and Psychiatry [2001] 71 (3) : 375-382 (R.M.de Bie, P.R.Schuurman, D.A.Bosch, R.J.de Haan, B. Schmand, J.D.Speelman)

[8] Journal of Neurosurgery [2001] 94 (1) : 43-49 (A.Alkhani, A.M. Lozano)

[9] Journal of Neurology, Neurosurgery, and Psychiatry [2000] 69 (3) : 326-336 (G.M.Rettig, M.K.York, E.C.Lai, J.Jankovic, J.K.Krauss, R.G. Grossman, H.S.Levin)

[10] Neurosurgery [2000] 46 (2) : 344-353; discussion 353-355 (J. Favre, K.J.Burchiel, J.M.Taha, J.Hammerstad)

[11] Lancet [1999] 354 (9191) : 1665-1669 (R.M.de Bie, R.J.de Haan, P.C.Nijssen, A.W.Rutgers, G.N.Beute, D.A.Bosch, R.Haaxma, B. Schmand, P.R.Schuurman, M.J.Staal, J.D.Speelman)

[12] Archives of Neurology [1999] 56 (11) : 1361-1365 (M.E.Melnick, G.A.Dowling, M.J.Aminoff, N.M.Barbaro)

[13] Journal of Neurology, Neurosurgery, and Psychiatry [1999] 67 (4) : 511-517 (A.Schrag, M.Samuel, E.Caputo, T.Scaravilli, M.Troyer, A. D.Marsden, D.G.Thomas, A.J.Lees, D.J.Brooks, N.P.Quinn)

[14] Journal of Neurosurgery [1998] 89 (2) : 194-199 (J.M.Desaloms, J.K.Krauss, E.C.Lai, J.Jankovic, R.G.Grossman)

[15] Brain : A Journal of Neurology [1998] 121 (Part 1) : 59-75 (M. Samuel, E.Caputo, D.J.Brooks, A.Schrag, T.Scaravilli, N.M. Branston, J.C.Rothwell, C.D.Marsden, D.G.Thomas, A.J.Lees, et al)

[16] Neurology [1997] 49 (4) : 1072-1077 (R.J.Uitti, R.E. Jr.Wharen, M.F.Turk, J.A.Lucas, M.J.Finton, N.R.Graff-Radford, K.B.Boylan, S.J. Goerss, B.A.Kall, C.H.Adler, J.N.Caviness, E.J.Atkinson)

[17] Brain : A Journal of Neurology [1997] 120 (Part 8) : 1301-1313 (M.Samuel, A.O.Ceballos-Baumann, N.Turjanski, H.Boecker, A. Gorospe, G.Linazasoro, A.P.Holmes, M.R.DeLong, J.L.Vitek, et al)

[18] Neurology [1995] 45 (4) : 753-761 (M.Dogali, E.Fazzini, E. Kolodny, D.Eidelberg, D.Sterio, O.Devinsky, A.Beric)

[19] Neurologia i Neurochirurgia Polska [2003] 37 Supplement 5 : 251-262 (M.Sobstyl, M.Zabek, H.Koziara, B.Kadziolka)

[20] Neurologia i Neurochirurgia Polska [2003] 37 Supplement 5 : 221-230 (M.Sobstyl, M.Zabek, H.Koziara, B.Kadziolka)

[21] Acta Neurochirurgica Supplement [1997] 68 : 14-17 (P.R. Schuurman, R.M.de Bie, J.D.Speelman, D.A.Bosch)

[22] Neurosurgery [2001] 48 (2) : 263-271 ; discussion 271-273 (G.Van Horn, S.J.Hassenbusch, G.Zouridakis, N.A.Mullani, M.C. Wilde, A.C.Papanicolaou)

[23] Journal of Neurology, Neurosurgery, and Psychiatry [1997] 62 (2) : 125-132 (F.Johansson, J.Malm, E.Nordh, M.Hariz)

[24] Surgical Neurology [2009] 71 (5) : 551-558 (A.M.Strutt, E.C.Lai, J.Jankovic, F.Atassi, E.M.Soety, H.S.Levin, R.G.Grossman, M.K. York)

[25] Acta Neurochirurgica [2007] 149 (9) : 857-866; discussion 866 (M.K.York, E.C.Lai, J.Jankovic, A.Macias, F.Atassi, H.S.Levin, R.G. Grossman)

[26] European Neurology [2006] 56 (2) : 113-118 (S.J.Chung, S.H. Hong, S.R.Kim, M.C.Lee, S.R.Jeon)

[27] Movement Disorders [2006] 21 (8) : 1252-1254 (W.G.Ondo, Y. Silay, M.Almaguer, J.Jankovic)

[28] Journal of Neurosurgery [2000] 92 (3) : 375-383 (E.N.Eskandar, L.A.Shinobu, J.B.Jr.Penney, G.R.Cosgrove, T.J.Counihan)

[29] New England Journal of Medicine [2000] 342 (23) : 1708-1714 (J.Fine, J.Duff, R.Chen, B.Chir, W.Hutchison, A.M.Lozano, A.E.Lang)

[30] Movement Disorders [2000] 15 (1) : 65-70 (P.Martínez-Martín, F. Valldeoriola, J.L.Molinuevo, F.A.Nobbe, J.Rumià, E.Tolosa)

[31] Movement Disorders [1999] 14 (6) : 951-957 (R.M.de Bie, P.R. Schuurman, P.S.de Haan, D.A.Bosch, J.D.Speelman)

[32] Neurologia [1999] 14 (2) : 53-61 (G.Linazasoro, A.Gorospe, M.C. Rodríguez, J.Guridi, E.Ramos, A.Mozo, J.A.Obeso)

[33] Journal of Neurosurgery [1999] 90 (2) : 197-202 (D.Kondziolka, E.Bonaroti, S.Baser, F.Brandt, Y.S.Kim, L.D.Lunsford)

[34] Neurology [1998] 50 (2) : 434-438 (K.M.Shannon, R.D.Penn, J.S. Kroin, C.H.Adler, K.A.Janko, M.York, S.J.Cox)

[35] Neurology [1998] 50 (1) : 266-270 (W.G.Ondo, J.Jankovic, E.C. Lai, C.Sankhla, M.Khan, L.Ben-Arie, K.Schwartz, R.G.Grossman, J.K. Krauss)

[36] Zentralblatt fur Neurochirurgie [1997] 58 (4) : 153-162 (J.K. Krauss, R.G.Grossman, E.C.Lai, K.Schwartz, J.Jankovic)

[37] Journal of Neurology, Neurosurgery, and Psychiatry [2000] 69 (3) : 337-344 (P.K.Pal, A.Samii, A.Kishore, M.Schulzer, E.Mak, S. Yardley, I.M.Turnbull, D.B.Calne)

[38] Acta Neurochirurgica [2000] 142 (2) : 169-175 (E.J.Herrera, J.C. Viano, M.Cáceres, G.Costello, M.Suárez, J.C.Suárez)

[39] Neurosurgery Clinics of North America [1998] 9 (2) : 325-336 (A.M.Lozano, A.E.Lang)

[40] Axone [1997] 18 (4) : 85-89 (J.Duff, E.Sime)

[41] Journal of the Neurological Sciences [1999] 167 (1) : 62-67 (J. Jankovic, E.Lai, L.Ben-Arie, J.K.Krauss, R.Grossman)

[42] Brain : A Journal of Neurology [1999] 122 (Part 3) : 417-425 (A. Samii, I.M.Turnbull, A.Kishore, M.Schulzer, E.Mak, S.Yardley, D.B. Calne)

[43] Movement Disorders [2010] 25 (10) : 1496-1498 (G.Kleiner-Fisman, A.Lozano, E.Moro, Y.Y.Poon, A.E.Lang)

[44] Movement Disorders [2003] 18 (9) : 1008-1017 (A.J.Bastian, V.E. Kelly, J.S.Perlmutter, J.W.Mink)

[45] Archives of Neurology [2000] 57 (2) : 198-204 (K.L.Siegel, L.V. Metman)

[46] The American Surgeon [1994] 60 (10) : 777-782 (R.P.Iacono, R. R.Lonser, G.Mandybur, J.D.Morenski, S.Yamada, F.Shima)

[47] Journal of Neurosurgery [1999] 91 (2) : 198-201 (C.R.Honey, A.J. Stoessl, J.K.Tsui, M.Schulzer, D.B.Calne)

[48] Movement Disorders [2003] 18 (5) : 515-523 (R.Hayashi, T. Hashimoto, T.Tada, S.Ikeda)

[49] Brain : A Journal of Neurology [1999] 122 (Part 5) : 895-906 (T. E.Kimber, C.S.Tsai, J.Semmler, B.P.Brophy, P.D.Thompson)

[50] Neurology [2000] 54 (5) : 1058-1064 (B.Schmand, R.Mde Bie, M. Koning-Haanstra, J.S.de Smet, J.D.Speelman, A.H.van Zomeren)

[51] Neurology [2002] 58 (7) : 1008-1012 (R.M.de Bie, R.J.de Haan, P.R.Schuurman, R.A.Esselink, D.A.Bosch, J.D.Speelman)

[52] Brain and Cognition [2000] 42 (3) : 313-323 (L.V.Laitinen)

ProSavin

Method : ProSavin (OXB-101) uses LentiVector gene delivery technology to deliver genes for three enzymes they claim to be required for the biosynthesis of dopamine : AADC (aromatic amino acid decarboxylase), TH (tyrosine hydroxylase), and also CH1 (GTP-cyclohydrolase 1). Only two of the three genes are actually needed for dopamine biosynthesis. The product is administered locally to the relevant region of the brain in order to increase the brain's own capacity for the formation of dopamine [1]. Stimulating gene and enzyme levels artificially reduces a person's own formation of those genes and enzymes.

Efficacy : In a Phase I/II clinical trial assessing three dosages 1x, 2x and 5x, the degree of efficacy was quite moderate, with an average 27% improvement after 3 months, peaking at 31% after 6 months, and declining to 23% after 2 years. Efficacy declined when the 5x dosage was used. An enhanced administration procedure, which facilitates higher dosing was used with some patients, but failed to demonstrate any additional benefit [2]. Clinical trials are proceeding with the use of OXB-102, which is potentially far more potent than Prosavin (OXB-101) [1].

Adverse effects : The safety profile was described as being favourable with no serious adverse effects. However, the details of the side effects were not provided [2].

[1] http://www.oxfordbiomedica.co.uk

[2] Lancet [2014] 383 (9923) : 1138-1146 (S.Palfi, J.M.Gurruchaga, G. S.Ralph, H.Lepetit, S.Lavisse, P.C.Buttery, C. Watts, J.Miskin, M. Kelleher, S.Deeley, et al)

Retinal Cell Therapy

Method : Retinal Cell Therapy (Spheramine) consists of an active component of cultured human retinal pigment epithelial (RPE) cells, attached to an excipient part of cross-linked porcine gelatin microcarriers. Spheramine is administered by stereotactic implantation into the striatum of Parkinson's Disease patients. Human RPE cells produce L-dopa. This constitutes the rationale to use Spheramine for the treatment of Parkinson's Disease [1].

Efficacy : A pilot study appeared to show promising results [2]. However, in subsequent clinical trials, Retinal Cell Therapy failed to demonstrate any efficacy [3].

Adverse effects : The adverse effects were the same as when undergoing sham surgery [4].

[1] Neurotherapeutics [2008] 5 (2) : 252-259 (N.P.Stover, R.L.Watts)

[2] Frontiers in Bioscience [2004] 9 : 592-602 (R.A.Bakay, C.D.Raiser, N.P.Stover, T.Subramanian, M.L.Cornfeldt, A.W.Schweikert, R.C. Allen, R.Watts)

[3] http://www.michaeljfox.org

[4] Lancet Neurology [2011] 10 (6) : 509-519 (R.E.Gross, R.L.Watts, R.A.Hauser, R.A.Bakay, H.Reichmann, R.von Kummer, W.G.Ondo, E.Reissig, W.Eisner, H.Steiner-Schulze, H.Siedentop, K.Fichte, et al)

SPINAL CORD STIMULATION

Method : Spinal cord stimulation (SCS) is a minimally invasive method that uses Spinal cord stimulators, which are implantable medical devices [1].

Efficacy : After three months and twelve months, pain was reduced and gait improved. Posture and postural stability improved after three months. Spinal cord stimulation is expected to lead to both amelioration of pain and improvement of motor function in advanced Parkinson's Disease [2]. In another evaluation, 18 out of 24 patients improved their Parkinson's Disease symptoms and 6 patients remained unchanged [3].

Adverse effects : Adverse events are divided into hardware-related complications and biological complications. The commonest hardware related complication is lead migration. Other lead related complications such as failure or fracture, and dislodgement of the electrodes have also been reported. Common biological complications include infection and pain over the implant [4, 5, 6].

[1] Spinal Cord Stimulation: Percutaneous Implantation Techniques [2009] (Paul Kreis, Scott Fishman)

[2] Neurologia Medico-Chirurgica (Tokyo) [2012] 52 (7) : 470-474 (T. Agari, I.Date)

[3] Neurosurgical Review [2016] 39 (1) : 27-35 (E.M.de Andrade, M.G.Ghilardi, R.G.Cury, E.R.Barbosa, R.Fuentes, M.J.Teixeira, E.T. Fonoff)

[4] Pain Medicine [2016] 17 (2) : 325-336 (S.Eldabe, E.Buchser, R.V. Duarte)

[5] Cochrane Database of Systematic Reviews [2015] 6 : CD009389 (L.Peng, S.Min, Z.Zejun, K.Wei, M.I.Bennett)

[6] Journal of Neurosurgery Spine [2006] 5 (3) : 191-203 (K.Kumar, J.R.Wilson, R.S.Taylor, S.Gupta)

STEM CELL THERAPY

Method : Stem cell therapy aims to promote the reparative response of diseased, dysfunctional or injured tissue using stem cells or their derivatives. Researchers grow stem cells in a laboratory. The stem cells are manipulated to specialise into specific types of cells, such as dopaminergic neurons. The specialised cells can then be surgically implanted into the appropriate part of a person's brain [1]. Stem cells derived from human tissue are able to multiply via cell division. Stem cell operations, in which stem cells are placed inside the brain in order to replace lost cells, are claimed to be necessary for Parkinson's Disease because it is assumed that there is massive loss of the dopaminergic neurons (the cells involved in Parkinson's Disease). The theoretical basis of stem cell surgery in Parkinson's Disease is based on a fallacy, because no studies have ever shown that there is a massive loss of the dopaminergic neurons in Parkinson's Disease. It is inevitable that any new cells will eventually function at the same insufficient rate as the existing cells, because their biochemical environment would be identical.

Efficacy : When stem cell surgery underwent formal clinical trials there was found to be little or no effect. [2, 3, 4]. In a later study, a patient who underwent adult neural stem cell transplantation appeared to significantly reduce their symptoms, but after five years they had symptoms that were worse than when they started, and were deteriorating rapidly [5]. In a subsequent study, involving the use of bone marrow derived mesenchymal stem cells, there was also little or no effect [6]. Human retinal pigment epithelial (RPE) cells in the eyes also produce L-dopa. However, their injection in to the brain made no difference [7]. A previous study found that the transplanted retinal cells simply failed to survive [8]. Stem cells have been delivered intranasally in rats as a means of trying to treat Parkinson's Disease. The ease of intranasal administration would open up the possibility of chronic stem cell treatment. The stem cells rapidly migrated to the damaged areas. It is claimed that the method substantially improved motor function in Parkinson's Disease. However, the study was only carried out on rats that did not actually have Parkinson's Disease [9]. Transplanted cells eventually cease to function normally anyway and still develop changes that are characteristic of Parkinson's Disease [10, 11], confirming that Parkinson's Disease is a biochemical state that can affect any cells - those that were already there, and those that are placed there.

Adverse effects : There were no serious adverse effects [2, 6].

[1] Stem Cells : An Insider's Guide [2013] (Paul Knoepfler)

[2] Neurology [2000] 54 (5) : 1042-1050 (J.M.Schumacher, S.A. Ellias, E.P.Palmer, H.S.Kott, J.Dinsmore, P.K.Dempsey, A.J.Fischman, C. Thomas, R.G.Feldman, S.Kassissieh, R.Raineri, C.Manhart, et al)

[3] New England Journal of Medicine [2001] 344 (10) : 710-719 (C.R. Freed, P.E.Greene, R.E.Breeze, W.Y.Tsai, W.DuMouchel, R.Kao, S. Dillon, H.Winfield, S.Culver, J.Q.Trojanowski, D.Eidelberg, S.Fahn)

[4] Annals of Neurology [2003] 54 (3) : 403-414 (C.W.Olanow, C.G. Goetz, J.H.Kordower, A.J.Stoessl, V.Sossi, M.F.Brin, K.M.Shannon, G.M.Nauert, D.P.Perl, J.Godbold, T.B.Freeman)

[5] The Open Stem Cell Journal [2009] 1 : 20-29 (M.F.Lévesque, T. Neuman, M.Rezak)

[6] Translational Research [2010] 155 (2) : 62-70 (N.K. Venkataramana, S.K.Kumar, S.Balaraju, R.C.Radhakrishnan, A.Bansal, A.Dixit, D.K. Rao, M.Das, M.Jan, P.K.Gupta, S.M.Totey)

[7] Lancet Neurology [2011] 10 (6) : 509-519 (R.E.Gross, R.L.Watts, R.A.Hauser, R.A.Bakay, H.Reichmann, R.von Kummer, W.G.Ondo, E.Reissig, W.Eisner, H.Steiner-Schulze, H.Siedentop, K.Fichte, et al)

[8] Neurology [2009] Sep 2 [Epub ahead of print] (E.S.Farag, H.V. Vinters, J.Bronstein)

[9] Rejuvenation Research [2011] 14 (1) : 3-16 (L.Danielyan, R. Schäfer, A.von Ameln-Mayerhofer, F.Bernhard, S.Verleysdonk, M. Buadze, A.Lourhmati, T.Klopfer, F.Schaumann, B.Schmid, et al)

[10] Nature Medicine [2008] 14 (5) : 501-503 (Jia-Yi Li1, E.Englund, J.L.Holton, D.Soulet, P.Hagell, A.J.Lees, T.Lashley, N.P.Quinn, S. Rehncrona, A.Björklund, H.Widner, T.Revesz, O.Lindvall, P.Brundin)

[11] Nature Medicine [2008] 14 (5) : 504-506 (J.H.Kordower, Yaping Chu, R.A.Hauser, T.B.Freeman, C.W.Olanow)

Stereotactic radio surgery (SRS)

Method : Stereotactic radiosurgery (SRS) is a precise form of radiation therapy used primarily to treat tumors and other abnormalities of the brain. It is a non-surgical procedure that delivers a single high dose of precisely targeted radiation using highly focused gamma-ray or x-ray beams. The beams converge on the area of the brain where the abnormality resides. Only a single or few treatments are necessary [1].

Efficacy : In a long term study amongst hard-to-treat tremors caused by Parkinson's Disease, 83% of patients had significant or complete resolution of tremors [2].

Adverse effects : Some of the patients experienced adverse effects including edema, transient hemiparesis and speech difficulty, which were mostly resolved by taking high doses of steroids. There were no cases of hemorrhage, infection, or death [2].

[1] Principles and Practice of Stereotactic Radiosurgery [2015] (Lawrence Chin, William F.Regine)

[2] Gamma Knife Radiosurgery (GKRS) in the management of Parkinson's Disease and Essential Tremor : Long-term follow up report of 183 cases (S.Johnson, H.Smith, R.Mark, D.Jacques, R. Young, B.Copcutt, C.Chen, P.Anderson, M.Nair)

Subthalamotomy

Method : Subthalamotomy is a type of brain surgery in which the subthalamis nucleus is destroyed. Before surgery brain scans are carried out to identify the precise location for treatment. During the surgery the patient is awake but the scalp area where instruments are inserted is numbed with a local anesthetic. The surgeon inserts a hollow probe through a small hole drilled in the skull to the target location. An extremely cold substance, liquid nitrogen, is circulated inside the probe. The cold probe destroys the targeted brain tissue. The probe is then removed and the wound is closed [1].

Efficacy : In response to unilateral subthalamotomy UPDRS motor scores improved significantly [2-5]. L-dopa daily doses were significantly reduced [5], but the reduction decreased with time [2, 3]. Axial motor features, gait, postural stability, off period tremor, and motor fluctuation improved at 6 and 12 months but showed a decline in benefits at 18 months [3]. There was a significant reduction in both UPDRS parts II and III in the "off" state at 1, 6, and 12 month follow up [5, 6]. This effect was maintained in four patients for up to 24 months [6].

Adverse effects : Operation-induced dyskinesia (OID) occurs in approximately 10% to 15% of patients submitted to subthalamotomy [2, 6, 7]. Drug-induced dyskinesias improved significantly after a year [4, 5]. Some people developed severe generalised chorea that gradually resolved within the next 3 to 6 months [5]. Some people experienced severe and persistent postoperative dysarthria [5].

[1] Parkinson's Disease and other Movement Disorders [2012] (Daniel Tarsy, Jerrold L.Vitek, Andres M.Lozano)

[2] Journal of Neurology, Neurosurgery and Psychiatry [2009] 80 (9) : 979-985 (L.Alvarez, R.Macias, N.Pavón, G.López, M.C. Rodríguez-Oroz, R.Rodríguez, M.Alvarez, I.Pedroso, J.Teijeiro, et al)

[3] Movement Disorders [2003] 18 (5) : 531-538 (P.C.Su, H.M. Tseng, H.M.Liu, R.F.Yen, H.H.Liou)

[4] British Journal of Neurosurgery [2008] 22 (3) : 415-422 (M. Merello, E.Tenca, S.Pérez Lloret, M.E.Martín, V.Bruno, S.Cavanagh, J.Antico, D.Cerquetti, R.Leiguarda)

[5] Brain [2005] 128 (Part 3) : 570-583 (L.Alvarez, R.Macias, G. Lopez, E.Alvarez, N.Pavon, M.C.Rodriguez-Oroz, J.L.Juncos, C. Maragoto, J.Guridi, I.Litvan, E.S.Tolosa, W.Koller, J.Vitek, et al)

[6] Movement Disorders [2001] 16 (1) : 72-78 (L.Alvarez, R.Macias, J.Guridi, G.Lopez, E.Alvarez, C.Maragoto, J.Teijeiro, A.Torres, N. Pavon, M.C.Rodriguez-Oroz, L.Ochoa, H.Hetherington, J.Juncos, et al)

[7] Stereotactic and Functional Neurosurgery [2013] 91(5) : 323-327 (O.Vilela-Filho, D.J.Silva, B.A.Morais, J.T.Souza, P.C.Ragazzo)

THALAMOTOMY

Method : Thalamotomy is a type of brain surgery in which the thalamus, a tiny area of the brain, is destroyed. Before surgery, detailed brain scans are done to identify the precise location for treatment. Surgery on one side of the brain affects the opposite side of the body. The procedure can be repeated on the other side of the brain if needed, but it greatly increases the risk of speech and cognitive problems after surgery has been carried out. Thalamotomy is usually reserved for people younger than 65 years old who have normal intellectual function and normal recent memory. During the surgery, the patient is awake, but the scalp area where instruments are inserted is numbed with a local anesthetic. The surgeon inserts a hollow probe through a small hole that is drilled in the skull to the target location. An extremely cold substance, liquid nitrogen, is then circulated inside the probe. The cold probe destroys the targeted brain tissue. The probe is then removed, and the wound is closed. [1].

Efficacy : Thalamotomy considerably improved tremor in most people [2-15] and modestly improved rigidity [2, 3], but had limited effect on akinesia [2], and no effect on bradykinesia, balance or gait disturbance [3]. In some people there is no further progression of Parkinson's Disease after surgery [16].

Adverse effects : Immediate complications of thalamotomy were common, occurring in 58% of patients. The most common complications were contralateral weakness (34%), dysarthria (29%), and confusion (23%). These complications generally resolved rapidly during the postoperative period [15].

[1] Parkinson's Disease and other Movement Disorders [2012] (Daniel Tarsy, Jerrold L.Vitek, Andres M.Lozano

[2] Neurologia Medico-Chirurgica [1999] 39 (5) : 350-356; discussion 356-357 (E.Moriyama, H.Beck, T.Miyamoto)

[3] Neurologia i Neurochirurgia Polska [2006] 40 (2) : 119-126 (M. Sobstyl, M.Zabek, H.Koziara, B.Kadziolka, Z.Mossakowski)

[4] Stereotactic and Functional Neurosurgery [1993] 61 (Supplement 1) : 65-92 (R.W.Rand, D.B.Jacques, R.W.Melbye, B.G.Copcutt, M.R. Fisher, M.N.Levenick)

[5] Neurosurgery Clinics of North America [1998] 9 (2) : 317-324 (V. L.Perry, F.A.Lenz)

[6] Clinical Neurophysiology [2005] 116 (6) : 1391-1399 (C.Duval, A. P.Strafella, A.F.Sadikot)

[7] Neurosurgery [2012] 70 (3) : 526-535; discussion 535-536 (C.Ohye, Y.Higuchi, T.Shibazaki, T.Hashimoto, T.Koyama, T.Hirai, S.Matsuda, T.Serizawa, T.Hori, M.Hayashi, T.Ochiai, H.Samura, K.Yamashiro)

[8] Stereotactic and Functional Neurosurgery [1997] 69 (Part 2) : 1-4 (B.P.Brophy, T.J.Kimber, P.D.Thompson)

[9] Journal of Neurosurgery [2000] 93 (Supplement 3) : 120-127 (C. Ohye, T.Shibazaki, J.Ishihara, J.Zhang)

[10] Surgical Neurology [1998] 49 (2) : 145-153; discussion 153-154 (R.R.Tasker)

[11] Journal of Neurosurgery [1998] 89 (2) : 183-193 (R.F.Young, A. Shumway-Cook, S.S.Vermeulen, P.Grimm, J.Blasko, A.Posewitz, W. A.Burkhart, R.C.Goiney)

[12] Neurosurgery [2000] 46 (2) : 390-395; discussion 395-398 (M.N. Linhares, R.R.Tasker)

[13] New England Journal of Medicine [2000] 342 (7) : 461-468 (P.R. Schuurman, D.A.Bosch, P.M.Bossuyt, G.J.Bonsel, E.J.van Someren, R.M.de Bie, M.P.Merkus, J.D.Speelman)

[14] Journal of Neurosurgery [1998] 88 (6) : 1044-1049 (C.M.Duma, D.B.Jacques, O.V.Kopyov, R.J.Mark, B.Copcutt, H.K.Farokhi)

[15] Neurosurgery [1995] 37 (4) : 680-686; discussion 686-687 (J. Jankovic, F.Cardoso, R.G.Grossman, W.J.Hamilton)

[16] Journal of Neurosurgery [1984] 60 (5) : 1033-1044 (K.Matsumoto, F.Shichijo, T.Fukami)

CHAPTER 48

NATURAL TREATMENTS OF PARKINSON'S DISEASE

BIOCHEMISTRY

Natural treatments aim to improve Parkinson's Disease without the side effects that usually accompany drug treatments of Parkinson's Disease. They attempt to do this by intending to assist the natural biochemical processes purported to be involved in Parkinson's Disease. However, some of the natural treatments of Parkinson's Disease have pharmacological effects.

NATURAL TREATMENTS

Natural treatments of Parkinson's Disease are largely nutrients, and the use of natural substances. The nutrients and natural substances include cannabis [PAGE 765], coenzyme Q10 [PAGE 766], creatine [PAGE 767], curcumin [PAGE 768], glutathione [PAGE 769], GM1 ganglioside [PAGE 770], inosine [PAGE 770], mannitol [PAGE 771], mitoquinone [PAGE 772], molecular hydrogen water [PAGE 772], herbal medicines [PAGE 773], thiamine [PAGE 773] and vitamins A, C, E [PAGE 774]. Another option in Parkinson's Disease is to remain untreated.

UNTREATED

The symptoms of those people with Parkinson's Disease that remained untreated did not deteriorate in their symptoms over the two years after their diagnosis [1]. However, those people with Parkinson's Disease that did start treatment within the first year actually had higher symptom scores than those people that remained untreated [1]. Some people with Parkinson's Disease reported that their motor functions got better and came nearer to their "on" level after the effect of L-dopa wears off [2].

[1] Journal of Neurology Neurosurgery and Psychiatry [2008] 79 (6) : 716-718 (P.Asimakopoulos, R.Caslake, C.E.Harris, J.C.Gordon, K.S. Taylor, C.Counsell)

[2] Parkinsonism & Related Disorders [2007] (H.J.Kim, J.Y.Kim, S.Ha Paek, B.S.Jeon)

CANNABIS

Biochemistry : Cannabis is a genus of flowering plant. Different parts of the plant that are used for pharmacological purposes are cannabis, marijuana and hashish. The main pharmacological constituents are Cannabinoids [1], which act on cannabinoid receptors in cells that repress neurotransmitter release in the brain [2].

Efficacy : A lot of people with Parkinson's Disease have used cannabis. Nearly half of them described beneficial effects [3]. Cannabis improved pain and motor symptoms [4]. The motor Unified Parkinson Disease Rating Scale score improved significantly. There were improvements in tremor, rigidity, and bradykinesia, and in sleep and pain, without significant adverse effects [5]. In another study, cannabis had no effect on either Parkinson's Disease or dyskinesia [6].

[1] Life Sciences [2005] 78 (5) : 539-548 (M.A.Elsohly, D.Slade)

[2] Royal Society, Philosophical Transactions [2001] 356 (1407) : 381-408 (M.R.Elphick, M.Egertová)

[3] Movement Disorders [2004] 19 (9) : 1102-1106 (K.Venderová, E. Ruzicka, V.Vorísek, P.Visnovský)

[4] European Journal of Pain [2016] Oct 10 [Epub ahead of print] (A.Shohet, A.Khlebtovsky, N.Roizen, Y.Roditi, R.Djaldetti)

[5] Clinical Neuropharmacology [2014] 37 (2) : 41-44 (I.Lotan, T.A. Treves, Y.Roditi, R.Djaldetti)

[6] Neurology [2004] 63 (7) : 1245-1250 (C.B.Carroll, P.G.Bain, L. Teare, X.Liu, C.Joint, C.Wroath, S.G.Parkin, P.Fox, D.Wright, J. Hobart, J.P.Zajicek)

Coenzyme Q10

Biochemistry : The mitochondria is the part of the cells that produces energy. The first step in producing energy in the mitochondria is Complex I (NADH : ubiquinone oxidoreductase). In people with Parkinson's Disease, Complex I is reduced in activity in the substantia nigra, which is the part of the brain primarily affected in Parkinson's Disease. Complex I needs Coenzyme Q10 in order to function properly [1], and Coenzyme Q10 tends to be deficient in Parkinson's Disease [2]. However, energy production has no direct effect on increasing dopamine formation. It is claimed that Coenzyme Q10 is a potent antioxidant that can partially recover the function of dopaminergic neurons.

Efficacy : Coenzyme Q10 was found to be completely ineffective in Parkinson's Disease [3, 12], in daily doses of 200mg [4], 300mg [5, 6], 400mg [7], 600mg [7], and 800mg [7]. Only one Coenzyme Q10 study has ever shown any improvement in Parkinson's Disease, using 360mg, but the effects were mild and were only assessed for four weeks [8]. Daily doses of 300mg, 600mg and 1200 mg failed to improve the symptoms of Parkinson's Disease, but reduced the rate of deterioration [9]. A daily dose of 1600mg for 16 months in a small sample improved ADL (activities of daily living) [10]. Coenzyme Q10 was safe to use in doses of 1200mg [9, 11] 1800mg [11], 2400 [11], and 3000 mg [11]. Plasma levels of Coenzyme Q10 did not increase in doses above 2400mg [11].

[1] Brain Research [2008] 1189 : 215-218 (W.D.Parker Jr, J.K.Parks, R.H.Swerdlow)

[2] Journal of Neurological Science [2012] 318 (1-2) : 72-75 (L.K. Mischley, J.Allen, R.Bradley)

[3] CNS and Neurological Disorders Drug Targets [2016] 15 (1) : 45-53 (A.Negida, A.Menshawy, G.El Ashal, Y.Elfouly, Y.Hani, Y.Hegazy, S.El Ghonimy, S.Fouda, Y.Rashad)

[4] Molecular Aspects of Medicine [1997] (18 Supplement) : S237-S240 (E.Strijks, H.P.Kremer, M.W.Horstink)

[5] Archives of Neurology [2007] 64 (7) : 938-944 (A.Storch, W.H. Jost, P.Vieregge, J.Spiegel, W.Greulich, J.Durner, T.Muller, A. Kupsch, H.Henningsen, W.H.Oertel, G.Fuchs, W.Kuhn, et al)

[6] Parkinsonism & Related Disorders [2015] 21 (8) : 911-916 (A. Yoritaka, S.Kawajiri, Y.Yamamoto, T.Nakahara, M.Ando, K. Hashimoto, M.Nagase, Y.Saito, N.Hattori)

[7] Neurology [1998] 50 (3) : 793-795 (C.W.Shults, M.F.Beal, D. Fontaine, K.Nakano, R.H.Haas)

[8] Neuroscience Letters [2003] 341 (3) : 201-204 (T.Müller, T. Büttner, A.F.Gholipour, W.Kuhn)

[9] Archives of Neurology [2002] 59 (10) : 1541-1550 (C.W.Shults, D.Oakes, K.Kieburtz, M.F.Beal, R.Haas, S.Plumb, J.L.Juncos, J.Nutt, I. Shoulson, J.Carter, K.Kompoliti, J.S.Perlmutter, S.Reich, et al)

[10] Cochrane Database Systematic Reviews [2011] 12 : CD008150 (J. Liu, L.Wang, S.Y.Zhan, Y.Xia)

[11] Experimental Neurology [2004] 188 (2) : 491-494 (C.W.Shults, M.Flint Beal, D.Song, D.Fontaine)

[12] Neurological Sciences [2017] 38 (2) : 215-224 (Z.G.Zhu, M.X. Sun, W.L.Zhang, W.W.Wang, Y.M.Jin, C.L.Xie)

CREATINE

Biochemistry : Creatine is a substance that the body normally produces itself in order to supply energy to muscle cells. Creatine does not have any direct effect on dopamine formation.

Efficacy : Creatine improved mood in people with Parkinson's Disease and led to a smaller increase of dopaminergic therapy but had no effect on Parkinson's Disease symptoms [1]. In rats treated with L-dopa, there were significant reductions in abnormal involuntary movements in the creatine supplemented group, without any worsening of Parkinson's Disease symptoms [2]. However, there was no significant effect on Parkinson's Disease symptoms in humans [3]. There was no clear evidence of an effect on motor function or quality of life after one or two years of treatment [4]. In people taking creatine, higher caffeine intake was associated with faster progression of symptoms [5].

[1] Neurology [2006] 67 (7) : 1262-1264 (A.Bender, W.Koch, M. Elstner, Y.Schombacher, J.Bender, M.Moeschl, F.Gekeler, B.Müller-Myhsok, T.Gasser, K.Tatsch, T.Klopstock)

[2] Behavioural Brain Research [2009] 197 (1) : 90-96 (B.Valastro, A. Dekundy, W.Danysz, G.Quack)

[3] CNS & Neurological Disorders Drug Targets [2016] Nov 4 [Epub ahead of print] (A.Attia, H.Ahmed, M.Gadelkarim, M.Morsi, K.Awad, M.Elnenny, E.Ghanem, S.El-Jafaary, A.Negida)

[4] Cochrane Database Systematic Reviews [2014] (Y.Xiao, M.Luo, H. Luo, J.Wang)

[5] Clinical Neuropharmacology [2015] 38 (5) : 163-169 (D.K.Simon, C.Wu, B.C.Tilley, A.M.Wills, M.J.Aminoff, J.Bainbridge, R.A.Hauser, J.S.Schneider, S.Sharma, C.Singer, C.M.Tanner, D.Truong, P.S.Wong)

Curcumin

Biochemistry : Curcumin is derived from the root of the plant Curcuma longa, which is usually called turmeric. Turmeric is a spice commonly used in Indian cooking. Its medicinal uses have been described for over 5000 years [1].

Efficacy : Neuroprotective properties in Parkinson's Disease have been claimed for curcumin [2, 3]. The effects of curcumin are attributed to its antioxidative properties [4]. However, there are no clinical studies demonstrating that curcumin has any degree of efficacy in Parkinson's Disease.

[1] The Molecular Targets and Therapeutic Uses of Curcumin in Health and Disease [2007] (Bharat B.Aggarwal, Young-Joon Surh, S. Shishodia)

[2] Free Radical Research [2005] 39 (10) : 1119-1125 (V.Zbarsky, K.P. Datla, S.Parkar, D.K.Rai, O.I.Aruoma, D.T.Dexter)

[3] Antioxidants and Redox Signalling [2007] 9 (3) : 399-408 (R.B. Mythri, B.Jagatha, N.Pradhan, J.Andersen, M.M.Bharath)

[4] Biochemical Pharmacology [2009] 78 (2) : 178-183 (J.Wang, X.X. Du, H.Jiang, J.X.Xie)

GLUTATHIONE

Biochemistry : Glutathione is a naturally occurring combination of three amino acids (glutamic acid, cysteine, glycine). When taken orally, glutathione separates in to the three amino acids, although there are biochemical means by which they can reform to some extent. Glutathione is most effectively administered intravenously because it avoids this problem altogether. Glutathione is an antioxidant, which is claimed to reduce cell damage. Glutathione also facilitates entry of the dopamine precursors in to the dopaminergic neurons in order to make dopamine.

Efficacy : In a small study, intravenous glutathione moderately reduced the Parkinson's Disease symptoms of all patients tested. The effect continued for a few months after ceasing the glutathione [1]. However, in a more comprehensive clinical trial, symptoms moderately improved whilst taking glutathione but worsened soon after [2]. Intra nasal glutathione moderately improved Parkinson's Disease [3].

[1] Progress in Neuro-psychopharmacology & Biological Psychiatry [1996] 20 (7) : 1159-1170 (G.Sechi, M.G.Deledda, G.Bua, W.M. Satta, G.A.Deiana, G.M.Pes, G.Rosati)

[2] Movement Disorders [2009] 24 (7) : 979-983 (R.A.Hauser, K.E. Lyons, T.McClain, S.Carter, D.Perlmutter)

[3] Journal of Parkinsons Disease [2017] Apr 20 [Epub ahead of print] (L.K.Mischley, R.C.Lau, E.G.Shankland, T.K.Wilbur, J.M. Padowski)

GM1 Ganglioside

Biochemistry : Gangliosides are components of the cell plasma membrane, mainly in the nervous system. The precise means of effect is not known but it has been suggested what effects it has are "neuroprotective".

Efficacy : In a 16 week clinical trial after having received IV infusion of 1000mg GM1 ganglioside and then self administering 200mg GM1 ganglioside per day, there was an improvement in : UPDRS motor scores, activities of daily living, performance of timed motor tests including tests of arm, hand, and foot movements, and walking [1]. GM1 ganglioside was well tolerated [1, 2]. In a 120 week clinical trial of the use of GM1 ganglioside there was significant improvement in Parkinson's Disease motor symptoms. There was only a reduced worsening of symptoms after 120 weeks. So it was slowing deterioration rather than ridding symptoms [3]. In a five year clinical trial people with Parkinson's Disease who took GM1 ganglioside generally had lower UPDRS motor scores. A similar result was found for UPDRS Activities of Daily Living scores [4].

[1] Neurology [1998] 50 (6) : 1630-1636 (J.S.Schneider, D.P. Roeltgen, E.L.Mancall, J.Chapas-Crilly, D.S.Rothblat, G.T.Tatarian)

[2] Neurology [1995] 45 (6) : 1149-1154 (J.S.Schneider, D.P. Roeltgen, D.S.Rothblat, J.Chapas-Crilly, L.Seraydarian, J.Rao)

[3] Journal of Neurological Science [2013] 324 (1-2) : 140-148 (J.S. Schneider, S.M.Gollomp, S.Sendek, A.Colcher, F.Cambi, W.Du)

[4] Journal of Neurological Science [2010] 292 (1-2) : 45-51 (J.S. Schneider, S.Sendek, C.Daskalakis, F.Cambi)

Inosine

Biochemistry : Inosine is a nucleoside. Nucleosides are able to form nucleotides, which are the molecular building blocks of the nucleic acids DNA and RNA. Inosine can give rise to urate in the body, and thereby increase levels of urate, which is a natural metabolite and antioxidant in humans.

Efficacy : Higher dietary urate is associated with a lower risk of Parkinson's Disease [1-6], and slower progression of Parkinson's Disease symptoms [7]. However, instead of urate reducing Parkinson's Disease, L-dopa lowers urate levels [8].

[1] American Journal of Epidemiology [2008] 167 (7) : 831-838 (X. Gao, H.Chen, H.K.Choi, G.Curhan, M.A.Schwarzschild, A.Ascherio)

[2] Movement Disorders [2010] 25 (7) : 932-936 (A.Winquist, K. Steenland, A.Shankar)

[3] American Journal of Epidemiology [2008] 167 (7) : 831-838 (M.G. Weisskopf, E.O'Reilly, H.Chen, M.A.Schwarzschild, A. Ascherio)

[4] American Journal of Epidemiology [2007] 166 (5) : 561-567 (X. Gao, H.Chen, H.K.Choi, G.Curhan, M.A.Schwarzschild, A.Ascherio)

[5] Annals of Neurology [2005] 58 (5) : 797-800 (L.M.de Lau, P.J. Koudstaal, A.Hofman, M.M.Breteler)

[6] American Journal of Epidemiology [1996] 144 (5) : 480-484 (J.W. Davis, A.Grandinetti, C.I.Waslien, G.W.Ross, L.R.White, D.M. Morens)

[7] Archives of Neurology [2009] 66 (12) : 1460-1468 (A.Ascherio, P. A.LeWitt, K.Xu, S.Eberly, A.Watts, W.R.Matson, C.Marras, K. Kieburtz, A.Rudolph, M.B.Bogdanov, S.R.Schwid, M.Tennis, et al)

[8] Life Sciences [1994] 55 (13) : 991-997 (M.Pinheiro-Carrera, C. Tomaz, J.P.Huston, H.Dai, R.J.Carey)

Mannitol

Biochemistry : Mannitol, which is used in medicine, is derived from mannose, which is a sugar. It has been proposed as a potential means of treating Parkinson's Disease because of the dual mechanisms it has in the brain : to interfere with the aggregation of alpha-synuclein, and its ability to disrupt the blood-brain barrier. Alpha-synuclein can accumulate in the brains of people with Parkinson's Disease and some other medical disorders but can also be absent in Parkinson's Disease.

Efficacy : The effect of mannitol was demonstrated on alpha-synuclein by various means, and a decrease in alpha-synuclein accumulation. However, the research was only carried out on mice and flies, who did not have Parkinson's Disease and who were not able to be rid of its symptoms [1].

[1] Journal of Biological Chemistry [2013] 288 (24) : 17579-17588 (R. Shaltiel-Karyo, M.Frenkel-Pinter, E.Rockenstein, C.Patrick, M.Levy-Sakin, A.Schiller, N.Egoz-Matia, E.Masliah, D.Segal, E.Gazit)

Mitoquinone

Biochemistry : Mitoquinone (MitoQ) is a highly potent derivative of Coenzyme Q10. Mitoquinone (MitoQ) combines ubiquinone, which is the anti-oxidant portion of the coenzyme Q10 molecule, with a lipophilic triphenyl- phosphonium cation.

Efficacy : Mitoquinone caused side effects, and was completely ineffective in treating people with Parkinson's Disease [1, 2].

[1] Neurology [2008] 70 : A483-A484 (B.Snow)

[2] Movement Disorders [2010] 25 (11) : 1670-1674 (B.J.Snow, F.L. Rolfe, M.M.Lockhart, C.M.Frampton, J.D.O'Sullivan, V.Fung, R.A. Smith, M.P.Murphy, K.M.Taylor)

Molecular Hydrogen Water

Biochemistry : Molecular hydrogen water is water in which molecular hydrogen (H_2) has been dissolved.

Efficacy : Drinking molecular hydrogen dissolved water had reduced oxidative stress and improved Parkinson's Disease features in animals.

People with Parkinson's Disease who were taking L-dopa drank either a litre a day of molecular hydrogen water or only water. Parkinson's Disease symptom scores improved in those people who drank molecular hydrogen water and worsened in those people who only drank normal water instead. Molecular hydrogen water was safe and well tolerated [1]. A full scale clinical trial is being arranged [2].

[1] Movement Disorders [2013] 28 (6) : 836-839 (A.Yoritaka, M. Takanashi, M.Hirayama, T.Nakahara, S.Ohta, N.Hattori, D.Weintraub, K.Papay, A.Siderowf)

[2] BMC Neurology [2016] 16 (1) : 66 (A.Yoritaka, T.Abe, C.Ohtsuka, T.Maeda, M.Hirayama, H.Watanabe, H.Saiki, G.Oyama, J.Fukae, Y. Shimo, T.Hatano, S.Kawajiri, Y.Okuma, Y.Machida, H.Miwa, et al)

Herbal medicines

Biochemistry : Most herbal medicines are effectively drugs in a natural form and have a pharmacological action.

Efficacy : A systematic review evaluated the current evidence of herbal medicines for treating Parkinson's Disease. Specific effects were not observed that were clearly in favour of herbal medicines. Comparison with conventional drugs suggested that there was no evidence of a better effect for herbal medicines. Many studies compared combination therapy with individual drugs. These showed significant improvement in Parkinson's Disease related outcomes and decreases in the doses of Parkinson's Disease drugs with low rates of adverse effects rate [1].

[1] PLoS One [2012] 7 (5) : e35695 (T.H.Kim, K.H.Cho, W.S.Jung, M. S.Lee)

Thiamine (Vitamin B1)

Biochemistry : Thiamine is the most active form of Vitamin B1. It is essential for the formation of the coenzyme Thiamine Pyrophosphate.

Efficacy : Thiamine reduced motor and non motor Parkinson's Disease symptom scores over three months and the symptoms remained stable over time [1]. Parenteral therapy of thiamine led to improvements in Parkinson's Disease symptoms [2, 3]. Plasma thiamine deficiency is associated with Alzheimer's Disease but not with Parkinson's Disease [4].

[1] Journal of Alternative and Complementary Medicine [2015] 21 (12) : 740-747 (A.Costantini, M.I.Pala, E.Grossi, S.Mondonico, L.Ercoli Cardelli, C.Jenner, S.Proietti, M.Colangeli, R.Fancellu)

[2] BMJ Case Reports [2013] Aug 28 (A.Costantini, M.I.Pala, L. Compagnoni, M.Colangeli)

[3] CNS Neuroscience and Therapeutics [2013] 19 (7) : 461-468 (K.V. Luong, L.T.Nguyen)

[4] Metabolic Brain Disease [1998] 13 (1) : 43-53 (M.Gold, R.A. Hauser, M.F.Chen)

VITAMINS A, C, E

Biochemistry : Superoxide anion can be formed when L-dopa is not formed properly. Superoxide anion is broken down by the enzymes superoxide dismutase and catalase, which require Vitamin C and Vitamin E. Vitamin C and Vitamin E are antioxidants as is Vitamin A.

Efficacy : Vitamin A levels generally are not lower in Parkinson's Disease [1-4], but some forms of vitamin A are [21]. Higher intakes are associated with a reduced risk of Parkinson's Disease [5]. Vitamin C deficiency was associated with a higher risk of Parkinson's Disease in one study [6], but not in another [7]. Dietary vitamin C intake was significantly associated with a reduced risk of Parkinson's Disease, down to 80%, but this was not long term [19]. Higher intakes of Vitamin C on its own were not associated with a lower risk of Parkinson's Disease [8, 9, 10]. Vitamin E levels were lower in Parkinson's Disease in some studies [11, 12] but not in others [13, 14, 15]. Higher intakes were associated with a reduced risk of Parkinson's

Disease [5, 16], but could not prevent the development of Parkinson's Disease [17]. Vitamin E, when taken with omega-3 fatty acids, moderately reduced Parkinson's Disease symptoms [20]. Progression of Parkinson's Disease can be slowed down by the administration of Vitamin C and Vitamin E [18].

[1] Journal of Neurological Science [2003] 215 (1-2) : 51-55 (G.P. Paraskevas, E.Kapaki, O.Petropoulou, M.Anagnostouli, V.Vagenas, C. Papageorgiou)

[2] Neuroscience Letters [1993] 157 (1) : 103-106 (F.J.Jiménez-Jiménez, J.A.Molina, P.Fernández-Calle, A.Vázquez, F.Cabrera-Valdivia, M.J.Catalán, E.García-Albea, F.Bermejo, R.Codoceo)

[3] Postgraduate Medical Journal [1992] 68 (802) : 634-637 (D.King, J.R.Playfer, N.B.Roberts)

[4] Journal of Neurological Science [1992] 111 (1) : 73-76 (F.J. Jiménez-Jiménez, J.A.Molina, P.Fernández-Calle, A.Vázquez, M. Pondal, T.del Ser, A.Gómez-Pastor, R.Codoceo)

[5] European Journal of Neurology [2011] 18 (1) : 106-113 (Y.Miyake, W.Fukushima, K.Tanaka, S.Sasaki, C.Kiyohara, Y.Tsuboi, T.Yamada, T.Oeda, T.Miki, N.Kawamura, N.Sakae, H.Fukuyama, H.Hirota, et al)

[6] Public Health [1992] 106 (5) : 393-395 (S.C.Yapa)

[7] Postgraduate Medical Journal [1992] 68 (802) : 634-637 (D.King, J.R.Playfer, N.B.Roberts)

[8] European Journal of Neurology [2011] 18 (1) : 106-113 (Y.Miyake, W.Fukushima, K.Tanaka, S.Sasaki, C.Kiyohara, Y.Tsuboi, T.Yamada, T.Oeda, T.Miki, N.Kawamura, N.Sakae, H.Fukuyama, Y.Hirota, et al)

[9] Lancet Neurology [2005] 4 (6) : 362-365 (M.Etminan, S.S.Gill, A. Samii)

[10] Journal of Neurological Science [1993] 118 (1) : 25-28 (P. Férnandez-Calle, F.J.Jiménez-Jiménez, J.A.Molina, F.Cabrera-Valdivia, A.Vázquez, D.García Urra, F.Bermejo, et al)

[11] Journal of Neurological Science [2012] 318 (1-2) : 72-75 (L.K. Mischley, J.Allen, R.Bradley)

[12] Indian Journal of Clinical Biochemistry [2009] 24 (1) : 98-101 (S. Nikam, P.Nikam, S.K.Ahaley, A.V.Sontakke)

[13] Archives of Gerontology and Geriatrics [2001] 33 (1) : 7-12 (G. Nicoletti, L.Crescibene, M.Scornaienchi, L.Bastone, A.Bagalà, I.D. Napoli, M.Caracciolo, A.Quattrone)

[14] Postgraduate Medical Journal [1992] 68 (802) : 634-637 (D.King, J.R.Playfer, N.B.Roberts)

[15] Neurology [1992] 42 (5) : 1064-1066 (P.Férnandez-Calle, J.A. Molina, F.J.Jiménez-Jiménez, A.Vázquez, M.Pondal, P.J. García-Ruiz, D.G.Urra, J.Domingo, R.Codoceo)

[16] Lancet Neurology [2005] 4 (6) : 362-365 (M.Etminan, S.S.Gill, A. Samii)

[17] Pharmacy World and Science [1993] 15 (4) : 146-150 (L.Bischot, G.Van den Brink, A.J.Porsius)

[18] Annals of Neurology [1992] (32 Supplement) : S128-S132 (S.Fahn)

[19] Movement Disorders [2016] Oct 27 [Epub ahead of print] (K.C. Hughes, X.Gao, I.Y.Kim, E.B.Rimm, M.Wang, M.G.Weisskopf, M.A. Schwarzschild, A.Ascherio)

[20] Neurochemistry International [2017] Mar 22 [Epub ahead of print] (M.Taghizadeh, O.R.Tamtaji, E.Dadgostar, R.D.Kakhaki, F. Bahmani, J.Abolhassani, M.H.Aarabi, E.Kouchaki, M.R.Memarzadeh, et al)

[21] Nutrition Research and Practice [2017] 11 (2) : 114-120 (J.H.Kim, J.Hwang, E.Shim, E.J.Chung, S.H.Jang, S.B.Koh)

CHAPTER 49

EXERCISE METHODS FOR PARKINSON'S DISEASE

PHYSIOLOGY

Parkinson's Disease causes excessive muscle contraction. Although the initial effect of exercise is to increase muscle contraction, the after effect of exercise is to reduce muscle contraction. This has the same type of effect on the muscles as most Parkinson's Disease drugs. However, exercise does not raise dopamine levels and thereby improve other Parkinson's Disease symptoms.

EXERCISE METHODS

Forms of exercise that have been used to try to lessen the muscular effects of Parkinson's Disease include general exercise [PAGE 777], progressive resistance exercise training [PAGE 780], treadmill training [PAGE 781], balance training [PAGE 784], aquatic exercise [PAGE 784], physiotherapy [PAGE 785], cycling [PAGE 786], dancing [PAGE 787], the traditional practice of Qigong [PAGE 788], the Chinese martial art of Tai Chi [PAGE 789], and the Hindu discipline Yoga [PAGE 790].

GENERAL EXERCISE

Method : Exercise is physical activity that maintains physical fitness. General exercise usually involves repeating the physical action and concentrating on particular muscles during each exercise. The exercises most relevant to Parkinson's Disease concern the muscles because the most prominent symptoms seen in Parkinson's Disease are muscular [1, 2].

Efficacy : In people with Parkinson's Disease, exercise can improve physical performance [3-8], the quality of life [9], and significantly improves instability, especially if it specifically addresses balance dysfunction [19]. Different means of exercising can be beneficial [10], including exercise as part of training for sports [11, 12, 13, 20]. In Parkinson's Disease there was a striking reduction in physical activity but not a complete abandonment of sports [14]. Participating in competitive sports prior to the age of 25 nearly halved the risk of developing Parkinson's Disease [15]. Higher levels of regular moderate to vigorous activity when somebody is in their late thirties and in the past ten years reduces the risk of Parkinson's Disease by 40%. Moderate to vigorous activities at earlier ages (prior to their late thirties), or light activity had no effect on the likelihood of developing Parkinson's Disease [16] but this was not always the case [15]. People who had consistently engaged in overall physical activity at high levels, before they were 65, had half the risk of developing Parkinson's Disease [15]. Occupational physical activity did not lessen the risk of Parkinson's Disease [15]. Current physical activity moderately reduced the risk of Parkinson's Disease [17, 18].

[1] Delay the Disease - Functional Fitness for Parkinson's [2012] (David Zid, Jackie Russell)

[2] Parkinson's Disease & the Art of Moving [2000] (John Argue)

[3] Clinical Practice and Epidemiology in Mental Health [2014] 10 : 126-128 (E.Lattari, P.P.Pereira-Junior, G.A.Neto, M.K.Lamego, A.M. Moura, A.S.de Sá, R.R.Rimes, J.P.Manochio, O.Arias-Carrión, et al)

[4] Clinical Journal of Sport Medicine [2006] 16 (5) : 422-425 (A.M. Crizzle, I.J.Newhouse)

[5] Physical Therapy [2012] 92 (11) : 1395-1410 (M.Schenkman, D.A. Hall, A.E.Barón, R.S.Schwartz, P.Mettler, W.M.Kohrt)

[6] Parkinsonism & Related Disorders [2014] 20 (11) : 1221-1225 (O. Oguh, A.Eisenstein, M.Kwasny, T.Simuni)

[7] NeuroRehabilitation [2014] 35 (4) : 789-794 (L.Cugusi, P.Solla, F. Zedda, M.Loi, R.Serpe, A.Cannas, F.Marrosu, G.Mercuro)

[8] Archives of Physical Medicine and Rehabilitation [2008] 89 (7) : 1221-1229 (B.E.Fisher, A.D.Wu, G.J.Salem, J.Song, C.H.Lin, J.Yip, S. Cen, J.Gordon, M.Jakowec, G.Petzinger)

[9] Journal of Aging and Physical Activity [2016] Jan 11 [Epub ahead of print] (F.C.da Silva, R.Iop Rda, P.D.Dos Santos, L.M.Bezerra, P.J.Gutierres, R.da Silva)

[10] Cochrane Database of Systematic Reviews [2012] 8 : CD002817 (C.L.Tomlinson, S.Patel, C.Meek, C.E.Clarke, R.Stowe, L.Shah, C.M. Sackley, K.H.Deane, C.P.Herd, K.Wheatley, N.Ives)

[11] Scandinavian Journal of Medicine and Science in Sports [2016] Feb 2 [Epub ahead of print] (E.P.Monteiro, L.T.Franzoni, D.M. Cubillos, A.de Oliveira Fagundes, A.R.Carvalho, H.B.Oliveira, et al)

[12] Physical Therapy [2011] 91 (1) : 132-142 (S.A.Combs, M.D. Diehl, W.H.Staples, L.Conn, K.Davis, N.Lewis, K.Schaneman)

[13] Movement Disorders [2008] 23 (15) : 2239-2243 (F.J.Van Eijkeren, R.S.Reijmers, M.J.Kleinveld, A.Minten, J.P.Bruggen, B.R. Bloem)

[14] Journal of Neural Transmission [1993] 5 (2) : 157-161 (E.Fertl, A.Doppelbauer, E.Auff)

[15] Parkinsonism & Related Disorders [2016] 28 : 112-117 (I.F.Shih, Z.Liew, N.Krause, B.Ritz)

[16] Neurology [2010] 75 (4) : 341-348 (Q.Xu, Y.Par, X.Huang, A. Hollenbeck, A.Blair, A.Schatzkin, H.Chen)

[17] Journal of Neurology, Neurosurgery and Psychiatry [2006] 77 (12) : 1318-1322 (G.Logroscino, H.D.Sesso, R.S.Paffenbarger Jr, I.M.Lee)

[18] Parkinsonism & Related Disorders [2015] 21 (10) : 1227-1231 (J.Snider, M.L.Müller, V.Kotagal, R.A.Koeppe, P.J.Scott, K.A.Frey, R.L.Albin, N.I.Bohnen)

[19] Journal of Neurologic Physical Therapy [2016] 40 (1) : 3-14 (S.Klamroth, S.Steib, S.Devan, K.Pfeifer)

[20] Parkinsonism and Related Disorders [2017] Feb 6 [Epub ahead of print] (F.Bombieri, F.Schena, B.Pellegrini, P.Barone, M.Tinazzi, R.Erro)

PROGRESSIVE RESISTANCE EXERCISE TRAINING

Method : Progressive resistance exercise training involves programmes of exercises that build muscular strength through the lifting of progressively heavier weights [1]. Progressive resistance exercise training is also referred to as body building.

Efficacy : In people with Parkinson's Disease, progressive resistance exercise training : reduces Parkinson's Disease symptom scores [2], reduces motor symptoms [3], improves balance [3], increases muscle strength [3, 4, 5], improves mobility [5], increases leg strength [6], improves walking capacity [7], reduces falls [8], and improves attention and working memory in people without dementia [9].

[1] Jim's Weight Training & Bodybuilding Workout Plan [2015] (James Atkinson)

[2] Movement Disorders [2013] 28 (9) : 1230-1240 (D.M.Corcos, J.A. Robichaud, F.J.David, S.E.Leurgans, D.E.Vaillancourt, C.Poon, M.R. Rafferty, W.M.Kohrt, C.L.Comella)

[3] Clinical Rehabilitation [2016] 30 (1) : 11-23 (C.L.Chung, S. Thilarajah, D.Tan)

[4] Medicine and Science in Sports and Exercise [2016] Apr 6 [Epub ahead of print] (C.Silva-Batista, D.M.Corcos, H.Roschel, H. Kanegusuku, L.T.Gobbi, M.E.Piemonte, E.C.Mattos, et al)

[5] Journal of American Medical Directors Association [2013] 14 (4) : 236-241 (L.A.Brienesse, M.N.Emerson)

[6] Frontiers in Aging Neuroscience [2015] 7 : 40 (A.Tillman, M. Muthalib, A.M.Hendy, L.G.Johnson, T.Rantalainen, D.J.Kidgell, P.G. Enticott, W.P.Teo)

[7] Journal of Physiotheray [2013] 59 (1) : 7-13 (L.O.Lima, A. Scianni, F.Rodrigues-de-Paula)

[8] Neurorehabilitation and Neural Repair [2015] 29 (8) : 777-785 (M.E.Morris, H.B.Menz, J.L.McGinley, J.J.Watts, F.E.Huxham, A.T. Murphy, M.E.Danoudis, R.Iansek)

[9] Movement Disorders [2015] 30 (12) : 1657-1663 (F.J.David, J.A. Robichaud, S.E.Leurgans, C.Poon, W.M.Kohrt, J.G.Goldman, C.L. Comella, D.E.Vaillancourt, D.M.Corcos)

Treadmill training

Method : A treadmill is an exercise machine for running or walking while staying in one place. It provides a moving platform with a wide conveyor belt driven by an electric motor. The belt moves to the rear requiring the user to walk or run at a speed matching that of the belt. The speed is adjustable to enable use at various speeds. Split-belt treadmills feature two separate belts running alongside each other, one for each leg. The two belts can move together or at independent speeds.

Efficacy : Treadmill training can improve walking ability in people with Parkinson's Disease [1-18] including : increased walking distance [1, 19], increased stride length [1-5, 11, 12, 17, 18, 20, 21, 22], increased walking speed [1, 3, 4, 5, 9, 11, 12, 15, 17-24, 29], reduced stride time variability [6, 7, 19, 24], reduced freezing of gait [15, 20]. It reduces the overall Parkinson's Disease symptoms [3, 8, 9, 12, 13, 23, 25, 26, 27], and reduces gait disturbances [28]. An additional load to increase the person's weight had no additional effect [30].

[1] Cochrane Database of Systematic Reviews [2010] (1) : CD007830 (J.Mehrholz, R.Friis, J.Kugler, S.Twork, A.Storch, M.Pohl)

[2] Gait Posture [2010] 32 (1) : 118-123 (O.Bello, G.Marquez, M. Camblor, M.Fernandez-Del-Olmo)

[3] Archives of Physical Medicine and Rehabilitation [2000] 81 (7) : 849-852 (I.Miyai, Y.Fujimoto, Y.Ueda, H.Yamamoto, S.Nozaki, T. Saito, J.Kang)

[4] Archives of Physical Medicine and Rehabilitation [2002] 83 (10) : 1370-1373 (I.Miyai, Y.Fujimoto, H.Yamamoto, Y.Ueda, T.Saito, S. Nozaki, J.Kang)

[5] Archives of Physical Medicine and Rehabilitation [2003] 84 (12) : 1760-1766 (M.Pohl, G.Rockstroh, S.Rückriem, G.Mrass, J. Mehrholz)

[6] Movement Disorders [2005] 20 (9) : 1109-1114 (S.Frenkel- Toledo, N.Giladi, C.Peretz, T.Herman, L.Gruendlinger, J.M. Hausdorff)

[7] Journal of Neuroengineering and Rehabilitation [2005] 2 : 23 (S. Frenkel-Toledo, N.Giladi, C.Peretz, T.Herman, L.Gruendlinger, J.M. Hausdorff)

[8] Neurological Science [2009] 30 (6) : 499-504 (E.Pelosin, E.Faelli, F.Lofrano, L.Avanzino, L.Marinelli, M.Bove, P.Ruggeri, G. Abbruzzese)

[9] Archives of Physical Medicine and Rehabilitation [2007] 88 (9) : 1154-1158 (T.Herman, N.Giladi, L.Gruendlinger, J.M.Hausdorff)

[10] Clinical Rehabilitation [2007] 21 (8) : 698-705 (B.D.Cakit, M. Saracoglu, H.Genc, H.R.Erdem, L.Inan)

[11] Movement Disorders [2008] 23 (9) : 1243-1249 (O.Bello, J.A. Sanchez, M.Fernandez-del-Olmo)

[12] Archives of Physical Medicine and Rehabilitation [2008] 89 (7) : 1221-1229 (B.E.Fisher, A.D.Wu, G.J.Salem, J.Song, C.H.Lin, J.Yip, S. Cen, J.Gordon, M.Jakowec, G.Petzinger)

[13] Archives of Physical Medicine and Rehabilitation [2007] 88 (9) : 1154-1158 (T.Herman, N.Giladi, L.Gruendlinger, J.M.Hausdorff)

[14] Journal of Neural Transmission [2009] 116 (3) : 307-318 (T. Herman, N.Giladi, J.M.Hausdorff)

[15] Movement Disorders [2009] 24 (8) : 1139-1143 (G.Frazzitta, R. Maestri, D.Uccellini, G.Bertotti, P.Abelli)

[16] NeuroRehabilitation [2005] 20 (4) : 307-322 (T.Toole, C.G. Maitland, E.Warren, M.F.Hubmann, L.Panton)

[17] American Journal of Physical Medicine and Rehabilitation [2015] 94 (10 Supplement 1) : 830-837 (L.C.Trigueiro, G.L.Gama, C.R.Simão, A. V.Sousa, C.O.Godeiro Júnior, A.R.Lindquist)

[18] Cochrane Database of Systematic Reviews [2015] (8) : CD007830 (J.Mehrholz, J.Kugler, A.Storch, M.Pohl, B. Elsner, K.Hirsch)

[19] Medical and Science in Sports and Exercise [2014] 46 (4) : 645-655 (A.Nadeau, E.Pourcher, P.Corbeil)

[20] Journal of Neuroengineering and Rehabilitation [2010] 7 (1) : 51 (A.C.Lo, V.C.Chang, M.A.Gianfrancesco, J.H.Friedman, T.S. Patterson, D.F.Benedicto)

[21] European Journal of Physical and Rehabilitation Medicine [2016] Mar 4 [Epub ahead of print] (J.Mehrholz, J.Kugler, A.Storch, M.Pohl, K.Hirsch, B.Elsner)

[22] PM & R [2016] May 10 [Epub ahead of print] (M.S.Bryant, C.D. Workman, J.G.Hou, H.K.Henson, M.K.York)

[23] Journal of Rehabilitation, Research and Development [2008] 45 (1) : 117-124 (F.M.Skidmore, S.L.Patterson, L.M.Shulman, J.D.Sorkin, R.F.Macko)

[24] Gait Posture [2016] 50 : 102-108 [Epub ahead of print] (S. Klamroth, S.Steib, H.Gaßner, J.Goßler, J.Winkler, B.Eskofier, J. Klucken, K.Pfeifer)

[25] Revista Brasileira de Fisioterapia [2010] 14 (4) : 344-350 (N.T. Filippin, P.H.Lobo da Costa, R.Mattioli)

[26] Archives of Physical Medicine and Rehabilitation [2015] 96 (9) : 1557-1565 (M.Ganesan, T.N.Sathyaprabha, P.K.Pal, A.Gupta)

[27] NeuroRehabilitation [2016] Jun 30 [Epub ahead of print] (C.Ayan, S.Varela, M.H.Vila, M.Seijo, J.M.Cancela)

[28] European Journal of Physical and Rehabilitation Medicine [2016] Jul 19 [Epub ahead of print] (E.Pelosin, L.Avanzino, R.Barella, C.Bet, E.Magioncalda, C.Trompetto, P.Ruggeri, M.Casaleggio, et al)

[29] Functional Neurology [2016] 31 (1) : 25-31 (A.Picelli, V.Varalta, C.Melotti, V.Zatezalo, C.Fonte, S.Amato, L.Saltuari, A.Santamato, P.Fiore, N.Smania)

[30] Journal of Bodywork and Movement Therapies [2017] 21 (1) : 93-100 (L.C.Trigueiro, G.L.Gama, T.S.Ribeiro, L.G.Ferreira, É.R. Galvão, E.M.Silva, C.O.Júnior, A.R.Lindquist)

Balance training

Method : Balance training trains the body to maintain postural control throughout a series of demands while standing still or through advanced transitional movements. The simplest exercises focus on stabilisation such as by standing on one leg. The exercise can be made more challenging by adding specific upper or lower body movements while balancing on one leg that is unsupported or by balancing on an unstable surface. Finally, there are more dynamic movements such as steps, hops, and jumps that end up with the person being in a balanced finish position.

Efficacy : The effect of balance training was evaluated in people with Parkinson's Disease using the following scales : Berg Balance Scale (BBS), Activities-Specific Balance Confidence Scale (ABC), postural transfer test, self-destabilisation of the centre of foot pressure test, number of falls, Unified Parkinson's Disease Rating Scale (UPDRS), modified Hoehn and Yahr (H&Y) Staging Scale, and the Geriatric Depression Scale (GDS). Those people with Parkinson's Disease who underwent balance training had improvements in all of the measures, except for the UPDRS and the H&Y scale [1]. They also improved on the Sensory Orientation Test. Consequently, for weeks after balance training they could balance for longer before falling [2].

[1] Neurorehabilitation and Neural Repair [2010] 24 (9) : 826-834 (N.Smania, E.Corato, M.Tinazzi, C.Stanzani, A.Fiaschi, P.Girardi, M. Gandolfi)

[2] Archives of Physical Medicine and Rehabilitation [2003] 84 (8) : 1109-1117 (M.A.Hirsch, T.Toole, C.G.Maitland, R.A.Rider)

Aquatic exercise

Method : Aquatic exercise is exercising in water, usually in a swimming pool. Aquatiuc exercise is a low-impact activity that takes the pressure off bones, joints and muscles. Water also offers natural resistance, which can help strengthen the muscles [1].

Efficacy : Aquatic exercise reduced motor disability quantified by the Unified Parkinson Disease Rating Scale (UPDRS III), but did not improve gait variability, freezing of gait or quality of life [1]. Aquatic exercise significantly improved walking speed, and stride length [2]. Patients improved according to the Berg Balance Scale (BBS), and the the UPDRS [3].

[1] Archives of Physical Medicine and Rehabilitation [2016] Jan 11 [Epub ahead of print] (L.M.Carroll, D.Volpe, M.E.Morris, J.Saunders, A.M.Clifford)

[2] Revista da Neurologia [2013] 56 (6) : 315-320 (P.Rodriguez, J.M. Cancela, C.Ayan, C.do Nascimento, M.Seijo-Martínez)

[3] Archives of Physical Medicine and Rehabilitation [2011] 92 (8) : 1202-1210 (J.Vivas P.Arias, J.Cudeiro)

Physiotherapy

Method : Physiotherapy involves rehabilitation that remediates impairments and promotes mobility and function, through examination, diagnosis, prognosis, and physical intervention using therapy involving mechanical force and movements. It is usually carried out by physiotherapists.

Efficacy : An analysis was carried out of all the published studies concerning the use of physiotherapy in Parkinson's Disease showed that physiotherapy was beneficial using most methods in the short term (less than three months). The benefit was significant when using the following tests : velocity, step length, two-minute or six-minute walk tests, Timed Up & Go, Functional Reach Test, Berg Balance Scale and clinician-rated UPDRS. However, for some outcomes (velocity, Berg Balance Scale and UPDRS), the differences observed were at, or approaching, minimally clinical important changes. There was no evidence of very significant differences in the effect between the types of physiotherapy used [1]. Physiotherapy did not improve activities of daily living (ADL) or quality of life (QOL) [2]. Physiotherapy was more effective than general exercise [3].

[1] Cochrane Database Systematic Reviews [2012] 7 : CD002817 (C.L. Tomlinson, S.Patel, C.Meek, C.P.Herd, C.E.Clarke, R.Stowe, L.Shah, C.M.Sackley, K.H.Deane, K.Wheatley, N.Ives)

[2] JAMA Neurology [2016] 73 (3) : 291-299 (C.E.Clarke, S.Patel, N.Ives, C.E.Rick, F.Dowling, R.Woolley, K.Wheatley, M.F.Walker, C.M.Sackley)

[3] Journal of Parkinsons Disease [2017] Jan 17 [Epub ahead of print] (S.Dipasquale, R.Meroni, F.Sasanelli, I.Messineo, D.Piscitelli, C.Perin, C.M.Cornaggia, C.G.Cerri)

Cycling

Method : Cycling training involves cycling over various speeds, times and distances that can also include cycling uphill.

Efficacy : A six week programme of cycle ergometry training for thirty minutes per week did not significantly influence exercise tolerance in people with Parkinson's Disease but improved balance, functional ability and Parkinson's Disease related disability [1]. A programme of cycle ergometry training for one hour per day resulted in improvement in speed, step length, cadence of gait, and the UPDRS [2]. Using a using stationary bicycle can also be beneficial [3].

[1] Disability and Rehabilitation - Assistive Technology [2013] 35 (5) : 382-387 (P.Lauhoff, N.Murphy, C.Doherty, N.F.Horgan)

[2] Restorative Neurology and Neuroscience [2015] Dec 12 [Epub ahead of print] (I.Arcolin, F.Pisano, C.Delconte, M.Godi, M. Schieppati, D.Picco, M.Grasso, A.Nardone)

[3] Frontiers in Human Neuroscience [2017] 10 : 690 (A.Nadeau, O. Lungu, C.Duchesne, M.E.Robillard, A.Bore, F.Bobeuf, R.Plamondon, A.L.Lafontaine, F.Gheysen, L.Bherer, J.Doyon)

DANCING

Method : Several forms of dancing have been assessed for their benefits in improving Parkinson's Disease symptoms, including Argentine Tango [1-9], ballroom dancing [9, 10], ballet [11], and Irish set dancing [12, 13].

Efficacy : Argentine Tango was found to be feasible [1] and improved motor disability [2, 3], gait [2, 4], mobility [5], and especially balance [2, 4, 7, 8, 9]. Ballroom dancing improved balance [9]. Ballet improved balance [11]. Irish set dancing improved motor disability [12], freezing of gait [12], and balance [12, 13], and can improve quality of life [15]. Dancing generally improved motor impairment and balance [14].

[1] Frontiers in Neurology [2015] 6 : 122 (L.M.Blandy, W.A.Beevers, K.Fitzmaurice, M.E.Morris)

[2] BMC Neurology [2015] 15 : 226 (D.Lötzke, T.Ostermann, A. Büssing)

[3] Neurorehabilitation and Neural Repair [2012] 26 (2) : 132-143 (R.P.Duncan, G.M.Earhart)

[4] Complementary Therapies in Medicine [2015] 23 (2) : 175-184 (S. Rios Romenets, J.Anang, S.M.Fereshtehnejad, A.Pelletier, R. Postuma)

[5] Journal of Visualized Experiments [2014] (94) (M.E.Hackney, K. McKee)

[6] Archives of Physical Medicine and Rehabilitation [2013] 94 (2) : 240-249 (E.R.Foster, L.Golden, R.P.Duncan, G.M.Earhart)

[7] Neurorehabilitation and Neural Repair [2010] 24 (4) : 384-392 (M.E. Hackney, G.M.Earhart)

[8] Complementary Therapies in Medicine [2009] 17 (4) : 203-207 (M.E.Hackney, G.M.Earhart)

[9] Journal of Rehabilitation Medicine [2009] 41 (6) : 475-481 (M.E. Hackney, G.M.Earhart)

[10] JMIR Research Protocols [2014] 3 (3) : e34 (A.Ashburn, L. Roberts, R.Pickering, H.C.Roberts, R.Wiles, D.Kunkel, S.Hulbert, J. Robison, C.Fitton)

[11] Arts and Health [2013] 5 (2) : 103-119 (S.Houston, A.McGill)

[12] BMC Geriatrics [2013] 13 : 54 (D.Volpe, M.Signorini, A. Marchetto, T.Lynch, M.E.Morris)

[13] Complementary Therapies in Clinical Practice [2015] 21 (1) : 47-51 (J.Shanahan, M.E.Morris, O.N.Bhriain, D.Volpe, M.Richardson, A.M.Clifford)

[14] Archives of Physical Medicine and Rehabilitation [2015] 96 (1) : 141-153 (J.Shanahan, M.E.Morris, O.N.Bhriain, J.Saunders, A.M. Clifford)

[15] Archives of Physical Medicine and Rehabilitation [2017] Mar 21 [Epub ahead of print] (J.Shanahan, M.E.Morris, O.N.Bhriain, D.Volpe, T.Lynch, A.M.Clifford)

QIGONG

Method : Qigong is a traditional practice of aligning body, breath, and mind and a form of exercise for health, meditation, and martial arts training. It involves coordinated body posture and movement, breathing, and meditation [1].

Efficacy : Qigong improved some aspects of sleep quality [2, 3]. Fatigue remained unchanged. Gait function was improved by a significant reduction of stride time and a slight increase in stride length. These changes resulted in significant improvements to gait velocity [2, 3]. Qigong was applied as 90 minute weekly group instructions for 2 months followed by a 2 month pause and a second 2 month treatment period. People improved after 3 months, 6 months and 12 months when compared to the outset. Depression and several non-motor symptoms decreased [4]. There was not sufficient evidence to support or refute the effect of Qigong plus medication being beneficial for Parkinson's Disease [5].

[1] Qigong for Parkinsons : A conversation with Bianca about her complete healing (Bianca Molle, Robert Rodgers)

[2] International Journal of Neuroscience [2015] 125 (8) : 578-584 (D.J.Wassom, K.E.Lyons, R.Pahwa, W.Liu)

[3] Geriatrics and Gerontology International [2015] Aug 26 [Epub ahead of print] (C.M.Xiao, Y.C.Zhuang)

[4] Movement Disorders [2006] 21 (4) : 543-548 (T.Schmitz-Hübsch, D.Pyfer, K.Kielwein, R.Fimmers, T.Klockgether, U.Wüllner)

[5] PLoS One [2015] 10 (4) : e0122469 (Y.Yang, W.Q.Qiu, Y.L.Hao, Z.Y.Lv, S.J.Jiao, J.F.Teng)

Tai Chi

Method : Tai Chi is a traditional Chinese martial art and form of exercise that is often practiced for health reasons. Tai Chi involves : solo hand routines, weapons routines, breathing, movement and awareness exercises, meditation, response drills, and self defence techniques [1].

Efficacy : Out of the studies in the medical literature concerning Tai Chi and Parkinson's Disease, four were either non-randomised or uncontrolled clinical trials. Two failed to show any effect. Only one study showed Tai Chi to be superior to conventional exercise for Parkinson's Disease [2]. In more recent studies Tai Chi training appeared to reduce balance impairments and falls in people with mild-to-moderate Parkinson's Disease [3, 4, 5]. Tai Chi improved mobility and balance in people with Parkinson's Disease [6] on its own and also in combination with the use of Parkinson's Disease drugs [7, 8].

[1] Tai Chi : A practical approach to the ancient Chinese movement for health and well-being [2002] (Angus Clark)

[2] Parkinsonism & Related Disorders [2008] 14 (8) : 589-594 (M.S. Lee, P.Lam, E.Ernst)

[3] Journal of Physiotherapy [2103] 59 (1) : 55 (W.W.Tsang)

[4] New England Journal of Medicine [2012] 366 (6) : 511-519 (F.Li, P.Harmer, K.Fitzgerald, E.Eckstrom, R.Stock, J.Galver, G.Maddalozzo, S.S.Batya)

[5] Clinical Rehabilitation [2014] Feb 11 [Epub ahead of print] (Q.Gao, A.Leung, Y.Yang, Q.Wei, M.Guan, C.Jia, C.He)

[6] Evidence Based Complementary and Alternative Medicine [2015] : 593263 (J.Zhou, T.Yin, Q.Gao, X.C.Yang)

[7] PLoS One [2014] 9 (6) : e99377 (X.Ni, S.Liu, F.Lu, X.Shi, X.Guo)

[8] PLoS One [2015] 10 (4) : e0122469 (Y.Yang, W.Q.Qiu, Y.L.Hao, Z.Y.Lv, S.J.Jiao, J.F.Teng)

YOGA

Method : Yoga is an ancient Hindu discipline a part of which includes breath control, simple meditation, and the adoption of specific bodily postures, for health and relaxation [1, 2, 3].

Efficacy : Twice weekly yoga sessions for 12 weeks led to a significant improvement in Parkinson's Disease symptom scores that were assessed using the UPDRS. Positive trends of improvement were also noted in depression, forced expiratory volume, and a reduction in immediate tremor [4]. There was significant improvement in upper and lower limb bradykinesia, rigidity, and also muscle strength [5].

[1] Yoga and Parkinson's Disease : A Journey to Health and Healing [2013] (Scott Sherman)

[2] Yoga for Movement Disorders : Rebuilding Strength, Balance and Flexibility for Parkinson's Disease and Dystonia [2012] (Renee Le Verrier, Lewis Sudarsky)

[3] The Book of Exercise and Yoga for Those with Parkinson's Disease : Using Movement and Meditation to Manage Symptoms [2010] (Lori A.Newell)

[4] International Journal of Yoga [2015] 8 (1) : 74-79 (N.K.Sharma, K. Robbins, K.Wagner, Y.M.Colgrove)

[5] Complementary Therapies in Medicine [2016] 25 : 126-131 (M.Ni, K.Mooney, J.F.Signorile)

CHAPTER 50

TECHNOLOGICAL METHODS FOR PARKINSON'S DISEASE

PHYSIOLOGY

Technological devices are being used to try to improve Parkinson's Disease without the necessity for drugs or surgery. They aim to have effect by means that include : stimulating the brain, the spinal cord, or weak muscles, or stimulating the body generally, destroying abnormal neurons, using light exposure to raise dopamine levels, or to provide visual information.

TECHNOLOGICAL METHODS

The technological methods being used or developed in order to improve Parkinson's Disease include Focused Ultrasound [PAGE 792], Functional electrical stimulation [PAGE 793], Google Glass, [PAGE 794], Laser devices [PAGE 795], Light Therapy [PAGE 796], Magneceutical therapy [PAGE 796], Nexalin Therapy [PAGE 797], Spinal cord stimulation [PAGE 797], STIMband [PAGE 798], Transcranial direct current stimulation [PAGE 799], Transcranial magnetic stimulation [PAGE 800], Virtual reality [PAGE 802], and Whole body vibration [PAGE 803].

FOCUSED ULTRASOUND

Technology : Focused ultrasound is an incisionless method of thalamotomy for people who are not candidates for surgery or who do not want to undergo an invasive procedure. The procedure is performed with the patient awake and involves no anaesthesia, no incisions in the scalp, no burr holes through the skull or insertion of electrodes into the brain. Multiple intersecting beams of ultrasound energy are focused with a high degree of precision and accuracy on the target in the thalamus to heat and destroy the abnormal neurons without harming adjacent tissue. During treatment the target is visualised in real time using MR imaging. It is claimed that "multiple intersecting beams of ultrasound energy are focused with a high degree of precision and accuracy on the target in the thalamus to heat and destroy the abnormal neurons" [1]. However, the cells that produce dopamine (the dopaminergic neurons) are simply functioning at a far lower rate than normal. So the cells that produce less dopamine do not need destroying.

Efficacy : In a small study single use resulted in a 7% reduction in their UPDRS score (Parkinson's Disease symptom score) after three months whereas repeated use resulted in a 57% reduction in their UPDRS score after three months [2].

[1] Focused Ultrasound Foundation - Current and future applications of Focused Ultrasound 2012 (3rd International Symposium)

[2] Current and future applications of Focused Ultrasound 2012 (3rd International Symposium) Study on incisionless Transcranial Magnetic Resonance-guided Focused Ultrasound treatment of Parkinson's Disease : Safety, accuracy and clinical outcomes (D.Jeanmonod, D. Moser, A.Magara, M.Kowalski, R.Bühler, P.Pourtehrani, T.Coray, J. Vogel)

Functional Electrical Stimulation

Technology : The use of electrical impulses to stimulate weak or paralysed muscles, called Functional Electrical Stimulation (FES), is often used to help stroke or multiple sclerosis patients to walk. Two self adhesive patches (electrodes) are placed on the skin close to the nerve supplying the muscle and over the centre of the muscle. Leads connect the electrodes to a stimulator that produces the impulses [1].

Efficacy : A study was carried out that was aimed at investigating the effect of Functional Electrical Stimulation (FES) on walking ability in people with Parkinson's Disease. For eight weeks people with idiopathic Parkinson's Disease received electrical stimulation to the common peroneal nerve in order to improve heel strike and provide sensory stimulus during walking. An immediate improvement was demonstrated with the use of Functional Electrical Stimulation (FES) on distance and average stride length during a short walk during the treatment period but not on the number of steps and walking speed during a longer walk. A training effect was observed for all measures of walking ability. Fewer falls and episodes of freezing occurred during the treatment. However, the number of occasions on which patients fell returned to pre-treatment levels when the treatment was stopped [2].

[1] Functional electrical stimulation of denervated skeletal muscles : A basic comparison of electrode arrangements on and in the human thigh [2011] (Fadi Dohnal)

[2] Neuromodulation [2008] 11 (2) : 143-149 (G.E.Mann, S.M.Finn, P. N.Taylor)

Google Glass

Technology : Glass is a wearable computer being developed by Google that appears to be a pair of designer glasses. The system works like a hands-free smartphone that displays visual information on the lens of the Glass. The technology is voice-operated and is also linked to the internet [1]. The technology provides discreet prompts linked to key behaviours typical of Parkinson's Disease such as reminding the wearer to speak up or to swallow to prevent drooling. Glass can also be used as a reminder for things such as taking medication and making appointments. So if the wearer is alone they just have to look through the Glass so that carers or relatives are able to see exactly where they are. The wearer can also tell it to call someone and it rings them [2].

Efficacy : Google Glass is being investigated as an assistive aid in order to help people with Parkinson's Disease [2].

[1] http://www.techradar.com/reviews/gadgets/google-glass-1152283/review

[2] http://www.ncl.ac.uk/press.office/press.release/item/google-glass-puts-the-focus-on-parkinson-s

LASER DEVICES

Technology : The Laser Cane was designed to address freezing of gait episodes in Parkinson's Disease and other neurological disorders. Laser Canes display a beam on the ground, which effectively provides a target to step over to help overcome freezing episodes. The laser feature can be turned on and off with the push of a button. A weight activated rubber cane tip provides another on/off switch for the laser [1]. The Parkinson Walker (Zimmer Frame) comes with a laser attached to it. The laser is a red beam that shoots across the path of travel in order to help the patient walk faster [2]. Handheld laser pointers have also been used in order to assist people with Parkinson's Disease.

Efficacy : Laser light was associated with a modest reduction in freezing of gait and falls when used with a cane or walker [3]. The use of a visual laser beam stick (LBS) was no better concerning the freezing of gait than the use of a modified inverted stick (MIS) [4]. Laser light use on a U-Step walker did not improve either gait measures or safety [5]. Laser light used on the ground made little difference to the person's walking ability [6, 7], but could improve step length [8].

[1] In Step Mobility Products - http://www.ustep.com/cane.htm

[2] Accessible Design and Consulting - http://www.accessibleconstruct ion .com/ services/walkers/parkinson-walker.html

[3] Parkinsonism & Related Disorders [2011] 17 (4) : 240-245 (S. Donovan, C.Lim, N.Diaz, N.Browner, P.Rose, L.R.Sudarsky, D.Tarsy, S.Fahn, D.K.Simon)

[4] Movement Disorders [2000] 15 (2) : 309-312 (K.Kompoliti, C.G. Goetz, S.Leurgans, M.Morrissey, I.M.Siegel)

[5] Gait Posture [2012] 38 (1) : 20-24 (D.A.Kegelmeyer, S. Parthasarathy, S.K.Kostyk, S.E.White, A.D.Kloos)

[6] Journal of Clinical Neuroscience [2011] 18 (6) : 798-802 (C.A. Lebold, Q.J.Almeida)

[7] Parkinson's Disease [2010] : 732508 (C.A.Lebold, Q.J. Almeida)

[8] Physiotherapy Theory and Practice [2015] 31 (7) : 518-526 (C.J. Egerton, P.McCandless, B.Evans, J.Janssen, J.D.Richards)

Light therapy

Technology : Light therapy consists of daily exposure to daylight, brighter artificial light, or specific wavelengths of light for a prescribed amount of time [1]. Light suppresses melatonin formation, which lowers dopamine activity. As a lack of dopamine causes Parkinson's Disease, light is used to suppress the interfering effect of melatonin.

Efficacy : Light therapy was found to reduce to some extent a variety of Parkinson's Disease symptoms without appearing to cause any side effects [2, 3]. It had a positive effect on sleep, mood and motor function [4]. Besides its effects being moderate, it is assumed that the effect would only occur on the days it is used.

[1] A Clinician's Guide to Using Light Therapy [2009] (Raymond W. Lam, Edwin M.Tam)

[2] Chronobiology International [2007] 24 (3) : 521-537 (G.L.Willis, E. J.Turner)

[3] Movement Disorders [2007] 22 (10) : 1495-1498 (S.Paus, T. Schmitz-Hbsch, U.Wllner, A.Vogel, T.Klockgether, M.Abele)

[4] Parkinson's Disease [2012] : 767105 (S.Rutten, C.Vriend, O.A.van den Heuvel, J.H.Smit, H.W.Berendse, Y.D.van der Werf)

Magneceutical Therapy

Technology : Magneceutical Therapy involves the use of an extremely low-level electromagnetic field applied by a specially designed device, the Magnesphere, along with proprietary therapeutic protocols, that are intended to improve a number of the symptoms of Parkinson’s Disease and some other neurological disorders. Helmholtz coils immerse the entire patient in a low strength electromagnetic field [1].

Efficacy : In a small clinical trial using magneceutical therapy there was a mild beneficial effect [2].

[1] http://www.magneceutical.com/

[2] http://www.clinicaltrials.gov "Evaluation of Long-term Effect of Resonator Therapy on Parkinson's Disease (PD)" [2011]

Nexalin Therapy

Technology : Nexalin Therapy is a technology that uses a mild stimulation of the brain to treat a variety of mood disorders, specifically anxiety, depression, and insomnia. The wave form of Nexalin is administered by placing medical grade conductive pads produced specifically for the Nexalin device on the forehead and behind each ear, which are connected to the Nexalin device with thin cables. The patient is placed in a reclining chair for the duration of a treatment session. Treatment sessions typically last for approximately forty minutes. The intended effect appears to be like a milder version of Deep Brain Stimulation but without using surgery [1].

Efficacy : A formal clinical trial is currently being carried out by the Michael J.Fox Foundation [2].

[1] http://nexalintherapy.com

[2] The Michael J.Fox Foundation https://www.michaeljfox.org/foundation/grant-detail.php?grant_id=438

Spinal cord stimulation

Technology : Spinal cord stimulation (SCS) is a minimally invasive method that uses Spinal cord stimulators, which are implantable medical devices. Spinal cord stimulation, in the simplest form, consists of stimulating electrodes, an electrical pulse generator, conducting wires connecting the electrodes to the generator, and the generator remote control. Spinal cord stimulators are used to exert pulsed electrical signals to the spinal cord to control chronic pain. Further applications are in motor disorders [1].

Efficacy : After three months, and also twelve months, pain had reduced and gait had improved in people with Parkinson's Disease. Posture and postural stability improved after three months. Spinal cord stimulation is claimed to lead to the amelioration of pain and the improvement of motor function in advanced Parkinson's Disease [2].

[1] Spinal Cord Stimulation: Percutaneous Implantation Techniques [2009] (Paul Kreis, Scott Fishman)

[2] Neurologia medico-chirurgica (Tokyo) [2012] 52 (7) : 470-474 (T. Agari, I.Date)

STIMBAND

Technology : STIMband is a non-invasive brain stimulator being developed for the treatment of Parkinson's Disease. STIMband is a headband shaped device that is simply placed on the head. STIMband is based on transcranial direct current stimulation in which low-level current is passed through two electrodes placed over the head to tweak the electrical activity in specific areas of the brain. The prototype enables a patient to activate the battery powered treatment by touching an easy-to-press button. With patient safety in mind the prototype delivers current for only 20 minutes daily at a doctor prescribed level. It is inexpensive, safe and easy to administer without any side effects. It is easy to put on, comfortable to wear, and is positioned so that the electrodes remain stable and properly target the motor cortices areas of the brain. One addition may be a wireless connection to allow a doctor to adjust a patient's treatment level from a remote location [1].

Efficacy : STIMband has not undergone clinical trials but is based on transcranial direct current stimulation, which has undergone clinical trials.

[1] http://hub.jhu.edu/2015/06/10/stimband-brain-stimulator

TRANSCRANIAL DIRECT CURRENT STIMULATION

Technology : Transcranial direct current stimulation (tDCS) is a non-invasive brain stimulation technique that applies mild direct currents via the scalp to enhance or diminish neuronal excitability [1].

Efficacy : In people with Parkinson's Disease Transcranial direct current stimulation (tDCS) improved gait for a short time and improved bradykinesia in both the on and off states for longer than three months. There were no changes in overall Parkinson's Disease symptoms, reaction time, physical and mental well being, and self-assessed mobility [2]. Transcranial direct current stimulation (tDCS) improved levodopa-induced dyskinesias [3]. There was evidence of an effect on UPDRS part III motor subsection score [4]. In other studies there was no significant difference in : overall Parkinson's Disease symptoms [5], anxiety [5], geriatric depression [5], sleepiness [5], off time and on time with dyskinesia [4], and gait speed [4]. I one study there was no significant effect on change in global UPDRS score. However, there was evidence of an effect on UPDRS part III motor subsection score [6].

[1] Journal of Affective Disorders [2009] 117 (3) : 137-145 (A.P. Arul-Anandam, C.Loo)

[2] Journal of Neurology, Neurosurgery, and Psychiatry [2010] 81 (10) : 1105-1111 (D.H.Benninger, M.Lomarev, G.Lopez, E.M.Wassermann, X.Li, E.Considine, M.Hallett)

[3] Cerebellum [2016] 15 (1) : 43-47 (R.Ferrucci, F.Cortese, M. Bianchi, D.Pittera, R.Turrone, T.Bocci, B.Borroni, M. Vergari, F. Cogiamanian, G.Ardolino, A.Di Fonzo, A.Padovani, A. Priori)

[4] Movement Disorders [2011] 26 (8) : 1477-1480 (H.A.Shill, S. Obradov, Y.Katsnelson, R.Pizinger)

[5] European Journal of Physical and Rehabilitation Medicine [2016] Oct 4 [Epub ahead of print] (B.Elsner, J.Kugler, M.Pohl, J.Mehrholz)

[6] Cochrane Database Systematic Reviews [2016] 7 : CD010916 (B.Elsner, J.Kugler, M.Pohl, J.Mehrholz)

TRANSCRANIAL MAGNETIC STIMULATION

Technology : Transcranial magnetic stimulation (TMS) is a method of exciting neurons. The excitation is caused by weak electric currents induced in the tissue by rapidly changing magnetic fields. In this way brain activity can be affected without the need for surgery or external electrodes. The magnetic field is generated by passing current pulses through a conducting coil that is held close to the scalp so that the magnetic field is focused in the cortex and through the skull [1].

Efficacy : In people with Parkinson's Disease Transcranial magnetic stimulation resulted in mild to moderate improvements in motor symptoms [2-8], reduced depression [6, 9], reduced freezing of gait [10], reduced some of the Parkinson's Disease symptoms [9, 11, 12], improved handwriting [13], improved short term upper limb function [14], improved walking performance [14], and improved motor symptoms [15]. There is a significant correlation between Parkinson's Disease symptoms and serum dopamine levels [11, 13]. However, in some studies the method was found to be largely ineffective [16, 17]. Instead of Repetitive transcranial magnetic stimulation (rTMS), Intermittent theta-burst stimulation (iTBS) was not found to be effective for gait, upper extremity bradykinesia, or other motor symptoms [18]. The risk of adverse effects is low [19].

[1] Oxford Handbook of Transcranial Stimulation [2008] (Eric Wassermann, Charles Epstein, Ulf Ziemann, Vincent Walsh, Toms Paus, Sarah Lisanby)

[2] PM & R [2015] : S1934-S1482 (A.Wagle Shukla, J. Shuster, J.W. Chung, D.E.Vaillancourt, C.Patten, J.L.Ostrem, M.S.Okun)

[3] Restorative Neurology and Neuroscience [2015] 33 (4) : 521-530 (M.S.Kim, W.Hyuk Chang, J.W.Cho, J.Youn, Y.K.Kim, S.Woong Kim, Y.H.Kim)

[4] Acta Neuropsychiatrica [2015] 27 (2) : 82-89 (H.Zhu, Z.Lu, Y.Jin, X.Duan, J.Teng, D.Duan)

[5] Movement Disorders [2015] 30 (6) : 750-758 (A.Zanjani, K.K. Zakzanis, Z.J.Daskalakis, R.Chen)

[6] Neuropsychobiology [2016] 73 (3) : 169-177 (A.Makkos, E.Pál, Z.Aschermann, J.Janszky, É.Balázs, K.Takács, K.Karádi, S.Komoly, N.Kovács)

[7] JAMA Neurology [2015] 72 (4) : 432-440 (Y.H.Chou, P.T. Hickey, M.Sundman, A.W.Song, N.K.Chen)

[8] Brain Stimulation [2014] 7 (2) : 297-300 (F.Spagnolo, M.A. Volonté, M.Fichera, R.Chieffo, E.Houdayer, M.Bianco, E.Coppi, A. Nuara, L.Straffi, G.Di Maggio, L.Ferrari, D.Dalla Libera, et al)

[9] Movement Disorders [2010] 25 (14) : 2272-2273 (E.Pal, F.Nagy, Z. Aschermann, E.Balazs, N.Kovacs)

[10] Restorative Neurology and Neuroscience [2015] 33 (4) : 521-530 (S.Y.Lee, M.S.Kim, W.H.Chang, J.W.Cho, J.Y.Youn, Y.H. Kim)

[11] Movement Disorders [2007] 22 (7) : 1046-1050 (E.M.Khedr, J.C. Rothwell, O.A.Shawky, M.A.Ahmed, N.Foly, A.Hamdy)

[12] Movement Disorders [2006] 21 (12) : 2201-2205 (E.M.Khedr, J.C.Rothwell, O.A. Shawky, M.A.Ahmed, A.Hamdy)

[13] Parkinson's Disease [2013] : 751925 (B.K.Randhawa, B.G.Farley, L.A.Boyd)

[14] Brain Stimulation [2016] 9 (4) : 475-487 (C.L. Chung, M.K.Mak)

[15] Neurology [2016] 87 (18) : 1907-1915 (M.Brys, M.D.Fox, S. Agarwal, M.Biagioni, G.Dacpano, P.Kumar, E.Pirraglia, R.Chen, A. Wu, H.Fernandez, A.W.Shukla, J.S.Lou, Z.Gray, D.K.Simon, et al)

[16] Movement Disorders [2011] 26 (8) : 1477-1480 (H.A.Shill, S. Obradov, Y.Katsnelson, R.Pizinger)

[17] Neurorehabilitation and Neural Repair [2012] 26 (9) : 1096-1105 (D.H.Benninger, K.Iseki, S.Kranick, D.A.Luckenbaugh, E. Houdayer, M.Hallett)

[18] Neurology [2011] 76 (7) : 601-609 (D.H.Benninger, B.D.Berman, E.Houdayer, N.Pal, D.A.Luckenbaugh, L.Schneider, S.Miranda, M. Hallett)

[19] Parkinsonism & Related Disorders [2013] 19 (6) : 573-585 (M. Vonloh, R.Chen, B.Kluger)

VIRTUAL REALITY

Method : Virtual reality (VR) technology is a means of experiencing things through computers that don't really exist. It is a believable and interactive 3D computer-created world that you can explore so that you feel you really are there, both mentally and physically [1].

Efficacy : In people with Parkinson's Disease, virtual reality may lead to a moderate improvement in step and stride length [2]. Virtual reality and physiotherapy may have similar effects on gait, balance, and quality of life [2]. Treadmill training plus virtual reality led to reduced falling compared to treadmill training alone [3], and can significantly improve physical performance and gait [4]. The use of virtual reality games (exergaming) improved balance and postural control [5]. Virtual reality dance exercise has a positive effect on balance [6]. Virtual reality balance training and conventional balance training were approximately equally effective in improving balance [7, 8].

[1] The VR Book : Human-Centered Design for Virtual Reality Paperback [2015] (Jason Jerald)

[2] Cochrane Database Systematic Reviews [2016] 12 : CD010760 (K. Dockx, E.M.Bekkers, V.Van den Bergh, P.Ginis, L.Rochester, J.M. Hausdorff, A.Mirelman, A.Nieuwboer)

[3] Lancet [2016] 388 (10050) : 1170-1182 (A.Mirelman, L. Rochester, I.Maidan, S.Del Din, L.Alcock, F.Nieuwhof, M.O.Rikkert, B.R.Bloem, E.Pelosin, L.Avanzino, G.Abbruzzese, K.Dockx, et al)

[4] Journals of Gerontology : Series A Biological Sciences and Medical Sciences [2011] 66 (2) : 234-240 (A.Mirelman, I.Maidan, T.Herman, J.E.Deutsch, N.Giladi, J.M.Hausdorff)

[5] Frontiers in Aging Neuroscience [2015] 7 : 167 (D.M.Harris, T. Rantalainen, M.Muthalib, L.Johnson, W.P.Teo)

[6] Journal of Physical Therapy Science [2015] 27 (1) : 145-147 (N.Y. Lee, D.K.Lee, H.S.Song)

[7] Journal of Formosan Medical Association [2016] 115 (9) : 734-743 (W.C.Yang, H.K.Wang, R.M.Wu, C.S.Lo, K.H.Lin)

[8] Physical Therapy [2011] 91 (6) : 862-874 (C.Y.Yen, K.H.Lin, M.H. Hu, R.M.Wu, T.W.Lu, C.H.Lin)

Whole body vibration

Technology : Whole body vibration (WBV) is a mechanical stimulus characterised by oscillatory motion delivered to the entire body. The person stands, sits or lies on a machine with a vibrating platform. As the machine vibrates, it transmits energy to the body, forcing muscles to contract and relax. The devices currently available for use in Whole body vibration use two different systems : (1) a vertical vibration, meaning the whole plate oscillates uniformly up and down with only a vertical translation, and (2) reciprocating vertical displacements on the left and the right side of a fulcrum, increasing the lateral accelerations. Biochemical parameters included in Whole body vibration training are body position, amplitude, frequency, magnitude and duration [1].

Efficacy : Ever being occupationally exposed to Whole body vibration was inversely associated with Parkinson's Disease. More recent and higher intensities were even more associated [2]. In response to Whole body vibration in Parkinson's Disease there were improvements in : disturbances of balance and gait (but being no better than the effect of conventional physiotherapy) [3], bradykinesia [4], Parkinson's Disease symptoms (UPDRS) [4, 5], tremor [5, 6], rigidity [5, 6], increase in step length and improved speed on the grooved pegboard task [6], and postural stability [7]. However, other results showed : postural stability, speech and facial expression remaining unchanged [4], tremor and postural stability being reduced but not significantly [4], a significant improvement of gait not showing significant results in comparison with physical therapy [8], and making no difference at all [9].

[1] Using Whole Body Vibration in Physical Therapy and Sport [2009] (Alfio Albasini, Martin Krause, Ingo Volker)

[2] American Journal of Epidemiology [2012] 176 (4) : 299-307 (M.A. Harris, S.A.Marion, J.J.Spinelli, J.K.Tsui, K.Teschke)

[3] Archives of Physical Medicine Rehabilitation [2008] 89 (3) : 399-403 (G.Ebersbach, D.Edler, O.Kaufhold, J.Wissel)

[4] NeuroRehabilitation [2011] 28 (4) : 353-358 (O.Kaut, N.Allert, C. Coch, S.Paus, A.Grzeska, M.Minnerop, U.Wüllner)

[5] NeuroRehabilitation [2006] 21 (1) : 29-36 (C.T.Haas, S.Turbanski, K.Kessler, D.Schmidtbleicher)

[6] NeuroRehabilitation [2009] 25 (4) : 297-306 (L.K.King, Q.J. Almeida, H.Ahonen)

[7] Research in Sports Medicine [2005] 13 (3) : 243-256 (S.Turbanski, C.T.Haas, D.Schmidtbleicher, A.Friedrich, P.Duisberg)

[8] Cochrane Database Systematic Reviews [2012] 2 : CD009097 (M. Sitjà Rabert, D.Rigau Comas, A.Fort Vanmeerhaeghe, C.Santoyo Medina, M.Roqué i Figuls, D.Romero-Rodríguez, X.Bonfill Cosp)

[9] Movement Disorders [2009] 24 (6) : 891-898 (P.Arias, M.Chouza, J.Vivas, J.Cudeiro)

APPENDIX 1

PARKINSON'S DISEASE ORGANISATIONS

Worldwide

World Parkinson Disease Association
http://www.wpda.org

North America

U.S.A.

American Parkinson Disease Association
http://www.apdaparkinson.org

National Parkinson Foundation
http://www.parkinson.org

The Parkinson's Disease Foundation
http://www.pdf.org

The Michael J.Fox Foundation
https://www.michaeljfox.org

Canada

Parkinson Canada
http://www.parkinson.ca

Oceania

Australia

Parkinson's Australia
http://www.parkinsons.org.au

New Zealand

Parkinson's New Zealand
http://www.parkinsons.org.nz

EUROPE

European Parkinson's Disease Association
http://www.epda.eu.com/en

UNITED KINGDOM

Parkinson's UK
http://www.parkinsons.org.uk

IRELAND

Parkinson's Association of Ireland
http://www.parkinsons.ie

FRANCE

Association France Parkinson
http://www.franceparkinson.fr

GERMANY

Deutsche Parkinson Vereiigung Bundesverband
https://www.parkinson-vereinigung.de

AUSTRIA

Parkinson Selbsthilfe Österreich
http://www.parkinson-sh.at

SWITZERLAND

Parkinson Switzerland
http://www.parkinson.ch

SPAIN

Federación Española de Parkinson
http://www.fedesparkinson.org

PORTUGAL

Associação Portuguesa de Doentes de Parkinson
http://www.parkinson.pt

NETHERLANDS

Parkinson Vereniging
https://www.parkinson-vereniging.nl

BELGIUM

Vlaamse Parkinson Liga
http://www.parkinsonliga.be

LUXEMBOURG

Parkinson Luxembourg
http://www.parkinsonlux.lu

DENMARK

Parkinsonforeningen
http://www.parkinson.dk

FINLAND

Finlands Parkinson-förbund
http://www.parkinson.fi

SWEDEN

Parkinson Förbundet
http://www.parkinsonforbundet.se

NORWAY

Norges Parkinsonforbund
http://www.parkinson.no

ICELAND

Parkinsonsamtökin á Íslandi
https://www.facebook.com/parkinsonsamtokin

FAEROE ISLANDS

Parkinsonforeningen
http://www.parkinson.fo

ITALY

Parkinson Italia
http://www.parkinson-italia.it

MALTA

Malta Parkinson's Disease Association
http://www.maltaparkinsons.com

GREECE

Epikouros - Kinesis
http://www.parkinsonportal.gr

CROATIA

HUBPP
http://hubpp.mef.hr

SLOVENIA

Društvo Trepetlika
http://www.trepetlika.si

CZECH REPUBLIC

Spolecnost Parkinson
http://www.spolecnost-parkinson.cz

ROMANIA

Asociatia Antiparkinson
http://www.parkinson.devaonline.ro

HUNGARY

Delta Magyar Parkinson Egyesület
www.fogomakezed.hu

POLAND

Parkinson Fundacja
http://www.parkinsonfundacja.pl

Ukraine

Ukrainian Parkinson Disease Society
http://www.geront.kiev.ua

Estonia

Eesti Parkinsoniliit
http://www.parkinson.ee

Lithuania

Lietuvos Parkinsono ligos draugija
http://www.parkinsonas.org

Asia

India

Parkinson's Disease Foundation of India
http://www.parkinsonsdiseaseindia.com

Parkinson's Disease and Movement Disorder Society
http://www.parkinsonssocietyindia.com

Pakistan

Pakistan Parkinson's Society
http://www.parkinsons.org.pk

Japan

Japan Parkinson Disease Association
https://www.facebook.com/jpda.org

Hong Kong

Hong Kong Parkinson's Disease Association
http://www.hkpda.org

Hong Kong Parkinson's Disease Foundation
http://www.hkpdf.org.hk

MALAYSIA

Malaysian Parkinson's Disease Association
http://www.mpda.org.my

SINGAPORE

Parkinson Society Singapore
http://www.parkinsonsingapore.com

ISRAEL

Israel Parkinson Association
http://www.parkinson.org.il/English

AFRICA

Africa Parkinson's Disease Foundation
http://www.africaparkinsons.org

SOUTH AFRICA

Parkinson's Association South Africa
http://www.parkinsons.co.za

ETHIOPIA

Parkinson Patients Support Organization - Ethiopia
http://parkinsonsethiopia.org

SOUTH AMERICA

BRAZIL

Associação Brasil Parkinson
http://www.parkinson.org.br

ARGENTINA

Asociación Civil Enfermedad de Parkinson
http://aceparparkinson.wix.com/acepar

APPENDIX 2

PARKINSON'S DISEASE WEB SITES

Parkinson's Disease News

For keeping completely up to date with all new significant research, reports, books, and resources concerning Parkinson's Disease.
http://viartis.net/parkinsons.disease/news.htm

PubMed

The most comprehensive database of medical and biochemical studies. Studies are best searched by using several authors surnames.
http://www.ncbi.nlm.nih.gov/pubmed

Barnes and Noble

On this web page, the bookstore Barnes and Noble summarises all of the presently available books related to Parkinson's Disease.
http://www.barnesandnoble.com/s/parkinsons+disease

Science Daily

Science Daily's news page that is specifically for new Parkinson's Disease research and related medical conditions.
https://www.sciencedaily.com/news/health_medicine/parkinson's_disease

Google News

Google News has searchable news pages that, when searched under Parkinson's Disease detail news concerning Parkinson's Disease.
https://news.google.com/news/section?=1&q=parkinsonsdisease

Medical News Today

Medical News Today is a news page that is specifically for new Parkinson's Disease research and related medical conditions.
http://www.medicalnewstoday.com/categories/parkinsons_disease

MEDICAL DICTIONARY

Medline's Medical Dictionary enables the searching of medical and biological terms including those concerning Parkinson's Disease.
https://www.nlm.nih.gov/medlineplus/mplusdictionary.html

MEDICAL ENCYCLOPEDIA

Medline's Medical Encyclopedia includes thousands of articles about diseases, tests, and symptoms including Parkinson's Disease.
https://www.nlm.nih.gov/medlineplus/encyclopedia.html

PARKINSON'S DISEASE CLINICAL TRIALS

Details of clinical trials being arranged or taking place around the world and the possibilities of participating in those clinical trials.
http://www.nhs.uk/Conditions/Parkinsons-disease/Pages/clinical-trial.aspx

CLINICALTRIALS.GOV

Searchable database providing details of clinical trials being arranged or taking place around the world and possible involvement in them.
https://clinicaltrials.gov

MEDLINE PLUS

MedlinePlus provides the details of drugs available in the U.S.A. including all of those used for the treatment of Parkinson's Disease.
https://www.nlm.nih.gov/medlineplus/druginformation.html

DRUGS.COM

Searchable database providing details and reviews of available drugs including all of those for the treatment of Parkinson's Disease.
http://www.drugs.com

RXLIST

Searchable database providing details and reviews of available drugs including all of those for the treatment of Parkinson's Disease.
http://www.rxlist.com/script/main/hp.asp

APPENDIX 3

PARKINSON'S DISEASE NURSING

Comprehensive Nursing Care for Parkinson's Disease

Authors : Lisette K.Bunting-Perry, Gwyn M.Vernon
Publisher : Springer Publishing Company [2007]
Publisher's description : The authors have many years of experience working with Parkinson's patients and have put together a team of internationally renowned clinicians in order to provide a truly comprehensive review of the information you need for patient care.

Parkinson's Disease : Theory and Practice for Nurses

Author : Lesley Swinn
Publisher : Whurr Publishers [2005]
Publisher's description : The aim of this book is to provide nurses with a readable and succinct text that will help them to deliver evidence-based, patient-centred nursing care for patients and their families with Parkinson's disease.

Everything you need to know about caregiving for Parkinson's Disease

Author : Lianna Marie
Publisher : CreateSpace Independent Publishing Platform [2016]
Publisher's description : This book answers your most important questions about caring for someone with Parkinson's Disease. It will help guide you through all the many stages of caregiving.

Parkinson's Disease : 300 Tips for Making Life Easier

Author : Shelley Peterman Schwarz
Publisher : Demos Health [2006]
Publisher's description : Filled with creative tips and techniques, 300 Tips for making life easier contains a wealth of ideas and shortcuts for working, organizing, simplifying, and conserving time and energy while living with Parkinson's disease.

The Comfort of home for Parkinson Disease : A guide for caregivers

Authors : Maria M.Meyer, Paula Derr
Publisher : CareTrust Publications [2007]
Publisher's description : It's all here in an illustrated, easy-to-read format, including the decision to provide home care, preparing the home, assisting with daily activities, financial management, and strategies for avoiding caregiver burnout.

Parkinson's Disease and the Family : A New Guide

Authors : Nutan Sharma, Elaine Richman
Publisher : Harvard University Press [2005]
Publisher's description : The authors draw on the latest research and clinical practice to offer valuable suggestions for managing patient care and, perhaps more important, for healing the family unit.

Parkinson's Disease and Parkinsonism in the Elderly

Authors : Jolyon Meara, William C.Koller
Publisher : Cambridge University Press [2000]
Publisher's description : This book covers all of the clinical features, diagnosis and management of Parkinson's disease in elderly people. It particularly stresses rehabilitation and total patient care.

Living With Parkinson's

Author : Robert K.Zimmerman
Publisher : America Star Books [2015]
Publisher's description : This book is not a medical treatise but rather a book filled with suggestions that will help the reader cope with the disease over a long period of time.

Navigating Life with Parkinson Disease

Authors : Sotirios Parashos, Rose Wichmann
Publisher : Oxford University Press [2012]
Publisher's description : Navigating Life with Parkinson Disease discusses the available treatments and provides practical advice on how to manage the disease in the long term.

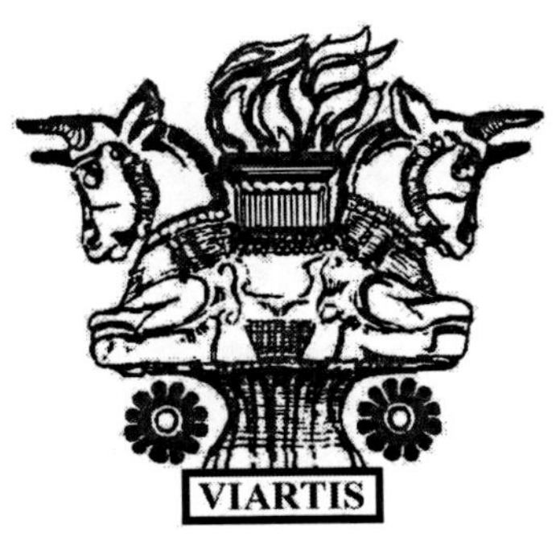
VIARTIS

CPSIA information can be obtained
at www.ICGtesting.com
Printed in the USA
LVOW10s2205110218
566157LV00021B/578/P

9 781906 421069